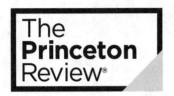

MCAT®

Physics and Math Review, 3rd Edition

The Staff of The Princeton Review

Penguin
Random
House

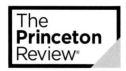

The Princeton Review, Inc.
24 Prime Parkway, Suite 201
Natick, MA 01760
E-mail: editorialsupport@review.com

Published in the United States by Penguin Random
House LLC, New York, and in Canada by Random
House of Canada, a division of Penguin Random House
Ltd., Toronto.

ISBN: 978-1-101-92059-6
ISSN: 2150-8895

MCAT is a registered trademark of the Association of
American Medical Colleges, which does not sponsor or
endorse this product.

The Princeton Review is not affiliated with Princeton
University.

Editor: Aaron Riccio
Production Artist: Deborah Silvestrini
Production Editors: Kiley Pulliam and Harmony Quiroz

Printed in the United States of America on partially
recycled paper.

10 9 8 7 6 5

3rd Edition

Editorial
Rob Franek, Senior VP, Publisher
Casey Cornelius, VP Content Development
Mary Beth Garrick, Director of Production
Selena Coppock, Managing Editor
Meave Shelton, Senior Editor
Colleen Day, Editor
Sarah Litt, Editor
Aaron Riccio, Editor
Callie McConnico, Editorial Assistant

Random House Publishing Team
Tom Russell, Publisher
Alison Stoltzfus, Publishing Manager
Melinda Ackell, Associate Managing Editor
Ellen Reed, Production Manager
Kristin Lindner, Production Supervisor
Andrea Lau, Designer

CONTRIBUTORS

Steven A. Leduc
      Senior Author

TPR MCAT Physics Development Team:
Jon Fowler, M.A., Senior Editor, Lead Developer
Chris Pentzell, M.S.
Carolyn J. Shiau, M.D.
Felicia Tam, Ph.D.

Edited for Production by:
Judene Wright, M.S., M.A.Ed.
      National Content Director, MCAT Program, The Princeton Review

The TPR MCAT Physics Team and Judene would like to thank the following people for their contributions to this book:

Khawar Chaudry, B.S., Doug Couchman, James Hudson, B.S., B.A., Ryan Katchky, Jason N. Kennedy, M.S., Brendan Lloyd, B.Sc., M.Sc., Travis Mackoy, B.S., Ashley Manzoor, Ph.D., Al Mercado, Gina Passante, Mark Shew, H.BSc, Gillian Shiau, M.D., Teri Stewart, B.S.E., Dylan Sweeney, Tom Watts, B.A., Barry Weliver, Hesham Zakaria.

Periodic Table of the Elements

1 H 1.0																	2 He 4.0
3 Li 6.9	4 Be 9.0											5 B 10.8	6 C 12.0	7 N 14.0	8 O 16.0	9 F 19.0	10 Ne 20.2
11 Na 23.0	12 Mg 24.3											13 Al 27.0	14 Si 28.1	15 P 31.0	16 S 32.1	17 Cl 35.5	18 Ar 39.9
19 K 39.1	20 Ca 40.1	21 Sc 45.0	22 Ti 47.9	23 V 50.9	24 Cr 52.0	25 Mn 54.9	26 Fe 55.8	27 Co 58.9	28 Ni 58.7	29 Cu 63.5	30 Zn 65.4	31 Ga 69.7	32 Ge 72.6	33 As 74.9	34 Se 79.0	35 Br 79.9	36 Kr 83.8
37 Rb 85.5	38 Sr 87.6	39 Y 88.9	40 Zr 91.2	41 Nb 92.9	42 Mo 95.9	43 Tc (98)	44 Ru 101.1	45 Rh 102.9	46 Pd 106.4	47 Ag 107.9	48 Cd 112.4	49 In 114.8	50 Sn 118.7	51 Sb 121.8	52 Te 127.6	53 I 126.9	54 Xe 131.3
55 Cs 132.9	56 Ba 137.3	57 *La 138.9	72 Hf 178.5	73 Ta 180.9	74 W 183.9	75 Re 186.2	76 Os 190.2	77 Ir 192.2	78 Pt 195.1	79 Au 197.0	80 Hg 200.6	81 Tl 204.4	82 Pb 207.2	83 Bi 209.0	84 Po (209)	85 At (210)	86 Rn (222)
87 Fr (223)	88 Ra 226.0	89 †Ac 227.0	104 Rf (261)	105 Db (262)	106 Sg (266)	107 Bh (264)	108 Hs (277)	109 Mt (268)	110 Ds (281)	111 Rg (272)	112 Cn (285)	113 Uut (286)	114 Fl (289)	115 Uup (288)	116 Lv (293)	117 Uus (294)	118 Uuo (294)

*Lanthanide Series:

58 Ce 140.1	59 Pr 140.9	60 Nd 144.2	61 Pm (145)	62 Sm 150.4	63 Eu 152.0	64 Gd 157.3	65 Tb 158.9	66 Dy 162.5	67 Ho 164.9	68 Er 167.3	69 Tm 168.9	70 Yb 173.0	71 Lu 175.0
90 Th 232.0	91 Pa (231)	92 U 238.0	93 Np (237)	94 Pu (244)	95 Am (243)	96 Cm (247)	97 Bk (247)	98 Cf (251)	99 Es (252)	100 Fm (257)	101 Md (258)	102 No (259)	103 Lr (260)

†Actinide Series:

MCAT PHYSICS CONTENTS

CONTENTS

MCAT MATH CONTENTS

Register Your

1 Go to **PrincetonReview.com/cracking**

2 You'll see a welcome page where you should register your book or boxed set of books using the ISBN. If you have a book, the ISBN can be found above the bar code on the back cover. If you have a boxed set, the ISBN can be found on the back of the box above the bar code.

3 After placing this free order, you'll either be asked to log in or to answer a few simple questions in order to set up a new Princeton Review account.

4 Finally, click on the "Student Tools" tab located at the top of the screen. It may take an hour or two for your registration to go through, but after that, you're good to go.

NOTE: If you are experiencing book problems (potential content errors), please contact EditorialSupport@review.com with the full title of the book, its ISBN number, and the page number of the error.

Experiencing technical issues? Please email TPRStudentTech@review.com with the following information:

- your full name
- e-mail address used to register the book
- full book title and ISBN
- your computer OS (Mac or PC) and Internet browser (Firefox, Safari, Chrome, etc.)
- description of technical issue

Book Online!

Once you've registered, you can...

· Take 3 full-length practice MCAT exams
· Find useful information about taking the MCAT and applying to medical school
· Check to see if there have been any updates to this edition

Offline Resources

If you are looking for more review or medical school advice, please feel free to pick up these books in stores right now!

· *Medical School Essays That Made a Difference*
· *The Best 167 Medical Schools*
· *The Princeton Review Complete MCAT*

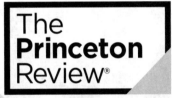

Chapter 1
MCAT Basics

SO YOU WANT TO BE A DOCTOR

So...you want to be a doctor. If you're like most premeds, you've wanted to be a doctor since you were pretty young. When people asked you what you wanted to be when you grew up, you always answered "a doctor." You had toy medical kits, bandaged up your dog or cat, and played "hospital." You probably read your parents' home medical guides for fun.

When you got to high school you took the honors and AP classes. You studied hard, got straight As (or at least really good grades!), and participated in extracurricular activities so you could get into a good college. And you succeeded!

At college you knew exactly what to do. You took your classes seriously, studied hard, and got a great GPA. You talked to your professors and hung out at office hours to get good letters of recommendation. You were a member of the premed society on campus, volunteered at hospitals, and shadowed doctors. All that's left to do now is get a good MCAT score.

Just the MCAT.

Just the most confidence-shattering, most demoralizing, longest, most brutal entrance exam for any graduate program. At about 7.5 hours (including breaks), the MCAT tops the list. Even the closest runners up, the LSAT and GMAT, are only about 4 hours long. The MCAT tests significant science content knowledge along with the ability to think quickly, reason logically, and read comprehensively, all under the pressure of a timed exam.

The path to a good MCAT score is not as easy to see as the path to a good GPA or the path to a good letter of recommendation. The MCAT is less about what you know, and more about how to apply what you know...and how to apply it quickly to new situations. Because the path might not be so clear, you might be worried. That's why you picked up this book.

We promise to demystify the MCAT for you, with clear descriptions of the different sections, how the test is scored, and what the test experience is like. We will help you understand general test-taking techniques as well as provide you with specific techniques for each section. We will review the science content you need to know as well as give you strategies for the Critical Analysis and Reasoning Skills (CARS) section. We'll show you the path to a good MCAT score and help you walk the path.

After all, you want to be a doctor. And we want you to succeed.

WHAT IS THE MCAT...REALLY?

Most test-takers approach the MCAT as though it were a typical college science test, one in which facts and knowledge simply need to be regurgitated in order to do well. They study for the MCAT the same way they did for their college tests, by memorizing facts and details, formulas and equations. And when they get to the MCAT they are surprised...and disappointed.

It's a myth that the MCAT is purely a content-knowledge test. If medical-school admission committees want to see what you know, all they have to do is look at your transcripts. What they really want to see is how you *think*, especially under pressure. *That's* what your MCAT score will tell them.

The MCAT is really a test of your ability to apply basic knowledge to different, possibly new, situations. It's a test of your ability to reason out and evaluate arguments. Do you still need to know your science content? Absolutely. But not at the level that most test-takers think they need to know it. Furthermore, your science knowledge won't help you on the Critical Analysis and Reasoning Skills (CARS) section. So how do you study for a test like this?

You study for the science sections by reviewing the basics and then applying them to MCAT practice questions. You study for the CARS section by learning how to adapt your existing reading and analytical skills to the nature of the test (more information about the CARS section can be found in the *MCAT Critical Analysis and Reasoning Skills Review*).

The book you are holding will review all the relevant MCAT Physics and Math content you will need for the test, and a little bit more. It includes hundreds of questions designed to make you think about the material in a deeper way, along with full explanations to clarify the logical thought process needed to get to the answer. It also comes with access to three full-length online practice exams to further hone your skills.

MCAT NUTS AND BOLTS

Overview

The MCAT is a computer-based test (CBT) that is *not* adaptive. Adaptive tests base your next question on whether or not you've answered the current question correctly. The MCAT is *linear*, or *fixed-form*, meaning that the questions are in a predetermined order and do not change based on your answers. However, there are many versions of the test, so that on a given test day, different people will see different versions. The following table highlights the features of the MCAT exam.

Registration	Online via www.aamc.org. Begins as early as six months prior to test date; available up until week of test (subject to seat availability).
Testing Centers	Administered at small, secure, climate-controlled computer testing rooms.
Security	Photo ID with signature, electronic fingerprint, electronic signature verification, assigned seat.
Proctoring	None. Test administrator checks examinee in and assigns seat at computer. All testing instructions are given on the computer.
Frequency of Test	Many times per year distributed over January, April, May, June, July, August, and September.
Format	Exclusively computer-based. NOT an adaptive test.
Length of Test Day	7.5 hours.
Breaks	Optional 10-minute breaks between sections, with a 30-minute break for lunch.
Section Names	1. Chemical and Physical Foundations of Biological Systems (Chem/Phys) 2. Critical Analysis and Reasoning Skills (CARS) 3. Biological and Biochemical Foundations of Living Systems (Bio/Biochem) 4. Psychological, Social, and Biological Foundations of Behavior (Psych/Soc)
Number of Questions and Timing	59 Chem/Phys questions, 95 minutes 53 CARS questions, 90 minutes 59 Bio/Biochem questions, 95 minutes 59 Psych/Soc questions, 95 minutes
Scoring	Test is scaled. Several forms per administration.
Allowed/Not allowed	No timers/watches. Noise reduction headphones available. An unopened package of foam earplugs is permitted. Scratch paper and pencils given at start of test and taken at end of test. Locker or secure area provided for personal items.
Results: Timing and Delivery	Approximately 30 days. Electronic scores only, available online through AAMC login. Examinees can print official score reports.
Maximum Number of Retakes	As of April 2015, the MCAT can be taken a maximum of three times in one year, four times over two years, and seven times over the lifetime of the examinee. An examinee can be registered for only one date at a time.

Registration

Registration for the exam is completed online at https://www.aamc.org/students/applying/mcat/reserving. The AAMC opens registration for a given test date at least two months in advance of the date, often earlier. It's a good idea to register well in advance of your desired test date to make sure that you get a seat.

Sections

There are four sections on the MCAT exam: Chemical and Physical Foundations of Biological Systems (Chem/Phys), Critical Analysis and Reasoning Skills (CARS), Biological and Biochemical Foundations of Living Systems (Bio/Biochem), and Psychological, Social, and Biological Foundations of Behavior (Psych/Soc). All sections consist of multiple-choice questions.

Section	Concepts Tested	Number of Questions and Timing
Chemical and Physical Foundations of Biological Systems	Basic concepts in chemistry and physics, including biochemistry; scientific inquiry; reasoning; research methods; and statistics.	59 questions in 95 minutes
Critical Analysis and Reasoning Skills	Critical analysis of information drawn from a wide range of social science and humanities disciplines.	53 questions in 90 minutes
Biological and Biochemical Foundations of Living Systems	Basic concepts in biology and biochemistry, scientific inquiry, reasoning, research methods, and statistics.	59 questions in 95 minutes
Psychological, Social, and Biological Foundations of Behavior	Basic concepts in psychology, sociology, and biology, research methods, and statistics.	59 questions in 95 minutes

Most questions on the MCAT (44 in the science sections, all 53 in the CARS section) are **passage-based**; the science sections have 10 passages each and the CARS section has 9. A passage consists of a few paragraphs of information on which several following questions are based. In the science sections, passages often include equations or reactions, tables, graphs, figures, and experiments to analyze. CARS passages come from literature in the social sciences, humanities, ethics, philosophy, cultural studies, and population health, and do not test content knowledge in any way.

Some questions in the science sections are *freestanding questions* (FSQs). These questions are independent of any passage information and appear in several groups of about four to five questions, interspersed throughout the passages. 15 of the questions in the science sections are freestanding, and the remainder are passage-based.

Each section on the MCAT is separated by either a 10-minute break or a 30-minute lunch break:

Section	Time
Test Center Check-In	Variable, can take up to 40 minutes if center is busy.
Tutorial	10 minutes
Chemical and Physical Foundations of Biological Systems	95 minutes
Break	10 minutes
Critical Analysis and Reasoning Skills	90 minutes
Lunch Break	30 minutes
Biological and Biochemical Foundations of Living Systems	95 minutes
Break	10 minutes
Psychological, Social, and Biological Foundations of Behavior	95 minutes
Void Option	5 minutes
Survey	5 minutes

The survey includes questions about your satisfaction with the overall MCAT experience, including registration, check-in, etc., as well as questions about how you prepared for the test.

Scoring

The MCAT is a scaled exam, meaning that your raw score will be converted into a scaled score that takes into account the difficulty of the questions. There is no guessing penalty. All sections are scored from 118–132, with a total scaled score range of 472–528. Because different versions of the test have varying levels of difficulty, the scale will be different from one exam to the next. Thus, there is no "magic number" of questions to get right in order to get a particular score. Plus, some of the questions on the test are considered "experimental" and do not count toward your score; they are just there to be evaluated for possible future inclusion in a test.

At the end of the test (after you complete the Psychological, Social, and Biological Foundations of Behavior section), you will be asked to choose one of the following two options: "I wish to have my MCAT exam scored" or "I wish to VOID my MCAT exam." You have five minutes to make a decision, and if you do not select one of the options in that time, the test will automatically be scored. If you choose the VOID option, your test will not be scored (you will not now, or ever, get a numerical score for this test), medical schools will not know you took the test, and no refunds will be granted. You cannot "unvoid" your scores at a later time.

So, what's a good score? The AAMC is centering the scale at 500 (i.e., 500 will be the 50th percentile), and recommends that application committees consider applicants near the center of the range. To be on the safe side, aim for a total score of around 510. Remember that if your GPA is on the low side, you'll need higher MCAT scores to compensate, and if you have a strong GPA, you can get away with lower MCAT scores. But the reality is that your chances of acceptance depend on a lot more than just your MCAT scores. It's a combination of your GPA, your MCAT scores, your undergraduate coursework, letters of recommendation, experience related to the medical field (such as volunteer work or research), extracurricular activities, your personal statement, etc. Medical schools are looking for a complete package, not just good scores and a good GPA.

GENERAL LAYOUT AND TEST-TAKING STRATEGIES

Layout of the Test

In each section of the test, the computer screen is divided vertically, with the passage on the left and the range of questions for that passage indicated above (e.g. "Passage 1, Questions 1–5"). The scroll bar for the passage text appears in the middle of the screen. Each question appears on the right, and you need to click "Next" to move to each subsequent question.

In the science sections, the freestanding questions are found in groups of 4–5, interspersed with the passages. The screen is still divided vertically; on the left is the statement "Questions [X–XX] do not refer to a passage and are independent of each other" and each question appears on the right as described above.

CBT Tools

There are a number of tools available on the test, including highlighting, strike-outs, the Mark button, the Review button, the Periodic Table button, and of course, scratch paper. The following is a brief description of each tool.

1) **Highlighting:** This is done in the passage text (including table entries and some equations, but excluding figures and molecular structures) and in the question stems by left-clicking and dragging the mouse across the words you wish to highlight; the selected words will then be highlighted in blue. When you release the mouse, a highlighting icon will appear; clicking on the icon will highlight the selected text in yellow. To remove the highlighting, left-click on the highlighted text.

2) **Strike-outs:** Right-clicking on an answer choice causes the entire text of that choice to be crossed out. The strike-out can be removed by right-clicking again. Left-clicking selects an answer choice; note than an answer choice that is selected cannot be struck out. When you strike out a figure or molecular structure, instead of being crossed out, the image turns grey.

3) **Mark button:** This allows you to flag the question for later review. When clicked, the flag on the "Mark" button turns red and says "Marked."

4) **Review button:** Clicking this button brings up a new screen showing all questions and their status (either "completed," "incomplete," or "marked"). You can choose to: "review all," "review incomplete," or "review marked." You can also double-click any question number to quickly return to that specific question. You can only review questions in the section of the MCAT you are currently taking, but the Review button can be clicked at any time during the allotted time for that section; you do NOT have to wait until the end of the section to click it.

5) **Periodic Table button:** Clicking this button will open a periodic table. Note that the periodic table is large, however it can be resized to see the questions and a portion of the periodic table at the same time.

6) **Scratch paper:** You will be given four pages (8 faces) of scratch paper at the start of the test. You can ask for more at any point during the test, and your first set of paper will be collected before you receive fresh paper. Scratch paper is only useful if it is kept organized; do not give in to the tendency to write on the first available open space! Good organization will be very helpful when/ if you wish to review a question. Indicate the passage number and the range of questions for that passage in a box near the top of your scratch work, and indicate the question you are working on in a circle to the left of the notes for that question. Draw a line under your scratch work when you change passages to keep the work separate. Do not erase or scribble over any previous work. If you do not think it is correct, draw one line through the work and start again. You may have already done some useful work without realizing it.

General Strategy for the Science Sections

Passages vs. FSQs in the Science Sections: What to Start With

Since the questions are displayed on separate screens, it is awkward and time-consuming to click through all of the questions up front to find the FSQs. Therefore, go through the section on a first pass and decide whether to do the passage now or to save it for later, basing your decision on the passage text and the first question. Tackle the FSQs as you come upon them. More details are below.

Here is an outline of the procedure:

1) For each passage, write a heading on your scratch paper with the passage number, the general topic, and its range of questions (e.g. "Passage 1, thermodynamics, Q 1–5" or "Passage 2, enzymes, Q 6–9). The passage numbers do not currently appear in the Review screen, thus having the question numbers on your scratch paper will allow you to move through the section more efficiently.

2) Skim the text and rank the passage. If a passage is a "Now," complete it before moving on to the next passage (also see "Attacking the Questions" below). If it is a "Later" passage, first write "SKIPPED" in block letters under the passage heading on your scratch paper and leave room for your work when you come back to complete that passage. (Note that the specific passages you skip will be unique to you; in the Bio/Biochem section, you might choose to do all Biology passages first, then come back for Biochemistry. Or in Chem/Phys you might choose to skip Experiment Presentation passages. Know ahead of time what type of passage you are going to skip and follow your plan.)

3) Next, click on the "Review" button at the bottom to get to the review screen. Double-click on the first question of the next passage; you'll be able to identify it because you know the range of questions from the passage you just skipped. This will take you to the next passage, where you will repeat steps 1–3.

4) Once you have completed the "Now" passages, go to the review screen and double-click the first question for the first passage you skipped. Answer the questions, and continue going back to the review screen and repeating this procedure for other passages you have skipped.

Attacking the Questions

As you work through the questions, if you encounter a particularly lengthy question, or a question that requires a lot of analysis, you may choose to skip it. This is a wise strategy because it ensures you will tackle all the easier questions first, the ones you are more likely to get right. If you choose to skip the question (or if you attempt it but get stuck), write down the question number on your scratch paper, click the Mark button to flag the question in the Review screen, and move on to the next question. At the end of the passage, click back through the set of questions to complete any that you skipped over the first time through, and make sure that you have filled in an answer for every question.

General Strategy for the CARS Section

Ranking and Ordering the Passages: What to Start With

Ranking: Since the questions are displayed on separate screens, it is awkward and time consuming to click through all of the questions before ranking each passage as "Now" (an easier passage), "Later" (a harder passage), or "Killer" (a passage that you will randomly guess on). Therefore, rank the passage and decide whether or not to do it on the first pass through the section based on the passage text, skimming the first 2–3 sentences.

Ordering: Because of the additional clicking through screens (or use of the Review screen) that is required to navigate through the section, the "Two-Pass" system (completing the "Now" passages as you find them) is likely to be your most efficient approach. However, if you find that you are continuously making a lot of bad ranking decisions, it is still valid to experiment with the "Three-Pass" approach (ranking all nine passages up front before attempting your first "Now" passage).

Here is an outline of the basic Ranking and Ordering procedure to follow.

1) For each passage, write a heading on your scratch paper with the passage number and its range of questions (e.g. Passage 1, Q 1–5). The passage numbers do not currently appear in the Review screen, thus having the question numbers on your scratch paper will allow you to move through the section more efficiently.

2) Skim the first 2–3 sentences and rank the passage. If the passage is a "Now," complete it before moving on to the next. If it is a "Later" or "Killer," first write either "Later" or "Killer" and "SKIPPED" in block letters under the passage heading on your scratch paper and leave room for your work if you decide to come back and complete that passage. Then click through each question, marking each one and filling in random guesses, until you get to the next passage.

3) Once you have completed the "Now" passages, come back for your second pass and complete the "Later" passages, leaving your random guesses in place for any "Killer" passages that you choose not to complete. You can go to the Review screen and use your scratch paper notes on the question numbers. Double-click on the number of the first question for that passage to go back to that question, and proceed from there. Alternatively, if you have consistently marked all the questions for passages you skipped in your first pass you can use "Review Marked" from the Review screen to find and complete your "Later" passages.

4) Regardless of how you choose to find your second pass passages, unmark each question after you complete it, so that you can continue to rely on the Review screen (and the "Review Marked" function") to identify questions that you have not yet attempted.

Previewing the Questions

The formatting and functioning of the tools makes previewing the questions effective! Having each question on a separate screen will encourage you to really focus on that question. Even more importantly, you can now highlight in the question stem (but still not in the answer choices).

Here is the basic procedure for previewing the questions:

1) Start with the first question, and if it has lead words referencing passage content, highlight them. You may also choose to jot them down on your scratch paper. Once you reach and preview the last question for the set on that passage, THEN stay on that screen and work the passage (your highlighting appears and stays on every passage screen, and persists through the whole 90 minutes).

2) Once you have worked the passage and defined the Bottom Line, work **backward** from the last question to the first. If you skip over any questions as you go (see "Attacking the Questions" below), write down the question number on your scratch paper. Then click **forward** through the set of questions, completing any that you skipped over the first time through. Once you reach and complete the last question for that passage, clicking "Next" will send you to the first question of the next passage. Working the questions from last to first the first time through the set will eliminate the need to click back through multiple screens to get to the first question immediately after previewing, and will also make it easier and more efficient to do the hardest questions last (see "Attacking the Questions" below).

Attacking the Questions

The question types and the procedure for actually attacking each type will be discussed later. However, it is still important **not** to attempt the hardest questions first (potentially getting stuck, wasting time, and discouraging yourself).

So, as you work the questions from last to first (see "Previewing the Questions" above), if you encounter a particularly difficult and/or lengthy question (or if you attempt a question but get stuck) write down the question number on your scratch paper (you may also choose to mark it) and move on backward to the next question you will attempt. Then click **forward** through the set and complete any that you skipped over the first time through the set, unmarking any questions that you marked that first time through and making sure that you have filled in an answer for every question.

Pacing Strategy for the MCAT

Since the MCAT is a timed test, you must keep an eye on the timer and adjust your pacing as necessary. It would be terrible to run out of time at the end only to discover that the last few questions could have been easily answered in just a few seconds each.

In the science sections you will have about one minute and thirty-five seconds (1:35) per question, and in the CARS section you will have about one minute and forty seconds (1:40) per question, not taking into account the time spent reading the passage before answering the questions.

Section	# of Questions in passage	Approximate time (including reading the passage)
Chem/Phys, Bio/Biochem, and Psych/Soc	4	6.5 minutes
	5	8 minutes
	6	9.5 minutes
CARS	5	8.5 minutes
	6	10 minutes
	7	11.5 minutes

When starting a passage in the science sections, make note of how much time you will allot for it, and the starting time on the timer. Jot down on your scratch paper what the timer should say at the end of the passage. Then just keep an eye on it as you work through the questions. If you are near the end of the time for that passage, guess on any remaining questions, make some notes on your scratch paper, Mark the questions, and move on. Come back to those questions if you have time.

For the CARS section, keep in mind that many people will maximize their score by *not* trying to complete every question or every passage in the section. A good strategy for test takers who cannot achieve a high level of accuracy on all nine passages is to randomly guess on at least one passage in the section, and spend your time getting a high percentage of the other questions right. To complete all nine CARS passages, you have about ten minutes per passage. To complete eight of the nine, you have about 11 minutes per passage.

To help maximize your number of correct answer choices in any section, do the questions and passages within that section in the order *you* want to do them in. See "General Strategy" above.

Process of Elimination

Process of elimination (POE) is probably the most useful technique you have to tackle MCAT questions. Since there is no guessing penalty, POE allows you to increase your probability of choosing the correct answer by eliminating those you are sure are wrong.

1) Strike out any choices that you are sure are incorrect or that do not address the issue raised in the question.
2) Jot down some notes to help clarify your thoughts if you return to the question.
3) Use the "Mark" button to flag the question for review. (Note, however, that in the CARS section, you generally should not be returning to rethink questions once you have moved on to a new passage.)
4) Do not leave it blank! For the sciences, if you are not sure and you have already spent more than 60 seconds on that question, just pick one of the remaining choices. If you have time to review it at the end, you can always debate the remaining choices based on your previous notes. For CARS, if you have been through the choices two or three times, have re-read the question stem and gone back to the passage and you are still stuck, move on. Do the remaining questions for that passage, take one more look at the question you were stuck on, then pick an answer and move on for good.
5) Special Note: if three of the four answer choices have been eliminated, the remaining choice must be the correct answer. Don't waste time pondering *why* it is correct, just click it and move on. The MCAT doesn't care if you truly understand why it's the right answer, only that you have the right answer selected.
6) More subject-specific information on techniques will be presented in the next chapter.

Guessing

Remember, there is NO guessing penalty on the MCAT. NEVER leave a question blank!

QUESTION TYPES

In the science sections of the MCAT, the questions fall into one of three main categories.

1) Memory questions: These questions can be answered directly from prior knowledge and represent about 25 percent of the total number of questions.
2) Explicit questions: These questions are those for which the answer is explicitly stated in the passage. To answer them correctly, for example, may just require finding a definition, or reading a graph, or making a simple connection. Explicit questions represent about 35 percent of the total number of questions.
3) Implicit questions: These questions require you to apply knowledge to a new situation; the answer is typically implied by the information in the passage. These questions often start "if…. then…." (for example, "if we modify the experiment in the passage like this, then what result would we expect?"). Implicit style questions make up about 40 percent of the total number of questions.

In the CARS section, the questions fall into four main categories:

1) Specific questions: These either ask you for facts from the passage (Retrieval questions) or require you to deduce what is most likely to be true based on the passage (Inference questions).
2) General questions: These ask you to summarize themes (Main Idea and Primary Purpose questions) or evaluate an author's opinion (Tone/Attitude questions).
3) Reasoning questions: These ask you to describe the purpose of, or the support provided for, a statement made in the passage (Structure questions) or to judge how well the author supports his or her argument (Evaluate questions).
4) Application questions: These ask you to apply new information from either the question stem itself (New Information questions) or from the answer choices (Strengthen, Weaken, and Analogy questions) to the passage.

More detail on question types and strategies can be found in Chapter 2.

TESTING TIPS

Before Test Day

- Take a trip to the test center at least a day or two before your actual test date so that you can easily find the building and room on test day. This will also allow you to gauge traffic and see if you need money for parking or anything like that. Knowing this type of information ahead of time will greatly reduce your stress on the day of your test.
- Don't do any heavy studying the day before the test. This is not a test you can cram for! Your goal at this point is to rest and relax so that you can go into test day in a good physical and mental condition.
- During the week before the test, adjust your sleeping schedule so that you are going to bed and getting up in the morning at the same times as on the day before and morning of the MCAT. Prioritize getting a reasonable amount of sleep during the last few nights before the test.
- Eat well. Try to avoid excessive caffeine and sugar. Ideally, in the weeks leading up to the actual test you should experiment a little bit with foods and practice tests to see which foods give you the most endurance. Aim for steady blood sugar levels during the test: sports drinks, peanut-butter crackers, trail mix, etc. make good snacks for your breaks and lunch.

General Test Day Info and Tips

- On the day of the test, arrive at the test center at least a half hour prior to the start time of your test.
- Examinees will be checked in to the center in the order in which they arrive.
- You will be assigned a locker or secure area in which to put your personal items. Textbooks and study notes are not allowed, so there is no need to bring them with you to the test center.

- Your ID will be checked, a digital image of your fingerprint will be taken, and you will be asked to sign in.
- You will be given scratch paper and a couple of pencils, and the test center administrator will take you to the computer on which you will complete the test. You may not choose a computer; you must use the computer assigned to you.
- Nothing, not even your watch, is allowed at the computer station except your photo ID, your locker key (if provided), and a factory sealed packet of ear plugs.
- If you choose to leave the testing room at the breaks, you will have your fingerprint checked again, and you will have to sign in and out.
- You are allowed to access the items in your locker, except for notes and cell phones. (Check your test center's policy on cell phones ahead of time; some centers do not even allow them to be kept in your locker.)
- Don't forget to bring the snack foods and lunch you experimented with in your practice tests.
- At the end of the test, the test administrator will collect your scratch paper and shred it.
- Definitely take the breaks! Get up and walk around. It's a good way to clear your head between sections and get the blood (and oxygen!) flowing to your brain.
- Ask for new scratch paper at the breaks if you use it all up.

A NOTE ABOUT FLASHCARDS

For most of the exams you've taken previously, flashcards were likely very helpful. This was because those exams mostly required you to regurgitate information, and flashcards are pretty good at helping you memorize facts. However, the most challenging aspect of the MCAT is not that it requires you to memorize the fine details of content knowledge, but that it requires you to apply your basic scientific knowledge to unfamiliar situations: flashcards alone may not help you there.

Flashcards can be beneficial if your basic content knowledge is deficient in some area. For example, if you don't know Big 5 kinematics equations, flashcards can certainly help you memorize these facts. Or, maybe you are unsure of the rules for waves. You might find that flashcards can help you memorize these. But unless you are trying to memorize basic facts in your personal weak areas, you are better off doing and analyzing practice passages than carrying around a stack of flashcards.

Chapter 2
Physics Strategy
for the MCAT

2.1 SCIENCE SECTIONS OVERVIEW

There are three science sections on the MCAT:

- Chemical and Physical Foundations of Biological Systems
- Biological and Biochemical Foundations of Living Systems
- Psychological, Social, and Biological Foundations of Behavior

The Chemical and Physical Foundations of Biological Systems section (Chem/Phys) is the first section on the test. It includes questions from General Chemistry (about 30%), Physics (about 25%), Organic Chemistry (about 15%), Biochemistry (about 25%), and Biology (about 5%). Further, the questions often test chemical and physical concepts within a biological setting; for example, pressure and fluid flow in blood vessels. A solid grasp of math fundamentals is required (arithmetic, algebra, graphs, trigonometry, vectors, proportions, and logarithms); however, there are no calculus-based questions.

The Biological and Biochemical Foundations of Living Systems section (Bio/Biochem) is the third section on the test. Approximately 65% of the questions in this section come from biology, approximately 25% come from biochemistry, and approximately 10% come from Organic and General Chemistry. Math calculations are generally not required on this section of the test; however, a basic understanding of statistics as used in biological research is helpful.

The Psychological, Social, and Biological Foundations of Behavior section (Psych/Soc) is the fourth and final section on the test. About 60% of the questions will be drawn from Psychology, about 30% from Sociology, and about 10% from Biology. As with the Bio/Biochem section, calculations are generally not required; however, a basic understanding of statistics as used in research is helpful.

Most of the questions in the science sections (44 of the 59) are passage-based, and each section has ten passages. Passages consist of a few paragraphs of information and include equations, reactions, graphs, figures, tables, experiments, and data. Four to six questions will be associated with each passage.

The remaining 25% of the questions (15 of 59) in each science section are freestanding questions (FSQs). These questions appear in approximately four groups interspersed between the passages. Each group contains four to five questions.

95 minutes are allotted to each of the science sections. This breaks down to approximately one minute and 35 seconds per question.

2.2 SCIENCE PASSAGE TYPES

The passages in the science sections fall into one of three main categories: Information and/or Situation Presentation, Experiment/Research Presentation, or Persuasive Reasoning.

Information and/or Situation Presentation

These passages either present straightforward scientific information or describe a particular event or occurrence. Generally, questions associated with these passages test basic science facts or ask you to predict outcomes given new variables or new information. Here is an example of an Information/Situation Presentation passage:

Figure 1 shows a portion of the inner mechanism of a typical home smoke detector. It consists of a pair of capacitor plates which are charged by a 9-volt battery (not shown). The capacitor plates (electrodes) are connected to a sensor device, D; the resistor R denotes the internal resistance of the sensor. Normally, air acts as an insulator and no current would flow in the circuit shown. However, inside the smoke detector is a small sample of an artificially produced radioactive element, americium-241, which decays primarily by emitting alpha particles, with a half-life of approximately 430 years. The daughter nucleus of the decay has a half-life in excess of two million years and therefore poses virtually no biohazard.

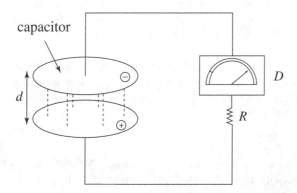

Figure 1 Smoke detector mechanism

The decay products (alpha particles and gamma rays) from the ^{241}Am sample ionize air molecules between the plates and thus provide a conducting pathway which allows current to flow in the circuit shown in Figure 1. A steady-state current is quickly established and remains as long as the battery continues to maintain a 9-volt potential difference between its terminals. However, if smoke particles enter the space between the capacitor plates and thereby interrupt the flow, the current is reduced, and the sensor responds to this change by triggering the alarm. (Furthermore, as the battery starts to "die out," the resulting drop in current is also detected to alert the homeowner to replace the battery.)

$$C = \varepsilon_0 \frac{A}{d}$$

Equation 1

where ε_0 is the universal permittivity constant, equal to $8.85 \times 10^{-12} \ C^2/(N \ m^2)$. Since the area A of each capacitor plate in the smoke detector is 20 cm^2 and the plates are separated by a distance d of 5 mm, the capacitance is $3.5 \times 10^{-12} \ F = 3.5$ pF.

Experiment/Research Presentation

These passages present the details of experiments and research procedures. They often include data tables and graphs. Generally, questions associated with these passages ask you to interpret data, draw conclusions, and make inferences. Here is an example of an Experiment/Research Presentation passage:

The development of sexual characteristics depends upon various factors, the most important of which are hormonal control, environmental stimuli, and the genetic makeup of the individual. The hormones that contribute to the development include the steroid hormones estrogen, progesterone, and testosterone, as well as the pituitary hormones FSH (follicle-stimulating hormone) and LH (luteinizing hormone).

To study the mechanism by which estrogen exerts its effects, a researcher performed the following experiments using cell culture assays.

Experiment 1:

Human embryonic placental mesenchyme (HEPM) cells were grown for 48 hours in Dulbecco's Modified Eagle Medium (DMEM), with media change every 12 hours. Upon confluent growth, cells were exposed to a 10 mg per mL solution of green fluorescent-labeled estrogen for 1 hour. Cells were rinsed with DMEM and observed under confocal fluorescent microscopy.

Experiment 2:

HEPM cells were grown to confluence as in Experiment 1. Cells were exposed to Pesticide A for 1 hour, followed by the 10 mg/mL solution of labeled estrogen, rinsed as in Experiment 1, and observed under confocal fluorescent microscopy.

Experiment 3:

Experiment 1 was repeated with Chinese Hamster Ovary (CHO) cells instead of HEPM cells.

Experiment 4:

CHO cells injected with cytoplasmic extracts of HEPM cells were grown to confluence, exposed to the 10 mg/mL solution of labeled estrogen for 1 hour, and observed under confocal fluorescent microscopy.

The results of these experiments are given in Table 1.

Table 1 Detection of Estrogen (+ indicates presence of Estrogen)

Experiment	Media	Cytoplasm	Nucleus
1	+	+	+
2	+	+	+
3	+	+	+
4	+	+	+

After observing the cells in each experiment, the researcher bathed the cells in a solution containing 10 mg per mL of a red fluorescent probe that binds specifically to the estrogen receptor only when its active site is occupied. After 1 hour, the cells were rinsed with DMEM and observed under confocal fluorescent microscopy. The results are presented in Table 2.

The researcher also repeated Experiment 2 using Pesticide B, an estrogen analog, instead of Pesticide A. Results from other researchers had shown that Pesticide B binds to the active site of the cytosolic estrogen receptor (with an affinity 10,000 times greater than that of estrogen) and causes increased transcription of mRNA.

Table 2 Observed Fluorescence and Estrogen Effects (G = green, R = red)

Experiment	Media	Cytoplasm	Nucleus	Estrogen effects observed?
1	G only	G and R	G and R	Yes
2	G only	G only	G only	No
3	G only	G only	G only	No
4	G only	G and R	G and R	Yes

Based on these results, the researcher determined that estrogen had no effect when not bound to a cytosolic, estrogen-specific receptor.

Persuasive (Scientific) Reasoning

These passages typically present a scientific phenomenon along with a hypothesis that explains the phenomenon, and may include counter-arguments as well. Questions associated with these passages ask you to evaluate the hypothesis or arguments. Persuasive Reasoning passages in the science sections of the MCAT tend to be less common than Information Presentation or Experiment-based passages. Here is an example of a Persuasive Reasoning passage:

Two theoretical chemists attempted to explain the observed trends of acidity by applying two interpretations of molecular orbital theory. Consider the pK_a values of some common acids listed along the conjugate base:

acid	pK_a	conjugate base
H_2SO_4	< 0	HSO_4^-
H_2CrO_4	5.0	$HCrO_4^-$
H_2PO_4	2.1	$H_2PO_4^-$
HF	3.9	F^-
HOCl	7.8	ClO^-
HCN	9.5	CN^-
HIO_3	1.2	IO_3^-

Recall that acids with a $pK_a < 0$ are called strong acids, and those with a $pK_a > 0$ are called weak acids. The arguments of the chemists are given below.

Chemist #1:

"The acidity of a compound is proportional to the polarization of the H—X bond, where X is some nonmetal element. Complex acids, such as H_2SO_4, $HClO_4$, and HNO_3 are strong acids because the H—O bonding electrons are strongly drawn towards the oxygen. It is generally true that a covalent bond weakens as its polarization increases. Therefore, one can conclude that the strength of an acid is proportional to the number of electronegative atoms in that acid."

Chemist #2:

"The acidity of a compound is proportional to the number of stable resonance structures of that acid's conjugate base. H_2SO_4, $HClO_4$, and HNO_3 are all strong acids because their respective conjugate bases exhibit a high degree of resonance stabilization."

MAPPING A PASSAGE

"Mapping a passage" refers to the combination of on-screen highlighting and scratch paper notes that you take while working through a passage. Typically, good things to highlight include the overall topic of a passage, unfamiliar terms and their definitions, familiar terms in unfamiliar contexts, repeated phrases in a paragraph (highlight the first instance), extreme or exclusive terms (most/least, maximum/minimum, always/never, except, etc.), italicized terms and their definitions, numerical values floating in text, hypotheses or causal terms, and results or effects terms. Scratch paper notes can be used to copy given equations and equations from memory (when none are given), to copy and label simplified figures or to draw diagrams of something described in words but not pictured, to summarize the paragraphs, and to jot down important facts and connections that are made when reading the passage. More details on passage mapping will be presented in Section 2.5.

2.3 SCIENCE QUESTION TYPES

Each question in the science sections is generally one of three main types: Memory, Explicit, or Implicit.

Memory Questions

These questions can be answered directly from prior knowledge, with little need to reference the passage or question text. Memory questions represent approximately 25 percent of the science questions on the MCAT. Usually, Memory questions are found as FSQs, but they can also be tucked into a passage. Here's an example of a Memory question:

Which of the following acetylating conditions will convert diethylamine into an amide at the fastest rate?

A) Acetic acid / HCl
B) Acetic anhydride
C) Acetyl chloride
D) Ethyl acetate

2.3

Explicit Questions

Explicit questions can be answered primarily with information from the passage, along with basic prior knowledge. They may require data retrieval, graph analysis, or making a simple connection. Explicit questions make up approximately 35–40 percent of the science questions on the MCAT; here's an example (taken from the Information/Situation Presentation passage above):

The sensor device D shown in Figure 1 performs its function by acting as:

A) an ohmmeter.
B) a voltmeter.
C) a potentiometer.
D) an ammeter.

Implicit Questions

These questions require you to take information from the passage, combine it with your prior knowledge, apply it to a new situation, and come to some logical conclusion. They typically require more complex connections than do Explicit questions, and may also require data retrieval, graph analysis, etc. Implicit questions usually require a solid understanding of the passage information. They make up approximately 35–40 percent of the science questions on the MCAT; here's an example (taken from the Experiment/Research Presentation passage above):

If Experiment 2 were repeated, but this time exposing the cells first to Pesticide A and then to Pesticide B before exposing them to the green fluorescent-labeled estrogen and the red fluorescent probe, which of the following statements will most likely be true?

A) Pesticide A and Pesticide B bind to the same site on the estrogen receptor.
B) Estrogen effects would be observed.
C) Only green fluorescence would be observed.
D) Both green and red fluorescence would be observed.

The Rod of Asclepius

You may notice this Rod of Asclepius icon as you read through the book. In Greek mythology, the Rod of Asclepius is associated with healing and medicine; the symbol continues to be used today to represent medicine and healthcare. You won't see this on the actual MCAT, but we've used it here to call attention to medically related examples and questions.

2.4   PHYSICS ON THE MCAT

Of all the sciences on the MCAT, Physics relies the least on information recall and the most on problem-solving and reading comprehension skills. This is in part because the subject matter lends itself to these kinds of problems. Perhaps more importantly, though, the subject content in Physics pertains less to the material you will ultimately study in medical school, whereas the critical thinking that Physics demands fits with what you will encounter (particularly during your clinical years). In many ways, your ability to formulate an "approach" to a tough problem is one of the most useful skills you can develop along the path to medicine.

The science sections of the MCAT have 10 passages and 15 freestanding questions (FSQs). Physics makes up about 25% of the questions in the Chemical and Physical Foundations of Biological Systems section (Chem/Phys). The remaining 75% of the questions are divided up as General Chemistry (30%), Organic Chemistry (15%), Biochemistry (25%), and Biology (5%) questions.

2.5   TACKLING A PASSAGE

Passage Types as They Apply to Physics

Information/Situation Presentation

These passages tend to fall into two types for Physics. The first type consists of straightforward descriptions of phenomena you should already understand well, such as a passage comparing the function of a nerve cell to a DC circuit with a battery, a capacitor, a couple of switches, and a few resistors in parallel combinations. Common question types include solving unknown variables using memorized formulas, true-or-false questions about physical laws, and comparisons of the "real" to the "ideal."

The second type of passage consists of technical elaborations of phenomena you know something about, such as a passage about an electrocardiogram circuit with resistors, a capacitor, and a number of operational amplifiers (circuit elements that multiply input voltage) that provides equations for the time-dependent voltage input from the body and output by the device. Such technical passages are often marked by several new equations and possibly graphs, followed by paragraphs defining the variables and constants. Common question types for technical passages include algebraic manipulation questions, functional dependence or proportionality questions, and graph generation or interpretation questions.

Experiment or Research Presentation

These passages often include data tables; if there's a table, the passage probably covers an experiment or multiple experiments. The subject matter in experimental passages is typically familiar, though the concepts might be extended somewhat beyond basic knowledge, for example, measuring the viscosity in a fluid or the resistance of a conducting wire as a function of temperature. These passages tend *not* to push your understanding of content as much as the technical passages or heavily conceptual passages. Rather, the implicit questions found in experiment presentation passages are usually of the form, "If another trial were conducted changing [some set of parameters], then the resulting value of [another parameter] would be…." Such questions require you to read numbers from the tables and determine their functional dependence on the altered parameters. In other words, you need to write down an equation for the value of the parameter, and to check whether the altered variables affect that value and how.

Persuasive (Scientific) Reasoning

Persuasive reasoning passages on the Physics portion of the MCAT are largely conceptual: They describe some particular phenomenon about which you most likely have no prior knowledge, offering one or more theories as to its causes and effects, and they do so almost entirely with words (as opposed to using figures, equations, and numbers). These are generally the hardest passages for most people, as they rely heavily on reading comprehension as well as the ability to recall and synthesize physics concepts and equations from different topics (e.g., atomic structure, magnetism, and standing waves). You can expect questions in which both the question text and the answer choices are themselves entirely in words. This means you must be comfortable translating sentences into proportions, ratios, or equations, and then translating them back into sentences. Moreover, it may not be enough to be a careful reader with a good memory for formulas: Conceptual passages will test whether you know the conditions under which equations apply (such as the conditions for an ideal fluid or when to hold Q or V constant in $Q = CV$).

Reading a Physics Passage

Don't let our heading here deceive you; "reading" in the sense we commonly use the word is seldom the best way to use physics passages effectively. A kind of "informed skimming" is usually the best strategy. A quick holistic scan of the passage, including reading its first sentence, should be enough to tell you its topic and type; this will help you decide whether to do it now or postpone it until you've tackled easier passages (for example, if you dislike circuits, or if a lot of reading comprehension slows you down, by all means leave those passages until later!). Once you decide to do a passage, use the following techniques to find what you need to know quickly.

1. Read the first sentence again carefully. It will probably define the main idea of the passage and might inform your answer to one of the questions directly. Similarly, if the passage describes a set of experimental procedures, read the first sentences in each subsection so you understand precisely what is being done and why.

2. Look for the familiar Physics terms within the passage and highlight them. Remember that the questions on the MCAT can come directly from anything mentioned by the AAMC topics list, or they can come from a reading-comprehension topic in a passage. And in fact, many Physics passages may not seem to be about a particular Physics topic at first glance. For example, a passage about ultrasound scans may be about waves, or sound, or fluid dynamics, or all of those topics at the same time! If you can identify the relevant physics within the passage text, you can focus in on that text and topic rather than getting stuck on the paragraph about, say, the historical perspective of how we measure heart rate.

3. Look for any new terms. These are often italicized but not always, so scan for long unfamiliar phrases (phrases like "aeroelastic flutter" stick out in a paragraph even in plain type). Highlight them along with their definitions.

2.5

4. Find the equations and figures. The text immediately before or after them tends to define terms or provide numerical values (measurements in a diagram or values of constants in an equation). If the diagrams are basically complete or the equations make sense to you, *skip this text*: There's no good reason to read a paragraph describing the circuit diagram for a defibrillator if the picture already tells the whole story.

5. Look for numbers. These are sometimes worth highlighting or jotting down on your scratch paper and they are easy to find (however, if a passage gives you a whole pile of values, just highlight them so you can find those you need for the questions). There are a couple of key things to remember about numbers:

    a. Numbers on the MCAT are always accompanied by their units, either immediately following the number, or in the heading of the table where the numbers appear. If there are no units, the number must be unitless.

    b. Highlighting can be done with a left-click and drag, then clicking the highlighting icon, but keep in mind that numbers in figures may not be in a format that allows for highlighting. In these cases, use scratch paper to note numbers.

6. Finally, for lengthy Persuasive (Scientific) Reasoning passages, you may need to spend time fruitfully highlighting the text and dealing with complicated figures by redrawing a simplified version or carefully studying it on the screen. The fact that this will take longer is a legitmate reason to leave conceptual passages for last, but don't make the common error of thinking you have to understand everything you read! This is a multiple choice test, not an essay exam: you often don't need to understand this sort of question to be able to eliminate all but one answer choice.

Mapping a Physics Passage

Physics work should be done on paper; there are very few answers on the test that can be found without writing something down. Thus, your scratch paper is your primary tool, whether solving FSQs or mapping a passage. As suggested above, there are a few specific reasons to use the highlighting tool, but apart from that you want to rely on your scratch paper. "Mapping" involves jotting down a schematic of the passage that will help you to answer the questions efficiently without having to fish for information. Here are some mapping strategies:

1. Label your scratch paper with the passage number and question numbers. Staying organized saves time and avoids errors.

2. Write down any given equations with space below to work on them. The chances that you will *not* end up using some equation given to you in a passage are low, so it's worth the time to prepare for the algebra and estimation the questions will require. Moreover, merely copying the equations helps you to understand them better than you would just looking at them.

3. If there are any simple diagrams, copy them down and label any values (some will be given in the text around the diagram and not labeled directly in the version on your screen). Again, you might resist this as a potential waste of time, but it is important to be able to manipulate the figures to answer the questions. For example, in a passage where forces are important (e.g., for most of mechanics, buoyancy in fluids, charges interacting with electric or magnetic fields, or simple harmonic oscillators), you should put the forces on your diagram *before* you do the questions. By doing so, you will probably anticipate the answers to one or more questions even before they are asked. Overall, this should both save you time and increase your percentage of right answers.

4. If the passage is conceptual or has conceptual parts to it, translate any mathematical statements written as sentences into symbols and treat those as you would equations given in a more technical passage. For example, if you were reading a passage on Poiseuille's law applied to blood flow and came across the sentence, "Poiseuille's law shows that the flow rate of a viscous fluid through a pipe with circular cross section is inversely proportional to the fourth power of its radius," you would jot down $f \propto 1/r^4$.

5. Especially for passages that don't include many diagrams or equations, write down the equations and basic ideas you recall about the passage topic. This will give you something tangible with which to tackle the questions. For example, a passage might describe a perfectly inelastic collision between two masses, and you might write down $\mathbf{p} = m\mathbf{v}$, $\mathbf{p}_i = \mathbf{p}_f$, and "momentum conserved, KE not."

Practice all of these strategies with the passages in this book to see which work best for you; then make those strategies a part of your standard repertoire. Give yourself about 90 seconds to map a passage before you look at the questions. Many passage maps will take less time than this, a few might take longer. Don't worry that you're spending time not answering questions; practice will make you more efficient.

Another, more advanced study technique you might use once you feel more comfortable about your passage mapping is to map a couple of passages, put those maps aside for an hour or so while you do something else (practice FSQs), then go back to the passages, cover up their text, and try to do the questions with just your map. You shouldn't necessarily be able to answer all the questions without referring to the passage, but if you find that you're unable to answer any but those that rely on memory of basic concepts, then you need to improve your mapping technique. Below is an example of these strategies applied to a passage.

Blood flow through the vascular system of the human body is controlled by several factors. The rate of flow, Q, is directly proportional to the pressure differential, ΔP, between any two points in the system and inversely proportional to the resistance, R, of the system:

$$Q = \Delta P/R$$

Equation 1

The resistance, R, is dependent on the length of the vessel, L, the viscosity of blood, η, and the vessel's radius, r according to the equation

$$R = \frac{8\eta L}{\pi r^4}$$

Equation 2

Under normal conditions, vessel length and blood viscosity do not vary significantly. However, certain conditions can cause changes in blood content, thereby altering viscosity. Veins are generally more compliant than arteries due to their less muscular nature. The flow of blood through the major arteries can be approximated by the equations of ideal flow.

The dynamics of fluid movement from capillaries to body tissue and back to capillaries is also driven by pressure differentials. The net filtration pressure is the difference between the hydrostatic pressure of the blood in the capillaries, P_c, and the hydrostatic pressure of tissue fluid outside the capillaries, P_i. The oncotic pressure is the difference between the osmotic pressure of the capillaries, Π_c (approximately 25 torr), and the osmotic pressure of the tissue fluids, Π_i (negligible). Whether fluid moves into or out of the capillary network depends on the magnitudes of the net filtration and oncotic pressures. The direction of fluid movement can be determined by calculating the following pressure differential:

$$\Delta P = (P_c + \Pi_i) - (P_i + \Pi_c)$$

Equation 3

The sum in the first set of parentheses gives the pressure acting to move fluid out of the capillaries, while the sum in the second set of parentheses gives the pressure acting to move fluid into the capillaries.

Capillaries are porous, and the blood pressure on the arterial end of a capillary bed is enough to push fluid out of the capillaries and into the surrounding tissues. However, blood proteins and cells are too big to fit through the pores. Consequently, as the blood travels across the capillary bed, it becomes relatively more concentrated in proteins and cells; this leads to an osmotic influx of fluid on the venous side of the capillary bed. Note, however, that the volume of fluid lost to the tissues due to pressure is greater than the volume of fluid returned to the blood due to osmosis, so there is a net outward flow of fluid to the tissues. This excess fluid is recaptured and returned to the cardiovascular system via the lymphatic vessels.

Sample Passage Analysis and Mapping

Highlight the key phrase, "blood flow." Note that this passage is heavily laden with equations (three), has several potentially unfamiliar terms, and has no tabular data. This is best characterized as a technical Information Presentation passage, not as obscure as some if you understand the underlying biology and physics, but still challenging.

The overall lack of numbers is obvious, so just highlight the 25 torr for the osmotic pressure of the capillaries and be done with it. Some people might be more comfortable drawing a simple figure of blood moving from capillaries to tissues to capillaries and including pressures there, but that's up to you: this isn't a case in which a force diagram or simplified circuit will shed tremendous light on the phenomenon.

A few possibly unfamiliar terms like "net filtration pressure" and "oncotic pressure" appear and should be highlighted with their definitions. The definitions of some given variables are worth highlighting both because the symbols can be confusing (Q for flow rate, R for flow resistance) and in case you encounter a question that uses the words without the algebraic symbols. You should copy the three given equations on your scratch paper, noting mentally the difference between this flow rate equation and the one you know from memory ($f = Av$). Remember, a new equation in a passage is always more important than a memorized equation for any questions that deal explicitly with the phenomenon described in the passage. At this point it may also be worthwhile to write down the continuity equation ($A_1v_1 = A_2v_2$). You should have committed to memory the rules for ideal fluid flow (including negligible viscosity) and know therefore that Bernoulli's equation would not apply except to the case of "major arteries."

The third paragraph presents perhaps the greatest mapping challenge for this passage. You might be tempted to highlight the entire paragraph because it describes an unfamiliar phenomenon. However, highlighting is not the same as comprehension; further, none of the terminology here is specialized. Thus, it's better to skip highlighting the paragraph entirely or to follow the rule to highlight causal phrases (as shown). It's worth noting that the passage doesn't actually mention what "certain conditions" are, so this paragraph lacks the information necessary to answer Explicit questions.

Your scratch paper map should thus look something like this:

$$Q = \Delta P/R \qquad R = \frac{8\eta L}{\pi r^4} \qquad \Delta P = (P_c + \Pi_i) - (P_i + \Pi_c)$$

$$\Pi_c = 25 \text{ torr}, \Pi_i = 0.$$

2.6 PHYSICS QUESTION TYPES

As stated previously, the questions in this section of the MCAT fall into one of three main categories:

1. **Memory questions**: Answered from concepts and equations you know walking into the test with just brute facts from the questions or passage, such as numbers or vector directions.
2. **Explicit questions**: Answered from information stated explicitly in the passage. To answer them correctly may require finding a definition, reading a graph, or manipulating a given equation.
3. **Implicit questions**: Answered by applying knowledge to a new situation or making more complex connections. Often the answer is implied by the information in the passage but requires logical reasoning on your part.

Note that the way you categorize questions on the MCAT will depend on how much knowledge you bring to the test in the first place. The more confident you are about the basic material outlined in the list of Physics topics, the less you will have to rely on the passage and question text to answer questions. This will ultimately save you those few precious seconds that can be better used for answering the tougher questions. For example, a passage may explicitly state the formula for the relationship of potential difference to the electric field and physical parameters of a parallel plate capacitor (i.e., $V = Ed$), but if you already know this formula, you will not need your map of the passage to find it when you need it to answer a question. That changes the type of question for you from Explicit to Memory.

Physics Memory Questions

These questions are often the easiest to answer. They follow a format that is more familiar for most students; typical Physics course work requires the memorization of formulas and facts, as well as their applications. Since Memory questions rely minimally if at all on information from the passage, they are similar to the freestanding questions on the MCAT.

Consider a question about the flow speed of blood in the major arteries taken from the previous blood flow passage. The following is an example of a Memory question.

2.6

The cross sectional area of the aorta is approximately 4 cm^2 and the total cross sectional area of the major arteries is 20 cm^2. If the speed of the blood in the aorta is 30 cm/sec, what is the average blood speed in the major arteries?

A) 5 cm/sec
B) 6 cm/sec
C) 120 cm/sec
D) 150 cm/sec

The equation to solve this question ($A_1v_1 = A_2v_2$) is not included in the passage.

Physics Explicit Questions

You need information directly from the passage in order to answer Explicit questions. It is critical to have a solid passage map so that information from the passage is easy to find and use. Even when you have inherent knowledge about the topic, it is important to read for information more specific to the precise situation in question.

Here's an example of an Explicit question from the blood flow passage:

Blood flow to the various systems in the body is regulated by the dilation and constriction of the blood vessels. After a person has eaten a large meal, the blood vessels supplying the digestive system dilate, increasing their radii by 50%. As a result of this blood vessel dilation, the flow of blood to the digestive system will:

A) increase to 500% of the original flow.
B) increase to 225% of the original flow.
C) increase to 150% of the original flow.
D) decrease to 50% of the original flow.

The equation needed to answer this question is given in the passage (Equation 2) and should be one that you recorded in your map. Note that you will always have to include information from the passage for an Explicit question.

Sometimes Explicit questions require more basic facts or principles from memory. In order to get the correct answer, you need to merge information from the passage with information you already know. For example, the passage gives an equation for a familiar variable in a new situation, and that must be blended with an understanding of the significance of that variable generally, or of other equations featuring that variable. These questions can appear straightforward but may be deceptively difficult, and it would certainly be justifiable to think of them as Implicit questions in some cases (the lines between the types are sometimes blurry).

The following is an example of an Explicit question using the blend of passage information and a bit of knowledge from memory:

> At the venular end of skeletal muscle capillaries, the hydrostatic pressure of the capillary is 17 torr and the hydrostatic pressure of the surrounding tissue is 1 torr. Fluid movement is from:
>
> A)   the capillary to the tissue, at a rate proportional to 7 torr.
> B)   the tissue to the capillary, at a rate proportional to 7 torr.
> C)   the capillary to the tissue, at a rate proportional to 9 torr.
> D)   the tissue to the capillary, at a rate proportional to 9 torr.

This asks about the pressure differential and the direction of fluid flow. This requires remembering that fluids move from high to low pressure (or correctly interpreting the final paragraph), but also requires using Equation 3 from the passage and the given values of osmotic pressures to solve for the numerical rate.

Physics Implicit Questions

This is the most difficult question type. Implicit questions often require information from memory, combined with information from the passage, and all applied to a new situation. They rely most heavily on critical reasoning skills, but also require a solid map, since information from the passage is usually needed. Most often, the answer choices for these questions contain a lot of words, but they can also sometimes be algebraic expressions or graphs. Note also that for many of these questions, you might be able to devise sound explanations that are not among the answer choices. However, there is always only *one* answer choice that *best* answers the question of all the options.

On Information and/or Situation passages, Implicit questions are often of the form "Which of the following best describes how [a parameter not mentioned in the passage] would change the [real world parameter described in the passage] from its present value?" The answers are verbal descriptions of increasing and decreasing values. Consider this example from the blood flow passage:

Adaptation to life at high altitudes is characterized by polycythemia (high red blood cell count). Excluding other physiological compensations, what is the effect of this change on the flow of blood?

A) Flow is decreased because viscosity is decreased.
B) Flow is increased because viscosity is decreased.
C) Flow is decreased because viscosity is increased.
D) Flow is increased because viscosity is increased.

The correct answer would be selected by using background knowledge about viscosity and applying it to Equation 2, which describes the flow rate.

On Experiment/Research passages, Implicit questions are often of the form "Which of the following changes to the experiment would result in a change to [an experimental parameter]?" and are followed by verbal descriptions of changes to the apparatus, process, or mechanism of the experiment described in the passage. Suppose the following paragraph were added to the end of the Experiment/Research Presentation Passage example in Section 2.2.

Confocal fluorescent microscopy relies on a light source of frequency tuned to the absorption frequencies of fluorescing compounds in the sample, focused through a pinhole using a converging mirror. This light illuminates the sample at specific focal planes, which are determined by a lens that focuses light both at the sample and eyepiece. Filters remove wavelengths other than those emitted by the fluorophores, and a semi-reflective mirror diverts the light to a pinhole, which is used in order to eliminate out-of-focus light from the image detector.

The following then is an example of an Implicit question in which the change to the apparatus is described in the answer choices:

Which of the following changes if made without any additional changes would be LEAST LIKELY to affect the observed results of the experiments described in the passage?

A) Using a fluorescing compound with a different wavelength dependence.
B) Changing the index of refraction of the lens without changing its curvature or position.
C) Decreasing the frequency of the light source from blue to yellow.
D) Rotating the sample 180°.

This question requires recall of the principles of optics and properties of fluorescence, as well as some understanding of the apparatus described in the passage addendum.

On Persuasive or Scientific Reasoning passages, Implicit questions are often of the form "Which of the following phenomena best exemplifies or analogizes to the [physics concept]?" and are followed by verbal descriptions of physics phenomena. Often selecting the right answer requires a combination of eliminating wrong answers by logical reasoning (or common sense) and revisiting the passage for the precise definition of the principle in question. Consider the blood flow passage: it's really more of a technical Information Presentation passage than a Persuasive or Scientific Reasoning passage, but this example suits either. An example of an Implicit question is

According to the following schematic diagram of systemic circulation, which of the following is true?

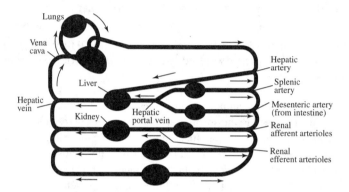

A) Vascular architecture of organs is in series so total peripheral resistance is greater than the resistance of individual organs.

B) Vascular architecture of organs is in parallel so total peripheral resistance is greater than the resistance of individual organs.

C) Vascular architecture of organs is in series so total peripheral resistance is less than the resistance of individual organs.

D) Vascular architecture of organs is in parallel so total peripheral resistance is less than the resistance of individual organs.

This question requires both understanding the analogy between resistance in blood flow and resistance in circuits and remembering the rules for adding resistors.

The physics question types discussed so far categorize questions based on where to find the information for the answer. There is another way to categorize questions based on *how* you achieve the answer once you have the information.

Question Types by Technique

Algebraic Manipulation questions: These require use of one or several equation(s) to solve algebraically for a variable. Typically they have either numeric answer choices (e.g., "5 newtons") or algebraic equations for answer choices (i.e. "$F_c = F_G + F_N$"). Another twist on algebraic manipulation questions would be a question that asks for the units of an unfamiliar term (e.g., "What are the units for viscosity?") followed by answer choices with a variety of units of measure.

Approximation/Computation questions: Are there numerical answer choices? It's likely you need to do some computation/approximation with a given or memorized equation (though *not necessarily:* be on the lookout for numbers directly implied by the scenario, such as the work done by a magnetic field always being zero). Just remember when you start plugging in numbers to check for shortcuts. Do all the answer choices have the same coefficient multiplied by different powers of ten? Then focus on the powers of ten and assume the coefficient comes out as given! Is your calculation coming out at 100 – (something hard to estimate)? Then the answer is <100 and all other choices can be eliminated. You can find more on approximation in chapter 15.

Functional Dependence/Proportionality questions: These require the use of one or more equations, graphs, or data tables to calculate proportions and changes in variables or values. These can have numeric answer choices, algebraic answer choices (e.g., "$a_{car} = -2a_{truck}$"), or verbal answer choices (e.g., "The radius doubles," or "The range increases from launch angle of 0° to launch angle of 45°, then decreases from launch angle of 45° to launch angle of 90°.").

Graph Generation or Interpretation questions: These require use of one or more equations, graphs, or data tables to create a graph of two variables; or they require you to locate points on a curve, the slope of a curve, or the area under a curve.

Conceptual questions: Is the question a paragraph and are all of the answer choices sentences? Such questions often require you to narrow down your choices by eliminating choices that express nonphysical scenarios, like gravity having a horizontal component or a resistor dissipating more energy than was output by the only battery in its circuit.

2.7 SUMMARY OF THE APPROACH TO PHYSICS

As with all the science sections, when tackling the Chemical and Physical Foundations of Biological Systems section of the MCAT, it is best to do the easy questions first; typically, the freestanding questions are easier Memory questions, so when you get to them as you progress through the test, do them all. As mentioned previously, the best strategy for tackling passages is probably to decide quickly whether each passage in sequence is a "Do Now" or a "Do Later." Skip the "Do Later" ones, note on your scratch paper the question numbers corresponding to that passage so you can be sure to come back to it, then come back to them once you've gotten to the end of the test. Within each passage, again, save especially difficult questions until last, and make sure to fill in answers for ALL the questions before moving to the next passage. If you find a question or two especially difficult, make your best guess and be sure to click the "Mark" button so that you can review the question later.

Since you will be skipping some questions within the test, it is important to keep your scratch paper organized. Clearly indicate the passage and question number beside the work that you do for that question. If you think you've made an error in calculation, do not waste time erasing, just draw a line through your work and start again.

Notes

After reading the text of the question, you may need to draw a quick sketch or diagram. This step is particularly useful for freestanding questions. Don't waste time or space on ornate drawings; just sketch enough to record the basic vectors and the positive direction, and make sure that your drawing is big enough for you to add vectors or numbers to it.

Try to predict the physics formula you'll need to answer the question before looking at the answer choices. This will either be an equation from memory or from the passage. Write this formula (or formulas) on your scratch paper by the label for the question. This will help when you want to review a previously marked question. Instead of having to search for the information all over again, you have an indicator on your scratch paper of where to start.

Avoid Confusion

When analyzing a question, remember that the situation will be ideal only when stated. Most of the concepts and equations you have memorized are for the ideal world. If the question asks for an approximation, the ideal world formulas are valid. If the question asks you to take the real world into consideration, look for a new formula or description in the passage that addresses the issue.

Remember to use the correct units! All calculations should be done with the "m.k.s." unit system (meters, kilograms, and seconds) unless otherwise specified. If you can't remember the formula, a unit analysis can help you regenerate or confirm the correct formula (for example, if you are solving a uniform circular motion question and you can't remember if velocity or radius is squared in the centripetal force equation, a quick unit analysis will show that velocity must be squared and the radius must *not* be squared in order to get an answer in newtons). Also, evaluating units may help you to quickly eliminate choices that have the wrong units. Finally, don't forget the "powers of 10": you may calculate the correct answer in meters, but if the answer choices are in millimeters, you will need to convert your results.

It can be helpful to form your own idea of the answer before looking at the choices. The MCAT tries to offer you similar-sounding answer choices that can muddle your thinking. Knowing what you are looking for before you read the answer choices keeps your POE focused.

Process of Elimination

Process of Elimination (POE) is paramount! Use the strikeout tool to indicate answer choices you have eliminated. Aggressively use process of elimination to improve your chances of guessing a correct answer even if you are not able to narrow it down to one choice. Remember each of the following POE strategies:

1. Eliminate answer choices that are clearly false or that do not answer the question.
2. If you think an answer choice is correct, double-check the remaining choices to confirm that they are incorrect. There may be two true statements in the answer choices, but only one best answers the question; make sure the answer you choose addresses the issue in the question.
3. Remember that if two answer choices are essentially the same, neither can be correct, and both can be eliminated immediately.
4. Work backwards, trying each answer choice to see if it correctly answers the question. This is particularly useful for questions such as "An increase in which of the following results in an increase in [some parameter] except...." Track these on your scratch paper so you can see the work done for each answer choice tried.
5. If you have eliminated three answer choices, the fourth choice must be the correct choice. Don't waste time pondering why it is correct.

2.8 EXAMPLES OF STRATEGY IN USE

Below is an example of these strategies applied to the blood flow passage we mapped earlier.

1. The cross sectional area of the aorta is approximately 4 cm^2 and the total cross sectional area of the major arteries is 20 cm^2. If the speed of the blood in the aorta is 30 cm/sec, what is the average blood speed in the major arteries?

   A) 5 cm/sec
   B) 6 cm/sec
   C) 120 cm/sec
   D) 150 cm/sec

This is a memory computation question. Your initial reaction to the question might well be to check the given equations in the passage for a possible route, but you should quickly notice that none of them has a flow-speed term. The equation for flow speed in terms of area is the Continuity equation: $A_1 v_1 = A_2 v_2$. Solving for v_2 yields $\dfrac{A_1 v_1}{A_2} = \dfrac{\left(4 \text{ cm}^2\right)\left(30 \text{ cm/s}\right)}{\left(20 \text{ cm}^2\right)} = 6 \text{ cm/s}$. Nothing to it but plugging and chugging once you've identified that this might as well be a freestanding question. The correct answer is choice B.

2. Blood flow to the various systems in the body is regulated by the dilation and constriction of the blood vessels. After a person has eaten a large meal, the blood vessels supplying the digestive system dilate, increasing their radii by 50%. As a result of this blood vessel dilation, the flow of blood to the digestive system will:

   A) increase to 500% of the original flow.
   B) increase to 225% of the original flow.
   C) increase to 150% of the original flow.
   D) decrease to 50% of the original flow.

This is an explicit proportionality question. The question mentions a fractional change to the radius of the blood vessels and asks for a fractional change in blood flow rate (both expressed as percentages), which should immediately suggest to you that you want a proportion. Equations 1 and 2 combine to express just such a proportion, so directly under them on your mapping you can write $Q \propto 1/R$ and $R \propto 1/r^4$, thus $Q \propto r^4$. If r goes to 1.5 times its original value (immediately eliminating choice D), then Q goes to $(1.5)^4$ times its original value (eliminating choice C). Since $1.5^2 = 2.25$, choice B is eliminated, so the answer must be choice A.

3. Adaptation to life at high altitudes is characterized by polycythemia (high red blood cell count). Excluding other physiological compensations, what is the effect of this change on the flow of blood?

A) Flow is decreased because viscosity is decreased.
B) Flow is increased because viscosity is decreased.
C) Flow is decreased because viscosity is increased.
D) Flow is increased because viscosity is increased.

This is an implicit functional-dependence question with a 2x2 answer choice pattern, that is, two variables vary between two possible values or trends (flow and viscosity are increasing or decreasing). With such questions, it is best to focus on one variable at a time. In this case, the question implies by stating that red blood cell count increases that viscosity will increase (eliminating choices A and B): this relies on commonsense reasoning (more stuff floating around in the fluid will make it more viscous) more than explicit knowledge of the passage or memory of a specific equation. On an implicit question like this, you're being asked to rely on your intuition and logic when you have no specific equations or definitions to apply. If viscosity η increases, then according to Equations 1 and 2 combined (as with the previous question), Q will decrease (there's an inverse proportionality between flow rate and viscosity, $Q \propto 1/\eta$). Thus choice C is correct.

2.8

4. At the venular end of skeletal muscle capillaries, the hydrostatic pressure of the capillary is 17 torr and the hydrostatic pressure of the surrounding tissue is 1 torr. Fluid movement is from:

A) the capillary to the tissue, at a rate proportional to 7 torr.
B) the tissue to the capillary, at a rate proportional to 7 torr.
C) the capillary to the tissue, at a rate proportional to 9 torr.
D) the tissue to the capillary, at a rate proportional to 9 torr.

This is an explicit computation question, with some dependence on basic outside knowledge. Like question 3, it has a 2x2 pattern of answer choices. Applying Equation 3 (we recommend you do your work directly below where you wrote the equation on your mapping) with the numbers given in the question stem and the passage, we get $\Delta P = (17 + 0) - (1 + 25) = -9$ torr (eliminating choices A and B). If the pressure differential is negative, then there is greater pressure acting to move fluid into the capillaries (this is stated explicitly in the final paragraph, but you should also have basic knowledge that fluid naturally flows from high to low pressure). The correct answer is choice D.

5. According to the following schematic diagram of systemic circulation, which of the following is true?

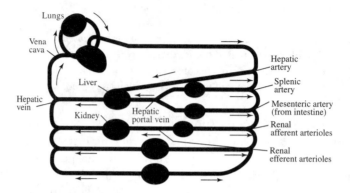

A) Vascular architecture of organs is in series so total peripheral resistance is greater than the resistance of individual organs.

B) Vascular architecture of organs is in parallel so total peripheral resistance is greater than the resistance of individual organs.

C) Vascular architecture of organs is in series so total peripheral resistance is less than the resistance of individual organs.

D) Vascular architecture of organs is in parallel so total peripheral resistance is less than the resistance of individual organs.

This is an implicit conceptual question. It requires you to make an analogy between fluid flow rate and current flow, an analogy justified by the similarity between Equation 1 and by Ohm's Law, $I = V/R$. The answer choices are once again in a 2x2 pattern, with the two variables being configuration (series or parallel) and total resistance (greater or less than the resistance of a single element, in this case an organ). Visual inspection of the provided diagram shows that the configuration (or "vascular architecture") is in parallel, because there are multiple paths the flow can take to get from and back to the heart. This eliminates choices A and C. At this point you must remember that resistors in parallel add reciprocally, so that the total resistance is always less than any given resistive element. Choice D is correct.

2.8

Chapter 3
Kinematics

3.1 UNITS AND DIMENSIONS

Before we begin our study of physics, we'll briefly go over metric units. Scientists —and the MCAT—use the <u>S</u>ystème <u>I</u>nternational d'Unités (the International System of Units), abbreviated **SI**, to express the measurements of physical quantities. The **base units** of the SI that we'll be interested in (at least for most of our study of MCAT Physics) are listed below:

SI base unit	abbreviation	measures	dimension
meter	m	length	L
kilogram	kg	mass	M
second	s	time	T

This system of units is also referred to as the **mks system** (<u>m</u> for meters, <u>k</u> for kilograms, and <u>s</u> for seconds). Each **dimension** is simply an abbreviation for the quantity that is being measured; it does not depend on the particular unit that's used. For example, we could measure a distance in miles, meters, or furlongs—to name a few—but in all cases, we're measuring a *length*. We say that distance has the dimensions of length, L. As another example, we could measure an object's speed in miles per hour, meters per second, or furlongs per fortnight; but regardless what units we use, we're always dividing a length by a time. Therefore, speed has dimensions of length per time (L/T).

Any physical quantity can be written in terms of the SI base units. Here are some examples:

quantity	symbol	units	dimensions
speed	v	m/s	L/T
density	ρ	kg/m^3	M/L^3
work	W	$kg{\cdot}m^2/s^2$	ML^2/T^2

Multiples of the base units that are powers of ten are often abbreviated and precede the symbol for the unit. For example, "n" is the symbol for nano-, which means 10^{-9} (one billionth). Thus, one billionth of a second, 1 nanosecond, would be written as 1 ns. The letter "M" is the symbol for mega-, which means 10^6 (one million), so a distance of one million meters, 1 megameter, would be abbreviated as 1 Mm.

Some of the most common power-of-ten prefixes are given in the following list:

prefix	symbol	multiple
pico-	p	10^{-12}
nano-	n	10^{-9}
micro-	μ	10^{-6}
milli-	m	10^{-3}
centi-	c	10^{-2}
kilo-	k	10^3
mega-	M	10^6
giga-	G	10^9

You should memorize this list.

On the MCAT, you won't need to convert between the American system of units (which uses things like inches, feet, yards, and pounds) and the metric system, so don't bother memorizing conversions like 2.54 cm = 1 inch or 39.37 inches = 1 meter, etc. You will need to be able to convert within the metric system using the powers-of-ten prefixes.

Example 3-1: Express a density of 5500 kg/m^3 in g/cm^3.

Solution: All we want to do with this physical measurement is to change the units in which it's expressed. For that, we need conversion factors. A **conversion factor** is simply a fraction whose value is 1, that multiplies a measurement in one set of units to give the equivalent measurement in a different set of units. In this case, we'd write

$$\rho = 5.5 \times 10^3 \, \frac{\text{kg}}{\text{m}^3} \times \left(\frac{10^3 \, \text{g}}{1 \, \text{kg}} \right) \times \left(\frac{1 \, \text{m}}{10^2 \, \text{cm}} \right)^3 = 5.5 \, \frac{\text{g}}{\text{cm}^3}$$

Notice that each of these conversion factors is written so that the unit we want to change (that is, the unit we want to eliminate) cancels out. The fraction

$$\frac{1 \, \text{kg}}{10^3 \, \text{g}}$$

is also a conversion factor for mass, but writing it like this would not have been helpful in this particular problem because then the "kg" would not have canceled.

Example 3-2: If a ball is dropped from a great height, then the force of air resistance it feels at any point during its descent is given by the equation $F = KD^2v^2$, where D is the diameter of the ball and v is its speed. If the units of F are kg·m/s^2, what are the units of K?

Solution: If the equation $F = KD^2v^2$ is to be valid, then the units of the left-hand side must be the same as the units of the right-hand side. To specify the unit of a quantity, we put brackets around it; for example, $[F]$ denotes the units of F; that is, $[F]$ = kg·m/s^2. So we need to make sure that $[F] = [KD^2v^2]$, which means

$$[F] = [K][D]^2[v]^2$$

$$\frac{\text{kg} \cdot \text{m}}{\text{s}^2} = [K] \cdot \text{m}^2 \cdot \left(\frac{\text{m}}{\text{s}} \right)^2$$

$$= [K] \cdot \frac{\text{m}^4}{\text{s}^2}$$

$$\text{kg} \cdot \text{m} = [K] \cdot \text{m}^4$$

$$\therefore [K] = \frac{\text{kg}}{\text{m}^3}$$

3.2 KINEMATICS

Kinematics is the description of motion in terms of an object's position, velocity, and acceleration. The MCAT will expect not only that you can answer mathematical questions about these quantities but also that you know the definitions of these quantities.

Displacement

The **displacement** of an object is its change in position. For example, let's say we were measuring an object moving along a straight line by laying a meter stick along the object's line of motion. If the object starts at, say, the *10 cm* mark on the meter stick and moves to the *70 cm* mark, then its position changed by 70 cm – 10 cm = 60 cm, so we'd say its displacement is 60 cm.

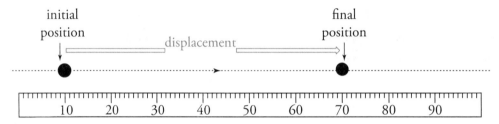

We find the displacement by subtracting the object's initial position from its final position:

$$\text{displacement} = \Delta(\text{position}) = \text{position}_{\text{final}} - \text{position}_{\text{initial}}$$

Now, what if the object moved from the *70 cm* mark on the meter stick to the *10 cm* mark? Then its displacement would be 10 cm – 70 cm = –60 cm.

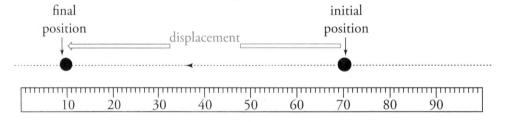

In both cases, the object moved a distance of 60 cm, but in the first case it moved to the right, and in the second case, it moved to the left. Displacement is a vector, so it takes direction into account. If we call *to the right* the positive direction (hence *to the left* automatically becomes the negative direction) then in the first case, we'd say the displacement is +60 cm, and in the second case, it's –60 cm.

The motion of the object can be more complicated. For example, what if the object started at the *10 cm* mark, moved to the *50 cm* mark, back to the *40 cm* mark, and then over to the *70 cm* mark?

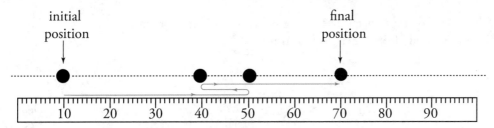

This example brings up a crucial point about displacement. The *total* distance that the object travels is (40 cm) + (10 cm) + (30 cm) = 80 cm, but the object's displacement is still

displacement $= \Delta(\text{position}) = \text{position}_{\text{final}} - \text{position}_{\text{initial}}$

$= (70 \text{ cm}) - (10 \text{ cm})$

$= +60 \text{ cm}$

Displacement gives us the *net* distance traveled by the object, which may very well be less than the total distance. So, the displacement is a vector that always points from the object's initial position to its final position, *regardless of the path the object took*, and whose magnitude is the *net* distance traveled by the object. There are multiple different symbols that are used to represent the displacement vector, such as $\Delta\mathbf{s}$, but the most common one is the single letter $\mathbf{d}$. Sometimes, we use $\Delta\mathbf{x}$ if we know the displacement is horizontal or $\Delta\mathbf{y}$ if we know the displacement is vertical. Be aware that the MCAT also uses the word *displacement* to mean just the magnitude of the displacement vector (that is, just the net distance traveled by the object without regard for direction); the question will make it clear which meaning is intended.

Displacement

$$\mathbf{d} = \text{position}_{\text{final}} - \text{position}_{\text{initial}} = \text{net distance plus direction}$$

For example, if a sprinter runs 400 meters around a circular track and returns to her starting point, she has covered a *total* distance of 400 meters, but her *displacement* is zero. If a sprinter runs 300 meters north, then 400 meters east, he's covered a total distance of 700 m, but his displacement is only 500 meters.

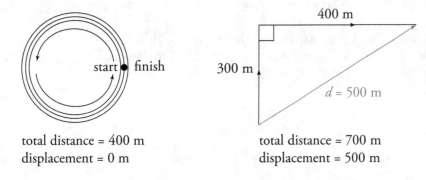

Example 3-3: Though the total length of all pathways of the human circulator system is on the order of 10^8 m, a typical red blood cell may complete a circuit of about 3 meters in one minute.

    a)   What is the total distance traveled by a red blood cell in an hour?
    b)   What is its total displacement in that time?

Solution:

    a)   If 3 m arc traveled in a minute, then 3 m/min × 60 min/hour = 180 m will be traveled in an hour.
    b)   Displacement is the net change in position. If a circuit is completed, regardless of the number of times, the displacement is 0 m.

Velocity

Displacement tells us how much an object's position changes. **Velocity** tells us how *fast* an object's position changes. If you're in a car traveling at 60 miles per hour along a long, straight highway, then this means your position changes by 60 miles every hour. To calculate velocity, simply divide how much the position has changed by how much time it took for it to change; in other words, divide displacement by time.

Average Velocity

$$\text{average velocity} = \frac{\text{displacement}}{\text{time}}$$

$$\bar{\mathbf{v}} = \frac{\Delta x}{\Delta t} = \frac{\mathbf{d}}{\Delta t}$$

This is actually the definition of **average velocity**, and we place a bar above the **v** to signify that it's an *average*. So, **v** is velocity and $\bar{\mathbf{v}}$ is average velocity. (If the velocity happens to be constant, then there's no distinction between *velocity* and *average velocity*, and we don't need the bar.) Notice right away that velocity is a vector; after all, we're dividing a vector (the displacement, **d**) by a number, so we're left with a vector. In fact, because Δt is always positive, $\bar{\mathbf{v}}$ always points in the same direction as **d**.

The magnitude of the velocity vector is called the **speed**. Speed is a scalar; it has no direction and can never be negative. (Notice that the speedometer in your car is well-named; it only tells you how fast the car is moving, not the direction of motion. It's not a "velocity-o-meter.") Velocity is a vector that specifies both speed and direction.

> ### Velocity
>
> $$\mathbf{v} = \text{speed \& direction}$$

In the figure below, each vector represents the car's velocity. Both cars have the same speed (let's say 20 m/s), so the magnitudes of their velocity vectors are the same. Nevertheless, they have different velocities, because the directions are different. (By the way, if the car on the right looks bigger than the car on the left, it's an optical illusion. Grab a ruler and check it for yourself. They're the same size!)

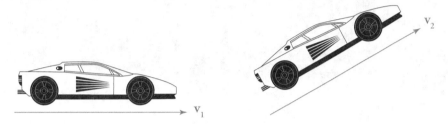

These two cars have the same speed but different velocities. Is it possible for two cars to have the same velocity but different speeds? No. Velocity is speed plus direction, so if the velocities are the same, then the speeds (and the directions) are the same.

Example 3-4: Though the total length of all pathways of the human circulatory system is on the order of 10^8 m, a typical red blood cell may complete a circuit of about 3 meters in one minute.

    a)   What is the average velocity of this red blood cell?
    b)   What is its average speed?

Solution:

    a)   In example 3-3(b) we determined that the displacement of the red blood cell was 0 m. Thus by definition the average velocity must be 0 m/s.

    b)   Average speed is not the magnitude of average velocity. (Confusing, though this example should make clear why this must be the case.) Rather, it is by definition the total distance traveled divided by time. In this case, v = (3 m/min)(1/60 min/sec) = 1/20 m/s or 0.05 m/s.

Example 3-5: A sprinter runs 300 meters north, then 400 meters east, which takes 100 seconds.

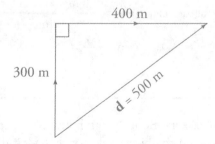

What was his average speed? What was the magnitude of his average velocity?

Solution: The sprinter's average speed was (700 m)/(100 s) = 7 m/s. However, because his displacement is 500 m, his average velocity has a magnitude of (500 m)/(100 s) = 5 m/s.

Example 3-6: An object moves from Point A to Point B in 4 seconds.

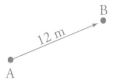

What was the object's velocity?

    A.   3 m/s
    B.   8 m/s
    C.   6 m/s
    D.   48 m/s

Solution: Notice that the question is asking for velocity (which is a vector) but all the choices are scalars. Strictly speaking, the answer should include the correct direction as well as the magnitude. However, the MCAT (as well as textbook authors and teachers) will often use the word *velocity* when they mean *speed*; usually, it won't cause confusion. From the choices given, we know it's the magnitude of the velocity that is the desired quantity, and this is

$$v = \frac{\Delta x}{\Delta t} = \frac{12 \text{ m}}{4 \text{ s}} = 3 \text{ m/s}$$

Choice A is the answer we'd choose.

Acceleration

Velocity tells us how fast an object's position changes. **Acceleration** tells us how fast an object's *velocity* changes.

Average Acceleration

$$\text{average acceleration} = \frac{\text{change in velocity}}{\text{time}}$$

$$\bar{a} = \frac{\Delta \mathbf{v}}{\Delta t}$$

Acceleration is a little trickier than velocity. Even though both involve how fast something changes, acceleration is how fast velocity changes, and an object's velocity changes if the speed *or* the direction changes. So, for example, an object can be accelerating even if its speed is constant. This is a very important point and a potential MCAT trap.

In everyday language, we use the word *acceleration* to describe what happens when we step on the gas pedal and go faster. Well, that's certainly an example of acceleration even from the "proper" physics perspective, but it isn't the only example of acceleration.

What happens when you step on the brake? You slow down. Is that acceleration? Yes, although we might also call it a *deceleration*, because our speed changes.

Now, imagine that you set the car on cruise control at, say, 60 miles per hour. Up ahead you see a curve in the road, so as you approach it, you slowly turn the wheel to stay on the road. Even though your speed remains constant, your direction of motion changes, which means your velocity vector changes. Thus, you experience an acceleration.

Let's try this one. Throw a baseball straight up into the air. It rises, gets to the top of its path, then falls back down. At the moment it's at the top of its path, its velocity is zero. What is the ball's acceleration at this point?

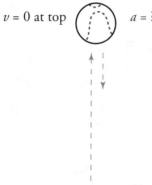

A common answer is, "If the velocity is 0, then the acceleration is 0 too." Let's see why this isn't the case here. What's happening to the baseball's velocity at the top of the path? Its direction is changing from up to *down*. The fact that the velocity is changing means there's an acceleration, so the acceleration can't be zero at the top of the path. Here's another way of looking at it: What if the acceleration *were* zero at the top? Zero acceleration means no change in velocity, so if $a = 0$ at a certain point, then whatever velocity there is at that point will stay constant. Does the velocity of the baseball remain zero? No, because the ball immediately starts to fall toward the ground.

Example 3-7: The velocity of an object moving along a straight line changes from $v_i = 4$ m/s at time $t_i = 0$ to $v_f = 10$ m/s at time $t_f = 2$ sec.

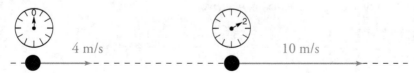

What was the object's average acceleration during this time interval?

Solution: By definition of average acceleration, we have

$$\overline{\mathbf{a}} = \frac{\Delta \mathbf{v}}{\Delta t} = \frac{\mathbf{v}_f - \mathbf{v}_i}{t_f - t_i} = \frac{10 \text{ m/s} - 4 \text{ m/s}}{(2 \text{ s}) - 0 \text{ s}} = 3 \text{ m/s}^2$$

Notice that $\overline{\mathbf{a}}$ is positive, which means that it points to the right, just like $\mathbf{v}_i$. If the acceleration points in the *same* direction as the initial velocity, then the object's speed is *increasing*.

Example 3-8: The velocity of an object moving along a straight line changes from $\mathbf{v}_i = 7$ m/s at time $t_i = 0$ to $\mathbf{v}_f = 1$ m/s at time $t_f = 3$ sec.

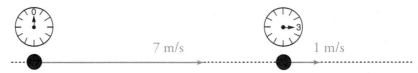

What was the object's average acceleration during this time interval?

Solution: By definition of average acceleration, we have

$$\overline{\mathbf{a}} = \frac{\Delta \mathbf{v}}{\Delta t} = \frac{\mathbf{v}_f - \mathbf{v}_i}{t_f - t_i} = \frac{1 \text{ m/s} - 7 \text{ m/s}}{(3 \text{ s}) - 0 \text{ s}} = -2 \text{ m/s}^2$$

Notice that $\overline{\mathbf{a}}$ is negative, which means that it points to the left, in the direction opposite to $\mathbf{v}_i$. If the acceleration points in the direction *opposite* to the initial velocity, then the object's speed is *decreasing*.

Example 3-9: The velocity of an object moving along a straight line changes from $\mathbf{v}_i = -2$ m/s at time $t_i = 0$ to $\mathbf{v}_f = -5$ m/s at time $t_f = 2$ sec.

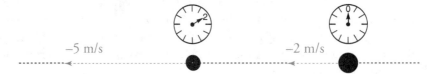

What was the object's average acceleration during this time interval?

Solution: By definition of average acceleration, we have

$$\overline{\mathbf{a}} = \frac{\Delta \mathbf{v}}{\Delta t} = \frac{\mathbf{v}_f - \mathbf{v}_i}{t_f - t_i} = \frac{-5 \text{ m/s} - (-2 \text{ m/s})}{(2 \text{ s}) - 0 \text{ s}} = -1.5 \text{ m/s}^2$$

Notice that $\overline{\mathbf{a}}$ is negative, which means that it points to the left, just like $\mathbf{v}_i$. If the acceleration points in the *same* direction as the initial velocity, then the object's speed is *increasing*.

Example 3-10: The velocity of an object changes from $\mathbf{v}_1$ at time $t_i = 0$ to $\mathbf{v}_2$ at time $t_f = 2$ sec.

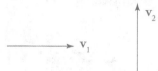

Which of the following best illustrates the object's average acceleration during this time interval?

A.

B.

C.

D.

Solution: By definition of average acceleration, we have

$$\overline{\mathbf{a}} = \frac{\Delta \mathbf{v}}{\Delta t} = \frac{\mathbf{v}_2 - \mathbf{v}_1}{t_f - t_i} = \frac{\mathbf{v}_2 - \mathbf{v}_1}{2\,\text{s}}$$

The direction of $\overline{\mathbf{a}}$ is (always) the same as the direction of $\Delta \mathbf{v} = \mathbf{v}_2 - \mathbf{v}_1 = \mathbf{v}_2 + (-\mathbf{v}_1)$. The following diagram shows how we find $\mathbf{v}_2 + (-\mathbf{v}_1)$:

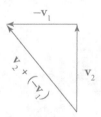

Therefore, choice B is the best answer.

The direction of **a** tells **v** how to change; the following diagrams summarize the possibilities:

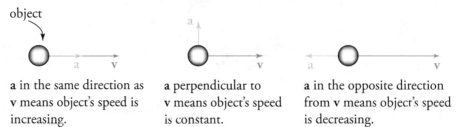

a in the same direction as
v means object's speed is
increasing.

a perpendicular to
v means object's speed
is constant.

a in the opposite direction
from v means object's speed
is decreasing.

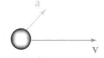

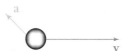

a at an angle between 0° and 90° to
v means object's speed is increasing
and direction of v is changing.

a at an angle between 90° and 180°
to v means object's speed is decreasing
and direction of v is changing.

Example 3-11: The velocity and acceleration of an object at a certain point are shown in the diagram below.

Describe the object's velocity a short time later.

Solution: We split the acceleration vector into components, one along the direction of **v** and one perpendicular to the direction of **v**:

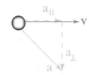

The component $a_\parallel$ points along the line of the object's motion, so the *speed* of the object will change; in particular, the speed will *increase*, since $a_\parallel$ points in the *same* direction as **v**. The component of **a** that's perpendicular to **v**, $a_\perp$, will make the *direction* of **v** change; in particular, it will turn downward (since $a_\perp$ points downward). Therefore, we'd expect the object to increase in speed as it turns downward.

3.3 UNIFORMLY ACCELERATED MOTION

In the last section, we defined the principal quantities of kinematics: displacement, velocity, and acceleration. In this section, we'll summarize the mathematical relationships between them in the special but important case of **uniformly accelerated motion**. This is motion in which the object's acceleration, **a**, is constant.

The definition of average velocity is $\bar{\mathbf{v}} = \Delta\mathbf{s}/\Delta t$. We can rewrite this equation without a fraction like this: $\Delta\mathbf{s} = \bar{\mathbf{v}}\Delta t$. To simplify the notation, let's agree to (1) use **d** for displacement, (2) use t, rather than Δt, for the time interval, and (3) abandon the bolding for vectors (although we'll still specify the direction of a vector by either a plus or a minus sign). With this change in notation, the equation reads simply $d = \bar{v}t$. In the case of uniformly accelerated motion (which means a is constant), the average velocity, $\bar{v}$ is just the average of the initial and final velocities: $\frac{1}{2}\left(v_i + v_f\right)$. Using t instead of Δt for the time interval means that we're setting the initial time, t_i, equal to 0 and that we're letting t stand for the final time, t_f (notice that $\Delta t = t_f - t_i = t - 0 = t$). The initial velocity is then the velocity at time 0, which we write as v_0 (pronounced "v zero" or "v naught") and the final velocity is v (dropping the subscript "f" on v_f just like we're dropping the subscript "f" on t_f). Therefore, the average velocity can be written as $\bar{v} = \frac{1}{2}\left(v_0 + v\right)$, and the equation for d becomes $d = \frac{1}{2}\left(v_0 + v\right)t$.

The definition of average acceleration is $\bar{a} = \Delta v/\Delta t$. We can rewrite this equation without a fraction like this: $\Delta v = \bar{a}\Delta t$. Now, since we are specifically looking at uniformly accelerated motion (motion in which the acceleration is constant), then there's no need for the bar on the **a**. After all, if **acceleration** is a constant, there's no distinction between **a** and $\bar{\mathbf{a}}$. So, removing the bar and using the simplified notation described in the last paragraph, the equation becomes $\Delta v = at$, or $v = v_0 + at$.

The two equations $d = \frac{1}{2}\left(v_0 + v\right)t$ and $v = v_0 + at$ follow directly from the definitions of average velocity and acceleration. There are three other equations that relate these quantities, but they would require more algebra to derive them. Instead of boring you with the details, we'll just state them. Since there are five equations, we call them **The Big Five**:

The Big Five

1. $d = \frac{1}{2}(v_0 + v)t$ missing a

2. $v = v_0 + at$ missing d

3. $d = v_0 t + \frac{1}{2}at^2$ missing v

4. $d = vt - \frac{1}{2}at^2$ missing v_0

5. $v^2 = v_0^2 + 2ad$ missing t

Notice that these equations involve *five* quantities—d, v_0, v, a, and t—and there are *five* equations. Each equation has exactly one of those quantities missing, and this is how you decide which equation to use in a particular problem. A quantity is *missing* from the problem if it's *not given and not asked for*. For example, if a question does not give or ask for v, then use Big Five #3; if a question does not give or ask for t, then use Big Five #5. On the MCAT, the Big Five equations that are used most frequently are #2, #3, and #5.

Example 3-12: An object has an initial velocity of 3 m/s and a constant acceleration of 2 m/s² in the same direction. What will the object's velocity be at $t = 6$ s?

Solution: We're given v_0, a, and t, and asked for v. Since the displacement, d, is neither given nor asked for, we use Big Five #2:

$$v = v_0 + at = 3 \text{ m/s} + (2 \text{ m/s}^2)(6 \text{ s}) = 15 \text{ m/s}$$

Example 3-13: A particle has an initial velocity of 10 m/s and a constant acceleration of 3 m/s² in the same direction. How far will the particle travel in 4 seconds?

Solution: We're given v_0, a, and t, and asked for d. Since the final velocity, v, is missing, we use Big Five #3:

$$d = v_0 t + \tfrac{1}{2} at^2 = (10 \text{ m/s})(4 \text{ s}) + \tfrac{1}{2}(3 \text{ m/s}^2)(4 \text{ s})^2 = 64 \text{ m}$$

Example 3-14: An object starts from rest and travels in a straight line with a constant acceleration of 4 m/s² in the same direction until its final velocity is 20 m/s. How far does it travel during this time?

Solution: We're given v_0, a, and v, and asked for d. Since the time, t, is neither given nor asked for, we use Big Five #5. Because the object starts from rest, we know that $v_0 = 0$, so we get

$$v^2 = v_0^2 + 2ad \;\rightarrow\; v^2 = 2ad \;\rightarrow\; d = \frac{v^2}{2a} = \frac{(20 \text{ m/s})^2}{2(4 \text{ m/s}^2)} = 50 \text{ m}$$

Example 3-15: A particular red blood cell traveling through the aorta has a peak speed of 92 cm/s after accelerating for 98 ms at a rate of 470 cm/s². What was its speed before undergoing this acceleration?

Solution: We're given a, v, and t, and asked for v_0. Since the displacement, d, is neither given nor asked for, we use Big Five #2:

$$v = v_0 + at \rightarrow v_0 = v - at = (92 \text{ cm/s}) - (470 \text{ cm/s}^2)(0.098 \text{ s}) \approx 45 \text{ cm/s}$$

3.4 KINEMATICS WITH GRAPHS

The MCAT expects you to be able to interpret graphs as well as to be able to apply equations. In general, you will need to be able to extract three forms of information from graphs: individual points, slopes, and areas. Below we consider these in two types of graphs: the **position vs. time** graph and the **velocity vs. time** graph.

Consider the following graph, which gives an object's position, x, as a function of time, t:

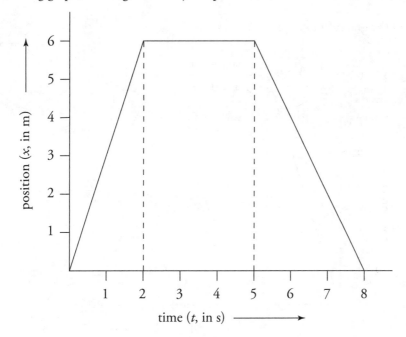

The object starts at $x = 0$, then moves to $x = 6$ m at $t = 2$ s. From $t = 2$ s to $t = 5$ s, it remains at position $x = 6$ m. Then, from $t = 5$ s to $t = 8$ s, the object moves from $x = 6$ m back to $x = 0$.

Let's figure out its velocity during these time intervals. From $t = 0$ to $t = 2$ s, its velocity is

$$v = \frac{\Delta x}{\Delta t} = \frac{x - x_0}{t_f - t_i} = \frac{(6\text{ m}) - (0\text{ m})}{2\text{ s}} = 3 \text{ m/s}$$

Note that Δx is the vertical change in this graph and Δt is the horizontal change, from $t = 0$ to $t = 2$ s. Dividing a vertical change by the corresponding horizontal change gives the *slope* of a graph. So, we have this rule:

> The slope of a position vs. time graph gives the velocity.

From $t = 2$ s to $t = 5$ s, the object remained at position $x = 6$ m. Since the object didn't move, we expect its velocity during this time interval to be zero. But notice that the graph is flat here, and the slope of a flat line is 0.

Finally, from $t = 5$ s to $t = 8$ s, the velocity is

$$v = \frac{\Delta x}{\Delta t} = \frac{x - x_0}{t_f - t_i} = \frac{(0 \text{ m}) - (6 \text{ m})}{(8 \text{ s}) - (5 \text{ s})} = -2 \text{ m/s}$$

This is the slope of the graph from $t = 5$ s to $t = 8$ s.

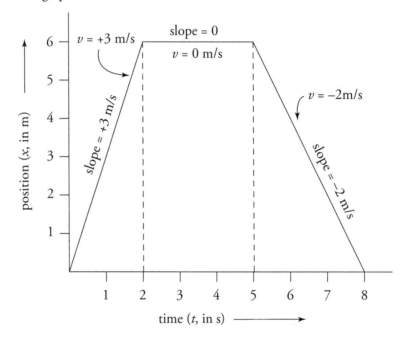

Now consider the following graph, which gives an object's velocity, v, as a function of time, t:

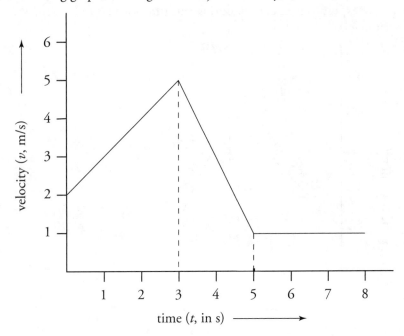

The object's velocity at $t = 0$ is $v = 2$ m/s, and steadily increases to $v = 5$ m/s at time $t = 3$ s. From $t = 3$ s to $t = 5$ s, the velocity decreases to $v = 1$ m/s. Then, from $t = 5$ s to $t = 8$ s, the object's velocity remains constant at $v = 1$ m/s.

Let's figure out the object's acceleration during these time intervals. From $t = 0$ to $t = 3$ s, its acceleration is

$$a = \frac{\Delta v}{\Delta t} = \frac{v - v_0}{t} = \frac{\left(5 \text{ m/s}\right) - \left(2 \text{ m/s}\right)}{3\,\text{s}} = 1 \text{ m/s}^2$$

Note that $\Delta \mathbf{v}$ is the vertical change in this graph and Δt is the horizontal change, from $t = 0$ to $t = 3$ s. Once again, dividing a vertical change by the corresponding horizontal change gives the slope of a graph. So, we have this rule:

> The slope of a velocity vs. time graph gives the acceleration.

From $t = 3$ s to $t = 5$ s, the acceleration is

$$a = \frac{\Delta v}{\Delta t} = \frac{v - v_0}{t_f - t_i} = \frac{\left(1 \text{ m/s}\right) - \left(5 \text{ m/s}\right)}{5\,\text{s} - 3\,\text{s}} = -2 \text{ m/s}^2$$

This is the slope of the graph from $t = 3$ s to $t = 5$ s.

Finally, from $t = 5$ s to $t = 8$ s, the object's velocity remained constant at $v = 1$ m/s. Since the object's velocity didn't change, we expect its acceleration during this time interval to be zero. The graph is flat here, and the slope of a flat line is 0.

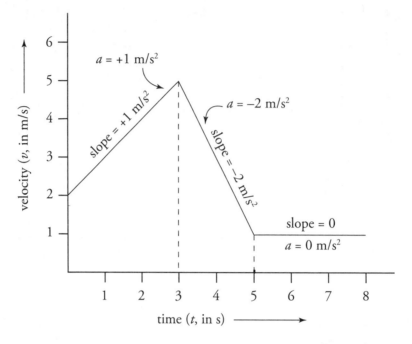

Besides asking about the object's acceleration, there's an additional type of question we could be asked given an object's velocity vs. time graph. For example, what was the object's *displacement* from $t = 5$ s to $t = 7$ s? Since the object's velocity was a constant $v = 1$ m/s, we just use the basic equation *distance* = *rate* × *time* (which is really just Big Five #1 in the case where v is constant) to find that $d = (1 \text{ m/s})(2 \text{ s}) = 2$ m. But if we look at the graph, we realize that what we've just found is the *area* under the graph from $t = 5$ s to $t = 7$ s. After all, the area under the graph is just a rectangle for which the height is a velocity and the base is a time. The area of a rectangle is *base* × *height* (bh), so we're multiplying velocity × time, and that gives us displacement. The same rule applies even if the graph isn't flat:

> The area under a velocity vs. time graph gives the displacement.

What is the object's displacement from $t = 0$ to $t = 3$ s? It will be the area under the velocity vs. time graph from $t = 0$ to $t = 3$ s. The figure below shows that we can split this area into two pieces: a triangle whose area is $\frac{1}{2}bh = \frac{1}{2}(3\text{s})(3 \text{ m/s}) = \frac{9}{2}$ m, and a rectangle whose area is $bh = (3\text{s})(2 \text{ m/s}) = 6$ m. Therefore, the object's displacement from $t = 0$ to $t = 3$ s, which is the *total* area under the graph between $t = 0$ and $t = 3$ s, is $\left(\frac{9}{2}\text{ m}\right) + \left(6\text{ m}\right) = 10.5$ m.

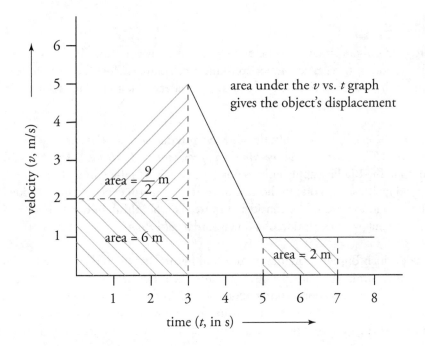

We can check this result using Big Five #1:

$$d = \frac{1}{2}(v_0 + v)t = \frac{1}{2}(2 \text{ m/s} + 5 \text{ m/s})(3\text{s}) = 10.5\text{m}$$

Example 3-16: For the object whose velocity vs. time graph is shown below, what is its displacement from $t = 2$ s to $t = 5$ s?

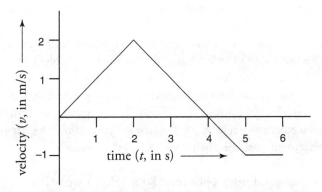

Solution: The area under the graph (or, more precisely, the area between the graph and the t-axis) gives the object's displacement. The area under the graph from $t = 2$ s to $t = 4$ s is $\frac{1}{2}bh = \frac{1}{2}(2\text{ s})(2\text{ m/s}) = 2$ m. After $t = 4$ s, the graph is *below* the t-axis, so any area here counts *negatively*. From $t = 4$ s to $t = 5$ s, the area is $\frac{1}{2}bh = \frac{1}{2}(1\text{ s})(-1\text{ m/s}) = -0.5$ m. Therefore, the total area between the graph and the t-axis, from $t = 2$ s to $t = 5$ s, is (2 m) + (−0.5 m) = 1.5 m.

3.5 FREE FALL

The Big Five are used only in situations where the acceleration is constant. The most important "real life" situation in which motion takes place under constant acceleration is **free fall**, which describes an object moving only under the influence of gravity (ignoring any effects due to the air, such as air resistance and buoyancy).

Near the surface of the earth, the magnitude of **g**, the **gravitational acceleration**, is approximately equal to 9.8 m/s². *For the MCAT, we can use the simpler approximation of 10 m/s².* The term "free fall" might make you think that The Big Five apply only to objects that are actually falling, but if we throw a baseball up into the air (and ignore effects due to the air), then the ball is still experiencing the downward acceleration due to gravity, so it, too, would be considered in free fall. So, think of free fall not as a description of a downward velocity but as a description of a downward *acceleration*.

The way we decide which Big Five equation to use is to figure out which one of the five kinematics quantities (d, v_0, v, a, or t) is missing from the question, and then use the equation that does not involve this missing quantity. Often, in questions asking about objects in free fall, the acceleration will not be given because it's known implicitly. As soon as you realize the question involves an object moving under the influence of gravity, then you know that a is automatically known; on Earth, the magnitude of this a is about 10 m/s².

However, there is one thing you will have to decide on once you've selected which Big Five equation to use. Gravitational acceleration, like any acceleration, is a vector, so it has magnitude and direction. We know the magnitude is 10 m/s² and the direction is downward, but is *down* the positive direction or the negative direction? The answer is: it's up to you. I suggest letting the direction of the object's displacement be the positive direction in every problem (this is almost always the simplest, most intuitive, decision). If the object's displacement is *down*, then call *down* the positive direction, and use $a = +g = +10$ m/s² in whichever Big Five equation you've selected. If the object's displacement is *up*, call *up* the positive direction (and thus *down* is automatically the negative direction) and use $a = -g = -10$ m/s².

It's important to remember that once you make your decision about which direction, up or down, is the positive direction, your decision applies to all other vectors in that problem: namely, v_0, v, and d. Therefore, if *down* is positive, for example, then in addition to the downward acceleration being positive, a downward initial velocity is positive, a downward final velocity is positive, and a downward displacement is positive. (This would mean that an upward initial velocity is negative, an upward final velocity is negative, and an upward displacement is negative.) Of course, if you follow the suggestion of always calling the direction of the displacement positive, then d will always be positive.

Example 3-17: An object is dropped from a height of 80 m. How long will it take to strike the ground?

Solution: We're given v_0, a, and d, and asked for t. Since the final velocity, v, is neither given nor asked for, we use Big Five #3. Because the object is falling, its displacement is downward, so let's call *down* the positive direction; this means that $a = +g = +10$ m/s². Since the term *dropped* means that the object's initial velocity is 0 m/s, we find that

$$d = v_0 t + \tfrac{1}{2}at^2 \rightarrow d = \tfrac{1}{2}at^2 \rightarrow t = \sqrt{\frac{2d}{a}} = \sqrt{\frac{2d}{+g}} = \sqrt{\frac{2(80 \text{ m})}{+10 \text{ m/s}^2}} = 4 \text{ s}$$

Example 3-18: An object is dropped from a height of 80 m. What is its velocity as it strikes the ground?

Solution: (Don't make the common mistake of thinking that the answer is 0 because once the object hits the ground, it stops. The question is really asking for the velocity of the object *as* it slams into the ground, and this won't be zero.) We're given v_0, a, and d, and asked for v. Since the time, t, is neither given nor asked for, we use Big Five #5. Because the object is falling, its displacement is downward, so let's call *down* the positive direction. This means that $a = +g = +10$ m/s². Since the term *dropped* means that the object's initial velocity is 0, we find that

$$v^2 = v_0^2 + 2ad \rightarrow v^2 = 2ad \rightarrow v = \sqrt{2ad} = \sqrt{2(+g)d} = \sqrt{2(+10 \text{ m/s}^2)(80 \text{ m})} = 40 \text{ m/s}$$

Example 3-19: A ball is thrown straight upward with an initial speed of 30 m/s. How high will it go?

Solution: We're given v_0, a, and v, and asked for d. (We know v because the question is asking how high the ball will go; at the top of the ball's path, its velocity at this point is 0.) Since the time, t, is missing, we use Big Five #5. Since we're interested only in the object's upward motion, let's call *up* the positive direction. This means that $v_0 = +30$ m/s and $a = -g = -10$ m/s². Because the velocity of the ball is 0 at its highest point, we find that

$$v^2 = v_0^2 + 2ad \rightarrow 0 = v_0^2 + 2ad \rightarrow d = -\frac{v_0^2}{2a} = -\frac{v_0^2}{2(-g)} = -\frac{(+30 \text{ m/s})^2}{2(-10 \text{ m/s})} = 45 \text{ m}$$

Notice that the displacement d turned out to be positive; that's because we chose *up* to be our positive direction, and the ball moves *up* to its highest position.

Example 3-20: A ball of mass 10 kg and a ball of mass 1 kg are dropped simultaneously from a tower of height 45 m. If air resistance could be ignored, which ball will hit the ground first and how long does it take?

Solution: We're given v_0, a, and d, and asked for t. Since the final velocity, v, is missing, we use Big Five #3. Because each object is falling, their displacement is downward, so let's call *down* the positive direction. This means that $a = +g = +10$ m/s². Remembering that the term *dropped* means that $v_0 = 0$, Big Five #3 becomes $d = \frac{1}{2}at^2$, so

$$t = \sqrt{\frac{2d}{a}} = \sqrt{\frac{2d}{+g}} = \sqrt{\frac{2(45 \text{ m})}{+10 \text{ m/s}^2}} = 3 \text{ s}$$

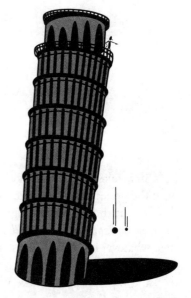

Because none of the Big Five equations involves the *mass* of the object, this is how long it takes *each* ball to strike the ground. The free-fall acceleration of an object does not depend on its mass (or size or shape), so in the absence of effects due to the air, both objects will hit the ground *at the same time.*

3.6 PROJECTILE MOTION

The examples we've worked through so far have involved objects that move along a straight line, either horizontal or vertical. However, if we were to throw a baseball up at an angle to the ground, the path the ball would follow (its **trajectory**) would not be a straight line. If we neglect effects due to the air, the path will be a *parabola*.

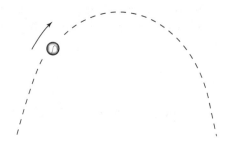

In this case, the motion of an object, experiencing only the constant, downward acceleration due to gravity (free fall), is called **projectile motion**. This is also a case of uniformly accelerated motion.

Because the projectile is experiencing both horizontal and vertical motion, we'll need to analyze both. But the trick is to analyze them *separately*. We'll use The Big Five to look at the horizontal motion, simply specializing the variables to horizontal motion; for example, we'll use x instead of d, we'll use v_{0x} and v_x instead of v_0 and v, and we'll use a_x instead of a. The same will be true for the vertical motion. We'll use The Big Five to look at the vertical motion, too, and simply specialize the variables to vertical motion; we'll use y instead of d, v_{0y} and v_y instead of v_0 and v, and a_y instead of a. In this case, a_y will be equal to the gravitational acceleration.

In order to make an object follow a parabolic path, we'll need to launch the object at an angle to the horizontal. Therefore, the initial velocity vector $\mathbf{v}_0$ will have a nonzero horizontal component (v_{0x}) *and* a nonzero vertical component (v_{0y}). In terms of the **launch angle**, θ_0, which is the angle the initial velocity vector makes with the horizontal, we have $v_{0x} = v_0 \cos \theta_0$ and $v_{0y} = v_0 \sin \theta_0$.

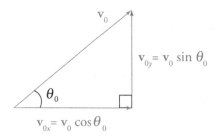

Let's first take care of the horizontal motion. This is the easier of the two for one important reason: once the projectile is launched, it no longer experiences a horizontal acceleration. That is, a_x will be zero throughout the projectile's flight. If the horizontal acceleration is zero throughout the projectile's flight, then *the horizontal velocity will be constant throughout the flight*. If the horizontal velocity does not change, then whatever it was initially is all it'll ever be; that is, the horizontal velocity of the projectile at any point during its flight will be equal to the initial horizontal velocity, v_{0x}. Finally, if a_x is always equal to 0, then by using Big Five #3, we have $x = v_{0x}t$ (this is just *distance = rate × time* in the case where the rate is constant).

For the vertical motion, we realize that there *is* an acceleration; after all, the gravitational acceleration is vertical. In order to write down the equations for the vertical motion, we need to make a decision about which direction is positive. Let's call *up* the positive direction, so that *down* is the negative direction; this will mean that $a_y = -g$. Big Five #2 now tells us that the vertical component of the velocity, v_y, will be $v_{0y} + a_y t = v_{0y} + (-g)t$ at time t. Big Five #3 tells us that the vertical displacement of the projectile, y, will be $v_{0y}t + \frac{1}{2}a_y t^2 = v_{0y}t + \frac{1}{2}(-g)t^2$.

Projectile Motion

	Horizontal Motion	Vertical Motion
displacement:	$x = v_{0x}t$	$y = v_{0y}t + \frac{1}{2}(-g)t^2$
velocity:	$v_x = v_{0x}$ (constant!)	$v_y = v_{0y} + (-g)t$
acceleration:	$a_x = 0$	$a_y = -g$
	$(v_{0x} = v_0 \cos\theta_0)$	$(v_{0y} = v_0 \sin\theta_0)$

In addition to these formulas (which are really nothing new, since they're just a few of the Big Five equations), there are a couple of other facts worth knowing. The first involves the projectile's velocity at the top of its trajectory. Since the top of the parabola is the parabola's turning point, and an object's velocity is always tangent to its path (whatever the shape of the trajectory), the projectile's velocity will be horizontal at the top of the parabola. This means that the vertical velocity is zero. (*Be careful* not to say that the velocity is zero at the top. For a projectile moving in a parabolic path, it's only the *vertical* velocity that's zero at the top; the horizontal velocity is still there!)

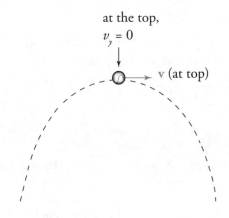

The second fact reflects the symmetry of the parabolic shape of the path. If we were to draw a vertical line up from the ground through the top point on the parabola, we'd notice that the left and right sides are just mirror images of each other. One of the consequences of this observation is that the time the projectile takes to reach the top will be the same as the time it takes to drop back down (to the same height from which it was launched). Therefore, *the projectile's total flight time will be twice the time required to reach the top*. So, for example, if the time it takes the projectile to reach the top of the parabola is 3 seconds, then the total flight time will be 6 seconds, because it'll take another 3 seconds to come back down.

3.6

Example 3-21: A cannonball is shot from ground level with an initial velocity of 100 m/s at an angle of 30° to the ground.

a) How high will the cannonball go?
b) What is the cannonball's velocity at the top of its path?
c) What will be the cannonball's total flight time?
d) How far will the cannonball travel horizontally?

Solution:

a) The maximum height reached by the projectile is the displacement y at the moment the cannonball is at the top of the parabola. What does it mean for the projectile to be at the top of the parabola? It means the vertical velocity is zero. So, we'll set the vertical velocity equal to zero. (Note that since we don't care about flight time for this particular question, we could ignore it and simply use Big Five #5.)

$$v_y = v_{0y} + (-g)t \text{ with } v_y = 0 \rightarrow v_{0y} + (-g)t = 0 \rightarrow t = \frac{v_{0y}}{g} = \frac{v_0 \sin\theta_2}{g}$$

This is how long it'll take the projectile to reach the top. If we plug in $v_0 = 100$ m/s, $\theta_0 = 30°$, and $g = 10$ m/s², we find that

$$t = \frac{v_0 \sin\theta_0}{g} = \frac{(100 \text{ m/s})\sin 30°}{10 \text{ m/s}^2} = 5 \text{ s}$$

So now the question is, "What is y when $t = 5$ s?" All we need to do is take the equation for the vertical displacement of the projectile and plug in $t = 5$ s:

$$y = v_{0y}t + \tfrac{1}{2}(-g)t^2$$
$$= (v_0 \sin\theta_0)t + \tfrac{1}{2}(-g)t^2$$

$$\therefore y \text{ (at } t = 5 \text{ s)} = (100 \text{ m/s} \cdot \sin 30°)(5 \text{ s}) + \tfrac{1}{2}(-10 \text{ m/s}^2)(5 \text{ s})^2 = 125 \text{ m}$$

b) At the top of its path, the cannonball's velocity is horizontal, and the horizontal velocity is the same throughout the flight, equal to the initial horizontal velocity:

$$v_x = v_{0x} = v_0 \cos\theta_0 = (100 \text{ m/s})\cos 30° \approx (100 \text{ m/s})(0.85) = 85 \text{ m/s}$$

c) The projectile's total flight time is just equal to twice the time required for it to reach the top. Since we found in part (a) that it takes 5 seconds for the cannonball to reach the top, its total flight time will be $2 \times (5 \text{ s}) = 10 \text{ s}$.

d) The question is asking for the horizontal displacement at the time when the cannonball strikes the ground. We found in part (b) that the cannonball's horizontal velocity is a constant 85 m/s, and we found in part (c) that the cannonball's total flight time is 10 seconds. Therefore, the total horizontal displacement is

$$x = v_{0x}t = (85 \text{ m/s})(10 \text{ s}) = 850 \text{ m}$$

(The total horizontal displacement is called the **range** of the projectile.)

Example 3-22: The archerfish is able to use a spit stream of water to knock insects off of branches overhanging the swamps and rivers they inhabit. Suppose the archerfish shoots at an insect with a spit speed of 8 m/s at a launch angle of 60°. What is the maximum height of the insect at which it could be knocked into the water?

Solution: The maximum height of a projectile occurs at the apex of the trajectory, at which point $v_y = 0$ m/s, and of course gravitational acceleration $a_y = -g = -10 \text{ m/s}^2$. The question implies the initial vertical velocity, $v_{0y} = v_0 \sin 60° = (8 \text{ m/s})\left(\dfrac{\sqrt{3}}{2}\right) = 4\sqrt{3} \text{ m/s}$. The question asks for vertical displacement y, and the missing variable is time t, so we use Big Five #5 adjusted for the vertical direction:

$$v_y^2 = v_{0y}^2 + 2a_y y \rightarrow y = \frac{v_y^2 - v_{0y}^2}{2a_y} = \frac{0 - \left(4\sqrt{3} \text{ m/s}\right)^2}{-20 \text{ m/s}} = \frac{48}{20} \approx 2.5 \text{ m}$$

Example 3-23: A rock is thrown horizontally, with an initial speed of 10 m/s, from the edge of a vertical cliff. It strikes the ground 5 s later.

a) How high is the cliff?

b) How far from the foot of the cliff does the rock land?

Solution:

a) The height of the cliff will be the vertical distance the rock falls. Because the rock is thrown horizontally, it has no initial vertical velocity: $v_{0y} = 0$. Therefore, the equation for the projectile's vertical displacement becomes $y = \frac{1}{2}(-g)t^2$. Considering the time it takes the rock to fall is $t = 5$ s, we have $y = \frac{1}{2}(-10 \text{ m/s}^2)(5 \text{ s})^2 = -125 \text{ m}$. This tells us that the rock falls 125 m in 5 s, so the height of the cliff is 125 m.

b) The horizontal displacement of the rock is given by the equation $x = v_{0x}t$. Since $v_{0x} = 10$ m/s and $t = 5$ s, we get $x = \left(10 \text{ m/s}\right)\left(5 \text{ s}\right) = 50 \text{ m}$

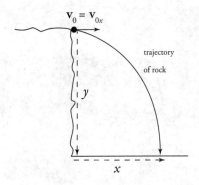

Summary of Formulas

displacement:
$\mathbf{d} - \Delta\mathbf{x} - $ (final position) – (initial position) = *net* distance (plus direction)

average velocity:
$$\bar{\mathbf{v}} = \frac{\Delta x}{\Delta t} = \frac{\mathbf{d}}{\Delta t}$$

average acceleration:
$$\bar{\mathbf{a}} = \frac{\Delta \mathbf{v}}{\Delta t}$$

The **BIG FIVE** (for Uniformly Accelerated Motion: $a = $ constant):

$$d = \frac{1}{2}\left(v_0 + v\right)t$$

$$v = v_0 + at$$

$$d = v_0 t + \frac{1}{2}at^2$$

$$d = vt - \frac{1}{2}at^2$$

$$v^2 = v_0^2 + 2ad$$

Position (x) vs. time (t) graph: slope = velocity (v)

Velocity (v) vs. time (t) graph: slope = acceleration (a)

area under graph = displacement (d)

Projectile Motion :

[Downward = Negative Direction]

	Horizontal Motion	**Vertical Motion**
displacement:	$x = v_{0x}t$	$y = v_{0y}t + \frac{1}{2}(-g)t^2$
velocity:	$v_{0x} = v_x$ [constant!]	$v_y = v_{0y} + (-g)t$
acceleration:	$a_x = 0$	$a_y = -g$
	$(v_{0x} = v_0\cos\theta_0)$	$(v_{0y} = v_0\sin\theta_0)$

$v_y = 0$ at the top of the trajectory

$v_x \neq 0$ at the top of the trajectory

Total flight time = [time from launch to top] + [time from top to landing]

CHAPTER 3 FREESTANDING PRACTICE QUESTIONS

1. In a crash simulation, a car traveling at x m/s can stop at a distance d m with a maximum deceleration. If the car is traveling at $2x$ m/s, which of the following statements is/are true, assuming a maximum deceleration?

    I. The stopping time is doubled.
    II. The stopping distance is doubled.
    III. The stopping distance is quadrupled.

A) I and II only
B) I and III only
C) II only
D) III only

2. A ball is thrown in a projectile motion trajectory with an initial velocity v at an angle θ above the ground. If the acceleration due to gravity is $-g$, which of the following is the correct expression of the time it takes for the ball to reach its highest point, y, from the ground?

A) $v^2 \sin\theta / g$

B) $-v\cos\theta / g$

C) $v\sin\theta / g$

D) $v^2 \cos\theta / g$

3. A surfer searching for the perfect wave paddles out to sea on her surfboard. She heads west from her beach spot and paddles at a rate of 8 meters per minute. There is a constant current in the water that day, pulling the surfer south at 6 meters per minute. After 5 minutes of paddling, how far is the surfer from her original beach spot?

A) 40 m west
B) 40 m southwest
C) 50 m southwest
D) 70 m southwest

4. A bubble in a glass of beer releases from rest at the bottom of the glass and rises at acceleration a to the surface in t seconds. If $t > 2$, how much farther does the bubble travel between times $t = 1$ s and $t = 2$ s than it does between times $t = 0$ s and $t = 1$ s?

A) $2a$ meters
B) $3a/2$ meters
C) a meters
D) $a/2$ meters

5. On Earth, a tennis player can hit a tennis ball normally, causing the ball to travel on a path that is a symmetrical parabola. A tennis player can also hit a tennis ball with a "slice" which causes the ball to spin and deviate to one side of its normal path. What is the best explanation for this deviation?

A) There is an additional acceleration on the ball.
B) The spin on the ball caused the acceleration from gravity to change direction.
C) The spin on the ball used energy so the ball could not travel in a straight line.
D) The gravitational field was not uniform.

6. An object is thrown with an initial speed of 7 m/s directed 45° above the horizontal from a cliff. After reaching the peak of its trajectory, it falls 20 m to the ground below. What is the approximate ratio of the time it takes to hit the ground from the peak of the trajectory to the time it takes from its release to the peak of the trajectory?

A) 0.5
B) 1
C) 2
D) 4

7. The position x of an object is plotted as a function of time t. What is the acceleration of the object from $t = 2$ s to $t = 4$ s?

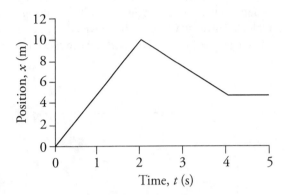

A) −2.5 m/s^2
B) 0 m/s^2
C) 2.5 m/s^2
D) 5 m/s^2

CHAPTER 3 PRACTICE PASSAGE

An airplane is susceptible to substantial deflection off course due to wind. A pilot calls the engines' contribution the *airspeed*. This motion relative to the air, combined with the wind velocity, results in the *ground speed*, or velocity relative to fixed terrestrial objects.

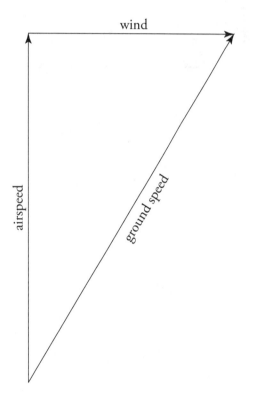

Figure 1

When a parachutist typically leaves an airplane, it is not so much a jump as a drop. He steps out of a door or lets go of a strut under the wing, not giving him any significant velocity relative to the airplane. He becomes subject to gravity without the lift of the wings. Air resistance allows the plane to get ahead of him. If we neglect this drag effect, then the parachutist's constant horizontal velocity and constant vertical acceleration gives him a trajectory resembling half of an inverted parabola. This is a reasonable assumption for the free fall before the parachute is engaged.

1. A pilot wanting to travel northeast in a wind blowing from the west at a speed similar to her airspeed should direct her airplane in which direction?

   A) north
   B) south
   C) east
   D) west

2. If an airplane has an airspeed of 100 km/hr southwest but is travelling 140 km/hr south relative to the ground, what is the wind velocity?

   A) 40 km/hr to the east
   B) 100 km/hr to the southeast
   C) 100 km/hr to the east
   D) 170 km/hr to the southeast

3. An airplane capable of an airspeed of 100 km/hr is 60 km off the coast above the sea. If the wind is blowing from the coast out to sea at 40 km/hr, what is the least amount of time it will take for the plane to get to shore?

   A) 26 minutes
   B) 36 minutes
   C) 60 minutes
   D) 100 minutes

4. Neglecting air resistance, if a parachutist drops from an airplane when it is flying horizontally at 100 m/s to the west at an altitude of 1 km, and the parachute never engages, what will be his final horizontal velocity?

   A) 0 m/s
   B) 100 m/s to the west
   C) 40 m/s to the west
   D) 170 m/s to the west

5. Neglecting air resistance, what is the total velocity of a parachutist just before engaging his parachute, 8 s after dropping from an airplane flying horizontally at 60 m/s?

A) 60 m/s
B) 80 m/s
C) 100 m/s
D) 140 m/s

6. Which graph correctly represents the vertical speed of a dropped object with respect to time?

A)

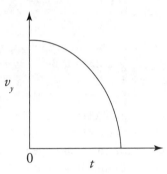

B)

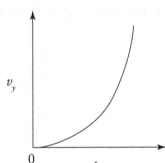

C)

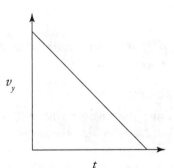

D)

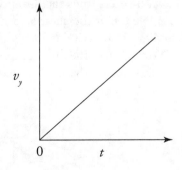

7. Relative to the typical dropping parachutist, one who thrusts himself downward on exiting the airplane (ignoring air resistance and assuming both parachutists open their parachutes after the same amount of time) will have:

A) lower acceleration but the same velocity just before engaging his parachute.
B) the same acceleration and the same velocity just before engaging his parachute.
C) the same acceleration but greater velocity just before engaging his parachute.
D) greater acceleration and greater velocity just before engaging his parachute.

SOLUTIONS TO CHAPTER 3 FREESTANDING PRACTICE QUESTIONS

1. **B** According to the formula $v^2 = v_0^2 + 2ad$, the initial velocity, v_0, can be related to the stopping distance, d. If v is zero, and the equation is rearranged for d, it becomes $d = v_0^2/2a$. Since the car is decelerating, a is negative. Therefore, if v_0 is doubled, the stopping distance, d, is quadrupled. To determine the relationship between v_0 and t, the formula $v = v_0 + at$ is used. Since v is zero, and the equation is rearranged for t, it becomes $t = -v_0/a$. Similar to the above scenario, a is negative. Therefore, if v_0 is doubled, the stopping time, t, is doubled. Only Items I and III are correct, and the correct answer is choice B.

2. **C** At the highest point from the ground, the ball has a velocity of zero. Therefore, applying the formula $v_y = v_{0y} + a_y t$ and rearranging for t, it becomes $t = -v_{0y}/-g$. Substituting $v_{0y} = v \sin \theta$ into the equation, $t = v \sin \theta / g$. Therefore the correct answer is C.

3. **C** The surfer is paddling west. That component of displacement can be calculated using the formula distance = (rate)(time) = (8 m/min)(5 min) = 40 m. So the surfer has travelled 40 m west on her own. The water current is constantly moving her south. That component of displacement can be calculated using the same formula, so distance = (6 m/min)(5 min) = 30 m. Each of these displacements are vectors and can be added together tip-to-tail. The result is a right triangle as shown below.

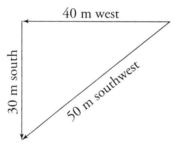

   The triangle is a 3-4-5 triangle, so the total displacement is 50 m southwest (the total distance can also be found using the Pythagorean theorem, where $c^2 = a^2 + b^2$). The correct answer is choice C.

4. **C** The distance travelled in the first second can be found using Big Five #3 with $v(0) = 0$ (because the bubble begins at rest) and $t = 1$ s, $d = (0)(1) + 1/2\, a(1)^2 = a/2$. The easiest way to find the distance traveled in the next second is to find the total distance traveled from $t = 0$ s to $t = 2$ s and to subtract the distance traveled during the first second, $a/2$. Again apply Big Five #3 with $v(0) = 0$ and $t = 2$ s, $d = (0)(2) + 1/2\, a(2)^2 = 2a$. Thus the distance traveled between $t = 1$ s and $t = 2$ s must be $2a - a/2 = 3a/2$. Note that the question asks how much *farther* the bubble travels between times $t = 1$ s and $t = 2$ s than it does between times $t = 0$ s and $t = 1$ s, which means we need a *difference*. Now subtract the distance traveled during the first second of travel from the distance traveled during the next second: $3a/2 - a/2 = a$. The correct choice is C.

5. **A** A projectile travelling in a uniform gravitational field, where the only acceleration is due to gravity, will travel in a symmetrical parabola. This describes the path of the ball when it is hit normally. The sliced ball travels off to the side, so there must be an acceleration causing the velocity change. Since gravity is always directed down toward Earth, there must be an additional acceleration from another source (other than gravity) causing the ball's velocity to deviate to the side. This is best described by choice A. Since the ball was hit on Earth, the direction of the acceleration due to gravity is always towards Earth, eliminating choice B. While the spin on the ball will use energy, it will not cause the ball to deviate off to one side, eliminating choice C. Unless there is a large change in the ball's distance from the center of the earth, the gravitational field on earth will always be uniform, eliminating choice D. The correct answer is choice A.

6. **D** To calculate the time it takes for the object to hit the ground from the peak, use $d = v_0 t + (\frac{1}{2})at^2 \rightarrow 20 = (0) + (\frac{1}{2})(10)t^2 \rightarrow 20 = 5t^2 \rightarrow t = 2$ s. To calculate the time it takes to reach the peak, use $v = v_0 + at \rightarrow 0 = 7 \sin 45° - 10t \rightarrow 10t = 5 \rightarrow t = 0.5$ s. So, the ratio of the time it takes to hit the ground from its peak to the time it takes to reach the peak is $2/0.5 = 4$.

7. **B** From $t = 2$ s to $t = 4$ s, the object is moving at a constant velocity, since the slope of the position vs. time graph does not change over this interval. Since the velocity of the object is constant, it is therefore not experiencing any acceleration.

SOLUTIONS TO CHAPTER 3 PRACTICE PASSAGE

1. **A** We are given the resultant airspeed and asked for a different component. You must subtract the wind velocity (or add its negative) to the desired ground speed. Alternatively, just draw out the vectors and reason which way would be required to get the addition resultant northeast. Beware that "from the west" means "pointing to the east."

2. **B** When you draw a vector diagram, remember that you are given the resultant and one of the components and asked for the other component. You must subtract the airspeed (or add its negative) to the resulting ground speed. This makes for a 1-1-$\sqrt{2}$ triangle, so the wind must also be 100 km/hr. It is southeast to counteract the westerly element of the airspeed and contribute more to the southerly component. There is more than just counteracting (like choices A or C). Mixing up the hypotenuse and sides might lead to choice D.

3. **C** The airspeed and opposing wind superimpose to result in a ground speed of 60 km/hr toward the coast, so the 60 km will take 1 hour (60 minutes) to traverse. If you add the velocity vectors to a total of 140 km/hr then you would calculate choice A. If you surmised that 100 km/hr was the relevant velocity, you would calculate choice B. If you thought the resultant velocity was 40 km/hr, you might select choice D.

4. **B**   The question states that air resistance can be neglected, so the horizontal velocity will be constant at the initial velocity inherited from when the parachutist was aboard the airplane. If air resistance brought him to rest in the horizontal, choice A would be the answer. One could calculate (using Big Five #5) the final velocity including the vertical acceleration as either choice C (starting from rest) or choice D (including the initial horizontal velocity), but these require mixing up the two coordinate axes.

5. **C**   This first requires the calculation of the vertical component of velocity starting from rest and accelerating at 10 m/s^2 for 8 s. According to Big Five #2, the parachutist will be falling at 80 m/s (choice B). Her horizontal velocity will be constant at 60 m/s (choice A). Adding these two components is easy if you recognize that it is a 3-4-5 triangle multiplied by 20, so the hypotenuse is 100 m/s. Both of the individual components are listed as distractions. Linear (rather than vector) addition would result in choice D.

6. **D**   Though the passage does say that the trajectory will be half of a parabola, this question is asking about velocity, not displacement. Do not be fooled by the quadratic forms of choices A and B. The question asks for the speed, or magnitude of velocity. This magnitude will increase linearly as the object falls. Choice C would be an object slowing down at a constant negative acceleration.

7. **C**   This parachutist gives himself higher initial vertical velocity, whereas the typical one starts from rest in the vertical. They will both be subject to the same acceleration due to gravity, so choices A and D can immediately be eliminated. Starting at a higher velocity will, however, result in a greater final velocity.

Chapter 4
Mechanics I

4.1 MASS, FORCE, AND NEWTON'S LAWS

In the preceding chapter, we studied kinematics, which is the description of motion in terms of an object's position, velocity, and acceleration. In this chapter, we'll begin our study of **dynamics**, which is the *explanation* of motion in terms of the forces that act on an object.

Simply put, a **force** is a push or pull exerted by one object on another. If you pull on a rope attached to a crate, you create a *tension* in the rope that pulls the crate. When a sky diver is falling through the air, the Earth exerts a downward pull called the *gravitational force*, and the air exerts an upward force called *air resistance*. When you stand on the floor, the floor provides an upward, supporting force called the *normal force*. If you slide a book across a table, the table exerts a *frictional force* against the book, so the book slows down and eventually stops. Static cling provides a simple example of the *electrostatic force*. (In fact, all of the forces mentioned above, with the exception of gravity, are due ultimately to the electromagnetic force.)

> **Newton's First Law**
>
> An object's state of motion—its *velocity*—will not change unless a net force acts on the object.
>
> That is, if no net force acts on an object, then:
>
> **if the object is at rest, it will remain at rest**
>
> *and*
>
> **if the object is moving, then it will continue to move with constant velocity**
>
> (constant speed in a straight line).
>
> Or, more simply: **no net force = no acceleration**.

How forces affect motion is described by three physical laws, known as **Newton's laws**. They form the foundation of mechanics, and you should memorize them.

The first law says that objects naturally resist changing their velocity. In other words, objects at rest don't just suddenly start moving all on their own. Some external source must exert a force to make them move. Also, an object that's already moving doesn't change its velocity. It doesn't go faster, or slower, or change direction all by itself; something must exert some force on it to make any of these changes happen. This property of objects, their natural resistance to change in their state of motion, is called **inertia**. In fact, the first law is often referred to as the *law of inertia*.

It's important to note that the first law applies when there is no *net* force on an object. This could mean there are no forces at all, though that couldn't happen in our universe; more commonly, it means the forces on an object balance out, in other words, the total of all the forces, in each dimension, is zero. We'll work examples of computing net force when we get to Newton's second law.

The **mass** of an object is the quantitative measure of its inertia; intuitively, mass measures how much matter is contained in an object. Mass is measured in *kilograms*, abbreviated kg. (Note: An object whose mass is 1 kg weighs a little more than 2 pounds on Earth, but be careful not to confuse mass with weight; they're different things.) Compared to an object whose mass is just 1 kg, an object whose mass is 100 kg has 100 times the inertia. Intuitively, we'd find it 100 times more difficult to cause the same change in its motion than we would with the 1 kg object. This point will be clearer after we state the second of Newton's laws.

Newton's Second Law

If $\mathbf{F}_{net}$ is the net—or total—force acting on an object of mass m, then the resulting acceleration of the object, $\mathbf{a}$, satisfies this simple equation:

$$\mathbf{F}_{net} = m\mathbf{a}$$

Notice that the first law is really just a special case of the second law: the case in which $\mathbf{F}_{net} = 0$.

Forces are represented by vectors, because a force has a magnitude and a direction. If two different forces (let's call them $\mathbf{F}_1$ and $\mathbf{F}_2$) act on an object, then the total—or *net*—force on the object is the sum of these individual forces: $\mathbf{F}_{net} = \mathbf{F}_1 + \mathbf{F}_2$. Since forces are vectors, they must be added as vectors; that is, their directions must be taken into account. The following figures show some examples of obtaining $\mathbf{F}_{net}$ from the individual forces that act on an object:

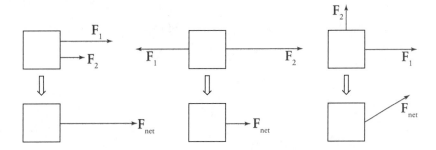

Note the following facts about the equation $\mathbf{F}_{net} = m\mathbf{a}$:

1. $\mathbf{F}_{net}$ is the sum of all the forces that act *on* the object; namely, the object whose mass, m, is on the other side of the equation. Any force exerted *by* the object is *not* included in $\mathbf{F}_{net}$.

2. Because m is a *positive* number, the direction of $\mathbf{a}$ is always the same as the direction of $\mathbf{F}_{net}$. Therefore, an object will accelerate in the direction of the net force it feels. This does not mean that an object will always *move* in the direction of $\mathbf{F}_{net}$. Be sure that this distinction makes sense, because it can be a source of confusion, and therefore a potential MCAT trap. Newton's second law tells us about the direction of an object's *acceleration* but does not define the direction of an object's velocity.

3. What if $\mathbf{F}_{net} = 0$? Then $\mathbf{a} = 0$. What does $\mathbf{a} = 0$ mean? It means that the object's velocity does not change, which is also what Newton's *first* law says. But how about this question: Does $\mathbf{F}_{net} = 0$ mean that $\mathbf{v} = 0$? Not necessarily! $\mathbf{F}_{net} = 0$ means that an object won't *accelerate*, not that it won't move. This is a key point and another potential MCAT trap. If the object is already moving at, say, 100 m/s toward the north, then it will continue to move at 100 m/s toward the north as long as the net force on the object remains zero.

4. Because $\mathbf{F}_{net} = m\mathbf{a}$ is a vector equation, it automatically means that the components of both sides must be the same. In other words, $\mathbf{F}_{net}$ could be written as the sum of a force in the horizontal direction, $(\mathbf{F}_{net,\,x})$ plus a force in the vertical direction $(\mathbf{F}_{net,\,y})$; these would be the horizontal and vertical components of $\mathbf{F}_{net}$. The equation $\mathbf{F}_{net} = m\mathbf{a}$ would then tell us that $\mathbf{F}_{net,\,x} = m\mathbf{a}_x$ and $\mathbf{F}_{net,\,y} = m\mathbf{a}_y$. So, dividing the horizontal component of the net force by m gives us the horizontal component of the object's acceleration, and dividing the vertical component of the net force by m gives us the vertical component of the object's acceleration.

5. The unit of force is equal to the unit of mass times the unit of acceleration:

$$[F] = [m][a] = kg \cdot m/s^2$$

A force of 1 kg·m/s² is called 1 **newton** (abbreviated N). A force of 1 N is about equal to a quarter of a pound, or about the weight of a medium-sized apple (on Earth).

Newton's Third Law

If Object 1 exerts a force, $\mathbf{F}_{1\text{-on-}2}$, on Object 2, then Object 2 exerts a force, $\mathbf{F}_{2\text{-on-}1}$, on Object 1. These forces, $\mathbf{F}_{1\text{-on-}2}$ and $\mathbf{F}_{2\text{-on-}1}$, have the same magnitude but act in opposite directions, so

$$\mathbf{F}_{1\text{-on-}2} = -\mathbf{F}_{2\text{-on-}1}$$

and they act on different objects. These two forces are said to form an **action–reaction pair**.

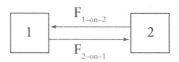

This is the law commonly stated as, "For every action, there is an equal but opposite reaction." Unfortunately, this popular version of Newton's third law can lead to confusion. Essentially, Newton's third law says that the *forces* in an action–reaction pair have the same magnitude and act in opposite directions (and on "opposite" objects). It does *not* say that the *effects* of these forces will be the same. For example, suppose that two skaters are next to and facing each other on a skating rink. Let's say that Skater 1 has a mass of 50 kg and Skater 2 has a mass of 100 kg. Now, what if Skater 1 pushes on Skater 2 with a force of 50 N? Then $\mathbf{F}_{1\text{-on-}2} = 50$ N and $\mathbf{F}_{2\text{-on-}1} = -50$ N, by Newton's third law.

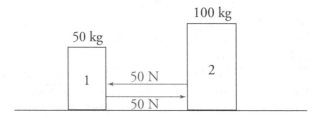

But will the *effects* of these equal-strength forces be the same? No, because the masses of the objects are different. The accelerations of the skaters will be

$$a_1 = \frac{F_{2\text{-on-}1}}{m_1} = \frac{-50\text{ N}}{50\text{ kg}} = -1\text{ m/s}^2 \quad \text{and} \quad a_2 = \frac{F_{1\text{-on-}2}}{m_2} = \frac{+50\text{ N}}{100\text{ kg}} = +0.5\text{ m/s}^2$$

So, Skater 2 will move away with an acceleration of 0.5 m/s², while Skater 1 moves away, in the opposite direction, with an acceleration of twice that magnitude, 1 m/s².

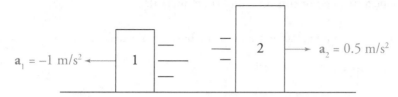

Therefore, while the forces are the same (in magnitude), the effects of these forces —that is, the resulting accelerations (and velocities)—are not the same, because the masses of the objects are different. Newton's third law says nothing about mass; it only tells us that the action and reaction forces will have the same magnitude. So, the point is not to interpret "equal but opposite reaction" as meaning "equal but opposite effect," because if the masses of the interacting objects are not the same, then the resulting accelerations (and velocities) of the objects will not be the same.

The key to distinguishing Newton's second law from Newton's third law is to focus on the description of the forces. In Newton's second law, all of the forces must be acting on a *single* object; thus, the net force on a single object is calculated by adding those vectors. However, in Newton's third law, each force must be acting on a *different* object in an action-reaction pair.

There are two aspects of Newton's third law that frequently give students trouble. First, just because two forces are equal and opposite does *not* mean they form an action-reaction pair; the forces also have to be from two objects acting on each other, not two objects acting on a third object. Second, the third law applies even when the objects are accelerating; even if one object is accelerating, the second object pushes or pulls just as hard on the first as the first pushes or pulls on the second.

Example 4-1: An object of mass 50 kg moves with a constant velocity of magnitude 1000 m/s. What is the net force on this object?

Solution: If the object moves with constant velocity, then the net force it feels must be zero, regardless of the object's mass or speed.

Example 4-2: The net force on an object of mass 10 kg is zero. What can you say about the speed of this object?

Solution: If the net force on an object is zero, all we can say is that it will not accelerate; its velocity may be zero, or it may not. Without more information, we cannot determine the object's speed; all we know is that whatever the speed is, it will remain constant.

Example 4-3: For 6 seconds, you push a 120 kg crate along a frictionless horizontal surface with a constant force of 60 N parallel to the surface. If the crate was initially at rest, what will its velocity be at the end of this 6-second time interval?

Solution: Using Newton's second law, we find that the acceleration of the crate is $a = F/m = (60 \text{ N})/(120 \text{ kg}) = 0.5 \text{ m/s}^2$. Using Big Five #2, we now find that $v = v_0 + at = 0 + (0.5 \text{ m/s}^2)(6 \text{ s}) = 3 \text{ m/s}$.

Example 4-4: For 6 seconds, you pull a 120 kg crate along a frictionless horizontal surface with a constant force of 60 N directed at an angle of 60° to the surface. If the crate was initially at rest, what will its horizontal velocity be at the end of this 6-second time interval?

Solution: To find the horizontal velocity, we need the horizontal acceleration.

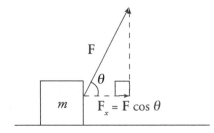

Using Newton's second law, we find that the horizontal acceleration of the crate is $a_x = F_x/m = (F\cos\theta)/m = (60\text{ N})(\cos 60°)/(120\text{ kg}) = (30\text{ N})/(120\text{ kg}) = 0.25\text{ m/s}^2$. Using Big Five #2, we now find that $v_x = v_{0x} + a_x t = 0 + (0.25\text{ m/s}^2)(6\text{ s}) = 1.5\text{ m/s}$.

Example 4-5: Two crates are moving along a frictionless horizontal surface. The first crate, of mass $M = 100$ kg, is being pushed by a force of 300 N. The first crate is in contact with a second crate, of mass $m = 50$ kg.

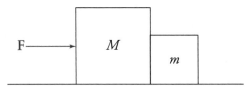

a) What's the acceleration of the crates?
b) What's the force exerted by the larger crate on the smaller one?
c) What's the force exerted by the smaller crate on the larger one?

Solution:

a) The force **F** is pushing on a combined mass of 100 kg + 50 kg = 150 kg, so by Newton's second law, the acceleration of both crates will be $a = (300\text{ N})/(150\text{ kg}) = 2\text{ m/s}^2$.

b) Because M and m are in direct contact, each is pushing on the other with a certain force. Let F_2 be the force that M exerts on m. Then we must have $F_2 = ma$, so $F_2 = (50\text{ kg})(2\text{ m/s}^2) = 100$ N.

c) By Newton's third law, if the force that M exerts on m is F_2, then the force that m exerts on M must be $-F_2$. So, if we call "to the right" our positive direction, then the force that m exerts on M is -100 N. We can check that this is correct by looking at all the forces acting on M. We have **F** pushing to the right and $-F_2$ pushing to the left. The net force on M is therefore $F_{\text{net on }M} = F + (-F_2) = (300\text{ N}) + (-100\text{ N}) = 200$ N. If this is correct, then $F_{\text{net on }M}$ should equal Ma. Since $M = 100$ kg and $a = 2\text{ m/s}^2$, we get $Ma = 200$ N, which does match what we found for $F_{\text{net on }M}$. (In effect, what's happening here is that M is using 200 N of the 300 N force from **F** for its own motion and passing the remaining 100 N along to m, so that both move together with the same acceleration.)

Example 4-6: Two forces act on an object of mass $m = 5$ kg. One of the forces has a magnitude of 6 N, and the other force, perpendicular to the first, has a magnitude of 8 N. What's the acceleration of the object?

Solution: Forces are vectors, and when we find the net force on this object, we see that it's the hypotenuse of a 6-8-10 right triangle.

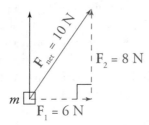

Since $F_{net} = 10$ N, the acceleration of the object will be $a = F_{net}/m = (10 \text{ N})/(5 \text{ kg}) = 2$ m/s^2.

Example 4-7: When a doctor injects someone with a hypodermic needle, she exerts about 15 N of force to pierce adult skin. Once the skin has been pierced, considerably less force is required to push the needle deeper. If a force of 5 N on the plunger is required to initiate the injection, how hard should one pull back on the barrel to minimize risk of hematoma to the patient once the needle is inserted into the vein?

Solution:

According to Newton's second law, $\mathbf{F}_{net} = m\mathbf{a}$. Minimizing risk of hematoma implies that the acceleration of the stationary needle should be zero (so it won't move deeper in or out of the vein during the injection). Thus $\mathbf{F}_{net} = 0$, and $F_{plunger} = F_{barrel}$, or $F_{barrel} = 5$ N.

Example 4-8: According to Newton's third law, every force is "accompanied by" an equal but opposite force. If this is true, shouldn't these forces cancel out to zero? How could we ever accelerate an object?

Solution: The answer does not involve the masses of the objects; Newton's third law says nothing about mass. The key is to remember what $\mathbf{F}_{net}$ means; it's the sum of all the forces that act *on* an object, not *by* the object. Let's say we have a pair of objects, 1 and 2, and an action–reaction pair of forces between them, and we wanted to find the acceleration of Object 2. We'd find all the forces that act on Object 2. One of these forces is $\mathbf{F}_{1\text{-on-}2}$. The reaction force, $\mathbf{F}_{2\text{-on-}1}$, is *not* included in $\mathbf{F}_{net\text{-on-}2}$ because it doesn't act on Object 2; it's a force *by* Object 2. So, the reason why the two forces in an action–reaction pair don't cancel each other is that we'd never add them in the first place because they don't act on the same object.

4.2 NEWTON'S LAW OF GRAVITATION

The mass of an object is a measure of its inertia, its resistance to acceleration. We'll now look at the related concept of an object's weight.

Although in everyday language the terms *mass* and *weight* are sometimes used interchangeably, in physics they have very different technical meanings. The **weight** of an object is the gravitational force exerted on it by the earth (or by whatever planet it happens to be on or near). **Mass** is an intrinsic property of an object and does not change with location. Put a baseball in a rocket and send it to the moon. The baseball's *weight* on the moon is less than its weight here on Earth, but you'd have as much "baseball stuff" there as you would here; that is, the baseball's *mass* would *not* change.

Since weight is a force, we can use $\mathbf{F} = m\mathbf{a}$ to compute it. What acceleration would the gravitational force (which is what *weight* means) impose on an object? The gravitational acceleration, of course! Therefore, setting $\mathbf{a} = \mathbf{g}$, the equation $\mathbf{F} = m\mathbf{a}$ becomes

$$\mathbf{w} = m\mathbf{g}$$

This is the equation for the weight, $\mathbf{w}$, of an object of mass m. (Weight is often symbolized by $\mathbf{F}_{grav}$, rather than $\mathbf{w}$; we'll use both notations.) Note that mass and weight are proportional but not identical. Furthermore, mass is measured in kilograms, while weight is measured in newtons.

Example 4-9:

  a) Find the weight of an object whose mass is 50 kg.
  b) Find the mass of an object whose weight is 50 N.

Solution:

  a) To find an object's weight, we multiply its mass by g. Using $g = 10$ m/s^2 (or, equivalently, $g = 10$ N/kg), we find that $w = mg = (50 \text{ kg})(10 \text{ N/kg}) = 500$ N.
  b) To find an object's mass, we divide its weight by g. With $g = 10$ N/kg, we find that $m = w/g = (50 \text{ N})/(10 \text{ N/kg}) = 5$ kg.

Most of the time, we'll use the formula $w = mg$ to find the weight of an object whose mass is m. However, the value of g can change, and if we're not near the surface of Earth (where we know that g is approximately 10 m/s^2), we may not know the value of g. In that case, we'll invoke another law discovered by Newton:

Newton's Law of Gravitation

Every object in the universe exerts a gravitational pull on every other object. The magnitude of this gravitational force is proportional to the product of the objects' masses and inversely proportional to the square of the distance between them. The constant of proportionality is denoted by G and known as Newton's universal gravitational constant.

$$F_{\text{grav}} = G\,\frac{Mm}{r^2}$$

distance between centers

The value of G is roughly 6.7×10^{-11} N·m²/kg², but don't bother memorizing this constant. The AAMC has removed gravitation from the list of topics subject to memory questions, so the main point of this section is to make connections between basic physics principles and to anticipate certain problem-solving techniques.

One of the most important features of Newton's law of gravitation is that it's an **inverse-square law**. This means that the magnitude of the gravitational force is *inversely* proportional to the *square* of the distance between the centers of the objects. Another important physical law, Coulomb's law (for the electrostatic force between two charges), which we'll see later, is also an inverse-square law.

Also notice that the forces illustrated in the box above form an action–reaction pair. Even if M and m are different, the gravitational force that M exerts on m has the same magnitude as the gravitational force that m exerts on M. (If the directions of the force vectors in the box above seem backward, remember that gravity is always a *pulling* force; therefore, in the figure above, $\mathbf{F}_{M\text{-on-}m}$ pulls to the left, toward M, while $\mathbf{F}_{m\text{-on-}M}$ pulls to the right, toward m.) Of course, the accelerations of the objects will have different magnitudes if the masses are different, as we discussed earlier when we studied Newton's third law.

Example 4-10: What will happen to the gravitational force between two objects if the distance between them is doubled? What if the distance is cut in half?

Solution: Since the gravitational force obeys an inverse-square law, if r increases by a factor of 2, then F_{grav} will *decrease* by a factor of $2^2 = 4$. On the other hand, if r decreases by a factor of 2, then F_{grav} will *increase* by a factor of $2^2 = 4$.

Notice that the two formulas given in this section, $w = mg$ and $F_{\text{grav}} = GMm/r^2$, are really formulas for the same thing. After all, weight *is* gravitational force. Therefore, we could set these expressions equal to each other:

$$mg = G\,\frac{Mm}{r^2}$$

Then, dividing both sides by m, we get

$$g = G\frac{M}{r^2}$$

This formula tells us how to find the value of the gravitational acceleration, g. On Earth, we know that $g \approx 10$ m/s^2. If we were to go to the top of a mountain, then the distance r to the center of the earth would increase, but compared to the radius of the earth, the increase would be very small. As a result, while the value of g *is* less at the top of a mountain than at the earth's surface, the difference is small enough that it can usually be neglected. However, at the position of a satellite orbiting the earth, for example, the distance to the center of the earth has now increased dramatically (for example, many satellites have an orbit radius that's over 6.5 times the radius of the earth), and the resulting decrease in g would definitely need to be taken into account.

This formula for g also shows us why g changes from planet (or moon) to planet. For example, on Earth's moon, the value of g is only about 1.6 m/s^2 (about a sixth of what it is on Earth) because the mass of the moon is so much smaller than the mass of the earth. It's true that the radius of the moon is smaller than the radius of the earth, which would, by itself, make g bigger, but M is *much* smaller, and this is why the value of g on the surface of the moon is smaller than its value on the surface of the earth. So, while big G is a universal gravitational constant, the value of little g depends on where you are.

Example 4-11: The radius of Earth is approximately 6.4×10^6 m. What's the mass of Earth?

Solution: We can use the formula $g = GM/r^2$ to solve for M:

$$M = \frac{gr^2}{G} = \frac{(10 \text{ m/s}^2)(6.4 \times 10^6 \text{ m})^2}{6.7 \times 10^{-11} \frac{\text{N·m}^2}{\text{kg}^2}} \approx 6 \times 10^{24} \text{ kg}$$

Example 4-12: The mass of Mars is about 1/10 the mass of Earth, and the radius of Mars is about half that of Earth. Is the value of g on the surface of Mars less than, greater than, or equal to the value of g on Earth?

Solution: We'll use the formula $g = GM/r^2$ to compare the two values of g:

$$\frac{g_{\text{Mars}}}{g_{\text{Earth}}} = \frac{G\dfrac{M_{\text{Mars}}}{r^2_{\text{Mars}}}}{G\dfrac{M_{\text{Earth}}}{r^2_{\text{Earth}}}} = \frac{M_{\text{Mars}}}{M_{\text{Earth}}} \cdot \left(\frac{r_{\text{Earth}}}{r_{\text{Mars}}}\right)^2 = \frac{1}{10} \cdot 2^2 = 0.4$$

Therefore, the value of g on Mars is only about 40% of its value here.

Example 4-13: A long, flat, frictionless table is set up on the surface of the moon (where $g = 1.6$ m/s^2). An object whose mass on Earth is 4 kg is also transported there.

   a)   What is the object's mass on the moon?
   b)   What is the object's weight on the moon?
   c)   If we drop this object from a height of $h = 20$ m, with what speed will it strike the lunar surface?
   d)   If we wish to push this object across the table to give it an acceleration of 3 m/s^2, how much force must we exert? Would this force be different if the table and object were back on Earth?

Solution:

   a)   The mass is the same, 4 kg.
   b)   The weight of the object on the moon is $w = m \cdot g_{moon} = (4 \text{ kg})(1.6 \text{ m/s}^2) = 6.4$ N. Notice that the object's weight on the moon is different from its weight on Earth.
   c)   Calling *down* the positive direction and using Big Five #5 with $v_0 = 0$ and $a = g_{moon} = 1.6$ m/s^2, we find that

$$v^2 = v_0^2 + 2ad \rightarrow v^2 = 2gh \rightarrow v = \sqrt{2gh} = \sqrt{2(1.6 \text{ m/s}^2)(20 \text{ m})} = 8 \text{ m/s}$$

   d)   Using $F = ma$, we get $F = (4 \text{ kg})(3 \text{ m/s}^2) = 12$ N. Since Newton's second law depends only on mass (not on weight, because there's no g in Newton's second law), we'd need this same force even if the object and table were back on Earth.

Example 4-14: The human body can only withstand a vertical *g-force* of about $5g$ before the body has difficulty pumping blood out of the feet and into the brain. Approximately how much upward force could be applied to a 60 kg person at sea level before that person risked fainting? (The phrase "g-force" is a misnomer, because it actually refers to acceleration: the real *force* involved is the normal force from the surface of contact. A person in free fall experiences "zero gees.")

Solution: A person standing motionless on flat ground experiences a normal force equal to his weight, mg. That corresponds to $1g$. Thus the additional upward force from the surface should provide an additional $4g$ of acceleration. According to Newton's second law $\mathbf{F}_{net} = m\mathbf{a} = 60 \text{ kg} \times 40 \text{ m/s}^2 = 2400$ N.

4.3 FRICTION

Some of the examples in the preceding sections described a frictionless surface. Of course, there's no such thing as a truly frictionless surface, but when a problem uses a term like *frictionless*, it simply means that friction is so weak that it can be neglected. Having frictionless surfaces also made those examples easier, so we could become comfortable with Newton's laws while first learning to apply them. However, there are cases in which friction cannot be ignored, so we need to learn how to handle such situations.

When two materials are in contact, there's an electrical attraction between the atoms of one surface with those of the other; this attraction will make it difficult to slide one object relative to the other. In addition, if the surfaces aren't perfectly smooth, the roughness will also increase the force required to slide the objects against each other. **Friction** is the term we use for the combination of these effects. Fortunately, the forces due to all those intermolecular forces and to the interactions of surface irregularities can be expressed by a single equation.

The MCAT will expect you to know about two big categories of friction; they're called **static friction** and **kinetic (or sliding) friction**.[1] When there's no relative motion between the surfaces that are in contact (that is, when there's no sliding) we have static friction; when there *is* relative motion between the surfaces (that is, when there *is* sliding) we have kinetic friction.

Now, in order to state the equations we'll use to figure out these frictional forces, we first need to discuss another contact force, the one known as the normal force.

Place a book on a flat table. Assuming that the book isn't too heavy and the tabletop isn't made of, say, tissue paper, the book will remain supported by the table. One force acting on the book is the downward gravitational force. If this were the only force acting on the book, then the book would fall through the table. Hence, there must be an upward force acting on the book that cancels out the book's weight. This supporting force, which acts perpendicular to the tabletop, is called the **normal force**. It's called the *normal* force because it is, by definition, perpendicular to the surface that exerts it. The word *normal* means *perpendicular*. We'll denote the normal force by **N** or by F_N. [Don't confuse **N** (or its magnitude, N) with the abbreviation for the newton, N.] In the case of an object simply lying on a flat surface, the magnitude of the normal force is just equal to the object's weight. As a result, the book feels a downward force of magnitude $w = mg$ and an upward force of magnitude $N = mg$, so the net force on the book is 0.

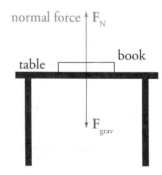

---

[1] Occasionally the MCAT may refer to **rolling resistance**. Rolling resistance is not technically friction; it is the force that resists an object's rolling motion. Do not confuse rolling resistance with kinetic friction; an object can roll without sliding (or skidding), and any friction at the contact point between the object and the surface will then be static, not kinetic.

Example 4-15: Do the normal force and the gravitational force described in the preceding paragraph form an action–reaction pair?

Solution: No. While these forces *are* equal but opposite, they do not form an action–reaction pair, because they act on the same object (namely, the book). The forces in an action–reaction pair always act on different objects. So, while it's true that the forces in an action–reaction pair are always equal but opposite, it is not true that any pair of equal but opposite forces must always form an action–reaction pair. The reaction force to $F_{\text{table-on-book}}$, which is the normal force, is $F_{\text{book-on-table}}$. The reaction force to $F_{\text{Earth-on-book}}$, which is the weight of the book, is $F_{\text{book-on-Earth}}$. The force $F_{\text{table-on-book}}$ is not the reaction to $F_{\text{Earth-on-book}}$.

For an object on a horizontal surface that feels no other vertical forces, the normal force will be equal to the weight of the object. However, there are many cases in which the normal force isn't equal to the weight of the object. For example, suppose we place a book against a vertical wall and push on the book with a horizontal force **F**. Then the magnitude of the normal force exerted by the wall will be equal to *F*, which may certainly be different from the weight of the book. Here's another example (which we'll look at in more detail in the next section): If we place a book on an inclined plane (e.g., a ramp), then the normal force exerted by the ramp on the book will not be equal to the weight of the book. What we can say is the general definition of the normal force: *The normal force is the perpendicular component of the contact force exerted by a surface on an object.*

We had to discuss the normal force here, because the force of friction exerted by a surface on an object in contact with is related to the normal force. In the case of sliding (kinetic) friction, the magnitude of the force of friction is directly proportional to the magnitude of the normal force. The constant of proportionality depends on what the surface is made of and what the object is made of; this constant is called the **coefficient of kinetic friction**, denoted by μ_k (the Greek letter *mu*, with subscript k), where the k denotes <u>k</u>inetic friction. For every pair of surfaces, the coefficient μ_k is an experimentally determined positive number with no units, and the greater its value, the greater the force of kinetic friction. For example, the value of μ_k for rubber-soled shoes on ice is only about 0.1, while for rubber-soled shoes on wood, the value of μ_k is much higher; it's about 0.7 for your sneakers, but could be greater than 1 if you walk around in rock-climbing shoes.

Notice carefully that this is *not* a vector equation. It is only an equation giving the *magnitude* of F_f in terms of the *magnitude* of F_N.

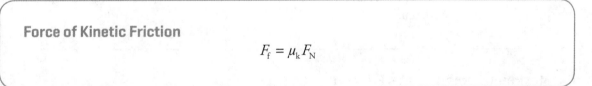

Force of Kinetic Friction

$$F_f = \mu_k F_N$$

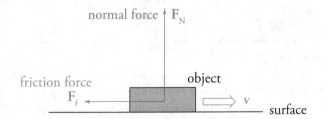

The magnitude of the force of kinetic friction is given by the equation $F_f = \mu_k F_N$. The direction of the force of kinetic friction is always parallel to the surface and in the opposite direction to the object's velocity (relative to the surface).

Example 4-16: A book of mass $m = 2$ kg slides across a flat tabletop. If the coefficient of kinetic friction between the book and table is 0.4, what's the magnitude of the force of kinetic friction on the book?

Solution: Because the magnitude of the normal force is $F_N = mg = (2 \text{ kg})(10 \text{ m/s}^2) = 20$ N, the magnitude of the force of kinetic friction is $F_f = \mu_k F_N = (0.4)(20 \text{ N}) = 8$ N.

The formula for static friction is similar to the one for kinetic friction, but there are two important differences. First, given a pair of surfaces, there's a **maximum coefficient of static friction** between them, μ_s (the subscript s now denotes static friction), and on the MCAT, it's always greater than the coefficient of kinetic friction. This is equivalent to saying that, in general, static friction is capable of being stronger than kinetic friction. To illustrate this, imagine there's a heavy crate sitting on the floor and you want to push the crate across the room. You walk up to the crate and push on it, harder and harder until, finally, it "gives" and starts sliding. Once the crate is sliding, it's easier to keep it sliding than it was to get it started in the first place. The friction that resisted your initial push to get the crate moving was static friction. Because it was easier to keep it sliding than it was to get it started sliding, kinetic friction must be weaker than the maximum static friction force.

The second difference between the formula for kinetic friction and the one for static friction is that there's actually no general formula for the force of static friction. All we have is a formula for the *maximum* force of static friction. It's important that you understand this distinction. Let's go back to that heavy crate sitting on the floor. Let's say you know by previous experience that it'll take 400 N of force on your part to get that crate sliding. So, what if you push with a force of 100 N? Well, obviously, the crate won't move. Therefore, there must be another 100 N acting on the crate, opposite to your push, to make the net force on the crate zero. Okay, what if you now push on the crate with a force of 200 N? The crate still won't move, so there must now be another 200 N acting on the crate, opposite to your push, to make the net force on the crate zero. Whatever force you exert on the crate, as long as it's less than 400 N, will cause the force of static friction to cancel you out. Static friction is capable of supplying any necessary force, but only up to a certain maximum. That's why we can't write down a general formula for the force of static friction, only a formula for the maximum force of static friction. The formula looks just like the one above, except we replace μ_k by μ_s, and add the word "max" to denote that all this formula gives is the maximum force of static friction.

Maximum Force of Static Friction

$$F_{f, \text{max}} = \mu_s F_N$$

The maximum magnitude of the force of static friction is given by the equation $F_{f, \text{max}} = \mu_s F_N$. The direction of the force of static friction (maximum or not) is always parallel to the surface and in the opposite direction to the object's intended velocity. The magnitude of the force of static friction is whatever value, up to the maximum given by the equation, it takes exactly to cancel out the force(s) that are trying to make the object slide.

Example 4-17: A crate that weighs 1000 N rests on a horizontal floor. The coefficient of static friction between the crate and the floor is 0.4. If you push on the crate with a force of 250 N, what is the magnitude of the force of static friction?

Solution: The answer is not 400 N. The *maximum* force of static friction that the floor could exert on the crate is $F_{f, max} = \mu_s F_N = (0.4)(1000 \text{ N}) = 400$ N. However, if you exert a force of only 250 N on the crate, then static friction will only be 250 N. (Just imagine what would happen to the crate if you pushed on it with a force of 250 N and the floor pushed it back toward you with a force of 400 N!)

Example 4-18: You push a 50 kg block of wood across a flat concrete driveway, exerting a constant force of 300 N. If the coefficient of kinetic friction between the wood and concrete is 0.5, what will be the acceleration of the block?

Solution: The normal force acting on the block has a magnitude of $F_N = mg = (50 \text{ kg})(10 \text{ m/s}^2) = 500$ N. Therefore, the force of kinetic friction acting on the sliding block has a magnitude of $F_f = \mu_k F_N = (0.5)(500 \text{ N}) = 250$ N. This means that the net force acting on the block (and parallel to the driveway) is equal to $F - F_f = (300 \text{ N}) - (250 \text{ N}) = 50$ N. If $F_{net} = 50$ N and $m = 50$ kg, then $a = F_{net}/m = (50 \text{ N})/(50 \text{ kg}) = 1 \text{ m/s}^2$.

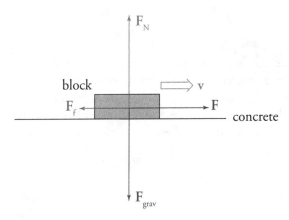

Example 4-19: Instead of pushing the block by a force that's parallel to the driveway, you wrap a rope around the block, sling the rope over your shoulder, and walk it across the driveway. If the rope makes an angle of 30° to the horizontal, and the tension in the rope is 300 N (the same force you exerted on the block in the last example), what will the block's acceleration be now?

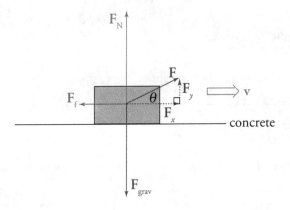

Solution: This is a tough question, but it uses a lot of the material we've covered so far. First, we'll need the normal force to find the friction force. The net vertical force on the block is 0 (because we're not lifting the block off the ground or watching it fall through the concrete). Therefore, $F_N + F_y = F_{grav}$, so $F_N = F_{grav} - F_y$. (Here's another example of the normal force not equaling the weight of the object.) Since $F_y = F \sin \theta = F \sin 30° = (300 \text{ N})(0.5) = 150 \text{ N}$, we have $F_N = (500 \text{ N}) - (150 \text{ N}) = 350 \text{ N}$. (Intuitively, the normal force is less than the weight of the block because the vertical component of the tension in the rope is "taking some of the pressure" off the surface.) Therefore, $F_f = \mu_k F_N = (0.5)(350 \text{ N}) = 175 \text{ N}$. Now, the horizontal force that you provide is $F_x = F \cos \theta = F \cos 30° \approx (300 \text{ N})(0.85) = 255 \text{ N}$. Therefore, the net force acting on the block, parallel to the driveway, is equal to $F_x - F_f = (255 \text{ N}) - (175 \text{ N}) = 80 \text{ N}$. If $F_{net} = 80 \text{ N}$ and $m = 50 \text{ kg}$, then $a = F_{net}/m = (80 \text{ N})/(50 \text{ kg}) = 1.6 \text{ m/s}^2$. (Notice that you get the block moving faster—even exerting the same force—by doing it this way!)

4.4 INCLINED PLANES

So far, we've had practice problems where the object is moving along a flat, horizontal surface. However, the MCAT will also expect you to handle questions in which the object is on a ramp, or, in fancier language, an **inclined plane**.

The figure below shows an object of mass m on an inclined plane; the angle the plane makes with the horizontal (the **incline angle**) is labeled θ. If we draw the vector representing the weight of the object, we notice that it can be written in terms of two components: one parallel to the ramp and one perpendicular to it. The diagram on the left shows that the magnitudes of the components of the object's weight, $\mathbf{w} = m\mathbf{g}$, are $mg \sin \theta$ (parallel to the ramp) and $mg \cos \theta$ (perpendicular to the ramp).

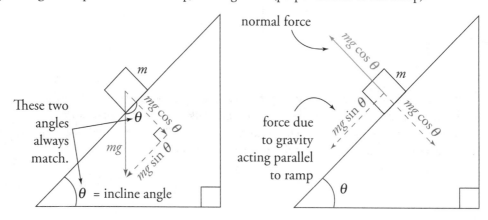

Therefore, as illustrated in the diagram on the right,

> the force due to gravity acting parallel to the inclined plane = $mg \sin \theta$
>
> the force due to gravity acting perpendicular to the inclined plane = $mg \cos \theta$

where θ is measured between the incline and horizontal. **You should memorize both of these facts.**

Incidentally, any time we see an angle in an MCAT problem we'll probably be breaking a vector (say a force, a velocity, or an acceleration) into components. When we looked at projectile motion we broke the projectile's initial velocity into horizontal and vertical components; here, we're breaking the force of gravity into a component parallel to and one perpendicular to the surface of the incline. Why the difference? In general, the components you'll use will be vertical and horizontal, *unless* the object can only move along one possible line; in that case, the components to use will be the direction of (possible) travel (in this case, parallel to the incline) and, the direction perpendicular to that.

Example 4-20: A block of mass $m = 4$ kg is placed at the top of a frictionless ramp of incline angle 30° and length 10 m.

   a)   What is the block's acceleration down the ramp?
   b)   How long will it take for the block to slide to the bottom?

Solution:

   a)   Because the force due to gravity acting parallel to the ramp is $F = mg \sin \theta$, the acceleration of the block down the ramp will be

$$a = \frac{F}{m} = \frac{mg \sin \theta}{m} = g \sin \theta = \left(10 \text{ m/s}^2\right) \sin 30° = 5 \text{ m/s}^2$$

   b)   Using Big Five #3 with $d = 10$ m, $v_0 = 0$, and $a = 5$ m/s², we find that

$$d = v_0 t + \frac{1}{2}at^2 = \frac{1}{2}at^2 \rightarrow t = \sqrt{\frac{2d}{a}} = \sqrt{\frac{2(10 \text{ m})}{5 \text{ m/s}^2}} = 2 \text{ s}$$

Notice that the block's mass was irrelevant to both of these questions. That's because all of the forces were directly proportional to mass, but so was the object's inertia; in effect, mass cancelled out of both sides of $F = ma$. This is common in problems in which the forces on an object are all functions of gravity.

Example 4-21: A block of mass m slides down a ramp of incline angle 60°. If the coefficient of kinetic friction between the block and the surface of the ramp is 0.2, what's the block's acceleration down the ramp?

Solution: There are now two forces acting parallel to the ramp: $mg \sin \theta$ (directed downward along the ramp) and F_f, the force of kinetic friction (directed upward along the ramp). Therefore, the net force down the ramp is $F_{net} = mg \sin \theta - F_f$. To find F_f, we multiply F_N by μ_k. Since $F_N = mg \cos \theta$, we have

$$F_{net} = mg \sin \theta - \mu_k mg \cos \theta$$

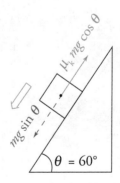

Dividing F_{net} by m gives us a:

$$a = \frac{F_{net}}{m} = \frac{mg \sin\theta - \mu_k mg \cos\theta}{m} = g(\sin\theta - \mu_k \cos\theta)$$

Putting in the numbers, we get

$$a = (10 \text{ m/s}^2)(\sin 60° - 0.2 \cos 60°) \approx (10 \text{ m/s}^2)(0.85 - 0.2 \cdot \tfrac{1}{2}) = 7.5 \text{ m/s}^2$$

Example 4-22: A block of mass m is placed on a ramp of incline angle θ. If the block doesn't slide down, find the relationship between μ_s (the coefficient of static friction) and θ.

Solution: If the block doesn't slide, then static friction is strong enough to withstand the pull of gravity acting downward parallel to the ramp. This means that the *maximum* force of static friction must be greater than or equal to $mg \sin\theta$. Since $F_{f(static),max} = \mu_s F_N$, and $F_N = mg \cos\theta$, we have $F_{f(static),max} = \mu_s mg \cos\theta$. Therefore,

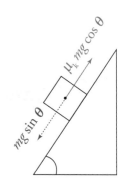

$$F_{f \text{ (static) max}} \geq mg \sin\theta$$

$$\mu_s mg \cos\theta \geq mg \sin\theta$$

$$\mu_s \cos\theta \geq \sin\theta$$

$$\mu_s \geq \frac{\sin\theta}{\cos\theta}$$

$$\therefore \mu_s \geq \tan\theta$$

4.5 PULLEYS

A **pulley** is a device that changes the direction of the **tension** (the force exerted by a stretched string, cord, or rope) that pulls on the object that the string is attached to. (We'll use $\mathbf{F_T}$ or $\mathbf{T}$ to denote a tension force.) For example, in the picture below, if we pull *down* on the string on the right with a force of magnitude F_T, then the tension force on the left side of the pulley will pull *up* on the block with the same magnitude of force, F_T.

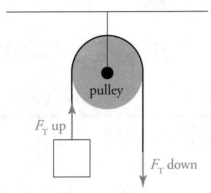

Pulleys can also be used to decrease the force necessary to lift an object. For example, consider the pulley system illustrated on the left below. If we pull down on the string on the right with a force of magnitude F_T, then we'll create a tension force of magnitude F_T throughout the entire string. As a result, there will be *two* tension forces, each of magnitude F_T, pulling up to lift the block (and the bottom pulley, too, but we assume that the pulleys are massless; that is, the mass of any pulley is small enough that it can be ignored). Therefore, we only need to exert half as much force to lift the block! This simple observation, that a pulley system (with massless, frictionless pulleys) causes a constant tension to exist through the entire string, which can lead to multiple tension forces pulling on an object, is the key to many MCAT problems on pulleys.

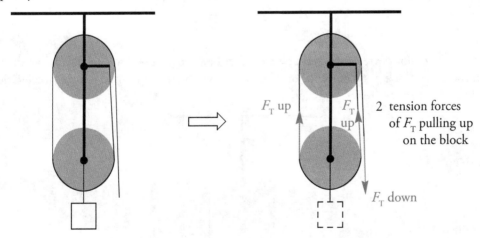

Pulley systems like this multiply our force by however many strings are pulling on the object.

Notice carefully that the tension force is applied wherever a string (or rope, or cable, or whatever) comes in contact with a pulley, which means that there will often be *two* tension forces on a single pulley, one on each side. You can see this in the right-hand diagram above.

Example 4-23: In the figure below, how much force would we need to exert on the free end of the cord in order to lift the plank (mass $M = 300$ kg) with constant velocity? (Ignore the masses of the pulleys.)

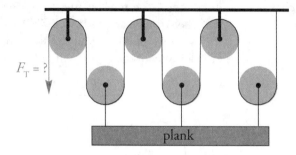

Solution: As a result of our pulling downward, there will be 6 tension forces pulling up on the plank:

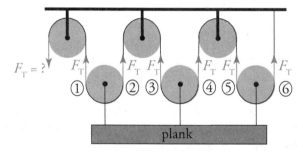

In order to lift with constant velocity (acceleration = zero), we require the net force on the plank to be zero. Therefore, the total of all the tension forces pulling up, $6F_T$, must balance the weight of the plank downward, Mg. This gives us

$$6F_T = Mg \rightarrow F_T = \frac{Mg}{6} = \frac{(300 \text{ kg})(10 \frac{\text{N}}{\text{kg}})}{6} = 500 \text{ N}$$

Example 4-24: Two blocks are connected by a cord that hangs over a pulley. One block has a mass, M, of 10 kg, and the other block has a mass, m, of 5 kg. What will be the magnitude of the acceleration of the system of blocks once they are released from rest?

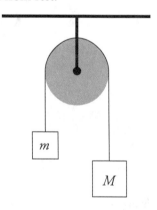

Solution: We'll solve this by a step-by-step approach using a **force diagram**. To apply Newton's second law, $\mathbf{F}_{net} = ma$, to any problem, we follow these steps:

Step 1: Draw all the forces that act *on* the object. (That is, draw the force diagram.)
Step 2: Choose a direction to call *positive* (simply take the direction of the object's motion to be positive; it's almost always the easiest, most natural decision).
Step 3: Find $\mathbf{F}_{net}$ and set it equal to ma.

We have effectively done these steps in the solutions to the examples we have seen already, but now that we have a situation involving two accelerating objects, it is even more important to make sure that we have a systematic plan of attack. When you have more than one object to worry about, just make sure that the Step-2 decision you make for one object is compatible with the Step-2 decision you make for the other one(s). On the left below are the force diagrams for the blocks on the pulley. Notice that we call *up* the positive direction for m (because that's where it's going), and we call *down* the positive direction for M (because that's where *it's* going); these decisions are compatible, because when m moves in its positive direction, so does M.

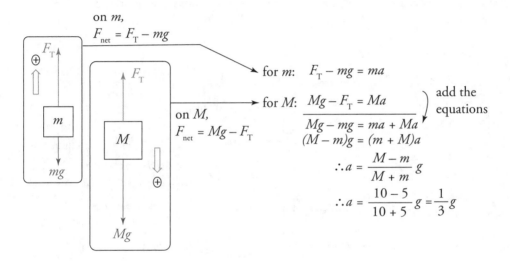

Because *up* is the positive direction for little m, the force F_T on m is positive and the force mg is negative; therefore, for little m, we have $F_{net} = F_T + (-mg) = F_T - mg$. Since *down* is the positive direction for big M, the force Mg on M is positive and the force F_T is negative; therefore, for big M, we have $F_{net} = Mg + (-F_T) = Mg - F_T$. On the right above, we've written down $F_{net} = $ mass $\times$ acceleration for each block. There are two equations, but we have two unknowns (F_T and a), so we *need* two equations. To solve the equations, the trick is simply to *add the equations*. Notice that this makes the F_T's drop out, so all we're left with is one unknown, a, which we can solve for immediately. The calculation shown above gives $a = g/3$, so we get $a = 3.3$ m/s^2.

If the question had asked for the tension in the cord, we could now use the value we found for a and plug it back into either of our two equations (we'd get the same answer no matter which one we used). Using $F_T - mg = ma$, we'd find that

$$F_T = ma + mg = m(a + g) = m(\tfrac{1}{3}g + g) = \tfrac{4}{3}mg = \tfrac{4}{3}(5 \text{ kg})(10 \tfrac{\text{N}}{\text{kg}}) = 67 \text{ N}$$

4.5

Example 4-25: In the figure below, the block of mass m slides up a frictionless inclined plane, pulled by another block of mass M that is falling. If $\theta = 30°$, $m = 20$ kg, and $M = 40$ kg, what's the acceleration of the block on the ramp?

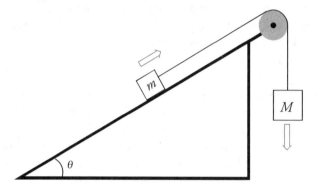

Solution: On the left below are the force diagrams for the blocks. Notice that we call *up the ramp* the positive direction for m (because that's where it's going), and we call *down* the positive direction for M (because that's where *it's* going); these decisions are compatible, because when m moves in its positive direction, so does M.

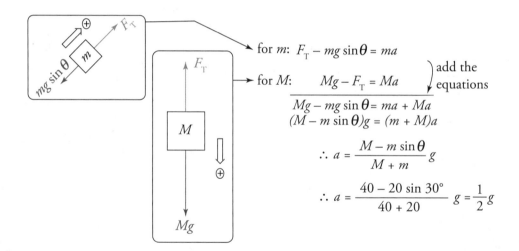

for m: $F_T - mg\sin\theta = ma$

for M: $Mg - F_T = Ma$ — add the equations

$$Mg - mg\sin\theta = ma + Ma$$
$$(M - m\sin\theta)g = (m + M)a$$

$$\therefore a = \frac{M - m\sin\theta}{M + m}g$$

$$\therefore a = \frac{40 - 20\sin 30°}{40 + 20}g = \frac{1}{2}g$$

Because *up the ramp* is the positive direction for little m, the force F_T on m is positive and the force due to gravity along the ramp, $mg\sin\theta$, is negative; therefore, for little m, we have $F_{net} = F_T + (-mg\sin\theta) = F_T - mg\sin\theta$. Since *down* is the positive direction for big M, the force Mg on M is positive and the force F_T is negative; therefore, for big M, we have $F_{net} = Mg + (-F_T) = Mg - F_T$. On the right above, we've written down F_{net} = mass × acceleration for each block. As in the preceding example, there are two equations, (and two unknowns, F_T and a). Again using the trick of adding the equations, the F_T's drop out, and all we're left with is one unknown, a, to solve for. The calculation shown above gives $a = g/2$, so we get $a = 5$ m/s^2.

Summary of Formulas

NEWTON'S LAWS:

First law: $\mathbf{F}_{net} = 0 \Leftrightarrow \mathbf{v}$ = constant

Second law: $\mathbf{F}_{net} = m\mathbf{a}$

Third law: $\mathbf{F}_{1\text{-on-}2} = -\mathbf{F}_{2\text{-on-}1}$

Weight: $\mathbf{w} = m\mathbf{g}$

Gravitational force: $F_{grav} = G\dfrac{Mm}{r^2}$ given that $w = F_{grav}$, we get $g = G\dfrac{M}{r^2}$.

Kinetic friction: $F_f = \mu_k F_N$

Static friction: $F_{f,max} = \mu_s F_N$

$$\mu_s > \mu_k$$

Direction of friction is opposite to the direction of motion (or intended direction of motion).

Force due to gravity acting parallel to inclined plane: $mg \sin \theta$

Force due to gravity acting perpendicular to inclined plane: $mg \cos \theta$, where θ is measured between the incline and horizontal.

CHAPTER 4 FREESTANDING PRACTICE QUESTIONS

1. The gravitational force the Sun exerts on Earth is F. Mars is 1.5 times further from the Sun than Earth and its mass is $\frac{1}{6}$ of Earth's mass. What is the gravitational force that the Sun exerts on Mars?

   A) $\frac{2}{27}\,F$

   B) $\frac{1}{9}\,F$

   C) $9\,F$

   D) $\frac{27}{2}\,F$

2. You have four frictionless, massless pulleys, arranged as shown below. If you have enough force to lift a 40 kg object without any pulleys, what is the maximum mass of the couch that can be raised with the pulley system?

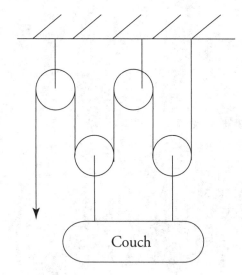

   A) 80 kg
   B) 120 kg
   C) 160 kg
   D) 240 kg

3. When an object falls from a very large height, it accelerates towards Earth because of the force of gravity. Air resistance also acts on the object as it falls, and the air resistance increases as the speed of the object increases. Eventually, the force due to air resistance equals that of gravity and the object reaches terminal velocity. What best describes this situation?

   A) The acceleration of the object at terminal velocity is the largest it will ever be.
   B) The speed of the object increases until it hits the ground.
   C) The speed of the object at terminal velocity is zero.
   D) The acceleration of the object at terminal velocity is zero.

4. A box of mass m is sitting on an incline of 45° and it requires an applied force F up the incline to get the box to begin to move. What is the maximum coefficient of static friction?

   A) $\left(\dfrac{\sqrt{2}F}{mg}\right)-1$

   B) $\left(\dfrac{\sqrt{2}F}{mg}\right)$

   C) $\left(\dfrac{\sqrt{2}F}{mg}\right)+1$

   D) $\left(\dfrac{2F}{mg}\right)-1$

5. A 100 g block is sitting at rest on a horizontal table. According to Newton's third law, which of the following indicates the correct action-reaction pair of the two forces?

   A) The gravitational force exerted by the table on the block and the normal force exerted by the block on the table
   B) The gravitational force exerted by the block on Earth and the normal force exerted by the table on the block
   C) The weight of the block and the normal force exerted by the table on the block
   D) The weight of the block and the gravitational force exerted by the block on Earth

6. A person is pulling a block of mass m with a force equal to its weight directed 30° above the horizontal plane across a rough surface, generating a friction f on the block. If the person is now pushing downward on the block with the same force 30° below the horizontal plane across the same rough surface, what is the friction on the block? (μ_k is the coefficient of kinetic friction across the surface.)

A) f
B) $1.5f$
C) $2f$
D) $3f$

7. A 2 kg ball is sliding east (without friction) down a hill that makes an angle of 30° with the horizontal. A child kicks the ball north with a force of 10 N. What is the net acceleration of the kicked ball?

A) $\left(5\sqrt{3}\right)/2$ m/s²
B) $5\sqrt{2}$ m/s²
C) $5\sqrt{3}$ m/s²
D) $10\sqrt{2}$ m/s²

CHAPTER 4 PRACTICE PASSAGE

When an object is falling through air, it experiences a drag force due to the frictional effects of the air. The drag force is always directed opposite the direction of motion of the object. For a spherical object, the drag force can be calculated using Stokes' law:

$$F_D = 6\pi\eta r v$$

Equation 1

where F_D is the drag force, η is the coefficient of viscosity of the air, r is the radius of the sphere, and v is the velocity of the sphere.

Since the drag force is related to the velocity of the sphere, as the sphere's velocity increases, so does the drag force. After a certain time, the drag force will be large enough that the net force acting on the sphere is zero. At this point, the sphere falls with a constant velocity, known as the terminal velocity, v_T.

A student experiments with different spherical objects falling on Earth in order to test Stokes' law. The experiment involves dropping a variety of spheres from the balcony of a building. The relative mass and radius for each sphere are listed in Table 1.

Object	Mass	Radius
Beach ball	m	$20r$
Bowling ball	$20m$	$10r$
Golf ball	m	r
Ping pong ball	$0.25m$	r

Table 1   Mass and radius of spheres

1. Ignoring air resistance, which ball will hit the ground first?

A) The beach ball, since it has the largest radius.
B) The bowling ball, since it has the largest mass.
C) The golf ball, since it has the smallest radius and more mass than the ping pong ball.
D) All the balls will hit at the same time.

2. Considering air resistance, which ball will take the longest time to reach the ground when dropped, assuming none of the balls reaches its terminal velocity?

A) Beach ball
B) Bowling ball
C) Golf ball
D) Ping pong ball

3. For the experiment conducted, let v_1 be the velocity of the golf ball after 10 seconds when dropped from height, h. Let v_2 be the velocity of the ping pong ball after 10 seconds when dropped from the same height, h. How do v_1 and v_2 compare?

A) $v_1 < v_2$
B) $v_1 = v_2$
C) $v_1 > v_2$
D) It cannot be determined without information on the drag force.

4. How does the drag force on the beach ball compare to the drag force on the bowling ball when the velocities of the two balls are the same?

A) The drag force on the beach ball is 20 times the drag force on the bowling ball.
B) The drag force on the beach ball is 2 times the drag force on the bowling ball.
C) The drag force on the beach ball is $\frac{2}{3}$ the drag force on the bowling ball.
D) The drag force on the beach ball is $\frac{1}{2}$ the drag force on the bowling ball.

5. Which of the following gives an equation for the terminal velocity for the balls?

A) $v_T = mg - 6\pi\eta r$

B) $v_T = mg + 6\pi\eta r$

C) $v_T = \dfrac{mg}{6\pi\eta r}$

D) $v_T = \dfrac{6\pi\eta r}{mg}$

6. Which ball has the greatest terminal velocity?

A)   Beach ball
B)   Bowling ball
C)   Golf ball
D)   Ping pong ball

SOLUTIONS TO CHAPTER 4 FREESTANDING PRACTICE QUESTIONS

1. **A** Given that the gravitational force of the Sun on the Earth is $F = GMm/r^2$, the force exerted on Mars is:

$$F_{\text{Mars}} = \frac{GM\left(\frac{1}{6}m\right)}{\left(\frac{3}{2}r\right)^2} = \frac{GMm\left(\frac{1}{6}\right)}{r^2\left(\frac{9}{4}\right)} = \frac{4}{54}F = \frac{2}{27}F$$

2. **C** With four pulleys you have four times the tension force acting upwards, allowing you to lift four times the weight. Since the maximum tension force is $(40 \text{ kg})(10 \text{ m/s}^2) = 400$ N, the maximum force that can be applied to the couch is 4×400 N $= 1600$ N. This corresponds to a mass of 160 kg.

3. **D** The net force on the object is the difference between the force due to gravity and the force due to air resistance. Therefore, as the force due to air resistance grows larger, the net force decreases, as does the acceleration, eliminating choice A. When the force due to air resistance equals that of gravity, the net force is zero, as is the acceleration (according to Newton's second law), which makes choice D correct. When there is zero acceleration, velocity is constant, eliminating choice B and the object does not stop moving once it reaches terminal velocity, eliminating choice C.

4. **A** The force of static friction and the force of gravity are acting down the incline in this situation. When the box just begins to move upwards the forces in both directions are equal and the force of static friction is at its maximum. Therefore, you have the equation $F = \mu_s \, mg \cos(45°) + mg \sin(45°)$. Solving for μ_s we find the correct answer to be choice A.

5. **D** Since the answers could be confusing, a good strategy would be to identify all the correct action–reaction pairs, and match them to the answer choices. Here are the correct action–reaction pairs in question:

   a. The weight of the block and the gravitational force exerted by the block on Earth
   b. The normal force exerted by the block on the table and the normal force exerted by the table on the block
   c. The gravitational force exerted by the table on the block and the gravitational force exerted by the block on the table

   Of all the answer choices, only choice D matches the pairs described above.

6. **D** The friction f on the block is represented by the formula $f = \mu_k N$, where N is the normal force acting on the block. When the force is applied 30° above the horizontal, $N = mg - mg \sin 30°$. Since $\sin 30°$ is 0.5, $N = mg - 0.5mg = 0.5mg$. Substituting N into the formula for friction, it becomes $f_1 = 0.5\mu_k mg$. When the force is applied 30° below the horizontal, $N = mg + mg \sin 30° = mg + 0.5mg = 1.5mg$. Substituting N into the formula for friction, it becomes $f_2 = 1.5\mu_k mg = 3f_1$.

Therefore, the correct answer is choice D.

7. **B** The force of gravity that is parallel to the surface of the hill $F_{G\text{-parallel}}$ is the initial force acting on the ball (there is no kinetic friction force acting on the ball). The F_G that is parallel to the surface of the hill can be calculated using $mg \sin \theta = (2 \text{ kg})(10 \text{ m/s}^2)\sin 30° = 20(\frac{1}{2}) = 10 \text{ N}$. This 10 N force is acting in the east direction. The child kicks the ball with a 10 N force in the north direction. These two forces are vectors and can be added tip-to-tail to find the resulting force vector. The three force vectors make an isosceles right triangle, so the hypotenuse must be equal to a leg of the triangle multiplied by $\sqrt{2}$, or in this case, $10\sqrt{2}$ N. (Another way to find the hypotenuse, c, is to use the Pythagorean theorem so $c^2 = 10^2 + 10^2 = 200$ and $c = 10\sqrt{2}$.)

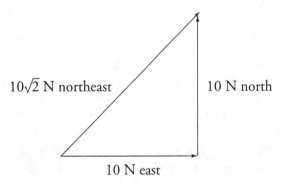

$10\sqrt{2}$ N northeast   10 N north

10 N east

The question is asking for the acceleration of the ball, and $a = F/m = (10\sqrt{2} \text{ N})/(2 \text{ kg}) = 5\sqrt{2} \text{ m/s}^2$. The correct answer is choice B.

SOLUTIONS TO CHAPTER 4 PRACTICE PASSAGE

1. **D**   For ideal conditions with no friction, the drag force will not exist (it is a frictional force). The acceleration of each ball can be calculated from $F_{net} = ma$. The only force acting on the ball is its weight, so $mg = ma$ and $a = g$ so the acceleration on each ball will be the acceleration from gravity, g. Since all balls are dropped from the same height and have the same acceleration, they will hit the ground at the same time.

2. **A**   The acceleration of each ball can be calculated from $F_{net} = ma$. Since the net displacement of the balls is down, F_G is in the positive direction and $F_G - F_D = ma$ so $mg - 6\pi\eta rv = ma$ and $a = g - 6\pi\eta rv/m$. The only values in the equation that change for the different balls are the mass and radius. The larger the ratio of r/m, the larger amount that is subtracted from g, and the slower the ball's acceleration. The question asks for the longest time, which is the slowest acceleration. The beach ball has the largest radius/mass ratio ($20r/m$) and so the slowest acceleration and the longest time.

3. **C**   The acceleration of each ball can be calculated from $F_{net} = ma$. Since the net displacement of the balls is down, F_G is in the positive direction and $F_G - F_D = ma$ so $mg - 6\pi\eta rv = ma$ and $a = g - 6\pi\eta rv/m$. The only value in the equation that changes for the different balls is the mass. The larger the mass, the smaller the amount that is subtracted from g, and the larger the ball's acceleration, so the larger the ball's velocity. Since the golf ball has the larger mass, it will have the larger velocity, v_1.

4. **B**   Using Equation 1, the drag force on the beach ball is F_D, beach ball $= 6\pi\eta(20r)v$. The drag force on the bowling ball is F_D, bowling ball $= 6\pi\eta(10r)v$. Thus, the drag force on the beach ball is twice the drag force on the bowling ball.

5. **C**   The passage states that terminal velocity is reached when the net force on the sphere is zero, so $F_{net} = 0$. The only two forces acting on the sphere are the force of gravity and the drag force, so these forces must be equal when the terminal velocity is reached. Starting with the equation $F_G = F_D$ and plugging in Equation 1 yields $mg = 6\pi\eta rv$. Solving this equation for the velocity, which in this case is the terminal velocity, yields $v = (mg)/(6\pi\eta r)$. Notice the equations in choices A and B include the sum and difference with the weight of the ball, which is not a velocity, so these two choices can be eliminated, leaving choice C as the correct answer.

6. **B**   The passage states that terminal velocity is reached when the net force on the sphere is zero, so $F_{net} = 0$. The only two forces acting on the sphere are the force of gravity and the drag force, so these forces must be equal when the terminal velocity is reached. Starting with the equation $F_G = F_D$ and plugging in Equation 1 yields $mg = 6\pi\eta rv$. Solving this equation for the velocity, which in this case is the terminal velocity, yields $v = (mg)/(6\pi\eta r)$. The sphere with the largest terminal velocity will have the largest ratio of mass/radius. The bowling ball has the largest mass/radius ratio ($2m/r$) and so will have the largest terminal velocity.

Chapter 5
Mechanics II

5.1 CENTER OF MASS AND GRAVITY

In the examples we looked at in the preceding chapter, objects were treated as though they were each a single particle. In fact, in the step-by-step solution to one of the pulley problems, we drew a force diagram showing all the forces acting on the objects in the system. To make that step go faster, we sometimes just represent each object by a dot and draw the force arrows on the dot. For example, the force diagram in the solution to Example 4-24 could have been drawn like this:

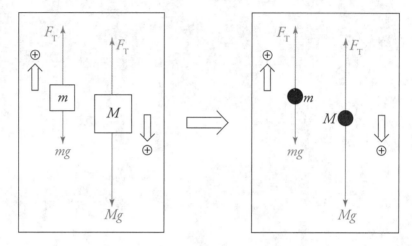

Each dot really denotes the *center of mass* of the object (or "center of gravity": the terms are interchangeable on the MCAT), which we'll now describe and define.

Imagine the following series of experiments. You walk into a large room with a friend, a hammer, and a glow-in-the dark (phosphorescent) sticker. After shining light on the sticker (so that it will glow), stick it on the metal head of the hammer. Hand the hammer to your friend, stand back, and turn off the light. Ask your friend to flip and toss the hammer across the room so that you can watch its trajectory. You'll see only the glow-in-the-dark sticker, and it will, in general, trace out some complicated loopy path as the hammer tumbles and flies through the air.

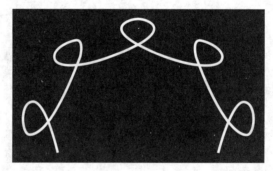

Repeat the experiment with the sticker attached to the end of the handle of the hammer. Once again, when your friend flips and tosses the hammer across the room so that you can watch it face on, you'll see only the glow-in-the-dark sticker, and it'll trace out another complicated loopy path.

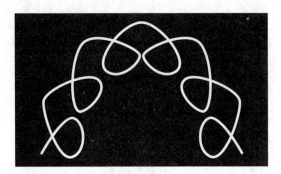

Now let's try this one more time, but rather than attaching the sticker at some random spot on the hammer, first find the point where the hammer just balances on the tip of your finger. Put the sticker on that spot and hand the hammer to your friend. Turn off the light, and watch as the hammer is tossed across the room. This time you'll see the sticker trace out a nice parabola, no loops.

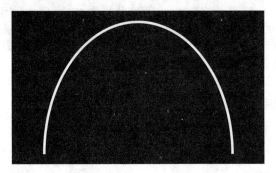

Apparently there was something special about the final location of the sticker. Most points on the hammer traced out complicated loopy trajectories, but this final point traced out a simple parabolic path, just as a single particle would. It is this one point that behaves as if the object (whether it's a block or a hammer or whatever) was a single particle. This special point is the **center of mass**. Another way of looking at it is to say that the center of mass is the point at which we could consider all the mass of the object to be concentrated. It's the dot in our simplified force diagrams.

For a simple object such as a sphere, block, or cylinder, whose density is constant (that is, for an object that's *homogeneous*), the center of mass is where you'd expect it to be—at its geometric center.

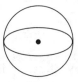 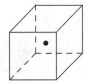 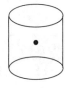

Note that in some cases, the center of mass isn't even located within the body of the object:

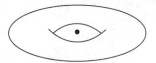

For a nonhomogeneous object, such as a hammer, whose density *does* vary from point to point, there's no single-step way mathematically to calculate the location of the center of mass.

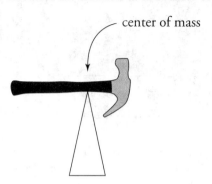

center of mass

However, there is a simpler type of problem on which the MCAT *will* expect you to locate the center of mass. The situation involves a series of masses arranged in a line. For example, imagine that you had a stick with several blocks hanging from it. Where should you attach a string to the stick so that this mobile would balance?

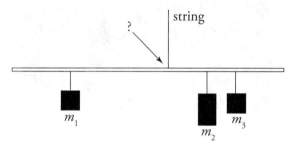

For a problem like this, in which each individual mass can be considered to be at a single point in space, here's the formula for the location of the center of mass:

Center of Mass for Point Masses

$$x_{CM} = \frac{m_1 x_1 + m_2 x_2 + m_3 x_3 \ldots}{m_1 + m_2 + m_3 \ldots}$$

(The location of the center of mass is often denoted by $\bar{x}$ as well. We'll use both notations.) To use this formula, follow these steps:

Step 1: Choose an origin (a reference point to call $x = 0$). The locations of the objects will be measured relative to this point. Often the easiest point to use will be at the location of the left-hand mass, but any point is fine; if a coordinate system is given in the problem, use it.

Step 2: Determine the locations (x_1, x_2, x_3, etc.) of the objects.

Step 3: Multiply each mass by its location ($m_1 x_1$, $m_2 x_2$, $m_3 x_3$, etc.) then add.

Step 4: Divide by the total mass ($m_1 + m_2 + m_3 + \ldots$).

Example 5-1: In the figure below, three blocks hang below a massless meter stick. Block m_1 hangs from the *20 cm* mark, block m_2 hangs from the *70 cm* mark, and block m_3 hangs from the *80 cm* mark. If $m_1 = 2$ kg, $m_2 = 5$ kg, and $m_3 = 3$ kg, at what mark on the meter stick should a string be attached so that this system would hang horizontally?

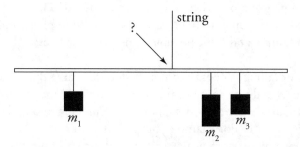

Solution: The first step is to choose an origin, a reference point to call $x = 0$. We are free to choose our zero mark anywhere we want, but the simplest choice here is the one implicitly mentioned in the question itself. The question wants to know at what mark on the meter stick we should attach the string; in other words, how far from the left end of the meter stick should we attach the string? Since the question asks essentially, "How far from the *left end...?*" the best place to choose our zero mark is at the *left end*. We now can write $x_1 = 20$ cm, $x_2 = 70$ cm, and $x_3 = 80$ cm. Using the formula above, we find that

$$x_{CM} = \frac{m_1 x_1 + m_2 x_2 + m_3 x_3}{m_1 + m_2 + m_3}$$

$$= \frac{(2 \text{ kg})(20 \text{ cm}) + (5 \text{ kg})(70 \text{ cm}) + (3 \text{ kg})(80 \text{ cm})}{(2 \text{ kg}) + (5 \text{ kg}) + (3 \text{ kg})}$$

$$= \frac{630 \text{ kg} \cdot \text{cm}}{10 \text{ kg}}$$

$$\therefore x_{CM} = 63 \text{ cm}$$

What if we had instead chosen the center of the meter stick (the *50 cm* mark) to be our origin? In that case, we would have found $x_1 = -30$ cm (because m_1 hangs from the *20 cm* mark, and *20 cm* is 30 cm to the *left*—hence the minus sign—of *50 cm*), $x_2 = 20$ cm, and $x_3 = 30$ cm. The formula would have told us that

$$x_{CM} = \frac{m_1 x_1 + m_2 x_2 + m_3 x_3}{m_1 + m_2 + m_3}$$

$$= \frac{(2 \text{ kg})(-30 \text{ cm}) + (5 \text{ kg})(20 \text{ cm}) + (3 \text{ kg})(30 \text{ cm})}{(2 \text{ kg}) + (5 \text{ kg}) + (3 \text{ kg})}$$

$$= \frac{130 \text{ kg} \cdot \text{cm}}{10 \text{ kg}}$$

$$\therefore x_{CM} = 13 \text{ cm}$$

Well, 13 cm to the *right* (because x_{CM} is *positive*) of the *50 cm* mark is the *63 cm* mark, the same answer we found before.

Example 5-2: Falls are one of the most serious medical issues among the elderly. Falls result when the center of mass of a person's body is not located over a base of support (determined largely by one's foot placement) and the person is unable to correct for the imbalance with sufficient speed and coordination. Center of mass when standing still is determined by body shape and weight distribution. It's important to keep in mind that when people move, they redistribute their body mass and thus change the location of their centers of mass. What are some likely physical (as opposed to physiological, neurological, or environmental) risk factors for falling, and some possible avoidance strategies?

Solution: One risk factor for falling is obesity: not only does this shift the center of mass while standing still, but because it can affect walking motion, the obese individual may be more likely to experience a shift of the center of mass outside the base of support while moving and be less able to prevent the fall once it begins. Another is posture. For example, people often develop a head protrusion and thoracic kyphosis (a hump in the upper back) as they age, shifting the center of mass forward.

Many ways of shifting the body's center of mass closer to the feet and thus making it more likely that the center of mass will remain above the base of support (at least while both feet are planted) are impractical: heavy shoes and pants, for example. However, apart from exercises and physical therapies to avoid or alleviate the risk factors mentioned above, one common risk avoidance strategy is to increase the size of the support base with a cane or a walker. Both of these have the effect of providing a larger total area that the center of mass can occupy without causing imbalance.

Example 5-3: An ammonia molecule (NH_3) contains 3 hydrogen atoms that are positioned at the vertices of an equilateral triangle. The nitrogen atom lies 38 pm (1 pm = 1 picometer = 10^{-12} m) directly above the center of this triangle. If the N:H mass ratio is 14:1, how far below the N atom is the center of mass of the molecule?

Solution: The objects in this system (the four atoms) are not arranged in a line, so how can we hope to determine the center of mass? The key to the answer is to realize that we don't need to include all four of these objects in a single calculation; we can divide the problem into stages. Since the three H atoms have equal masses and are symmetrically arranged at the corners of an equilateral triangle, the center of mass of just these 3 H's is at their geometric center: namely, the center of the triangle. Therefore, by definition of center of mass, the 3 H atoms behave as if all their mass were concentrated at the center of the triangle. This now turns the problem into computing the center of mass of 2 objects (which obviously lie on a line): the 3 H atoms at the center of the triangle and the N atom:

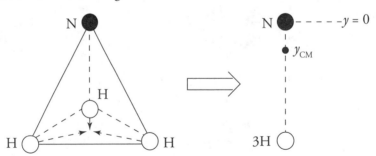

Because the question asks for the center of mass of the molecule relative to the N atom, we'll let the position of the N atom be our zero mark. (It's labeled y in the diagram on the right simply because the way the system is drawn, the objects are arranged along a *vertical* line.) The formula now gives us

$$y_{CM} = \frac{m_N x_N + m_{3H} x_{3H}}{m_N + m_{3H}}$$

$$= \frac{(14)(0 \text{ cm}) + (3 \cdot 1)(38 \text{ pm})}{(14) + (3 \cdot 1)}$$

$$= \frac{114 \text{ pm}}{17}$$

$$\therefore y_{CM} = 7 \text{ pm}$$

Therefore, the center of mass of the NH_3 molecule is 7/38, or about 1/6 of the way down from the nitrogen atom toward the plane of the hydrogens. Because the nitrogen atom is more massive than the hydrogens, we expect the center of mass to not be at the geometric center but, rather, much closer to the nitrogen atom. (This is just like the balancing point of the hammer: Since the metal head is much heavier [because it's denser] than the rest of the hammer, we expect the hammer's center of mass to be not at the geometric center, but, instead, closer to the heavier end.)

You may have noticed in Example 5-1 that we applied the point mass formula to a system that didn't include only point masses: The stick's mass was spread along its entire length. What we did in that problem is what we can *always* do with a collection of homogenous (i.e., constant density) masses: First, find the center of mass of each piece; second, apply the point mass formula, assuming that each piece's mass is concentrated at its own center of mass.

It's possible (though unlikely) that on the MCAT you'll have to find the center of mass of a two-dimensional collection of masses. In Example 5-3 on the previous page, we were able to simplify the problem to reduce it to a single dimension, but that might not always be the case. If you can't simplify the problem in this way, do what we always do with multidimensional problems: break it into components, and consider the components separately. In other words, first find the center of mass in, say, the x-direction, using only the x-components of position; then do the same in the y-direction.

5.2 UNIFORM CIRCULAR MOTION

So far, we've analyzed motion that takes place along a straight line (horizontal, vertical, or slanted) or along a parabola. The MCAT will also require that you know how to analyze an object that moves in a circular path.

The title of this section is Uniform Circular Motion (often abbreviated UCM). What does *uniform* mean here? When we talk about uniform acceleration, we mean constant acceleration; uniform density means constant density; *uniform* is a term used in physics to denote something that remains constant. What property of an object undergoing uniform circular motion is constant? The radius of its path is constant, but that's already in the definition of *circular*, so it must be something else.

> An object moving in a circular path is said to execute
>
> **uniform circular motion**
>
> if its *speed* is constant.

Notice right away that this does *not* mean the object's *velocity* is constant. Velocity is a vector: It has both speed and direction. If an object is moving in a circular path, then it's constantly turning, so its direction is constantly changing. A changing direction, even at constant speed, automatically means a changing velocity. An object's velocity vector is always tangent to its path, regardless of the shape of the path (parabola, circle, figure-8, or whatever) so in the figure below, you can see that the object will have a different velocity vector at every point on the circle, even though the magnitudes of these vectors are all the same.

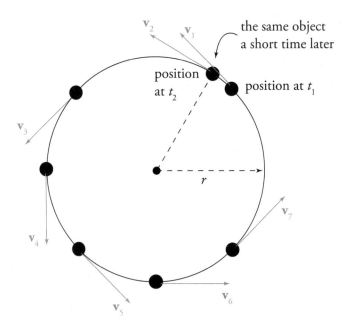

The first thing that should come to mind when you see an object's velocity changing is that the object is experiencing acceleration. The acceleration of an object undergoing uniform circular motion is not affecting the *speed* of the object; this acceleration is only changing the direction of the velocity in order to keep the object moving in a circle.

In the figure below, the velocity vectors of the object are drawn at two close points in its path; they're labeled v_1 and v_2. By definition, the direction of the acceleration is the same as the direction of the velocity change (remember the definition: $a = \Delta v/\Delta t$). So, the acceleration of the object has the same direction as $\Delta v = v_2 - v_1$. Notice that $v_2 - v_1$, which is $v_2 + (-v_1)$, points toward the center of the circle. Therefore, the acceleration of the object always points toward the center of the circle. (This will be true no matter where on the circle we look.)

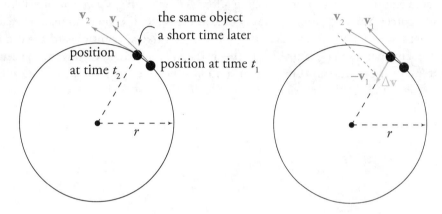

The acceleration of an object undergoing uniform circular motion always points toward the center of the circle. The term **centripetal** (from the Latin, meaning *to seek the center*) is therefore used to describe the acceleration of an object undergoing UCM. We'll denote centripetal acceleration by a_c.

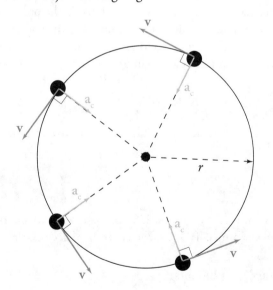

Since **v** is always tangent to the circle, and a_c always points to the center of the circle, **v** and a_c are always perpendicular to each other at any position of the object.

(*Note*: In the figure above, all the velocity vectors are different—because they point in different directions—so they really shouldn't all be labeled by the same v. The same is true for the centripetal acceleration vectors. However, adding subscripts to distinguish all the v vectors and all the a_c vectors would have made the picture look too confusing.)

We now know the *direction* of the centripetal acceleration at any point on the circle; what is its *magnitude*? If v is the speed of the object and r is the radius of the circular path, then the magnitude of the centripetal acceleration, a_c, is v^2/r.

Magnitude of Centripetal Acceleration

$$a_c = \frac{v^2}{r}$$

If an object is accelerating, then it must be feeling a force (after all, $\mathbf{F}_{net} = m\mathbf{a}$, so you can't have an acceleration without a force). Since $\mathbf{F}_{net}$ and $\mathbf{a}$ always point in the same direction, no matter what the path of the object, the net force on an object undergoing UCM must, like $\mathbf{a}$, point toward the center. So, guess what we call it? **Centripetal force** (denoted $\mathbf{F}_c$). This is the *net* force directed toward the center that acts on an object to make it execute uniform circular motion. And since $F_{net} = ma$, we'll have $\mathbf{F}_c = m\mathbf{a}_c$ and $F_c = ma_c$, so the magnitude of the centripetal force is mv^2/r, where m is the mass of the object that's moving around the circle.

Magnitude of Centripetal Force

$$F_c = ma_c = \frac{mv^2}{r}$$

Example 5-4: Separating blood plasma from the solid bodies in blood (blood cells and platelets) by rapid sedimentation requires use of a *centrifuge* to produce the necessary accelerations on the order of 5000g. In one approach, the blood is placed in a bag inside a rigid container and mounted to the end of a horizontal rotor (so that it extends out beyond the rotor), which then spins up to several thousands of revolutions per minute. Suppose the rotor has a radius of 30 cm and rotates at a maximum rate of 5000 rpm, and that the bag is 10 cm long. Note that translational velocity $v = r\omega$, where ω is in radians/second.

a) What will be the centripetal acceleration at the middle of the bag?
b) Will the centripetal acceleration increase or decrease for the blood further from the axis of rotation?

Solution:

a) First we convert rpm to rad/s: 5000 rev/min $\times$ 2π rad/rev $\times$ 1/60 min/s $\approx$ 500 rad/s. Now $v = r\omega = (0.30 \text{ m} + 0.05 \text{ m})(500 \text{ rad/s}) = 175 \text{ m/s}$. Thus for the centripetal acceleration we have

$$a_c = \frac{v^2}{r} = \frac{(175 \text{ m/s})^2}{0.35 \text{ m}} \approx \frac{(200 \text{ m/s})^2}{0.5 \text{ m}} = 8 \times 10^4 \text{ m/s}^2$$

This is 8000g, so more than enough acceleration to achieve separation of blood.

b) Your first instinct upon reading this question might be to say, "I know that centripetal acceleration is inversely proportional to the radius, so increasing the distance from the central axis should decrease the acceleration." That would be wrong: such reasoning implicitly (and falsely) assumes that speed is constant as radius increases, but for a *rigid rotator* like a centrifuge or a merry-go-round, translational speed is proportional to the radius according to the equation $v = r\omega$, (the constant is the angular speed ω). If you're having trouble picturing this, imagine what happens when you're on a merry-go-round: standing at the center, you are spinning in place and thus have a translational speed of zero (your position isn't changing with time). The further you get from the center, the faster you are moving. Thus because of the v^2 term in the numerator, $a_c \propto r$, and centripetal acceleration increases for blood further from the axis of rotation.

Example 5-5: If an object undergoing uniform circular motion is being acted upon by a constant force toward the center, why doesn't the object fall into the center?

Solution: Actually, it *is* falling toward the center, but because of its speed, the object remains in a circular orbit around the center. Remember: the direction of **v** is not necessarily the same as the direction of $\mathbf{F}_{net}$. So, just because $\mathbf{F}_{net}$ points toward the center does not mean that **v** must point toward the center. It's the direction of the *acceleration*, not the velocity that always matches the direction of $\mathbf{F}_{net}$. Let's look at the motion of the object at a certain point in its circular path:

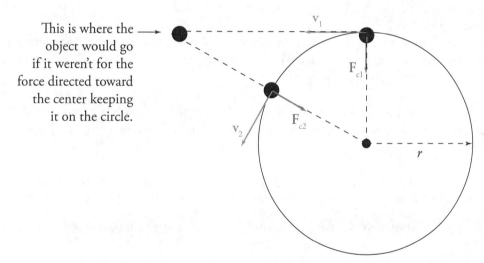

This is where the object would go if it weren't for the force directed toward the center keeping it on the circle.

In this figure, the net force on the object at Position 1 points downward (toward the center of the circle). Therefore, it's telling v_1 to move downward a little, so that at the next moment, at Position 2, the velocity will point downward slightly. Notice that this is just what we want in order to keep the object traveling in a circle! If it weren't for this force pointing toward the center (that is, if the centripetal force were suddenly removed), then the object's velocity wouldn't change. It would not continue to move in a circle but would instead fly off in a straight line, tangent to the circle at the point where the force was removed.

Example 5-6: How would the net force on an object undergoing uniform circular motion have to change if the object's speed doubled?

Solution: Centripetal force, mv^2/r, is proportional to the *square* of the speed. So, if the object's speed increased by a factor of 2, then the magnitude of $\mathbf{F}_c$ would have to increase by a factor of $2^2 = 4$.

Solving circular motion problems often involves something more than simply using the formulas $a_c = v^2/r$ or $F_c = mv^2/r$. The key to solving such problems is to answer this question:

What provides the centripetal force?

In other words, what force(s) act in the dimension toward the center of the circle?

Centripetal force is not some new kind of force like gravity or tension. It's simply the name for the net force directed toward the center of the circular path. The vector sum of forces such as gravity and tension is what gets *called* centripetal force, when those forces, or components of them, are directed toward the center of the circle. When drawing a force diagram for an object undergoing UCM, here are a couple of tips:

1. Do not add a force called $\mathbf{F}_c$ in your picture; forces such as gravity, tension, normal force, etc. *do* go in your picture, but $\mathbf{F}_c$ doesn't. Remember, $\mathbf{F}_c$ is what the forces toward the center have to add up to.
2. Always call *toward the center* the positive direction. Any forces toward the center are then positive forces, and any forces directed away from the center are negative. You'll need this to find F_{net} and then set the result equal to F_c.

Example 5-7: The moon orbits the earth in a (nearly) circular path at (nearly) constant speed. If M is the mass of the earth, m is the mass of the moon, and r is the radius of the moon's orbit, find an expression for the speed of the moon's orbit.

Solution: We begin by answering the question, *What provides the centripetal force?* The answer is the gravitational pull by the earth. We now simply translate our answer into an equation, like this:

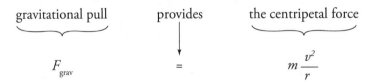

$$\underbrace{\text{gravitational pull}} \qquad \text{provides} \qquad \underbrace{\text{the centripetal force}}$$

$$F_{grav} \qquad\qquad = \qquad\qquad m\frac{v^2}{r}$$

Since we know $F_{grav} = GMm/r^2$, we get

$$F_{grav} = F_c \;\rightarrow\; G\frac{Mm}{r^2} = m\frac{v^2}{r} \;\rightarrow\; G\frac{M}{r} = v^2 \;\rightarrow\; \therefore v = \sqrt{G\frac{M}{r}}$$

Notice that the mass of the moon, m, cancels out. So, any object orbiting at the same distance from the earth as the moon must move at the same speed as the moon.

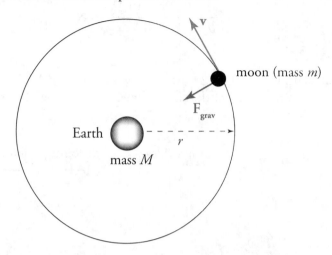

Example 5-8: A string is tied around a rock of mass 0.2 kg, and the rock is then whirled at a constant speed v in a horizontal circle of radius 0.4 m, as shown in the figure below. If $\sin\theta = 0.4$ and $\cos\theta = 0.9$, what's v?

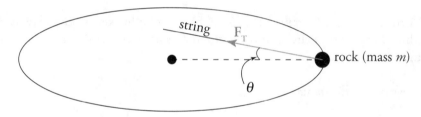

Solution: First, let's draw a bigger force diagram:

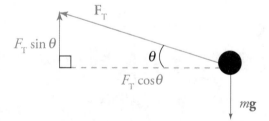

(This figure also shows why the end of the string is slightly above the center of the circle. The string has to point upward a little in order for there to be an upward component of the tension to cancel out the weight of the rock and allow the rock to revolve in a *horizontal* circle.) Because the rock is moving in a horizontal circle and not accelerating vertically, we know that the net vertical force must be zero. Therefore, the vertical component of the string's tension, $F_y = F_T \sin\theta$, must balance out the weight of the rock, mg:

$$F_T \sin\theta = mg$$

From this, we can figure out that

$$F_T = \frac{mg}{\sin\theta} = \frac{(0.2 \text{ kg})(10\frac{N}{kg})}{0.4} = 5 \text{ N}$$

Now, let's look at the circular motion: *What provides the centripetal force?* As the diagram shows, there's only one force directed toward the center of the circle (namely, the horizontal component of the tension, $F_x = F_T \cos\theta$) so this must be it:

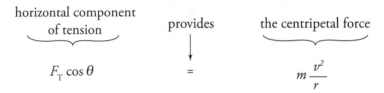

$$F_T \cos\theta \qquad\qquad = \qquad\qquad m\frac{v^2}{r}$$

We now just plug in the value we found for F_T to get v:

$$F_T \cos\theta = m\frac{v^2}{r} \rightarrow v = \sqrt{\frac{rF_T \cos\theta}{m}} = \sqrt{\frac{(0.4 \text{ m})(5 \text{ N})(0.9)}{0.2 \text{ kg}}} = 3 \text{ m/s}$$

Example 5-9: A rope of length 60 cm is tied to the handle of a bucket (whose mass is 3 kg), and the bucket is then whirled in a vertical circle. At the bottom of its path, the tension in the rope is 50 N. What is the speed of the bucket at this point?

Solution: First, let's draw a diagram.

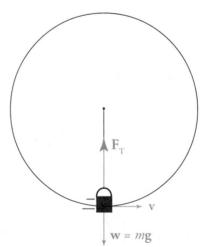

Because we call *toward the center* the positive direction when doing circular motion problems, we see that the tension, $\mathbf{F}_T$, is a positive force, and the bucket's weight, $\mathbf{w}$, is a negative force. (Because $\mathbf{w}$ points *away* from the center, we count it as negative.) Therefore, the net force on the bucket at this point is $F_T - w$. Because the net force directed toward the center is called the centripetal force, we'd write

$$F_T - w = F_c$$

Because $w = mg$ and $F_c = mv^2/r$, this equation becomes

$$F_T - mg = m\frac{v^2}{r}$$

We now just use this equation and the numbers we were given to figure out v, realizing that the radius of the circle is equal to the length of the rope (so $r = 0.6$ m):

$$v = \sqrt{\frac{r(F_T - mg)}{m}} = \sqrt{\frac{(0.6\text{ m})[50\text{ N} - (3\text{ kg})(10\frac{\text{N}}{\text{kg}})]}{3\text{ kg}}} = 2\text{ m/s}$$

Example 5-10: For the situation described in the preceding example, what is the tension force on the bucket when the bucket is at the position shown below?

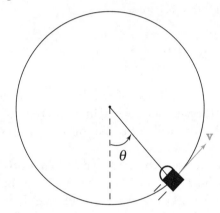

Solution: Here's the force diagram:

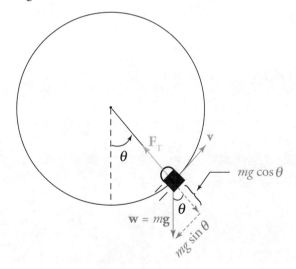

Because there's a force of F_T pointing toward the center and a force of $mg \cos\theta$ pointing *away* from the center, the net force toward the center of the circle (which is the centripetal force) is

$$F_{net\,toward\,center} = F_c = F_T - mg\cos\theta$$

Let's examine this situation a little more closely. Notice that at the position of the bucket shown, we also have a force component *tangent* to the circle ($mg \sin\theta$), which *opposes* the direction of the bucket's velocity. As a result, the bucket's speed will be reduced. Centripetal acceleration only makes an object turn so that it moves in a circular path; it does not change the speed. **Tangential** acceleration, on the other hand, *does* change the speed. Therefore, the bucket's speed will decrease as it rises to the top of the circle, and we wouldn't call the entire motion of the bucket "uniform." However, even if the speed of an object moving in a circle changes, there will always be a component of the net force that points toward the center of the circle; this is the centripetal force. The mathematical translation of the statement "the net force toward the center provides the centripetal force" becomes

$$F_T - mg\cos\theta = m\frac{v^2}{r} \rightarrow F_T = m\frac{v^2}{r} + mg\cos\theta$$

Because v decreases as the bucket rises (because of the downward tangential force, $mg \sin\theta$) and since $\cos\theta$ decreases as the bucket rises (because the angle θ increases from 0° to 180°), this final equation for F_T shows us that the tension in the rope will decrease as the bucket rises.

It's not often that we need to worry about both centripetal and tangential acceleration in an MCAT problem, but the example above shows how to deal with it when we do encounter such a situation: Ignore the tangential components of force and acceleration when calculating the centripetal force and acceleration. This is really just another example of the general principle: In MCAT-level Physics, you can always consider the components of motion separately.

5.3 TORQUE

We can tie a rope to a bucket and make it move in a circular path, but how would we make the bucket itself spin? One way would be to grab the handle and then rotate our hand, or we could place our hands on opposite sides of the bucket and then, by moving our hands in opposite directions, rotate the bucket. In order to make an object's center of mass accelerate, we need to exert a force. In order to make an object *spin*, we need to exert a *torque*.

Torque is the measure of a force's effectiveness at making an object spin or rotate. (More precisely, it's the measure of a force's effectiveness at making an object *accelerate* rotationally.) If an object is initially at rest, and then it starts to spin, something must have exerted a torque. And if an object is already spinning, something would have to exert a torque to get it to stop spinning. In this section, we'll begin by looking at two different (but entirely equivalent) ways of figuring out torque.

All systems that can spin or rotate have a "center" of turning. This is the point that does not move while the remainder of the object is rotating, effectively becoming the center of the circle. There are many terms used to describe this point, including **pivot point** and **fulcrum**.

Let's say we want to tighten a bolt with a wrench. The figure below illustrates the situation.

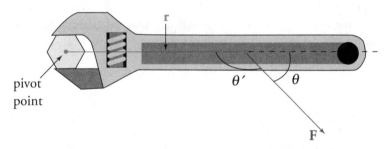

If we applied the force **F** to the wrench, would we make the wrench and the bolt rotate? Yes, because this force **F** has *torque*. (Notice: Torque is not a force; it's a property of a force.) To say how *much* torque **F** provides, we need a couple of preliminary definitions. First, the vector from the center of rotation (the **pivot point**) to the point of application of the force is called the **radius vector, r**. The angle between the vectors **r** and **F** is called θ. Now notice in the figure above that the angle between the vectors **r** and **F** at the point where they actually meet is denoted by θ'. This is because the angle between two vectors is actually the angle they make *when they start at the same point*. But in the figure, the vector **r** starts at the pivot point (which is where **r** always starts), and **F** starts at the *end* of **r** (which is where **F** always starts). One way to find the correct angle between these vectors is to imagine sliding **r** over so that it does start where **F** starts; the dashed line in the figure shows the line along which such a translated **r** vector would lie and the resulting correct angle θ. However, all this fuss about which angle is the correct one doesn't really matter, as you'll soon see.

The amount of torque a force **F** provides depends on three things: the magnitude of **F**, the length of **r**, and the angle θ.

Torque

$$\tau = rF \sin \theta$$

(The letter we use for torque is τ, the Greek letter *tau*.) From this equation, we can immediately figure out the unit of torque:

$$[\tau] = [r][F] = \text{m·N} = \text{N·m}$$

There's no special name for this unit; it's just a newton-meter.[1]

For example, let's say that $F = 20$ N, $r = 10$ cm, and $\theta = 30°$. Then the torque provided by this force would be $\tau = rF \sin \theta = (0.1 \text{ m})(20 \text{ N}) \sin 30° = 1$ N·m. Notice that if we had instead used θ', we would have gotten the same answer, since $\theta' = 150°$ and $\sin 150° = \sin 30°$. This is why we don't have to worry about which angle, θ or θ', is the true angle between **r** and **F** when we calculate torque, because θ and θ' will always be *supplements* (they'll add up to 180°) and the sine of an angle is always equal to the sine of its supplement. Therefore, $\tau = rF \sin \theta = rF \sin \theta'$.

Look at this force on the wrench:

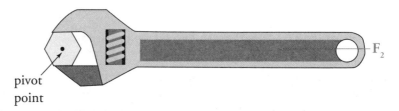

pivot
point

Our intuition tells us that this force would not make the wrench (or bolt) rotate. Therefore, we expect that this force has zero torque. Using the definition, we can see that this is true. If we were to draw the **r** vector from the pivot to the point where F_2 is applied, we'd see that the value of $\sin \theta$ is 0, so $\tau_2 = 0$. Forces with no torque (like this one) cannot increase (or decrease) the rotational speed of an object.

---

[1] In Chapter 6 we'll encounter another newton-meter and rename it the joule. What's the difference? Torque has a direction, like a vector (though technically it's what's called a pseudovector), while the joule, a unit of energy, is a scalar. For the MCAT, there's no need to worry about this; just calculate torque in newton-meters, and then label it clockwise or counterclockwise.

How about this force on the wrench?

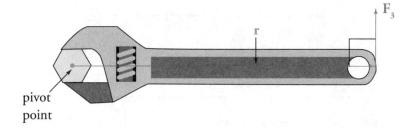

The force F_3 is perpendicular to its **r** vector, so $\theta = 90°$ and $\sin \theta = 1$, its maximum value. Therefore, when $\mathbf{r} \perp \mathbf{F}$, we get the maximum torque for a given r and F, and the equation for torque gives us simply $\tau_3 = rF_3$. (This situation is very common, by the way.)

$$\text{If } \mathbf{r} \perp \mathbf{F}, \text{ then } \tau = rF.$$

The force F_3 above would produce counterclockwise rotation, so we say that it produces a **counterclockwise (CCW) torque**. The force F_4 below would produce clockwise rotation, so we say it produces a **clockwise (CW) torque**.

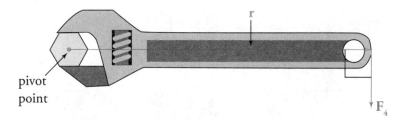

If $F_3 = F_4$, then these forces produce the same amount of torque, but one is clockwise and the other is counterclockwise. If we want to distinguish between them mathematically, we can say that $\tau_3 = +rF_3$ and $\tau_4 = -rF_4$, since it's customary to specify CCW rotation as positive and CW as negative.

The other method for calculating torque, which gives the same answer as the method we've just described, is based on the *lever arm* of a force. Let's look again at the first picture of our wrench:

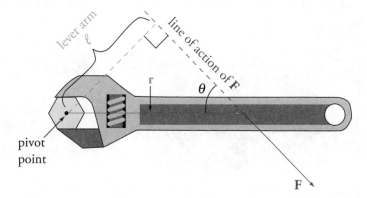

This time, however, rather than measuring the distance from the pivot to the *point* where the force is applied (the length r), we'll measure the shortest distance from the pivot to the *line* along which F is applied. This distance, which is always perpendicular to the line of action of F, is called the **lever arm** of F, written as ℓ or l.

Once we know the lever arm, ℓ, the definition of the torque of **F** is then simply $\tau = \ell F$.

> **Torque**
>
> $$\tau = \ell F$$

To see that this gives the same value for the torque as the formula $\tau = rF \sin \theta$, just notice that in the picture on the preceding page (bottom), the lever arm, ℓ, is the side opposite the angle θ in a right triangle whose hypotenuse is r; therefore, $\ell = r \sin \theta$. So, $\tau = \ell F$ is the same as $\tau = (r \sin \theta)F$. Because you can use either formula for calculating the torque, use whichever one is more convenient in a particular problem. In general, it's convenient to use the lever arm method if the length of the lever arm is obvious from the situation; otherwise, use $\tau = rF \sin \theta$.

For the force **F₅** shown on the next page, our intuition tells us that this force would not make the wrench (or bolt) rotate. Therefore, we expect that this force has zero torque. Using the definition of lever arm, we can see that this is true. The line of action of **F₅** passes right through the pivot point, so the level arm of the force is zero, and $\tau_5 = \ell_5 F_5 = (0)F_5 = 0$.

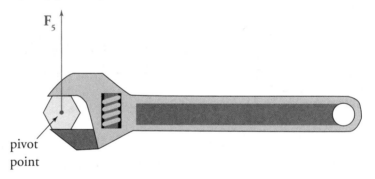

In general, if a force acts at the pivot or along a line through the pivot, then its torque is zero.

Example 5-11: A square metal plate (of side length s) rests on a flat table, and we exert a force **F** at one corner, parallel to one of the sides, as shown below. What is the torque of this force? (Use the center of the plate as the pivot point.)

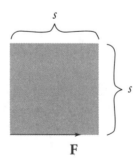

Solution: We'll calculate the torque of **F** by two different methods: first using the formula $\tau = rF \sin \theta$, and then using the formula $\tau = \ell F$.

Method 1. We draw in the **r** vector, which points from the pivot to the point where the force is applied. The angle between **r** and **F** can be taken to be $\theta = 45°$. If s is the length of each side of the square, then the length of **r** is $\frac{1}{2}s\sqrt{2}$ (because r is the hypotenuse of a 45°-45° right triangle, it's $\sqrt{2}$ times the length of each leg).

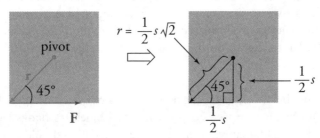

This gives $\tau = rF\sin\theta = \left(\frac{1}{2}s\sqrt{2}\right)(F)\sin 45° = \left(\frac{1}{2}s\sqrt{2}\right)(F)\left(\frac{\sqrt{2}}{2}\right) = \frac{1}{2}sF$.

Method 2. The line of action of the force **F** is simply the bottom side of the square. The perpendicular distance from the pivot to the side of the square is half the length of the square, $\frac{1}{2}s$, so this is the lever arm, ℓ.

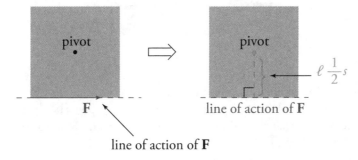

Therefore, $\tau = \ell F = \frac{1}{2}sF$.

In this situation, the formula using the lever arm is the easier way to calculate the torque. That's because you can look at the diagram and see the length of the lever arm right away. If you find yourself having to *calculate* the length of the lever arm, you probably should just be using $\tau = rF\sin\theta$.

Example 5-12: Which of the following best explains why people with bicep attachment points farther from their elbows tend to have greater elbow flexion strength, and thus an improved ability to perform a dumbbell curling exercise?

A. An attachment point that is farther from the elbow increases the force provided by muscle contraction.
B. An attachment point that is farther from the elbow decreases the force provided by muscle contraction.
C. An attachment point that is farther from the elbow results in a greater torque produced by the bicep as it contracts.
D. An attachment point that is closer to the hand results in a lesser torque produced by the bicep as it contracts.

Solution: The first two answer choices discuss a difference in the muscle's contraction force. This force is a function of the muscle fibers, not its point of attachment to the forearm, which eliminates choices A and B. An attachment point farther from the elbow increases r, the distance from the pivot point (elbow) to the where the force is applied (at the attachment), so according to the equation for torque, $\tau = rF\sin\theta$, this would increase the torque created by the biceps contraction, which makes choice C correct. The distance to the hand is a trap answer: there are two torques acting on someone curling a dumbbell or other mass, one provided by the contraction of the biceps muscle and an opposing one from the weight of the dumbbell acting downward at the hand. Both torques depend on the radial distance from the pivot point, which is the elbow.

Example 5-13: In the figure below, three blocks hang below a massless meter stick. Block m_1 hangs from the 20 cm mark, block m_2 hangs from the 70 cm mark, and block m_3 hangs from the 80 cm mark. If $m_1 = 2$ kg, $m_2 = 5$ kg, and $m_3 = 3$ kg, at what mark on the meter stick should a string be attached so that this system would hang horizontally?

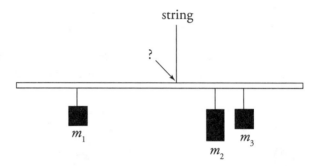

Solution: Look familiar? This is the same example we solved in the Center of Mass section. Let's see how we can answer this same question by balancing the torques. Let the pivot be the point where the string is attached to the stick. (Consider that the string is attached at the x cm mark, so that it's x cm from the left end of the stick.) Then the weight of mass m_1 produces a counterclockwise torque (τ_1), and the weights of m_2 and of m_3 each produce a clockwise torque (τ_2 and τ_3). If the counterclockwise torque (τ_1) balances the total clockwise torque ($\tau_2 + \tau_3$), the stick will remain level.

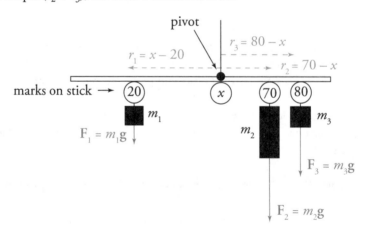

For each force, we need to find its corresponding r. For $\mathbf{F}_1$, we have $r_1 = (x - 20)$ cm; for $\mathbf{F}_2$, we have $r_2 = (70 - x)$ cm; and for $\mathbf{F}_3$, we have $r_3 = (80 - x)$ cm. The equation that balances the torques is

$$\tau_{\text{CW}} = \tau_{\text{CCW}}$$

$$r_1 \cdot m_1 g = r_2 \cdot m_2 g + r_3 \cdot m_3 g$$

$$r_1 m_1 = r_2 m_2 + r_3 m_3$$

$$(x - 20)(2 \text{ kg}) = (70 - x)(5 \text{ kg}) + (80 - x)(3 \text{ kg})$$

$$\therefore x = 63 \text{ cm}$$

This is the same answer we found before. (By the way, the torque exerted by the tension in the string is equal to zero [which is why we ignored it] because the tension acts *at* the pivot.)

Example 5-14: A homogeneous rectangular sheet of metal lies on a flat table and is able to rotate around an axis through its center, perpendicular to the table. Four forces, all of the same magnitude, are exerted on the sheet as shown below:

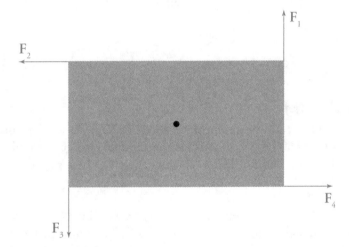

Which one of the following statements is true?

    A.   The net force is zero, but the net torque is not.
    B.   The net torque is zero, but the net force is not.
    C.   Neither the net force nor the net torque is zero.
    D.   Both the net force and the net torque equal zero.

Solution: There are two vertical forces that point in opposite directions (so they cancel), and two horizontal forces that point in opposite directions (so *they* cancel). Therefore, the net force, $\mathbf{F}_{\text{net}} = \mathbf{F}_1 + \mathbf{F}_2 + \mathbf{F}_3 + \mathbf{F}_4$, is zero. Eliminate choices B and C.

Now for the torques. In the figure below, each force has its corresponding lever arm. Notice that each force produces a counterclockwise (CCW) torque. As a result, the total, or net, torque cannot be zero. (The net torque is zero only when the total counterclockwise torque balances the total clockwise torque.) Therefore, the answer is A.

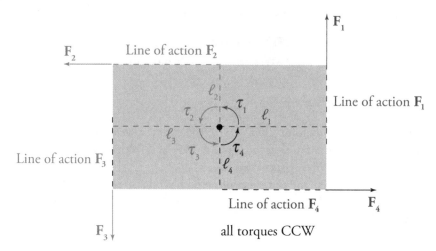

all torques CCW

5.4   EQUILIBRIUM

As it's used in physics, the term **equilibrium** means *zero acceleration*. Notice that this does not mean zero velocity. As long as the velocity of the system remains constant (no change in speed or direction), then we can say that the system is in equilibrium. If the velocity happens to be zero, then we say the system is in **static** equilibrium.

There are actually two kinds of equilibrium, because there are two kinds of acceleration. There's *translational* equilibrium and *rotational* equilibrium. A system is said to be in **translational equilibrium** if the forces cancel; if $F_{net} = 0$, then the translational acceleration (a) is zero. A system is in **rotational equilibrium** if the torques cancel; if $\tau_{net} = 0$, then the rotational acceleration (denoted by α, the Greek letter *alpha*) is zero. If the term *equilibrium* is used without specifying which type, then it's assumed that the system is in *both* translational and rotational equilibrium.

Example 5-13 (the blocks balancing on the stick) involved a system in equilibrium. We balanced the torques to ensure rotational equilibrium. We didn't explicitly analyze the translational equilibrium, but in the example of the blocks hanging from the stick, the upward tension in the supporting string balanced the total weight of the blocks.

We'll now look at a couple of other examples of systems in equilibrium.

5.4

Example 5-15: A barber pole of mass 10 kg hangs from the end of a homogeneous rod of mass 40 kg that sticks out horizontally from the side of a vertical wall. The end of the rod, where the barber pole is attached, is connected to the upper part of the wall by a taut cable. For the angle θ, it is known that $\sin \theta = 0.6$ and $\cos \theta = 0.8$.

a)   What's the tension in the cable?
b)   What force is exerted by the wall on the rod?

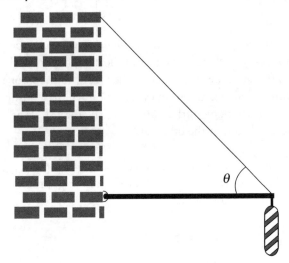

Solution:

a)   First, let's draw a diagram of all the forces acting on the rod.

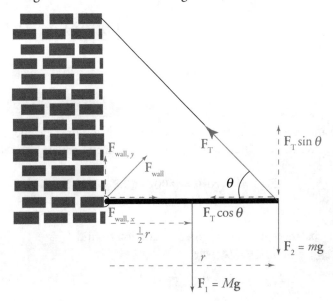

Notice that because the rod is in contact with the wall, the wall is exerting a force on the rod. However, at the start of the problem, we have no way of knowing what this force looks like (in other words, what either its magnitude or its direction are), so we break the force F_{wall} into a horizontal component and a vertical component. We do the same with the tension force, F_T, (which must act along the direction of the cable), and we can write these components as $F_{T,x} = F_T \cos\theta$ and $F_{T,y} = F_T \sin\theta$.

The system is in static equilibrium, so there must be no net torque and no net force. If we try to balance out all the forces, we find that we have too many unknowns. To balance the vertical forces, we'd write $F_{wall,y} + F_T \sin\theta = Mg + mg$, and to balance the horizontal forces, we'd write $F_{wall,x} = F_T \cos\theta$. We have three unknown ($F_{wall,x}$, $F_{wall,y}$, and F_T) but only two equations.

The trick is to balance the *torques* first and to choose our pivot to be the point of contact between the rod and wall. Notice that the torques of the components of the force exerted by the wall will both be zero (because they're applied *at* the pivot), so they won't even appear in the equation. As a result, our "balance-the-torques" equation will have just one unknown, F_T. That's why we chose to put the pivot point at the wall end of the rod: There are two unknown force components there, and only one at the other end.

So, with our pivot so chosen, we have three forces exerting torque: $\mathbf{F}_{T,y}$ produces a counter-clockwise torque, and each of the weight vectors, $M\mathbf{g}$ and $m\mathbf{g}$, produces a clockwise torque. These torques balance to keep the rod level.

$$\tau_{CW} = \tau_{CCW}$$

$$r \cdot F_T \sin\theta = \tfrac{1}{2} r \cdot Mg + r \cdot mg$$

$$F_T \sin\theta = \tfrac{1}{2} Mg + mg$$

$$F_T = \frac{(\tfrac{1}{2}M + m)g}{\sin\theta}$$

$$= \frac{(\tfrac{1}{2} \cdot 40 \text{ kg} + 10 \text{ kg})(10 \tfrac{N}{kg})}{0.6}$$

$$\therefore F_T = 500 \text{ N}$$

b) Now that we've answered part (a) and found F_T, the tension in the cable, we can now find $F_{wall,x}$ and $F_{wall,y}$. We use the "balance-the-horizontal-forces" equation, $F_{wall,x} = F_T \cos\theta$, to get

$$F_{wall,x} = F_T \cos\theta = (500 \text{ N})(0.8) = 400 \text{ N}$$

Then we use the "balance-the-vertical-forces" equation to find $F_{wall,y}$:

$$F_{wall,y} + F_T \sin\theta = Mg + mg$$

$$F_{wall,y} = Mg + mg - F_T \sin\theta$$

$$= (40 \text{ kg})(10 \tfrac{N}{kg}) + (10 \text{ kg})(10 \tfrac{N}{kg}) - (500 \text{ N})(0.6)$$

$$\therefore F_{wall,y} = 200 \text{ N}$$

Finally, the magnitude of the force exerted by the wall on the rod can be found using the Pythagorean theorem:

$$\left(F_{\text{wall}}\right)^2 = \left(F_{\text{wall, }x}\right)^2 + \left(F_{\text{wall, }y}\right)^2 \rightarrow F_{\text{wall}} = \sqrt{\left(F_{\text{wall, }x}\right)^2 + \left(F_{\text{wall, }y}\right)^2} \rightarrow F_{\text{wall}} = \sqrt{(400\ \text{N})^2 + (200\ \text{N})^2} \approx 447\ \text{N}$$

Whew! Let's now look at a problem that's more MCAT-like in terms of the amount of calculation:

Example 5-16: In the figure below, a block of mass 40 kg is held in place by two ropes exerting equal tension forces. If $\cos\theta = 2/3$, what's the tension in each rope?

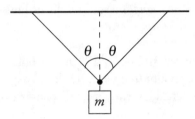

Solution: At the point where the mass is attached to the two ropes, we balance the forces. The horizontal forces automatically balance (we have $F_T \sin\theta$ pointing to the left and $F_T \sin\theta$ pointing to the right). For the vertical forces, we notice that there's the vertical component of the tension in the left-hand rope plus the vertical component of the tension in the right-hand rope ($F_T \cos\theta + F_T \cos\theta = 2F_T \cos\theta$), to balance out the weight of the block, mg. This gives us:

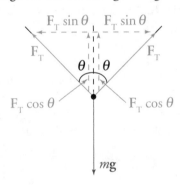

$$2F_T \cos\theta = mg$$

$$F_T = \frac{mg}{2\cos\theta}$$

$$= \frac{(40\ \text{kg})(10\ \tfrac{\text{N}}{\text{kg}})}{2\left(\tfrac{2}{3}\right)}$$

$$\therefore F_T = 300\ \text{N}$$

5.5 ROTATIONAL INERTIA

An object's mass, *m*, measures its inertia, or its resistance to acceleration. If Object 1 has a greater mass than Object 2, then it will be more difficult to accelerate Object 1 than Object 2. More precisely, a greater force will be required to give Object 1 the same acceleration as Object 2, or, equivalently, if the same force is applied to both objects, Object 1 will undergo a smaller acceleration. This all follows from $F = ma$.

Now that we've studied torque and rotation, we can talk about an object's **rotational inertia** (also known as its **moment of inertia**). Think of mass as *translational* inertia, since it measures an object's resistance to translational acceleration, *a*. Then, just as translational inertia tells us how resistant an object is to translational acceleration, an object's *rotational* inertia, *I*, tells us how resistant the object is to rotational acceleration (which we denote by α, the Greek letter *alpha*).

First, let's define rotational acceleration. In the "old" days, people listened to music on vinyl records, known as albums. They would place an album on a device known as a turntable. Initially, of course, the turntable was at rest. Once it was switched on, the turntable platter would start to rotate, faster and faster, until it reached a rotational speed of 33.3 rpm (rotations per minute). During the time that the turntable was rotating faster and faster, it was experiencing a positive rotational acceleration. Then, when the turntable was switched off, the rotational speed of the platter decreased, and it experienced negative rotational acceleration.

A torque is required to produce rotational acceleration, just as a force is required to produce translational acceleration. The rotational analog of the equation $F_{net} = ma$ is $\tau_{net} = I\alpha$. Notice that torque, τ, is to rotational motion what force, *F*, is to translational motion. Similarly, rotational inertia, *I*, is to rotational motion what translational inertia (mass, *m*) is to translational motion.

What does the equation $\tau_{net} = I\alpha$ tell us? It says that the larger *I* is, the smaller α will be for a given torque (just as $F = ma$ says that the larger *m* is, the smaller *a* will be for a given force). If Object 1 has a greater rotational inertia than Object 2, then it will be more difficult to rotate Object 1 than Object 2. More precisely, a greater torque will be required to give Object 1 the same rotational acceleration as Object 2, or, equivalently, if the same torque is applied to both objects, Object 1 will undergo a smaller rotational acceleration.

So, how do we find the rotational inertia of an object? It depends on the object's mass, but there's more to it than that. Two objects can have the same mass, but different rotational inertias. What rotational inertia depends on is how the object's mass is distributed with respect to the axis it rotates around; *the farther away the mass is from the axis of rotation, the greater the rotational inertia will be*. We can illustrate this with a simple example. Imagine a barbell with a weight near each end, and an identical barbell with the weights pushed near the middle of the bar. These two barbells have the same mass, but their rotational inertias are different. If we wanted to rotate each bar around its midpoint, the first barbell has its attached masses farther from the rotation axis than the second one. As a result, we would find it more difficult to rotate the first barbell than the second one. The first barbell has the greater value of *I*.

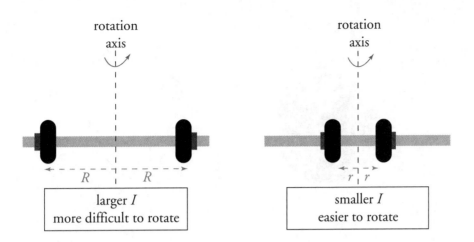

Consider a uniform metal bar of mass m. In the first situation illustrated below, we want to rotate the bar around its midpoint; in the second, we want to rotate it around one of its ends. For which configuration does the bar have the greater rotational inertia?

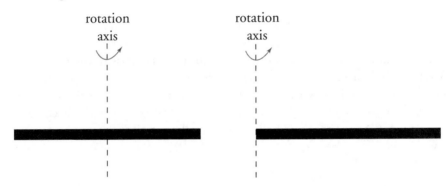

The answer is the second configuration, since, on average, the bar's mass here is farther from the axis of rotation than in the first configuration. Therefore, we'd find it more difficult to rotate the bar around one of its ends than around its middle. In this case, we didn't move any of the mass around, like we did with the weights on the barbell above; instead we considered two different rotation axes. Remember that the distribution of the object's mass relative to the axis of rotation is what determines the rotational inertia. This example illustrates a simple, useful fact: For a given object, the rotational inertia will be smallest when the rotation axis passes through the object's center of mass. So, if we want to rotate the metal bar around its midpoint (which, since the bar is uniform, *is* the location of the center of mass), the rotational inertia is the smallest in this case. In fact, this is the axis around which we would find it easiest to rotate.

Now, consider two spheres of the same size and mass, except one is solid and the other is hollow. If we wanted to rotate each of them around an axis through their centers, which one would be easier to rotate?

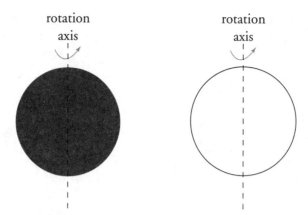

Since the spheres have the same mass (and, therefore, weight), if we picked them up, we wouldn't be able to tell the difference. However, if we rolled them across the floor, we'd know right away that they were different, because their rotational inertias are different. If we gave each ball the same push (and thus the same torque), the one with the smaller rotational inertia would roll more easily than the other one.

One way to determine which sphere has the smaller rotational inertia (and thus, which sphere would be easier to rotate) is to imagine how the hollow sphere became hollow. Suppose we had a copy of the solid sphere and could somehow stick our hands inside and push all the mass to the outside, thus creating a hollow ball. We haven't changed the mass, we've just redistributed it. To be specific, we've moved the mass away from the rotation axis, so we know that we've increased its rotational inertia. (Remember, the farther the mass is from the axis of rotation, the greater the rotational inertia.) Because the hollow ball has the greater rotational inertia, the solid ball has the smaller rotational inertia and would therefore rotate more easily.

Summary of Formulas

Center of mass: $\quad x_{CM} = \dfrac{m_1 x_1 + m_2 x_2 + m_3 x_3 \cdots}{m_1 + m_2 + m_3 \cdots}$

Center of gravity: $\quad x_{CG} = \dfrac{w_1 x_1 + w_2 x_2 + w_3 x_3 \cdots}{w_1 + w_2 + w_3 \cdots}$

in uniform gravitational field (g constant), $x_{CM} = x_{CG}$

Centripetal acceleration: $\quad a_c = \dfrac{v^2}{r}$ (directed toward center of circle)

Centripetal force: $\quad F_c = m a_c = \dfrac{mv^2}{r}$

$\qquad F_c = F_{\text{net towards center}}$

Torque: $\qquad \tau = rF \sin\theta$ (θ = angle between **r** and **F**)

$\qquad \tau = \ell F$ (ℓ = lever arm of force)

Equilibrium: $\quad F_{\text{net}} = 0$ (translational equilibrium)

$\qquad \tau_{\text{net}} = 0$ (rotational equilibrium)

static equilibrium means:

$\qquad F_{\text{net}} = 0$

$\qquad \tau_{\text{net}} = 0$

$\qquad \mathbf{v} = 0$

Rotational Inertia:

mass closer to rotation axis gives a smaller I

–easier to rotate

mass farther from rotation axis gives a larger I

–more difficult to rotate

CHAPTER 5 FREESTANDING PRACTICE QUESTIONS

1. A 100 kg skier's knee can withstand a lateral torque of 500 N·m before dislocating. As the skier loses control going around a corner, one ski comes up off the snow and the other boot and lower leg remain vertical, such that the knee starts to bend laterally. If the distance from the skier's knee to his center of mass is 1 m, at what angle θ from vertical will the knee dislocate due to the torque of gravity alone?

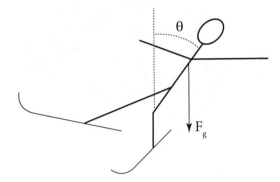

A) 30°
B) 45°
C) 60°
D) 90°

2. When rapidly turning a corner on a flat road, a cyclist leans into the center of the turn. The frame of the bike is nearly parallel to which vector?

A) The force of gravity on the bicycle and rider
B) The normal force on the pair
C) The centripetal force
D) The sum of the normal and friction forces

3. A 1000 kg gondola is operated on a cable between two towers 340 m apart. When the gondola is exactly between the towers, it is 100 m below their height. What is the tension in the cable at this midpoint?

A) 5 kN
B) 8 kN
C) 10 kN
D) 20 kN

4. Which of the following concerning uniform circular motion is true?

A) The centrifugal force is the action-reaction pair of the centripetal force.
B) Unlike the centrifugal force, the centripetal force is a type of force akin to that of friction, gravity, and tension forces.
C) The velocity of the object in motion changes, whereas the acceleration of the object is constant.
D) A satellite undergoing uniform circular motion is falling towards the center in a circular path.

5. When spinning a coin on a flat surface, two equal forces with opposite directions are applied to the opposite sides of a coin. Which of the following is true about the coin after it leaves the hand? (Assume ideal frictionless motion.)

A) The coin does not rotate because equal but opposite forces cancel each other out.
B) The coin does not rotate because equal but opposite torques cancel each other out.
C) The coin rotates and the rotational acceleration is zero.
D) The coin rotates and the rotational acceleration is equal to the nonzero net torque divided by the moment of inertia.

6. In human legs, 20% of the body's mass is in the upper legs (acting at 20 cm from the hip), 10% is in the lower legs (acting at 90 cm), and 3% is in the feet (acting at 120 cm). Find the center of mass of an outstretched leg for a person who is 70 kg.

A) 30 cm from the hip
B) 40 cm from the hip
C) 50 cm from the hip
D) 60 cm from the hip

7. A fully unraveled yo-yo is being swung around in a vertical circle (a trick known as "around the world"). The yo-yo is 100 g on a string that is 90 cm long. A yo-yo guru manages to make his yo-yo travel three complete circles in 1 second. Determine the centripetal acceleration on the yo-yo.

A) 28 m/s^2
B) 32 m/s^2
C) 284 m/s^2
D) 320 m/s^2

CHAPTER 5 PRACTICE PASSAGE

As part of a school project, a group of physics students goes on a trip to an amusement park. The students who went on the trip were told to enjoy all the rides, but to be prepared to explain the physics behind two particular rides.

The first ride is a rotating cylinder that spins the riders uniformly in a circle. The passengers initially stand along the outer rim of the cylinder, at a radius $r = 4$ m. When the ride is started up, the cylinder begins to rotate, with its axis of rotation at its center. When a certain speed (v) is achieved, the floor of the ride drops away entirely, leaving the riders suspended against the wall.

In order for the passengers to be suspended, the coefficient of static friction (μ_s) of the wall needs to be large. The larger the coefficient of static friction, the slower the ride needs to spin in order to keep the riders suspended. Normally, $\mu_s = 0.50$. Because of its unique mechanism of action, the riders do not need to be restrained to the wall during the ride (see Figure 1).

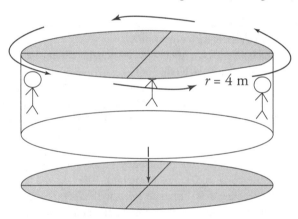

Figure 1 The first ride

The second ride consists of a carriage with mass 300 kg and with maximum occupancy of 300 kg. The carriage is attached to a mechanical arm of length $L = 5$ m that is capable of rotation. The arm is able to provide the torque necessary to swing the riders back and forth on a circular path. Initially, the trips back and forth are very small, but with each trip the swings become larger. Eventually, the riders have enough momentum to swing 360° around, performing a complete circle. In order to partake in this ride, the passengers must be restrained to their seats (see Figure 2).

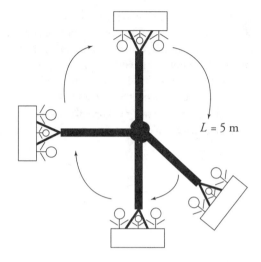

$L = 5$ m

Figure 2 The second ride

1. In the first ride, when the floor drops down and away, the passengers feel pushed up against the wall. Which of the following best explains this phenomenon?

A) The passengers experience a centrifugal force due to the rotation of the ride.
B) The passengers experience a centripetal force due to the circular configuration of the ride.
C) The passengers experience linear inertia that is opposed by the rotation of the ride.
D) The passengers experience rotational inertia that is opposed by the rotation of the ride.

2. In the first ride, what is the tangential speed required to suspend a 50 kg man?

A) 7 m/s
B) 8 m/s
C) 9 m/s
D) 10 m/s

3. In the first ride, when spinning at a speed v, a person with mass m is successfully suspended. If a person with mass $3m$ rides, the ride would have to spin at a speed of:

A) v
B) $3v$
C) $6v$
D) $9v$

4. With a full carriage, the second ride suffers a power outage with the mechanical arm parallel to the ground. How much torque must the mechanical arm provide in order to prevent the passengers from swinging down? (Assume the mechanical arm itself does not require any torque support.)

A) 0 N·m
B) 3×10^4 N·m
C) 18×10^4 N·m
D) 24×10^4 N·m

5. Assume the riders in the second ride are undergoing uniform circular motion. Which of the following is true?

A) The normal force and the centripetal force are at their maximum values at the bottom of the swing.
B) The normal force and the centripetal force are at their maximum values at the top of the swing.
C) The normal force is at maximum value at the bottom of the swing, while the centripetal force value does not change.
D) The normal force is at maximum value at the top of the swing, while the centripetal force is constantly changing.

6. With its carriage full, the second ride goes through the top of its swing. What is the value of the normal force if its speed is 20 m/s?

A) 42 kN
B) 48 kN
C) 54 kN
D) 60 kN

7. In the second ride, a mass of 200 kg is placed on the mechanical arm 3 meters from the center of rotation. In this setup, where is the center of mass relative to the center of rotation? (Assume that the mechanical arm itself has no mass and that the carriage is full.)

A) 3.5 m
B) 4.0 m
C) 4.25 m
D) 4.5 m

SOLUTIONS TO CHAPTER 5 FREESTANDING QUESTIONS

1. **A** Rearranging the formula for torque, we find that $\sin \theta = \tau/rF$. The force of gravity is acting at the center of mass, 1 m from the knee, which is the fulcrum. Substituting the values, being careful to use 1000 N of gravitational force rather than 100 kg, we find that $\sin \theta = 0.5$. Therefore, $\theta = 30°$.

2. **D** A free body diagram is a very important first step here. Gravity always acts downward meaning choice A cannot be correct. The normal force is always perpendicular to the surface, so up in this case, eliminating choice B. The centripetal force will be toward the center of the turn, which will be horizontal on a flat road, so choice C is wrong. The answer is choice D because the friction is the source of that horizontal centripetal force and the normal force is up. If you add them, the resultant will be similar to the angle at which the bike leans.

3. **C** A diagram is vital here. Looking at the symmetrical triangles formed by the cable, one finds that the top side is 170 m on each, while the vertical displacement of the gondola is 100 m. This is a 1-2-$\sqrt{3}$ triangle, so the hypotenuse must be 200 m, though the actual distance does not matter, just the proportion. We find that the gravitational force is 10,000 N, which is divided evenly between the vertical components of the two tensions, giving each a T_y of 5000 N. Do not stop here; that would give you choice A, which is wrong. Because of the nature of the triangle, we know that the total tension is twice the value of this vertical component. So each tension must be 10,000 N. Note that if you add up the tension of the two spans acting on the gondola, which is not what the question is asking, then you get choice D.

4. **D** This requires an understanding of the basic concepts of uniform circular motion and the forces at work. The centripetal force is a name given to the net force of an object undergoing uniform circular motion. Therefore, it is not a separate force and does not have an action-reaction pair. This eliminates choices A and B. The speed of the object in uniform circular motion is constant, but its direction changes, therefore the velocity changes with time. However, the acceleration also changes because the direction of the centripetal acceleration always points to the center of the circle. This eliminates choice C. A satellite undergoing uniform circular motion is in fact falling towards the center, but never accomplishes its goal due to its tangential velocity. Its velocity changes as a result, but it would always form a tangent to its circular path.

5. **C** This is a two-by-two question. Although two equal forces with opposite directions are applied, giving a zero translational acceleration, the net torque is the sum of the two torques, resulting in a rotation of the coin. This eliminates choices A and B. However, after the coin leaves the hand, it undergoes rotational equilibrium, as no net torque is applied. In this case, the rotational acceleration is zero, with the coin undergoing a constant angular rotation.

6. **C** Using the hip as the reference point, center of mass can be calculated using the formula: $x_{CM} = (m_1x_1 + m_2x_2 + \ldots + m_nx_n) / (m_1 + m_2 + \ldots + m_n)$.

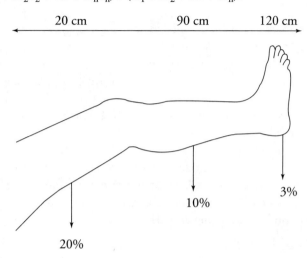

The points where the mass is centered for each body part can be used as the distances. Note that the mass of 70 kg does not affect the solution since it is in every term so it factors out of both the numerator and denominator.

$$x_{CM} = \frac{(0.03)(70)(120) + (0.1)(70)(90) + (0.2)(70)(20)}{(0.03)(70) + (0.1)(70) + (0.2)(70)} \approx 50 \text{ cm.}$$

7. **D** The formula for centripetal acceleration is: $a_c = v^2/r$. To determine the speed, we must know what distance the yo-yo traveled. The yo-yo makes one revolution in 1/3 s. Thus, $v = (2\pi r/t)$ = $2\pi(0.9)/(0.33)$ = 17 m/s. Given the speed of the yo-yo, the centripetal acceleration is given as $a_c = v^2/r = (17)^2/(0.9) \approx 320$ m/s^2.

SOLUTIONS TO CHAPTER 5 PRACTICE PASSAGE

1. **C** There is no net force towards the outside of the circle ("centrifugal"), so choice A can be eliminated. It is true that the centripetal force points toward the center of the circle, but the mere geometry of the ride does not explain why the passengers feel pushed up against the wall (eliminate choice B). Finally, the rotation of the ride is causing the rotational inertia, not opposing it; choice D can be eliminated, leaving choice C. The linear inertia of the passengers would cause them to move in a straight line, but this is opposed by the normal force of the wall of the ride.

2. **C** In the first ride, the riders are undergoing uniform circular motion, therefore $F_c = mv^2/r$. The cause of the centripetal force is actually the normal force F_N of the wall on the rider. Therefore, $F_c = F_N = mv^2/r$. To suspend the man, the force of gravity (F_G) must be counteracted by the force of static friction (F_f). Therefore,

$$F_f = F_G$$

$$F_N \cdot \mu_s = mg$$

$$\frac{mv^2}{r} \cdot \mu_s = mg$$

$$v = \sqrt{gr/\mu_s} = \sqrt{10 \cdot 4/0.5} = \sqrt{80} \cong 9 \text{ m/s}$$

3. **A** Since it is uniform circular motion, $F_c = mv^2/r$, with $F_N = F_c$. In order for the riders to be suspended, the force of gravity (F_G) and the friction force (F_f) must be equal to each other. Therefore:

$$F_f = F_G$$

$$F_N \cdot \mu_s = mg$$

$$\frac{mv^2}{r} \cdot \mu_s = mg$$

$$v = \sqrt{gr/\mu_s}$$

Thus, the equation for speed of spin is independent of mass. Therefore, a $3m$ person would only have to spin at speed v.

4. **B** If the arm is stuck parallel to the ground, then the mechanical arm must provide enough torque to cancel out the torque produced by the gravitational force.

$$\tau = rF\sin\theta = mgr = (m_{carriage} + m_{passengers})gr = (300 + 300) \times 10 \times 5 = 3 \times 10^4 \text{ N} \cdot \text{m}$$

5.   C   If the riders are undergoing uniform circular motion, then $F_c = mv^2/r$ with constant speed v. Since mass m and radius r are also constant, then F_c must also be constant, eliminating all options except choice C. Even though F_c may be constant during rotation, the normal force is not. The centripetal force is the sum of the forces radially, which include the tension force of the mechanical arm as well as the force of gravity. At the bottom of the swing, the normal force is opposite to the force of gravity, as opposed to at the top of the swing where the normal force and gravity are facing the same direction. Therefore, at the bottom of the swing, the normal force must be at a maximum, in order to cancel out the force of gravity, while at the top of the swing the normal force is at a minimum, because gravity is working with the normal force.

6.   A   At the top of the swing, $F_c = F_G + F_N$, since both are pointing radially and in the same direction. Therefore:

$$F_c = F_G + F_N = \frac{mv^2}{r}$$

$$6000 + F_N = \frac{600 \times 20^2}{5}$$

$$F_N = 48,000 - 6000 = 42 \text{ kN}$$

7.   D   For a two mass system, $x_{CM} = (m_1 x_1 + m_2 x_2)/(m_1 + m_2)$. For this question, we shall measure the position from the center of rotation (although other centers are usable as well). For the carriage (m_1), $x_1 = 5$ m. For the second mass (m_2), $x_2 = 3$. Thus,

$$x_{CM} = \frac{m_1 x_1 + m_2 x_2}{m_1 + m_2}$$

$$= \frac{600 \times 5 + 200 \times 3}{800}$$

$$= 4.5 \text{ m}$$

Chapter 6
Mechanics III

6.1 WORK

Imagine a constant force **F** pushing a crate through a displacement **d**, as shown below:

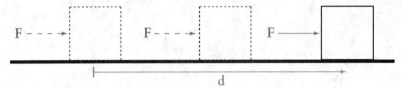

(Notice that the force **F** here doesn't just act momentarily at the initial position of the crate, with the crate then sliding across the floor with **F** removed; the force **F** is assumed to act constantly over the entire displacement.) We say that the **work** done by **F** is the product of *F* and *d*: Work $W = Fd$.

For example, if the magnitude of **F** is 20 N and the magnitude of **d** is 5 m, then the work done by the force **F** in the situation pictured above is (20 N)(5 m) = 100 N·m. When it's used to measure work, the newton-meter (N·m) is renamed the **joule**, abbreviated J. Therefore, we have $W = 100$ J.

The situation pictured above is quite special, however, because the vectors **F** and **d** point in the same direction. What if **F** and **d** do not point in the same direction? For example, what if we tie one end of a rope around the crate, sling the other end over our shoulder and pull the crate across the floor? Then our force **F** (which is actually the tension in the rope) will be at an angle to the displacement:

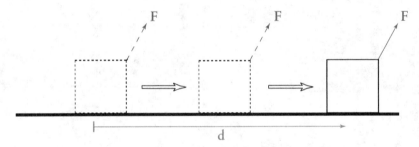

In this case, the work done by **F** is not the product of *F* and *d*. It's only the component of the force in the direction of **d** that does work. If θ is the angle between **F** and **d**, then the component of **F** that's parallel to **d** has magnitude $F \cos \theta$. Therefore, the work done by **F** is $(F \cos \theta)(d)$.

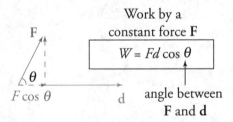

Work by a
constant force **F**

$$W = Fd \cos \theta$$

angle between
F and **d**

Work by a Constant Force, F

$$W = Fd \cos\theta$$

where θ = angle between **F** and **d**

Notice that the formula $W = Fd \cos \theta$ includes the formula $W = Fd$ as a special case. After all, if $\mathbf{F}$ and $\mathbf{d}$ do point in the same direction, then $\theta = 0°$, and $\cos \theta = \cos 0° = 1$, so $Fd \cos \theta$ becomes Fd. Therefore, the formula $W = Fd \cos \theta$ covers all cases of a constant force $\mathbf{F}$ acting through a displacement $\mathbf{d}$.

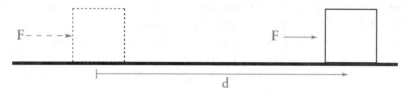

Example 6-1: In the situation pictured above, assume the mass of the crate, m, is 20 kg and the coefficient of kinetic friction between the crate and the floor is 0.4. If $F = 100$ N and $d = 6$ m,

a) How much work is done by $\mathbf{F}$?
b) How much work is done by the normal force?
c) How much work is done by gravity?
d) How much work is done by the force of friction?
e) What is the total work done on the crate?

Solution:

a) Because $\mathbf{F}$ is parallel to $\mathbf{d}$, the work done by $\mathbf{F}$ is simply $Fd = (100$ N$)(6$ m$) = 600$ J.
b) The normal force is perpendicular to the floor, and to $\mathbf{d}$. Since the angle between $\mathbf{F}_N$ and $\mathbf{d}$ is $\theta = 90°$, and $\cos 90° = 0$, the work done by $\mathbf{F}_N$ is zero.
c) The gravitational force is also perpendicular to the floor, and to $\mathbf{d}$. Because the angle between $\mathbf{F}_{grav}$ and $\mathbf{d}$ is $\theta = 90°$, and $\cos 90° = 0$, the work done by $\mathbf{F}_{grav}$ is zero, too.
d) First, since $F_N = mg = (20$ kg$)(10$ N/kg$) = 200$ N, we have $F_f = \mu_k F_N = (0.4)(200$ N$) = 80$ N. However, the direction of the vector $\mathbf{F}_f$ is opposite to the direction of $\mathbf{d}$, so the angle between $\mathbf{F}_f$ and $\mathbf{d}$ is $\theta = 180°$. Because $\cos 180° = -1$, the work done by the friction force is $(80$ N$)$ $(6$ m$)(-1) = -480$ J.
e) To find the total work done on the crate, we just add up the work done by each of the forces that acts on the crate. In this case, then, we'd have

$$W_{total} = W_{by\ F} + W_{by\ F_N} + W_{by\ F_{grav}} + W_{by\ F_f} = (600\ J) + (0\ J) + (0\ J) + (-480\ J) = 120\ J$$

Here are a couple of things to notice about Example 6-1:

1) Although work depends on two vectors for its definition (namely, $\mathbf{F}$ and $\mathbf{d}$), work itself is *not* a vector. *Work is a scalar.* W may be positive, negative, or zero, but work has no direction.
2) In this example, there were four forces acting on the crate: the pushing force $\mathbf{F}$, gravity, the normal force, and friction. Each force does its own amount of work, which is why each part had to specify for which force we wanted the work. Only in the last part, where the total work is desired, can we omit the specific force we're looking at (because we're considering them all).

Example 6-2: In the situation described in Example 6-1, what is the net force on the crate? How much work is done by $\mathbf{F}_{net}$?

Solution: The normal force cancels out the gravitational force, so the net force on the crate is just $\mathbf{F} + \mathbf{F}_f =$ (100 N) + (−80 N) = +20 N, where the + indicates that $\mathbf{F}_{net}$ points to the right. Now, since $\mathbf{F}_{net}$ is parallel to $\mathbf{d}$, the work done by $\mathbf{F}_{net}$ is just the product, $F_{net}d =$ (20 N)(6 m) = 120 J. Notice that this is the same as the total amount of work done on the crate, as we figured out in part (e) of Example 6-1. This wasn't a coincidence. The total work done (found by adding up the values of the work done by each force separately) is always equal to the work done by the net force.

Remember that work is a scalar and it can be positive, zero, or negative. Now here's how to know *when* W will be positive, zero, or negative. Because $W = Fd \cos \theta$, and F and d are magnitudes (which means they're positive), the sign of W depends entirely on the sign of $\cos \theta$.

The diagrams below show the three cases.

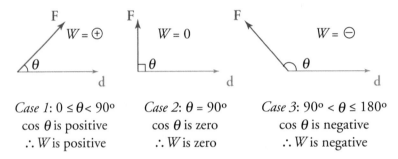

Case 1: $0 \le \theta < 90°$
$\cos \theta$ is positive
∴ W is positive

Case 2: $\theta = 90°$
$\cos \theta$ is zero
∴ W is zero

Case 3: $90° < \theta \le 180°$
$\cos \theta$ is negative
∴ W is negative

In Case 1, the angle between $\mathbf{F}$ and $\mathbf{d}$ is less than 90° (an acute angle); since the cosine of such an angle is positive, the work done by this force will be positive.

In Case 2, the angle between $\mathbf{F}$ and $\mathbf{d}$ is 90°; since the cosine of 90° is zero, the work done by this force will be zero.

In Case 3, the angle between $\mathbf{F}$ and $\mathbf{d}$ is greater than 90° (an obtuse angle); since the cosine of such an angle is negative, the work done by this force will be negative.

Example 6-1 illustrated all three cases. The force that pushed the crate across the floor did positive work, gravity and the normal force did zero work, and sliding friction did negative work.

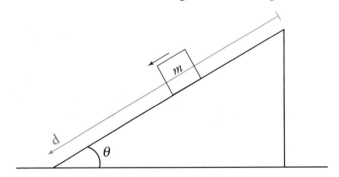

Example 6-3: In the situation pictured on the previous page, assume the mass of the block, *m*, is 20 kg and the coefficient of kinetic friction between the block and the ramp is 0.4. If *d* = 10 m and θ = 30°,

a) How much work is done by the normal force?
b) How much work is done by the force of friction?
c) How much work is done by gravity?
d) What is the total work done on the block?

Solution:

a) The normal force is perpendicular to the ramp, and to **d**. Since the angle between $\mathbf{F}_N$ and **d** is θ = 90°, and cos 90° = 0, the work done by $\mathbf{F}_N$ is zero. Forces acting perpendicular to the direction of travel always do zero work.

b) First, we know that since the block is on a ramp, we'll have $F_N = mg \cos \theta$, where θ is the incline angle of the ramp. The magnitude of $\mathbf{F}_f$, the force of kinetic friction, is $\mu_k F_N$, so we get F_f = (0.4)(20 kg)(10 N/kg) cos 30°, which is approximately (0.4)(200 N)(0.85) = 68 N. Now, since the vectors $\mathbf{F}_f$ and **d** point in opposite directions (because **d** points down the ramp and $\mathbf{F}_f$ points up the ramp), the work done by $\mathbf{F}_f$ will be $-F_f d$ = –(68 N)(10 m) = –680 J.

c) There are two ways we can answer this part. One way is to remember that the force due to gravity acting parallel to the ramp is $mg \sin \theta$, where θ is the incline angle. Since this component of the gravitational force is parallel to **d**, we can simply multiply $mg \sin \theta$ by *d* to find the work done by gravity: $W = (mg \sin \theta)(d)$ = (20 kg)(10 N/kg)(sin 30°)(10 m) = 1000 J. Here's another way: The force $\mathbf{F}_{grav} = m\mathbf{g}$ points straight down, and the angle between $\mathbf{F}_{grav}$ and **d** is β, where β is the angle shown below. It's the complement of the incline angle θ; that is, $\beta = 90° - \theta$.

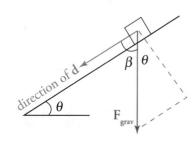

Since θ = 30°, we have β = 60°. Therefore, the work done by $\mathbf{F}_{grav}$ is $F_{grav} d \cos \beta = mgd \cos \beta$ = (20 kg)(10 N/kg)(10 m) (cos 60°) = 1000 J. You need to be very careful here; the formula for work reads, "$W = Fd \cos \theta$," but the θ in this formula is *not* the same as the θ labeled in the figure. The angle in the formula for *W* is the angle between **F** and **d**, and this is not the same as the incline angle.

d) To find the total work done on the block, we just add up the work done by each of the forces that acts on the block. In this case, then, we'd have

$$W_{total} = W_{by\ F_N} + W_{by\ F_f} + W_{by\ F_{grav}} = (0\ J) + (-680\ J) + (1000\ J) = 320\ J$$

The formula $W = Fd \cos\theta$ can only be used if the force is constant during the motion. What if the force changes? In general, calculus is required, which is not needed for the MCAT. However, if a graph of force vs. position is given (assuming $\theta = 0$), then the work done by that force is equal to the area *under the curve*.

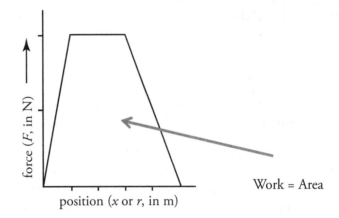

In Chapter 11, we will apply this to find the work required to compress or stretch a spring.

6.2 POWER

Power measures how fast work gets done. For example, if a force does 100 J of work in 20 seconds, then work is being done at a *rate* of

$$\frac{100 \text{ J}}{20 \text{ s}} = 5 \text{ J/s}$$

This is the power.

We use the letter P to denote power, and from the sample calculation above, we can see that the unit of power is the joule-per-second. This unit has its own name: the **watt**, abbreviated W. Therefore, power is measured in watts: $[P] = \text{J/s} = \text{W}$. (Don't confuse the abbreviation for the watt, W, with the usual variable used for work, W.)

The term *watt* makes most of us think of light bulbs, but the watt is used to measure the power of anything, not just light bulbs. After all, should the unit *horsepower* make us think that only horses can provide power? By the way, 1 hp (1 horsepower) is equal to about 750 W.

The sample calculation above also shows us how we should define P in general:

> **Power**
>
> $$P = \frac{\text{work}}{\text{time}} = \frac{W}{t}$$

What if 100 J of work is done over a time interval of just 2 seconds? Then the power would be 50 W; it's easy to see that the faster work gets done, the greater the power.

A handy formula that you can also use to calculate P uses the fact that $v = d/t$:

$$P = \frac{W}{t} = \frac{Fd}{t} = F\frac{d}{t} = Fv \rightarrow P = Fv$$

(We're assuming here that **F** is parallel to **d**, so that $W = Fd$, and that the object's speed, v, is constant.) To see how this formula would be used, let's answer this question: How much power must be provided to a model rocket of mass 50 kg to keep it moving upward at a constant speed of 40 m/s? Ignoring air resistance, the engine thrust must provide an upward force that's equal to the weight of the rocket: $F = mg = (50 \text{ kg})(10 \text{ N/kg}) = 500 \text{ N}$. Therefore, $P = Fv = (500 \text{ N})(40 \text{ m/s}) = 20{,}000 \text{ W} = 20 \text{ kW}$.

From the definition of power, we can see that

> $$W = Pt$$

This equation is used as often on the MCAT as the definition $P = W/t$. For example, if a machine has a power output of 200 W, how much work can it do in 1 hour? Multiplying power by time (and remembering to change 1 hour into $(60)(60) = 3600$ seconds) gives the work:

$$W = Pt = (200 \text{ W})(3600 \text{ s}) = 720{,}000 \text{ J} = 720 \text{ kJ}$$

Example 6-4: A force of magnitude 40 N pushes on an object of mass 8 kg through a displacement of 5 m for 10 seconds. What's the power provided by this force?

Solution: Power is equal to work divided by time, so

$$P = \frac{W}{t} = \frac{Fd}{t} = \frac{(40 \text{ N})(5 \text{ m})}{10 \text{ s}} = 20 \text{ W}$$

Example 6-5: You're lifting bricks, each with a mass of 2 kg, from the floor up to a shelf that is 1.5 m high.

a) How much work do you perform lifting each brick?
b) If you can place 20 bricks on the shelf every minute, what is your power output?
c) If you continue this effort for an hour, how many Calories of work will you do (1 Cal = 4184 J)?

Solution:

a) The force you must provide to lift a brick is equal to the weight of the brick, which is $mg = (2 \text{ kg})(10 \text{ N/kg}) = 20$ N. Since this force must act over a distance of 1.5 m to lift it up to the shelf, the work required is $W = Fd = (20 \text{ N})(1.5 \text{ m}) = 30$ J.

b) If you can place 20 bricks on the shelf every 60 seconds, then on average you're lifting one brick every 3 seconds. If the work performed in 3 seconds is 30 J—as we found in part (a)—then your power output is

$$P = \frac{W}{t} = \frac{30 \text{ J}}{3 \text{ s}} = 10 \text{ W}$$

c) In an hour a power of 10 W amounts to $W = Pt = 10 \text{ J/s} \times 3600 \text{ s/hr} = 36{,}000$ J. Unfortunately, that's only $36{,}000 \text{ J} \times 1/4184 \text{ Cal/J} \approx 9$ Cal. However, our bodies are far from perfectly efficient, so we have to burn many more Calories than that to achieve that much work output. Moreover, there's a lot more to making a human body move than ideal work done against gravity in a frictionless process. After all, if you run for an hour on a horizontal treadmill, you have accomplished zero physical work, but obviously you will burn a lot of Calories!

Example 6-6: A car of mass 2000 kg accelerates from rest to a speed of 30 m/s in 9 seconds. Given that the engine does a total of 900,000 J of work, what is the average power output of the car's engine?

Solution: Since we're given the amount of work done and the time interval, we can find the average power output of the engine simply by dividing work by time:

$$P = \frac{W}{t} = \frac{900{,}000 \text{ J}}{9 \text{ s}} = 100{,}000 \text{ W} = 100 \text{ kW}$$

Notice that neither the mass of the car, nor its final speed, were needed to answer the question because the required information (work and time) was given.

Example 6-7: One month, your electric bill states that you used 500 kWh of electricity, at a cost of 8¢ per kWh. What is a kWh, and how much is your electric bill that month?

Solution: A kilowatt (kW) is a thousand watts; it's a unit of power. An hour (h) is a time interval. Therefore, a kilowatt-hour, kWh, obtained by multiplying power times time, Pt, has units of work. (1 kWh = $(1000 \text{ W})(3600 \text{ s}) = 3.6 \times 10^6 \text{ J} = 3.6$ MJ.) The electric company performed 500 kWh of work pushing and pulling the electrons within the wires in your home to make electrical devices function, at a cost to you of $(500 \text{ kWh})(8\text{¢/kWh}) = \$40$.

6.3 KINETIC ENERGY

An intuitive way to describe **energy** is that it's the ability to do work. Objects that move have this ability, since they can crash into something and thus exert a force over a distance. Therefore, objects that move have energy; specifically, we say they have **kinetic energy**, the energy due to motion.

To figure out how much kinetic energy a moving object has, imagine that an object of mass m is initially at rest (and thus has no kinetic energy). To get it moving, we have to exert a force **F** on it, over some distance d. (Let's assume, to keep things simple, that **F** points in the same direction as **d**.) How fast will the object be moving as a result? The acceleration is a constant $a = F/m$, so, using Big Five #5, we get

$$v^2 = v_0^2 + 2ad \rightarrow v^2 = 2ad \rightarrow v^2 = 2\frac{F}{m}d$$

Therefore, the final speed, v, will be $\sqrt{2Fd/m}$

Now let's do a little algebra and rewrite the last equation above like this:

$$Fd = \tfrac{1}{2}mv^2$$

We recognize the product Fd as the work done by the force. So, we did work on the object to get it moving, and now because it's moving, it has kinetic energy. How much kinetic energy? This last equation tells us that we should consider the amount of kinetic energy to be $\frac{1}{2}mv^2$.

Kinetic Energy

$$KE = \frac{1}{2}mv^2$$

In words, this definition says that the kinetic energy of an object whose mass is m and whose speed is v is equal to one-half m times the square of the speed. Since $\frac{1}{2}mv^2$ is equal to the work Fd, we see right away that the unit of KE should also be the joule. In addition, like work, kinetic energy is a scalar.

Example 6-8: An object of mass 10 kg moves with a velocity of 4 m/s to the north. What is its kinetic energy? What would happen to the kinetic energy if the speed of the object doubled?

Solution: Kinetic energy is a scalar that cares only about the speed of an object; the direction of the object's velocity is irrelevant. So we find that

$$KE = \tfrac{1}{2}mv^2 = \tfrac{1}{2}(10 \text{ kg})(4 \text{ m/s})^2 = 80 \text{ J}$$

Because KE is proportional to v^2, if v were to increase by a factor of 2 then KE would increase by a factor of $2^2 = 4$.

The Work-Energy Theorem

The use of Big Five #5 on the previous page above (to motivate the definition $KE = \frac{1}{2}mv^2$) assumed that the initial speed of the object was zero. But what if the initial speed wasn't zero? Then we'd have

$$v^2 - v_0^2 = 2\frac{F}{m}d$$

$$v^2 = v_0^2 + 2ad \rightarrow v^2 - v_0^2 = 2ad \rightarrow \frac{1}{2}m(v^2 - v_0^2) = Fd$$

$$Fd = \frac{1}{2}mv^2 - \frac{1}{2}mv_0^2$$

$$W = KE_{final} - KE_{initial}$$

In other words, the total work done on the object is equal to the change in its kinetic energy. This fact is important enough that it's given a name:

Work-Energy Theorem

$$W_{total} = \Delta KE$$

This formula gives you another way to calculate work. You don't even need to know the force or the displacement! If you know the change in an object's kinetic energy, then you automatically know the total amount of work that was done on it.

Look back at the set of three diagrams showing when the work done by a force is positive, zero, or negative. In Case 1, the force is pulling in roughly the same direction as the object's displacement (more formally, the force **F** has a component that's in the same direction as **d**). We can think of such a force as "helping" the object move, and therefore causing its speed to increase. More technically, the work done on an object *transfers* energy from the environment into the object. In the case of positive work being done, and according to the work-energy theorem, positive work would automatically imply a positive change in kinetic energy. If the kinetic energy increases, then the speed increases.

In Case 3, the force is pulling in roughly the opposite direction from the object's displacement (more formally, the force **F** has a component that's in the opposite direction from **d**). We can think of such a force as "hindering" the object's motion, and therefore causing its speed to decrease. This is also consistent with the work-energy theorem because Case 3 was the case of negative work being done on the object, transferring energy out of the object into the environment. According to the work-energy theorem, negative work automatically implies a negative change in kinetic energy. If the kinetic energy decreases, then the speed decreases.

Example 6-9: An object of mass 10 kg whose initial speed is 4 m/s is accelerated until it achieves a final speed of 9 m/s.

    a)   How much work was done on this object?

    b)   If the acceleration took place over a displacement **d** of magnitude 13 m, and the force **F** exerted on it was constant and parallel to **d**, what was F?

Solution:

    a)   Although neither **F** nor **d** is given, we can still figure out the work done by using the work-energy theorem:

$$W_{total} = \Delta KE$$
$$= KE_f - KE_i$$
$$= \tfrac{1}{2}mv^2 - \tfrac{1}{2}mv_0^2$$
$$= \tfrac{1}{2}m(v^2 - v_0^2)$$
$$= \tfrac{1}{2}(10 \text{ kg})\left[\left(9 \text{ m/s}\right)^2 - \left(4 \text{ m/s}\right)^2\right]$$

$$\therefore W = 325 \text{ J}$$

    b)   Because **F** is parallel to **d**, we know that $W = Fd$. We just found W in part (a), and since we now know d, we can find F:

$$W = Fd \rightarrow F = \frac{W}{d} = \frac{325 \text{ J}}{13 \text{ m}} = 25 \text{ N}$$

Example 6-10: An object of mass 10 kg is moving at a speed of 9 m/s. How much work must be done on this object in order to stop it?

Solution: Once again, we're asked to find W without being given **F** and **d**, so we use the work-energy theorem. If we want to stop the object, we want to bring its final kinetic energy to zero. Therefore,

$$W = \Delta KE$$
$$= \tfrac{1}{2}mv^2 - \tfrac{1}{2}mv_0^2$$
$$= 0 - \tfrac{1}{2}mv_0^2$$
$$= -\tfrac{1}{2}(10 \text{ kg})(9 \text{ m/s})^2$$

$$\therefore W = -405 \text{ J}$$

The work that must be done on the object has to be negative, because only negative work causes a decrease in speed.

6.3

Example 6-11: Recall the centrifuge Example 5-4 from the preceding chapter. Suppose the mass of blood in one bag is 0.5 kg.

   a)   What's the magnitude of the net force on the blood?
   b)   How much work is done by the net force during each revolution of the centrifuge?

Solution:

   a)   The net force on an object undergoing uniform circular motion (UCM) is the centripetal force:

$$F_c = m\frac{v^2}{r} = (0.5 \text{ kg})\frac{(175 \text{ m/s})^2}{0.35 \text{ m}} \approx 4 \times 10^4 \text{ N}$$

   b)   We can answer this part in two ways. The centripetal force points toward the center of the circular path, so it's always perpendicular to the blood's velocity:

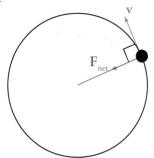

The work done by a force that's perpendicular to an blood's motion is *zero* (remember Case 2 depicted in Section 6.1: $\mathbf{F} \perp \mathbf{d}$ means $W = 0$.)

Another way is to use the work-energy theorem. Since the blood's speed is constant, its kinetic energy is constant, too. No change in kinetic energy means no work is being done.

Example 6-12: A box of mass 4 kg is initially at rest on a frictionless horizontal surface. A horizontal force **F** of magnitude 32 N is exerted on the object and then removed. If the speed of the object is then 2 m/s, over what distance did **F** act?

Solution: By the work-energy theorem, the work done by **F** was

$$W = \Delta KE = KE_f - KE_i = KE_f = \tfrac{1}{2}mv^2 = \tfrac{1}{2}(4 \text{ kg})(2 \text{ m/s})^2 = 8 \text{ J}$$

The question now is, "Given that **F** is parallel to **d** (so $W = Fd$), what's d?"

$$W = Fd \rightarrow d = \frac{W}{F} = \frac{8 \text{ J}}{32 \text{ N}} = 0.25 \text{ m}$$

Example 6-13: Consider the block described in Example 6-3. If the initial speed of the block was zero, what is the block's speed when it reaches the bottom of the ramp?

Solution: We figured out in part (d) of that example that the total work done on the block was 320 J. By the work-energy theorem, we find that

$$W = \Delta KE = KE_{\mathrm{f}} - KE_{\mathrm{i}} = KE_{\mathrm{f}} = \tfrac{1}{2}mv^2 \rightarrow v = \sqrt{\frac{2W_{\mathrm{total}}}{m}} = \sqrt{\frac{2(320\,\mathrm{J})}{20\,\mathrm{kg}}} = \sqrt{32\ \mathrm{m^2/s^2}} \approx 5.6\ \mathrm{m/s}$$

Example 6-14: Consider the crate described in Example 6-1.

a)   If the initial speed of the crate was zero, what was the speed once the force **F** was removed after acting through the given displacement **d**?
b)   How far would the crate slide before coming to rest?

Solution:

a)   We figured out in part (e) of that example that the total work done on the crate was 120 J. The work-energy theorem then tells us that

$$W = \Delta KE = KE_{\mathrm{f}} - KE_{\mathrm{i}} = KE_{\mathrm{f}} = \tfrac{1}{2}mv^2 \rightarrow v = \sqrt{\frac{2W_{\mathrm{total}}}{m}} = \sqrt{\frac{2(120\,\mathrm{J})}{20\,\mathrm{kg}}} = \sqrt{12\ \mathrm{m^2/s^2}} \approx 3.5\ \mathrm{m/s}$$

b)   Once the force **F** is removed, the only force acting on the crate that doesn't do zero work is friction. The work done by friction will be $-F_{\mathrm{f}}d'$, where d' is the distance the crate will slide before coming to rest. By the work-energy theorem, we have

$$W = \Delta KE = KE_{\mathrm{f}} - KE_{\mathrm{i}} = 0 - KE_{\mathrm{i}}$$
$$-KE_{\mathrm{i}} = -F_{\mathrm{f}}d'$$
$$F_{\mathrm{f}}d' = KE_{\mathrm{i}}$$
$$d' = \frac{KE_{\mathrm{i}}}{F_{\mathrm{f}}}$$

Since the crate had 120 J of kinetic energy right when the force **F** was removed, using the equation $F_{\mathrm{f}} = \mu_{\mathrm{k}}F_{\mathrm{N}} = \mu_{\mathrm{k}}mg$ gives us

$$d' = \frac{KE_{\mathrm{i}}}{F_{\mathrm{f}}} = \frac{KE_{\mathrm{i}}}{\mu_{\mathrm{k}}mg} = \frac{120\,\mathrm{J}}{(0.4)(20\ \mathrm{kg})(10\frac{\mathrm{N}}{\mathrm{kg}})} = 1.5\ \mathrm{m}$$

6.4 POTENTIAL ENERGY

In the preceding section, we defined kinetic energy as the energy an object has due to its motion. **Potential energy** is the energy an object has by virtue of its *position*. There are different "kinds" of potential energy because there are different kinds of forces. For example, in our study of MCAT physics, we'll look at three types of potential energy: gravitational, electrical, and elastic. In this chapter, we'll study the first of these: *gravitational* potential energy.

Imagine a brick lying on the ground. Now, pick it up and place it on a shelf. You've just changed the position of the brick, and, since potential energy is the energy an object has by virtue of its position, you might expect that you've changed the brick's potential energy as well. You did. The brick's gravitational potential energy has been changed, because its position in a gravitational field has changed.

Now, let's be more specific. By *how much* did the brick's gravitational potential energy change? To find the answer, we need to look at the work done by the gravitational force (this is gravitational potential energy, after all). While the brick was being lifted, gravity did work on the brick. Let m be the mass of the brick, and let h be the height from the ground up to the shelf. The gravitational force on the brick is $F_{grav} = m\mathbf{g}$, pointing downward; the displacement of the brick is h, upward.

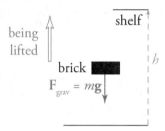

Because the force $\mathbf{F}_{grav}$ and the displacement $\mathbf{h}$ point in opposite directions, we know that the work done by $\mathbf{F}_{grav}$ will be the negative of F_{grav} times h: $W_{by\,F_{grav}} = -F_{grav}h = -mgh$. The change in gravitational potential energy is defined to be the opposite of the work done by the gravitational force:

$$\Delta PE_{grav} = -W_{by\,F_{grav}}$$

In this case, then, we have $\Delta PE_{grav} = -(-mgh) = mgh$. If the brick had *fallen* from the shelf to the floor, so that its height *decreased* by h, then we would have had $W_{by\,F_{grav}} = -F_{grav}h = mgh$ and $\Delta PE_{grav} = -mgh$. In summary, then, we have

Change in Gravitational Potential Energy

$$\Delta PE_{grav} = \begin{array}{l} +mgh, \text{ if the height of } m \text{ is increased by } h \\ -mgh, \text{ if the height of } m \text{ is decreased by } h \end{array}$$

where it's assumed that we're close enough to the surface of the earth that g can be considered a constant.

The formulas on the previous page give the *change* in the gravitational potential energy of an object of mass *m*. If we designate the ground as our "$PE_{grav} = 0$" level, then we can say that the gravitational potential energy of an object at height *h* is equal to *mgh*.

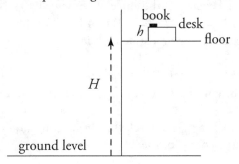

Potential energy is relative. Consider a book sitting on the desk in a second-floor office. Relative to the floor, the height of the book might be, say, half a meter. So, if the book has a mass of 1 kg, its gravitational potential energy is *mgh* = (1 kg)(10 N/kg)(0.5 m) = 5 J. But what if we were to measure the height of the book above the *ground*? Relative to the ground, the floor of the office might be at height *H* = 5 m, so the height of the book above the ground would be *H* + *h* = 5.5 m, and the book's gravitational potential energy is *mg*(*H* + *h*) = (1 kg)(10 N/kg)(5.5 m) = 55 J. Whenever we talk about "the" potential energy of an object, we must specify where we're choosing our "*PE* = 0" level.

The fact that potential energy is relative typically doesn't matter because only *changes* in potential energy are important and physically meaningful. Let's go back to our book on the office desk example. If the book falls off the desk to the floor, what is the change in its potential energy? To the person who calls the floor of the office their "*PE* = 0" level, the change in the book's potential energy will be

$$\Delta PE_{grav} = PE_f - PE_i = 0 - mgh = -mgh = -(1 \text{ kg})(10\tfrac{\text{N}}{\text{kg}})(0.5 \text{ m}) = -5 \text{ J}$$

Now, to the person who calls the ground their "*PE* = 0" level, the change in the book's potential energy will be the same:

$$\Delta PE_{grav} = PE_f - PE_i = mgH - mg(H + h) = -mgh = -(1 \text{ kg})(10\tfrac{\text{N}}{\text{kg}})(0.5 \text{ m}) = -5 \text{ J}$$

Both people will always agree on the *change* in an object's potential energy, even if they disagree about what the potential energy *is* at a certain height (because they choose different "*PE* = 0" levels).

Example 6-15: A brick that weighs 25 N is lifted from the ground to a shelf that's 2 m high. What is its change in gravitational potential energy?

Solution: Because *mg* = 25 N, we have ΔPE_{grav} = *mgh* = (25 N)(2 m) = 50 J. Notice that since the brick was lifted *up*, its change in gravitational potential energy is *positive*.

Example 6-16: A 1 N apple in a tree is at a height 4 m above the ground. The apple falls off its branch and lands on a branch that's only 1 m above the ground. What is the change in the apple's potential energy?

Solution: Because the apple *falls* a distance of $h = 4 - 1 = 3$ m, the change in its gravitational potential energy is $-mgh = -(1 \text{ N})(3 \text{ m}) = -3$ J. We could also have answered the question like this: First, we choose, say, the ground to be our "$PE = 0$" level. Then the initial potential energy of the apple is $PE_i = mgh_i = (1 \text{ N})(4 \text{ m}) = 4$ J, and the final potential energy of the apple is $PE_f = mgh_f = (1 \text{ N})(1 \text{ m}) = 1$ J. The change in the potential energy is, therefore, $\Delta PE = PE_f - PE_i = (1 \text{ J}) - (4 \text{ J}) = -3$ J. Note that because the apple *falls*, the change in its gravitational potential energy must be *negative*.

Example 6-17: Which has more gravitational potential energy: an object of mass 2 kg at a height of 50 m, or an object of mass 50 kg at a height of 2 m? (Set $PE_{grav} = 0$ at the ground for both objects.)

Solution: Since the ground is the $PE_{grav} = 0$ level, then at height h an object's gravitational potential energy is $PE_{grav} = mgh$. The potential energy of the 2 kg object is

$$PE_1 = m_1 g h_1 = (2 \text{ kg})(10 \tfrac{\text{N}}{\text{kg}})(50 \text{ m}) = 1000 \text{ J}$$

and the potential energy of the 50 kg object is

$$PE_2 = m_2 g h_2 = (50 \text{ kg})(10 \tfrac{\text{N}}{\text{kg}})(2 \text{ m}) = 1000 \text{ J}$$

Therefore, these two objects have the *same* gravitational potential energy relative to the ground.

Gravity is a Conservative Force

Suppose we want to move a brick from the floor up to a shelf. One way we could do it would be to simply lift the brick straight up. Another way would be to set up a ramp and then push the brick up the ramp to the shelf. Let's figure out how much work gravity does in each of these cases. We'll assume that the brick has a mass of 3 kg and that the shelf is 2 m high.

The first case is easy. The gravitational force on the brick is $mg = (3 \text{ kg})(10 \text{ N/kg}) = 30$ N, directed straight downward. Since the displacement **h** of the brick is straight upward (that is, in the opposite direction from F_{grav}), we know that the work done by gravity is negative F_{grav} times h:

$$W_{\text{by } F_{grav}} = -F_{grav} h = -(30 \text{ N})(2 \text{ m}) = -60 \text{ J}$$

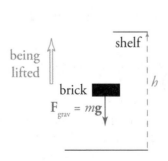

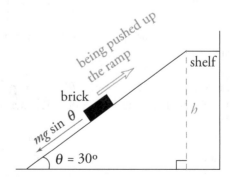

Now, let's look at the second case. Let's use a ramp whose incline angle θ is 30°. The gravitational force acting parallel to the ramp has magnitude $mg \sin \theta$, directed downward along the ramp. Because the displacement **d** is upward along the ramp (that is, in the opposite direction), we know the work done by gravity is negative, and equal to $-(mg \sin \theta)(d)$. Since the height of the shelf is $h = 2$ m, the length of the ramp (i.e., the hypotenuse of the right triangle) must be $d = h/(\sin \theta) = (2 \text{ m})/(\sin 30°) = 4$ m. Therefore, the work done by the gravitational force as the block is pushed up the ramp is

$$W_{\text{by } \mathbf{F}_{\text{grav}}} = -(mg \sin \theta)(d) = -(30 \text{ N})(\sin 30°)(4 \text{ m}) = -(15 \text{ N})(4 \text{ m}) = -60 \text{ J}$$

This is the same answer as we found before! Since the change in the gravitational potential energy is defined to be the opposite of the work done by the gravitational force, $\Delta PE_{\text{grav}} = -W_{\text{by } \mathbf{F}_{\text{grav}}}$, we can say that $\Delta PE_{\text{grav}} = -(-60 \text{ J}) = 60 \text{ J}$ in either case.

In the first case (lifting the brick straight upward), we exert a greater force over a smaller distance, while in the second case (moving the brick up a ramp), we exert a smaller force over a greater distance. However, the work done is the same in both cases.

These examples illustrate the following:

> *The work done by gravity*
>
> *depends only on the initial and final heights of the object,*
>
> *not on the path the object follows.*

Another way of saying this is to state that gravity is a **conservative** force. (In fact, it is the conservative nature of the gravitational force that allows us to define gravitational potential energy.)

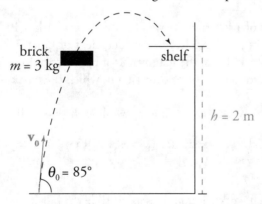

Example 6-18: In the situation pictured above, a brick is projected upward with an initial velocity $\mathbf{v}_0$ that makes an angle of 85° with the horizontal. The brick follows the path indicated and lands on the shelf. How much work did the gravitational force do on the brick?

Solution: The work done by gravity depends only on the initial and final positions of the object, not on the particular path the object takes. Since the initial height was $h_i = 0$ and the final height was $h_f = 2$ m, the change in the brick's gravitational potential energy is $\Delta PE_{grav} = mgh_f - mgh_i = mgh_f - 0 = mgh_f = (3\text{ kg})(10\text{ N/kg})(2\text{ m}) = 60$ J. Therefore, the work done by the gravitational force is

$$W_{\text{by } \mathbf{F}_{grav}} = -\Delta PE_{grav} = -60 \text{ J}$$

just as we found before.

Friction Is NOT a Conservative Force

Gravity is a conservative force because the work done by gravity depends only on the initial and final positions of the object, not on the path taken. We'll now show that friction is *not* a conservative force; the work done by kinetic friction *does* depend on the path taken.

Consider a flat tabletop and mark two points on it, A and B. We're going to slide a block from Point A to Point B along two different paths; the work done will be different for the two paths, which will show that friction is not a conservative force. The figure below shows the two points, A and B, separated by a distance of 5 m. Another way to get from A to B is to move from A to C and then from C to B; I've chosen a point C that's 3 m from A and 4 m from B.

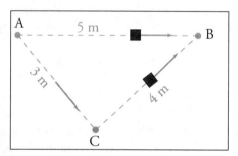

Assume the block has a mass of 1 kg; then its weight is $w = mg = (1\text{ kg})(10\text{ N/kg}) = 10$ N, so the normal force on the block has magnitude 10 N also. If the coefficient of kinetic friction between the block and tabletop is 0.4, then, as the block slides, the magnitude of the force of kinetic friction is $F_f = \mu_k F_N = (0.4)(10\text{ N}) = 4$ N, always directed opposite to the direction in which the block is sliding.

Let's first figure out how much work friction does as we slide the block directly from A to B:

$$W_{\substack{\text{by } F_f \\ A \to B}} = -F_f \cdot d_{A \to B} = -(4\text{ N})(5\text{ m}) = -20 \text{ J}$$

Now let's figure out how much work friction does as we slide the block from A to B by way of C:

$$W_{\substack{\text{by } F_f \\ A \to C \to B}} = W_{\substack{\text{by } F_f \\ A \to C}} + W_{\substack{\text{by } F_f \\ C \to B}} = (-F_f \cdot d_{A \to C}) + (-F_f \cdot d_{C \to B}) = (-4\text{ N})(3\text{ m}) + (-4\text{ N})(4\text{ m}) = -28 \text{ J}$$

Even though we started at A and ended at B in both cases, we got a different amount of work done by friction for two different paths from A to B. Therefore, friction is *not* a conservative force. This means that there's no such thing as "frictional potential energy," because potential energy can be defined only for conservative forces.

6.5 TOTAL MECHANICAL ENERGY

Now that we've defined kinetic energy and potential energy, we can define an object's **total mechanical energy**, E. It's just the sum of the object's kinetic energy and potential energy:

Total Mechanical Energy

$$E = KE + PE$$

For example, consider an object of mass m sitting on a shelf that's at height h above the floor. Then, relative to the floor (where we'll set PE_{grav} equal to 0), the object's total mechanical energy is

$$E = KE + PE = 0 + mgh = mgh$$

Now, what if this same object falls off the shelf? What is its total mechanical energy when its height is, say, $h/2$? If v is the object's speed at this point, then the object's total mechanical energy is

$$E = KE + PE = \tfrac{1}{2}mv^2 + mg\tfrac{h}{2}$$

Example 6-19: An object of mass m is projected straight upward with an initial speed of v_0 at time $t = 0$.

a) What is the object's total mechanical energy at time $t = 0$?
b) At what time t will the object reach its maximum height?
c) What is the maximum height?
d) What is the object's total mechanical energy at this point?

Solution:

a) If we take the object's height at $t = 0$ to be $h = 0$, then its initial total mechanical energy is

$$E = KE + PE = \tfrac{1}{2}mv_0^2 + mg(0) = \tfrac{1}{2}mv_0^2$$

b) When the object reaches the highest point in its vertical path, its velocity is 0. Using Big Five #2 with $a = -g$, we find that

$$v = v_0 + at \;\rightarrow\; 0 = v_0 + \left(-g\right)t \;\rightarrow\; t = \frac{v_0}{g}$$

c) Using Big Five #5, we can find the object's maximum height:

$$v^2 = v_0^2 + 2ad \rightarrow \quad (0)^2 = v_0^2 + 2(-g)d \quad \rightarrow \quad d = -\frac{v_0^2}{2(-g)} = \frac{v_0^2}{2g}$$

6.5

d) The object's total mechanical energy at this point is

$$E = KE + PE = \tfrac{1}{2}mv^2 + mgh = \tfrac{1}{2}m(0)^2 + mg\left(\tfrac{v_0^2}{2g}\right) = 0 + m\tfrac{v_0^2}{2} = \tfrac{1}{2}mv_0^2$$

Notice in this example that the answer to part (d) is the same as the answer to part (a): the object's total mechanical energy at its highest point is the same as it was at the object's initial point. This illustrates a very important concept: the **Conservation of Total Mechanical Energy**. If the only forces acting on an object during its motion are conservative (that means, for example, *no friction*), then the object's total mechanical energy will remain the same throughout the motion. Pick any two positions (or times) during the object's motion; for example, we could pick the initial position (initial time) and the final position (final time). Then

$$E_i = E_f$$

Writing E as $KE + PE$, we have

**Conservation of Total Mechanical Energy
(no nonconservative forces)**

$$KE_i + PE_i = KE_f + PE_f$$

Example 6-20: An object of mass m is projected straight upward with an initial speed of v_0 at time $t = 0$. Use Conservation of Total Mechanical Energy to find its maximum height.

Solution: If we take the object's height at $t = 0$ to be $h = 0$, then its initial total mechanical energy is

$$E = KE_i + PE_i = \tfrac{1}{2}mv_0^2 + mgh = \tfrac{1}{2}mv_0^2 + mg(0) = \tfrac{1}{2}mv_0^2$$

When the object reaches the highest point in its vertical path, its velocity is 0. Calling this height h, the object's total mechanical energy at this point is

$$E = KE_f + PE_f = \frac{1}{2}mv_0^2 + mgh = \frac{1}{2}m(0)^2 + mgh = mgh$$

Therefore, by Conservation of Total Mechanical Energy, we have

$$E_i = E_f$$
$$\tfrac{1}{2}mv_0^2 = mgh$$

$$\therefore h = \frac{v_0^2}{2g}$$

This is the same answer we found in Example 6-19(c) using the Big Five equations.

Another way to think about this problem is in terms of an energy *transformation*. At the moment the object was shot upward, it had only *KE*; at the top of its path, however, it has only *PE*. In other words, kinetic energy was transformed into gravitational potential energy:

$$KE \to PE \to \quad \frac{1}{2}mv_0^2 = mgh \quad \to \quad \therefore h = \frac{v_0^2}{2g}$$

It can be very helpful to think of Conservation of Total Mechanical Energy in terms of energy transformation between *KE* and *PE*. (The MCAT likes to ask questions about such energy transformations.)

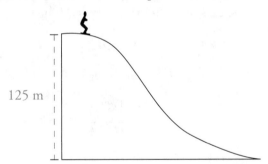

Example 6-21: A skier begins at rest at the top of a hill of height 125 m. If friction between her skis and the snow is negligible, what will be her speed at the bottom of the hill?

Solution: Let the bottom of the hill be $h = 0$, and call the top of the hill the skier's initial position and the bottom of the hill her final position. Then we have

$$KE_i + PE_i = KE_f + PE_f$$
$$0 + mgh = \tfrac{1}{2}mv^2 + 0$$
$$v = \sqrt{2gh}$$
$$= \sqrt{2(10 \text{ m/s}^2)(125 \text{ m})}$$
$$\therefore v = 50 \text{ m/s}$$

We could also think about this problem in terms of an energy transformation. At the top of the hill, the skier had only *PE*; at the bottom of the hill, she has only *KE*. In other words, gravitational potential energy was transformed into kinetic energy:

$$PE \rightarrow KE \rightarrow mgh = \frac{1}{2}mv_0^2 \rightarrow \therefore v = \sqrt{2gh}$$

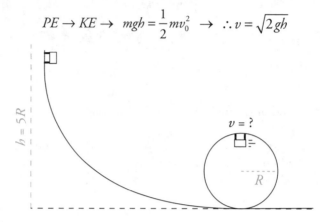

Example 6-22: A roller-coaster car drops from rest down the track and enters a loop. If the radius of the loop is R, and the initial height of the car is $5R$ above the bottom of the loop, how fast is the car going at the top of the loop? Assume that $R = 15$ m and ignore friction.

Solution: Let's call the bottom of the loop our $h = 0$ level. At the car's initial position, we have $h_i = 5R$ and $v_i = 0$ (so $KE_i = 0$). At the top of the loop (the "final" position, for purposes of this question), we have $h_f = 2R$. The question is to find the car's speed, v, at this point. Using Conservation of Total Mechanical Energy, we get

$$KE_i + PE_i = KE_f + PE_f$$
$$0 + mgh_i = \tfrac{1}{2}mv^2 + mgh_f$$
$$gh_i = \tfrac{1}{2}v^2 + gh_f$$
$$v = \sqrt{2g(h_i - h_f)}$$
$$= \sqrt{2g(5R - 2R)}$$
$$= \sqrt{2g \cdot 3R}$$
$$= \sqrt{2(10 \text{ m/s}^2) \cdot 3(15 \text{ m})}$$
$$\therefore v = 30 \text{ m/s}$$

For extra practice, show that the car's speed when it's at the "9 o'clock" position within the loop is $\sqrt{1200}$ m/s ≈ 35 m/s, and that the car's speed when it's at the bottom of the loop is $\sqrt{1500}$ m/s ≈ 39 m/s.[1]

---

[1] For even more practice, compute the centripetal acceleration at these points, and show that the amusement park operator is in danger of being sued. (As a benchmark, consider that fighter pilots with the benefit of pressurized suits risk blacking out at accelerations greater than about $9g \approx 88$ m/s^2.)

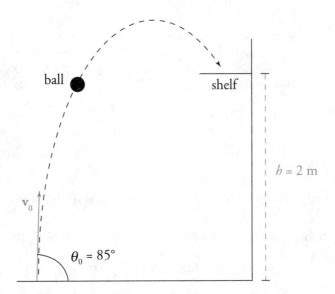

Example 6-23: In the situation pictured above, a ball is projected upward from the floor with an initial velocity v_0 of magnitude 12 m/s that makes an angle of 85° with the horizontal. The ball follows the path indicated and lands on the shelf. How fast is the ball traveling as it hits the shelf? (Ignore air resistance.)

Solution: Let's call the floor our $h = 0$ level. At the object's initial position, we have $h_i = 0$ (so $PE_i = 0$). At the shelf (the final position), we have $h_f = 2$ m. The question is to find the speed of the ball, v, at this point. Using Conservation of Total Mechanical Energy, we get

$$KE_i + PE_i = KE_f + PE_f$$

$$\tfrac{1}{2}mv_0^2 + 0 = \tfrac{1}{2}mv^2 + mgh_f$$

$$\tfrac{1}{2}v_0^2 = \tfrac{1}{2}v^2 + gh_f$$

$$v = \sqrt{v_0^2 - 2gh_f}$$

$$= \sqrt{(12 \text{ m/s}^2)^2 - 2(10 \text{ m/s}^2)(2 \text{ m})}$$

$$\therefore v \approx 10 \text{ m/s}$$

Notice that the direction of the initial velocity vector (given to be "at an angle of 85° with the horizontal") was irrelevant here. One of the most useful attributes of solving problems by Conservation of Total Mechanical Energy is that KE, PE, and E are all *scalars*. This makes it easier to solve questions because we don't have to worry about direction.

Using the Energy Method when There Is Friction

If friction acts during an object's motion, then total mechanical energy is no longer conserved. Consider this example: We give a block of mass 2 kg an initial speed of 6 m/s across a flat surface, where the coefficient of kinetic friction between the block and the surface is $\mu_k = 0.2$.

Kinetic friction will do work as the block slides. If d is the distance the block slides, then the work done by friction will be

$$W_{\text{by } F_f} = -F_f \cdot d = -\mu_k F_N d = -\mu_k mgd = -(0.4)(2 \text{ kg})(10 \tfrac{N}{kg})d = -(4 \text{ N})d$$

In particular, when $d = 9$ m, the work done by friction will be

$$W_{\text{by } F_f} = -(4 \text{ N})d = -(4 \text{ N})(9 \text{ m}) = -36 \text{ J}$$

Since the initial kinetic energy of the block was

$$KE_i = \tfrac{1}{2}mv_0^2 = \tfrac{1}{2}(2 \text{ kg})(6 \text{ m/s})^2 = 36 \text{ J}$$

then the work-energy theorem tells us that the final kinetic energy of the block will be 0:

$$W = \Delta KE = KE_f - KE_i \rightarrow KE_f = KE_i + W = \left(36 \text{ J}\right) + \left(-36 \text{ J}\right) = 0 \text{ J}$$

The block lost KE (and, therefore, E) as it moved because of friction. So, when friction acts, total mechanical energy is not a constant; in other words, it's not conserved.

Despite the fact that total mechanical energy is no longer conserved if friction acts, we can use a *modified* version of the Conservation of Total Mechanical Energy equation to handle questions with friction (or any force besides gravity). We can write this modified equation either in the form

$$E_i + W_{\text{by } \mathbf{F}} = E_f$$

or as:

**Conservation of Total Mechanical Energy
(with outside forces)**

$$KE_i + PE_i + W_{\text{by } \mathbf{F}} = KE_f + PE_f$$

Since $W_{\text{by } F_f}$ is negative, E_f will be less than E_i, just as we expect, since friction takes away mechanical energy.

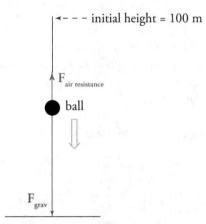

initial height = 100 m

$F_{\text{air resistance}}$

ball

F_{grav}

Example 6-24: A ball of mass 2 kg is dropped from a height of 100 m. As it falls, the ball feels an average force of air resistance of magnitude 4 N. What is the ball's speed as it strikes the ground?

Solution: Let's call the ground our $h = 0$ level. At the object's initial position, we have $h_i = 100$ m and $v_0 = 0$ (so $KE_i = 0$). As it hits the ground (the final position), we have $h_f = 0$ m (so $PE_f = 0$). The question is to find the speed of the ball, v, as it strikes the ground. Because the air resistance is given, and air resistance is friction exerted by the air on the moving object, we need to use the modified version of the energy equation, the one that includes the work done by friction.

Let's figure out the work done by the force of air resistance. Since the displacement of the ball is downward, the force of air resistance is upward; the opposite direction. This tells us that the work done by air resistance is negative, as we expect:

$$W_{\text{by } F_f} = -F_f \cdot h = -(4 \text{ N})(100 \text{ m}) = -400 \text{ J}$$

Therefore, using the modified equation for Conservation of Total Mechanical Energy, we find that

$$KE_i + PE_i + W_{\text{by } F_f} = KE_f + PE_f$$

$$0 + mgh + (-400 \text{ J}) = \tfrac{1}{2}mv^2 + 0$$

$$v = \sqrt{2gh - \frac{800 \text{ J}}{m}}$$

$$= \sqrt{2(10 \text{ m/s}^2)(100 \text{ m}) - \frac{800 \text{ J}}{2 \text{ kg}}}$$

$$= \sqrt{1600 \text{ m}^2/\text{s}^2}$$

Without air resistance, you can check that the ball's speed at impact would have been greater:

$$\sqrt{2000} \text{ m/s} \approx 45 \text{ m/s}$$

6.6 SIMPLE MACHINES AND MECHANICAL ADVANTAGE

Simple machines are tools that allow us to accomplish a variety of tasks with less applied force. Some examples of common simple machines are inclined planes, pulleys, levers, screws, and wheel and axle systems. These machines generally have few or no moving parts. If the simple machine is used in the "ideal world" where there are only conservative forces (i.e., no loss of energy to friction, heat, etc.), the work done to complete the task using the machine is equal to the work that would be required to complete the task without the machine. The difference is that with less applied or effort force, a larger distance must be covered to satisfy the work requirements.[2]

Let's consider the task of lifting a 3 kg brick up to a shelf that is 2 m above the ground.

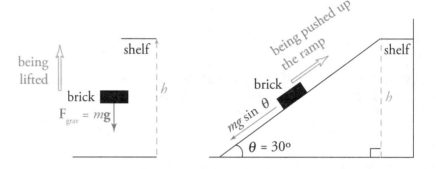

To move a mass straight upward, the applied force, $F_{app_{lift}}$, would need to be at least equal to the force of gravity acting on the mass. Thus, $F_{app_{lift}} \geq F_{grav} = mg = (3 \text{ kg})\left(10 \, \frac{\text{N}}{\text{kg}}\right) = 30 \text{ N}$. The minimum amount of work to lift the brick upward is

$$W_{lift} = F_{app_{lift}} \cdot d = mgh = 60 \text{ J}$$

Now, let's consider the inclined plane shown above. The plane allows us to push the brick up the ramp. If this is a frictionless ramp, the applied force on the ramp, $F_{app_{ramp}}$ would need to overcome the component of F_{grav} parallel to the plane. Thus,

$$F_{app_{ramp}} \geq mg \sin\theta = (3 \text{ kg})(10 \, \tfrac{\text{N}}{\text{kg}})(\sin 30°) = 15 \text{ N}$$

which will be less than $F_{app_{lift}} = mg$ (because the maximum value for sin θ is 1). However, compared to lifting the box straight up through a distance h, the ramp requires you to push the brick over a longer distance, $d = \dfrac{h}{\sin\theta}$. Therefore, the work done to push the brick up the ramp is

$$W_{ramp} = F_{app_{ramp}} \cdot d = (mg \sin\theta) \cdot \left(\frac{h}{\sin\theta}\right) = mgh = 60 \text{ J}$$

---

[2] Simple machines are also used to *increase* distance (and therefore speed) while *decreasing* force; this does not change the way we analyze the situation.

The work required to move a brick to a height of h is the same, regardless of whether you lift it straight upward or push it up a ramp.

The fact that the inclined plane allows your effort force or applied force to be decreased in comparison to the straight lift is called **mechanical advantage**. Mechanical advantage can be quantified into a factor that describes precisely how much less force is required when using that particular simple machine. In other words, mechanical advantage tells us the factor by which the mechanism multiplies the input or effort force.

Mechanical Advantage

$$\text{mechanical advantage } (MA) = \frac{\text{resistance force}}{\text{effort force}} = \frac{F_{\text{resistance}}}{F_{\text{effort}}}$$

Resistance force is the force that would be applied if no machine were being used, and *effort force* is the force applied with the machine. Mechanical advantage is also sometimes expressed as $F_{\text{out}} / F_{\text{in}}$.

For the previous example of the inclined plane, the mechanical advantage of the ramp would be

$$MA = \frac{F_{\text{resistance}}}{F_{\text{effort}}} = \frac{mg}{mg \sin \theta} = \frac{1}{\sin 30°} = \frac{1}{\frac{1}{2}} = 2$$

Therefore, this specific inclined plane with an angle of $\theta = 30°$ has a mechanical advantage of 2, allowing it to "multiply" the input force $F_{\text{app}_{\text{ramp}}} = 15 \text{ N}$ by a factor of 2 to give the force that would have been required without the machine, $F_{\text{app}_{\text{lift}}} = 30 \text{ N}$.

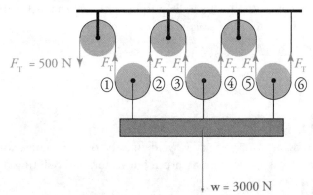

As another example, look back at Example 4-23 which shows a system consisting of 6 pulleys used to lift a plank. The plank weighs 3000 N, but we only have to exert a force of 500 N to lift it. The mechanical advantage is therefore equal to 3000 N/500 N = 6.

Efficiency

So far, we have described simple machines that are used in the ideal world. However, if the machine is used in the real world, we have to take into consideration the possibility of energy losses to the surroundings. In general, the actual mechanical advantage of a machine is less than its ideal mechanical advantage. The fact that the machine does not work as well in the real world leads us to the concept of **efficiency**. The efficiency of any machine measures the degree to which friction and other factors reduce the actual work output of the machine from its theoretical maximum. This can be calculated by examining the ratio of the useful energy output versus the supplied or input energy.

Efficiency

$$\text{Efficiency (\%)} = \frac{W_{\text{output}}}{\text{Energy}_{\text{input}}}$$

A machine that operates in the ideal world has an efficiency of 100% because it has no loss of energy to its surroundings. However, a machine with an efficiency of 50% has an output only one-half of its theoretical output. By calculating a machine's efficiency, we can determine what percentage of energy is being lost to heat, sound, light, etc.

How does an efficiency of less than 100% affect mechanical advantage? For the inclined plane example, the presence of friction would reduce the efficiency, since some of the work done to push the block up would be lost as heat. In terms of force, the minimum applied force (the effort force) would now have to be enough to balance the component of gravity down the inclined plane plus the force of kinetic friction.

$$F_{\text{effort}} = mg \sin\theta + F_{\text{f}} = mg \sin\theta + \mu_k mg \cos\theta$$

Since $MA = F_{\text{resistance}} / F_{\text{effort}}$, and the resistance force remains the same, the mechanical advantage will decrease. This makes sense conceptually, since the purpose of using the inclined plane is to reduce force. There will be less of an advantage to using a plane with friction.

6.7 MOMENTUM

For an object of mass m moving with velocity **v**, we define the object's **momentum**, **p**, as the product of m and **v**. Notice that because **v** is a vector, momentum is a vector, too, pointing in the same direction as **v** (because m is always a *positive* scalar).

Momentum

$$\mathbf{p} = m\mathbf{v}$$

The SI unit of momentum is just the kg·m/s; there's no special name for it.

Example 6-25: A car whose mass is 2000 kg is traveling at a velocity of 15 m/s due east. What is its momentum? How does its momentum compare to that of a car whose mass is 2000 kg traveling at a velocity of 15 m/s due west?

Solution: Since $\mathbf{p} = m\mathbf{v}$, we have $\mathbf{p} = (2000 \text{ kg})(15 \text{ m/s, east}) = 30{,}000 \text{ kg·m/s, east}$. If we call *east* the positive direction, then we can write $\mathbf{p} = +30{,}000 \text{ kg·m/s}$. For the car traveling west, the magnitude of its momentum will be the same, 30,000 kg·m/s, but the direction of its momentum will be to the west. So, if *east* is again the positive direction, then *west* is the negative direction, and we'd write $\mathbf{p} = -30{,}000 \text{ kg·m/s}$. Remember, momentum is a vector, and its direction must be taken into account.

$\mathbf{p} = -30{,}000 \text{ kg·m/s}$ $\mathbf{p} = +30{,}000 \text{ kg·m/s}$

Example 6-26: An object of mass m is moving with velocity $\mathbf{v}$. What will happen to its momentum if v doubles? What will happen to its kinetic energy?

Solution: Momentum has something in common with kinetic energy: namely, only moving objects have it. Also, the more massive an object, or the greater its velocity, the greater its momentum (and kinetic energy). However, there are two important differences. First, kinetic energy is a scalar, while momentum is a vector. Second, kinetic energy is proportional to v^2 whereas the magnitude of momentum is proportional only to v. So, if the object's speed doubles, then its momentum doubles while its kinetic energy increases by a factor of 4.

Now that we've defined momentum, let's see how it applies to the MCAT.

Impulse

Let's say we exert a force $\mathbf{F}$ on an object of mass m over a time interval Δt. We can use Newton's second law, $\mathbf{F} = m\mathbf{a}$, to predict the effect of this force. Because $\mathbf{a} = \Delta\mathbf{v}/\Delta t$, we can rewrite $\mathbf{F} = m\mathbf{a}$ as

$$\mathbf{F} = m\frac{\Delta\mathbf{v}}{\Delta t}$$

Multiplying both sides by Δt gives

$$\mathbf{F}\Delta t = m\Delta\mathbf{v}$$

If the object's mass remains constant, then $m\Delta\mathbf{v}$ is the same as $\Delta(m\mathbf{v})$, so we get

$$\mathbf{F}\Delta t = \Delta(m\mathbf{v})$$

We now recognize the quantity on the right-hand side as $\Delta\mathbf{p}$, the change in momentum. The quantity on the left-hand side, force multiplied by time, is called **impulse**, denoted by $\mathbf{J}$. (Don't confuse the variable for impulse, $\mathbf{J}$, with the abbreviation for the joule, J.) So, this last equation can be written simply as $\mathbf{J} = \Delta\mathbf{p}$. This alternative way of expressing Newton's second law is known as the "Impulse-Momentum Theorem."

6.7

> **Impulse-Momentum Theorem**
>
> $$\mathbf{J} = \Delta\mathbf{p} = \Delta(m\mathbf{v}) = \mathbf{F}\Delta t$$

Example 6-27: A batter strikes a pitched baseball (mass = 0.15 kg) that was moving horizontally at 40 m/s, and it leaves his bat moving at a speed of 50 m/s directly back toward the pitcher. The bat was in contact with the baseball for 15 ms.

- a) What's the baseball's change in momentum?
- b) What's the impulse of the force exerted by the batter?
- c) What's the magnitude of the average force exerted by the bat on the ball?

Solution:

a) Since we're dealing with momentum, which is a vector, we need to define our positive direction. Let's choose *toward the pitcher* as the positive direction. This means that the initial momentum of the baseball (the momentum it had on its way from the pitcher to the batter) was negative, and the final momentum of the baseball (which is its momentum after the batter hits it) is positive. This gives

$$\mathbf{p}_i = m\mathbf{v}_i = \left(0.15 \text{ kg}\right)\left(-40 \text{ m/s}\right) = -6 \tfrac{\text{kg·m}}{\text{s}} \text{ and } \mathbf{p}_f = m\mathbf{v}_f = \left(0.15 \text{ kg}\right)\left(+50 \text{ m/s}\right) = 7.5 \tfrac{\text{kg·m}}{\text{s}}$$

So the change in the baseball's momentum is

$$\Delta\mathbf{p} = \mathbf{p}_f - \mathbf{p}_i = \left(+7.5 \tfrac{\text{kg·m}}{\text{s}}\right) - \left(-6 \tfrac{\text{kg·m}}{\text{s}}\right) = +13.5 \tfrac{\text{kg·m}}{\text{s}}$$

b) Impulse is equal to force multiplied by the time during which it acts. However, we are not told what the force is; in fact, we're asked that in part (c). So we need another way of figuring out the impulse. The impulse-momentum theorem tells us that the impulse is equal to the change in momentum, which we just computed in part (a). Since $\Delta\mathbf{p}$ = +13.5 kg·m/s, this is also the impulse of the force. (We can also write the unit as a newton-second, N·s, which is the most natural unit for impulse: $J = F\Delta t$ implies that $[J] = [F][\Delta t]$ = N·s. However, the unit of momentum, kg·m/s, is the same as the unit of impulse, N·s, so we could say that J = +13.5 N·s.)

c) Now that we know J, we can use the definition $J = F\Delta t$ to find F:

$$J = F\Delta t \rightarrow \quad F = \frac{J}{\Delta t} = \frac{13.5 \text{ N·s}}{0.015 \text{ s}} = 900 \text{ N}$$

Because F usually varies while it acts, this is actually the *average* force exerted by the bat.

To be more precise, we should place a bar over the F and write the definition of impulse as $J = \overline{F}\Delta t$.

Example 6-28: The graph at the right shows how a force **F** acting on an object of mass $m = 1$ kg varies as a function of time.

a) What is the magnitude of the impulse of this force?
b) If the object's initial velocity is +2 m/s, what will be the object's velocity after this force acts?

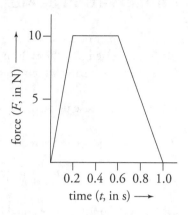

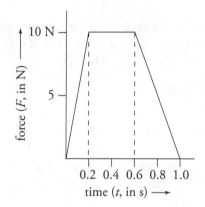

Solution:

a) Because impulse is equal to force × time, the area under a force vs. time graph gives the impulse. (Compare this to the fact mentioned earlier in the chapter that work is equal to the area under a force vs. position graph.) The area under the graph shown can be split into two right triangles and a rectangle, so the total area under the graph is

area = (first triangle) + (rectangle) + (second triangle)

$$= \tfrac{1}{2}(0.2 \text{ s})(10 \text{ N}) + (0.6 \text{ s} - 0.2 \text{ s})(10 \text{ N}) + \tfrac{1}{2}(1 \text{ s} - 0.6 \text{ s})(10 \text{ N})$$

$$= (1 \text{ N} \cdot \text{s}) + (4 \text{ N} \cdot \text{s}) + (2 \text{ N} \cdot \text{s})$$

$$\therefore J = 7 \text{ N} \cdot \text{s}$$

b) The impulse-momentum theorem says $\mathbf{J} = \Delta\mathbf{p} = \mathbf{p}_f - \mathbf{p}_i$, so

$$\mathbf{p}_f - \mathbf{p}_i = \mathbf{J} \rightarrow m\mathbf{v}_f = m\mathbf{v}_i + \mathbf{J}$$

$$\mathbf{v}_f = \mathbf{v}_i + \frac{\mathbf{J}}{m}$$

$$= (+2 \text{ m/s}) + \frac{7 \text{ N} \cdot \text{s}}{1 \text{ kg}}$$

$$= (+2 \text{ m/s}) + (7 \text{ m/s})$$

$$\therefore \mathbf{v}_f = +9 \text{ m/s}$$

Conservation of Momentum

Consider a pair of objects, 1 and 2, that exert forces (an action/reaction pair) on each other. Let $\mathbf{F}_{\text{1-on-2}}$ be the force exerted by Object 1 on Object 2, let $\mathbf{F}_{\text{2-on-1}}$ be the force exerted by Object 2 on Object 1, and let Δt be the time during which these forces act.

What's the impulse delivered by $\mathbf{F}_{\text{1-on-2}}$? It's $\mathbf{J}_{\text{1-on-2}} = \mathbf{F}_{\text{1-on-2}}\Delta t$

What's the impulse delivered by $\mathbf{F}_{\text{2-on-1}}$? It's $\mathbf{J}_{\text{2-on-1}} = \mathbf{F}_{\text{2-on-1}}\Delta t$

Now, since $\mathbf{F}_{\text{1-on-2}} = -\mathbf{F}_{\text{2-on-1}}$ by Newton's third law, we'll automatically have $\mathbf{J}_{\text{1-on-2}} = -\mathbf{J}_{\text{2-on-1}}$

Okay, so the impulses are equal but opposite. What will that do? By the impulse-momentum theorem, we know that $\mathbf{J}_{\text{1-on-2}} = \Delta\mathbf{p}_2$, where $\Delta\mathbf{p}_2$ is the change in momentum of Object 2, and that $\mathbf{J}_{\text{2-on-1}} = \Delta\mathbf{p}_1$, where $\Delta\mathbf{p}_1$ is the change in momentum of Object 1. So, because $\mathbf{J}_{\text{1-on-2}} = -\mathbf{J}_{\text{2-on-1}}$, we have

$$\Delta\mathbf{p}_2 = -\Delta\mathbf{p}_1$$

Therefore, the momentum changes of the two objects are equal but opposite too.

Now what if we ask, what's the change in momentum of both objects *together*? That is, what's $\Delta(\mathbf{p}_1 + \mathbf{p}_2)$? Well, if $\Delta\mathbf{p}_1$ and $\Delta\mathbf{p}_2$ are equal but opposite, then the total change in momentum is zero:

$$\Delta\mathbf{p}_2 + \Delta\mathbf{p}_1 \rightarrow \Delta\mathbf{p}_1 + \Delta\mathbf{p}_2 = 0 \rightarrow \Delta(\mathbf{p}_1 + \mathbf{p}_2) = 0$$

If the total momentum, $\mathbf{p}_1 + \mathbf{p}_2$, doesn't change, then it's a constant. We say that the total momentum is *conserved*.

In summary, what is shown above is simply that Newton's third law implies that when two objects interact only with each other, their total momentum doesn't change. That is, the total momentum *of the system* doesn't change. In fact, we could have any number of mutually interacting objects, not just two, and the result would be the same: The total momentum of the system will remain constant. This fact has the same stature as the Law of Conservation of Total Mechanical Energy, and it's called the Law of Conservation of Momentum:

Law of Conservation of Momentum

$$\Delta\mathbf{p}_{\text{system}} = 0$$

or

$$\text{total } \mathbf{p}_i = \text{total } \mathbf{p}_f$$

This law says that if a system of interacting objects feels no net external force (that is, if the forces the objects feel are only from other objects within the system) then the total momentum of the system will remain constant. The *individual* momenta of the objects in the system certainly can change, but always in such a way that their sum, the total momentum of all the objects, *doesn't* change. The second form of the law, total $\mathbf{p}_i$ = total $\mathbf{p}_f$, simply says that if we find the total momentum of an isolated system at one moment and then find the total momentum of the system at some later time, we'll get the same answer. We'll usually find it more convenient to use this second form when we solve problems, but of course, the two forms of the law say exactly the same thing.

Strictly speaking, the quantity $\mathbf{p}$ = $m\mathbf{v}$ is known as **linear momentum**, so the law "$\Delta\mathbf{p}_{system} = 0$" or "total $\mathbf{p}_i$ = total $\mathbf{p}_f$" is known as the Law of Conservation of Linear Momentum. (There's another kind of momentum studied in physics: *angular momentum*. Since we rarely worry about this type of momentum for the MCAT, we just use the word "momentum" for "linear momentum.")

Example 6-29: An astronaut (total mass, body + suit + equipment = 100 kg) is floating at rest in deep space near her ship, when she notices that the cord that's supposed to keep her connected to the ship has broken. She reaches into her pocket, finds a metal tool of mass 1 kg and throws it out into space with a velocity of 10 m/s, directly away from the ship. If she's 5 m away from the ship, how long will it take her to reach it?

Solution: Consider the astronaut and the metal tool as the system. Initially, both are at rest, so their total momentum is zero. Because of the Law of Conservation of Momentum, $\Delta\mathbf{p}_{system} = 0$, we know that after the astronaut throws the tool, the total momentum will still be zero:

$$m_{astronaut}\mathbf{v}'_{astronaut} + m_{tool}\mathbf{v}'_{tool} = 0$$

We can now solve for the astronaut's velocity after throwing the tool:

$$m_{astronaut}\mathbf{v}'_{astronaut} = -m_{tool}\mathbf{v}'_{tool}$$
$$\mathbf{v}'_{astronaut} = -\frac{m_{tool}\mathbf{v}'_{tool}}{m_{astronaut}}$$
$$= -\frac{(1 \text{ kg})(-10 \text{ m/s})}{100 \text{ kg}}$$
$$\therefore \mathbf{v}'_{astronaut} = 0.1 \text{ m/s}$$

The minus sign on $\mathbf{v}'_{tool}$ simply indicates that we're calling *away from the ship* the negative direction; as a result, the astronaut's velocity is in the opposite direction, toward the ship and positive. Now, the question is, traveling at a rate of 0.1 m/s, how long will it take her to move the 5 m to the ship? Using distance = rate × time, we find that

$$t = \frac{d}{v} = \frac{5 \text{ m}}{0.1 \text{ m/s}} = 50 \text{ s}$$

6.7

Example 6-30: A radioactive atom of polonium-204, initially at rest, undergoes alpha decay. Show that, as a result of ejecting the alpha particle, the daughter nucleus recoils with a speed equal to 2% of the speed of the alpha particle.

Solution: Initially, the parent nucleus is at rest, so its total momentum is zero. Because of the Law of Conservation of Momentum, $\Delta\mathbf{p}_{system} = 0$, we know that after the decay, the total momentum of the daughter atom (actually, ion, but we'll ignore the electrons because they're such a small portion of the mass) and the alpha particle will still be zero; that is, $m_D\mathbf{v}_D + m_\alpha\mathbf{v}_\alpha = 0$, where D represents the daughter. This gives

$$m_D\mathbf{v}_D = -m_\alpha\mathbf{v}_\alpha \quad \rightarrow \quad \mathbf{v}_D = -\frac{m_\alpha}{m_D}\mathbf{v}_\alpha \quad \rightarrow \quad v_D = -\frac{m_\alpha}{m_D}v_\alpha$$

Now, since the daughter atom has a mass number that's 4 less than that of the parent, we'll have $m_D = 204 - 4 \approx 200$ u; and, since we know that $m_\alpha \approx 4$ u, we find that

$$v_D = -\frac{m_\alpha}{m_D}v_\alpha = -\frac{4\text{ u}}{200\text{ u}}v_\alpha = -\frac{1}{50}v_\alpha = -2\% \cdot v_\alpha$$

Collisions

Conservation of momentum is used to analyze collisions between objects. For example, consider this situation:

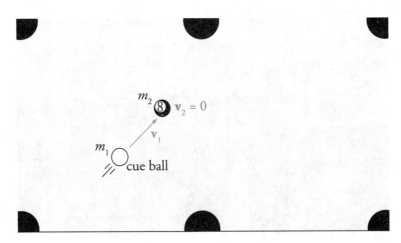

Let the cue ball and the 8-ball constitute our *system*, that is, the objects whose impending collision we're going to analyze. Before the collision, the cue ball is moving toward the 8-ball with a certain velocity, $\mathbf{v}_1$, and the 8-ball is at rest ($\mathbf{v}_2 = 0$). After the collision, the individual velocities of the objects change, to $\mathbf{v}_1'$ and $\mathbf{v}_2'$, respectively,

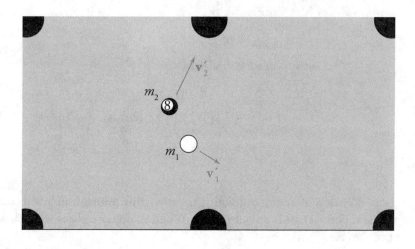

but in such a way that the *total* momentum *doesn't* change, because we must have $\Delta\mathbf{p}_{\text{system}} = 0$. Equivalently, we can say that $\mathbf{p}_{\text{total}}$ before the collision is equal to $\mathbf{p}_{\text{total}}$ after the collision:

$$\mathbf{P}_{\text{total before}} = \mathbf{P}_{\text{total after}}$$
$$m_1\mathbf{v}_1 + m_2\mathbf{v}_2 = m_1\mathbf{v}_1' + m_2\mathbf{v}_2'$$
$$m_1\mathbf{v}_1 = m_1\mathbf{v}_1' + m_2\mathbf{v}_2'$$

In this case, $\mathbf{v}_2 = 0$, which is why the term $m_2\mathbf{v}_2$ dropped out of the last equation.

Let's look at a simpler collision, one in which the motion of the objects is along a straight line.

Example 6-31: Ball 1 rolls with velocity $\mathbf{v}_1 = 5\frac{m}{s}$ toward Ball 2, which is initially at rest. Ball 1 has a mass of $m_1 = 1\ \text{kg}$, and Ball 2 has a mass of $m_2 = 4\ \text{kg}$. After the collision, Ball 2 is observed to move with a velocity of $\mathbf{v}_2' = 2\ \text{m/s}$. What's the velocity of Ball 1 after the collision?

before the collision

$\mathbf{v}_2 = 0$

$\mathbf{v}_1 = 5$ m/s

(1) (2)

after the collision

$\mathbf{v}_1' = ?$

$\mathbf{v}_2' = 2$ m/s

(1)(2)

Solution: Using Conservation of Momentum, we get

$$\mathbf{P}_{\text{total before}} = \mathbf{P}_{\text{total after}}$$

$$m_1\mathbf{v}_1 + m_2\mathbf{v}_2 = m_1\mathbf{v}_1' + m_2\mathbf{v}_2'$$

$$m_1\mathbf{v}_1 = m_1\mathbf{v}_1' + m_2\mathbf{v}_2'$$

$$(1 \text{ kg})(5 \text{ m/s}) = (1 \text{ kg})\mathbf{v}_1' + (4 \text{ kg})(2 \text{ m/s})$$

$$\therefore \mathbf{v}_1' = -3 \text{ m/s}$$

Notice that the velocity of Ball 1 after the collision is negative; this means it points to the left (since we called velocities to the right positive). This isn't surprising. When an object collides with a heavier object, the lighter object often bounces backward.

after the collision

$$\mathbf{v}_1' = -3 \text{ m/s} \qquad \mathbf{v}_2' = 2 \text{ m/s}$$

Example 6-32: Ball 1 and Ball 2 are rolling toward each other at the same speed, 5 m/s. Ball 1 has a mass of $m_1 = 8$ kg, and Ball 2 has a mass of $m_2 = 2$ kg. After the collision, Ball 1 is observed to move with a velocity of 2 m/s in the same direction as $\mathbf{v}_1$. What's the velocity of Ball 2 after the collision?

before the collision

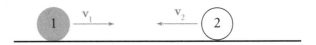

after the collision

$$\mathbf{v}_2' = ?$$
$$\mathbf{v}_1' = 2 \text{ m/s}$$

Solution: Since $\mathbf{v}_1$ and $\mathbf{v}_2$ point in opposite directions, we need to choose which direction to call positive. Let's choose *to the right* as our positive direction; then $\mathbf{v}_1 = +5$ m/s and $\mathbf{v}_2 = -5$ m/s. Now, using Conservation of Momentum, we get

$$\mathbf{P}_{\text{total before}} = \mathbf{P}_{\text{total after}}$$

$$m_1\mathbf{v}_1 + m_2\mathbf{v}_2 = m_1\mathbf{v}_1' + m_2\mathbf{v}_2'$$

$$(8 \text{ kg})(+5 \text{ m/s}) + (2 \text{ kg})(-5 \text{ m/s}) = (8 \text{ kg})(+2 \text{ m/s}) + (2 \text{ kg})\mathbf{v}_2'$$

$$30\tfrac{\text{kg·m}}{\text{s}} = 16\tfrac{\text{kg·m}}{\text{s}} + (2 \text{ kg})\mathbf{v}_2'$$

$$14\tfrac{\text{kg·m}}{\text{s}} = (2 \text{ kg})\mathbf{v}_2'$$

$$\therefore \mathbf{v}_2' = +7 \text{ m/s}$$

6.7

Notice that the velocity of Ball 2 after the collision is positive; this means it points to the right (since we called velocities to the right positive). This isn't surprising. When a heavy object collides with a lighter one, the lighter object often gets pushed forward.

after the collision

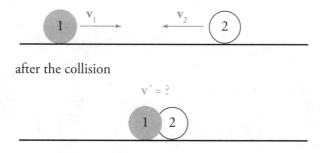

Now that we've looked at some collisions, it's time to classify them. Collisions can be grouped into two major types: elastic and inelastic. A collision is said to be **elastic** if the total *kinetic* energy is conserved also. (Notice I say "also," because total *momentum* is already conserved.) A collision is said to be **inelastic** if total kinetic energy is *not* conserved. Further, as a subcategory of inelastic collisions, we have **perfectly** (or **completely**) **inelastic** collisions; on the MCAT, these are collisions in which the objects stick together afterwards.[3] *Perfectly inelastic collisions are the MCAT's favorite type.*

> **Elastic Collision:** Total momentum *and* total kinetic energy are conserved.
> **Inelastic Collision:** Total momentum is conserved but total kinetic energy is not.
> **Perfectly Inelastic:** An inelastic collision in which the objects stick together afterwards.

Example 6-33: Ball 1 and Ball 2 are rolling toward each other at the same speed, 5 m/s. Ball 1 has a mass of $m_1 = 8$ kg, and Ball 2 has a mass of $m_2 = 2$ kg. After the collision, Ball 1 and Ball 2 stick together and slide frictionlessly across the table. What's their common velocity after the collision?

before the collision

after the collision

---

[3] Technically, a perfectly inelastic collision is one in which the loss of kinetic energy is as great as possible (consistent with Conservation of Momentum). Luckily, we don't need to worry about this definition, because collisions in which the objects stick together are always perfectly inelastic.

Solution: Choosing *to the right* as our positive direction, we have $\mathbf{v}_1 = +5$ m/s and $\mathbf{v}_1 = -5$ m/s. Now, using Conservation of Momentum, we get

$$\mathbf{P}_{\text{total before}} = \mathbf{P}_{\text{total after}}$$

$$m_1 \mathbf{v}_1 + m_2 \mathbf{v}_2 = (m_1 + m_2) \mathbf{v}'$$

$$(8 \text{ kg})(+5 \text{ m/s}) + (2 \text{ kg})(-5 \text{ m/s}) = (8 \text{ kg} + 2 \text{ kg}) \mathbf{v}'$$

$$30 \tfrac{\text{kg·m}}{\text{s}} = (10 \text{ kg}) \mathbf{v}'$$

$$\therefore \mathbf{v}' = +3 \text{ m/s}$$

6.7

The MCAT likes these collisions because the math is easier; after the collision, we have just one object, with a combined mass of $m_1 + m_2$, moving with a *single* velocity, $\mathbf{v}'$.

after the collision

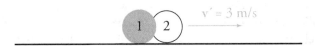

Example 6-34: Recall Example 6-31: Ball 1 rolled with velocity $\mathbf{v}_1 = 5$ m/s toward Ball 2, which was initially at rest. Ball 1's mass was $m_1 = 1$ kg, and Ball 2's mass was $m_2 = 4$ kg. After the collision, Ball 2 moved with a velocity of $v_2' = 2$ m/s. We found that the velocity of Ball 1 after the collision was $v_1' = -3$ m/s. Was this collision elastic or was it inelastic?

before the collision

after the collision

Solution: We need to decide whether total kinetic energy was conserved. Consider the following:

$$KE_{\text{before collision}} = \tfrac{1}{2} m_1 v_1^2 + \tfrac{1}{2} m_2 v_2^2 = \tfrac{1}{2}(1 \text{ kg})(5 \text{ m/s})^2 + 0 = \tfrac{25}{2} \text{ J}$$

and

$$KE_{\text{after collision}} = \tfrac{1}{2} m_1 v_1'^2 + \tfrac{1}{2} m_2 v_2'^2 = \tfrac{1}{2}(1 \text{ kg})(3 \text{ m/s})^2 + \tfrac{1}{2}(4 \text{ kg})(2 \text{ m/s})^2 = \tfrac{25}{2} \text{ J}$$

Since the kinetic energy was conserved in this case, we can conclude that this collision was elastic.

Example 6-35: Recall Example 6-32: Ball 1 and Ball 2 were rolling toward each other at the same speed, 5 m/s. Ball 1's mass was $m_1 = 8 \text{ kg}$, and Ball 2's mass was $m_2 = 2 \text{ kg}$. After the collision, Ball 1 moved with a velocity of 2 m/s in the same direction as $\mathbf{v}_1$. We found that the velocity of Ball 2 after the collision was 7 m/s. Was this collision elastic or was it inelastic?

Solution: We need to check whether total kinetic energy was conserved. Consider the following:

$$KE_{\text{before collision}} = \tfrac{1}{2}m_1 v_1^2 + \tfrac{1}{2}m_2 v_2^2 = \tfrac{1}{2}(8 \text{ kg})(5 \text{ m/s})^2 + \tfrac{1}{2}(2 \text{ kg})(5 \text{ m/s})^2 = 125 \text{ J}$$

and

$$KE_{\text{after collision}} = \tfrac{1}{2}m_1 v_1'^2 + \tfrac{1}{2}m_2 v_2'^2 = \tfrac{1}{2}(8 \text{ kg})(2 \text{ m/s})^2 + \tfrac{1}{2}(2 \text{ kg})(7 \text{ m/s})^2 = 65 \text{ J}$$

6.7

Since the kinetic energy was not conserved in this case, we can conclude that this collision was inelastic. This is what happens with macroscopic objects that collide. Some of the initial kinetic energy is converted to other forms: heat (mostly) and sound. The objects may also suffer some permanent deformation, which can also use up some of the pre-collision kinetic energy.

Example 6-36: In the process of phagocytosis, a neutrophil collides with a potentially harmful bacterium in the blood and completely envelops it. Suppose the bacterium with about one hundredth the mass of the neutrophil was stationary when absorbed by the neutrophil moving at speed v. What kind of collision is this, and what percentage of its kinetic energy did the neutrophil lose in the collision?

Solution: First, if one object is absorbed by the other in a collision, this clearly must be a perfectly inelastic collision: only one mass emerges! The final velocity of the neutrophil will be given by the conservation of momentum: $mv + 0 = (m + 0.01m)v_f$, so $v_f = (1/1.01)v \approx 0.99v$. The change in kinetic energy then is given by

$$\Delta KE = \frac{1}{2}(1.01)m(0.99v)^2 - \frac{1}{2}mv^2 \approx \frac{1}{2}(0.99mv^2 - mv^2) = -0.01\left(\frac{1}{2}mv^2\right)$$

In other words, a loss of about 1% of the initial kinetic energy results from this perfectly inelastic collision. If one object is much more massive than another, it won't lose much if it collides with the smaller object, unless that object is moving relatively fast in the opposite direction. Completely inelastic collisions always result in the maximum possible loss of kinetic energy.

After our work on the Conservation of Total Mechanical Energy, you might be tempted to solve collision problems by Conservation of Energy. *Don't.* Total kinetic energy is conserved only for elastic collisions, and these are very special. In the everyday world of macroscopic-sized objects, collisions result in a loss of energy due to heat, sound, and deformation, so all such collisions are, by definition, *not* elastic. (In the subatomic domain, when particles such as neutrons and protons run into each other, elastic collisions are common.) So, the moral is: Unless the question specifically says, "Assume the collision is elastic," or "Assume that energy losses are negligible," then you should never assume that a collision between macroscopic-sized objects is elastic. And even if a collision is (or can be treated as) elastic, you can still use Conservation of Momentum, because total momentum is conserved in both types of collisions, elastic *and* inelastic.

Example 6-37: A fast-moving neutron collides with another neutron initially at rest. Could such a collision be elastic? If so, describe what would happen.

Solution: Yes, a collision between subatomic particles could be elastic. Assume that before the collision, the moving neutron had velocity **v** and the target neutron was at rest. If the resulting collision is elastic, the moving neutron hits the target and stops, and the target neutron moves away with the same velocity, **v**, that the first one had coming in to the collision. In other words, the moving neutron gives up all its momentum and kinetic energy to the target neutron. This conserves both total momentum and kinetic energy, and describes an elastic collision.

before the collision   after the collision

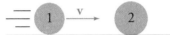 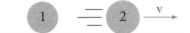

6.8

6.8   A NOTE ON ANGULAR MOMENTUM

In Section 5.5, we introduced moment of inertia, I, as the rotational analog (or rotational version) of mass, m. Similarly, torque is viewed as the rotational version of force. The rotational version of Newton's second law, $F_{net} = ma$, is then $\tau_{net} = I\alpha$, where α is the rotational acceleration.

We can also study the rotational version of linear momentum; it's known as **angular momentum**. Just as torque is defined with respect to some reference point (the pivot), an object's angular momentum must also be defined relative to some reference point. Consider a particle of mass m and velocity **v**. If P is some reference point, let ℓ be the "lever arm" from P to the particle such that ℓ is perpendicular to **v**. The particle's angular momentum, usually denoted by the letter L, is then defined to be ℓmv.

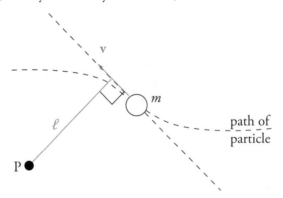

It may be helpful to notice that angular momentum is ℓp, where p is linear momentum. That is, to figure out the rotational version of linear momentum, we just multiply by ℓ. This is just like the formula for torque: to calculate the rotational version of force, we just multiply by ℓ: $\tau = \ell F$.

Example 6-38: A particle of mass 3 kg moves with speed 5 m/s around a circle of radius 60 cm. What is the magnitude of its momentum? Its angular momentum?

Solution: The magnitude of the particle's linear momentum is

$$p = mv = (3 \text{ kg})(5 \text{ m/s}) = 15 \tfrac{\text{kg} \cdot \text{m}}{\text{s}}$$

Now, for an object of mass m moving at speed v around a circle of radius r, its angular momentum relative to the center of the circle is rmv, since the lever arm ℓ will always be equal to r, the radius of the circle (see the figure below). Therefore,

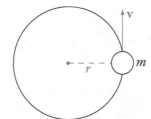

$$L = rmv = (0.6 \text{ m})(3 \text{ kg})(5 \text{ m/s}) = 9 \tfrac{\text{kg} \cdot \text{m}^2}{\text{s}}$$

Another way to determine an object's angular momentum is to form the rotational version of the equation $p = mv$. We already know the rotational version of m; it's I, the moment of inertia. The rotational version of v is ω, the angular velocity. (Angular velocity is measured in radians per second because it tells us how fast the object's *angular* position is changing.) Therefore, $L = I\omega$.

Angular Momentum

$$L = \ell mv = I\omega$$

Example 6-39: The moment of inertia of a solid sphere of mass m and radius r is $\tfrac{2}{5}mr^2$, and the moment of inertia of a hollow sphere of mass m and radius r is $\tfrac{2}{3}mr^2$. Which has more angular momentum: a solid bowling ball of mass 7 kg rolling with an angular velocity of 10 rad/s, or a hollow bowling ball of the same radius but mass 4 kg rolling with an angular velocity of 12 rad/s?

Solution: We use the equation $L = I\omega$ to compare the angular momenta of the two bowling balls:

$$\frac{L_{\text{solid}}}{L_{\text{hollow}}} = \frac{I_{\text{solid}}\omega_{\text{solid}}}{I_{\text{hollow}}\omega_{\text{hollow}}} = \frac{\tfrac{2}{5}mr^2 \cdot \omega_{\text{solid}}}{\tfrac{2}{3}mr^2 \cdot \omega_{\text{hollow}}} = \frac{3}{5} \cdot \frac{7 \text{ kg}}{4 \text{ kg}} \cdot \frac{10 \tfrac{\text{rad}}{\text{s}}}{12 \tfrac{\text{rad}}{\text{s}}} = \frac{210}{240} < 1$$

This means that $L_{\text{solid}} < L_{\text{hollow}}$, so the hollow ball has the greater angular momentum.

The impulse-momentum theorem (which is equivalent to Newton's second law) says $\mathbf{J} = \Delta\mathbf{p}$. That is, the change in momentum of an object is equal to the impulse delivered to it. So, the greater the desired change in momentum, the greater the impulse required, and this means we must either apply a stronger force, or apply the force for more time. The impulse-momentum theorem can also be written in another way:

$$\mathbf{J} = \Delta\mathbf{p} \;\rightarrow\; \mathbf{F}\Delta t = \Delta\mathbf{p} \;\rightarrow\; \mathbf{F} = \frac{\Delta\mathbf{p}}{\Delta t}$$

In this last form, the equation says that force is the rate of change of linear momentum. The rotational version of this statement would be:

$$\text{torque is the rate of change of angular momentum: } \tau = \frac{\Delta L}{\Delta t}$$

Example 6-40: Consider the two bowling balls described in the preceding example. If we want to stop each ball from rolling by applying a torque for 1 second, which ball would require more torque?

Solution: Since the rate of change of angular momentum is equal to the torque, the fact that the hollow ball has more angular momentum means that we'd have to exert a greater torque on the hollow ball to stop it from rotating.

Finally, one of the most important consequences of the impulse-momentum theorem and Newton's third law was the Law of Conservation of Total Linear Momentum; namely, if the net force on a system is zero, then the total momentum doesn't change. The rotational version of this statement is the Law of Conservation of Total Angular Momentum: If the net torque on a system is zero, then the total angular momentum doesn't change. For a single rotating object, the mathematical statement of this law can be written as $L_i = L_f$, or $I_i\omega_i = I_f\omega_f$. In this form, we can see that if I changes by a certain factor, then ω must change inversely by the same factor.

The classic (and often cited) example of this law is the spinning of an ice skater. Suppose a skater is initially spinning with her arms outstretched. Then, if she brings her hands in toward her body, her moment of inertia decreases (because the mass that used to be far from the axis of rotation is now closer to it); as a result, the skater's angular velocity must increase, and she spins faster. The same phenomenon happens with collapsing stars; as a dying star collapses, its radius decreases and its moment of inertia decreases too. The result: greater rotational speed.

6.8

Summary of Formulas

Work: $W = Fd\cos\theta$ [$\theta =$ angle between $\mathbf{F}$ and $\mathbf{d}$]

Power: $P = \dfrac{W}{t}$

$P = Fv$ if $\mathbf{F}$ is parallel to $\mathbf{v}$ and constant

Kinetic Energy: $KE = \dfrac{1}{2}mv^2$

Work-energy theorem: $W_{total} = \triangle KE$

Gravitational Potential Energy: $\triangle PE_{grav} = -W_{by\,F_{grav}} = +mg\triangle h$ [if g is constant]

Gravity is a conservative force [path independent]

Friction is NOT a conservative force [path dependent]

Total Mechanical Energy: $E = KE + PE$

Conservation of Total Mechanical Energy: $KE_i + PE_i = KE_f + PE_f$

If non-conservative forces [i.e., friction] act: $KE_i + PE_i + W_{other} = KE_f + PE_f$

Simple Machines:

Mechanical Advantage $= \dfrac{F_{resistance}}{F_{effort}}$

Efficiency [%] $= \dfrac{W_{output}}{Energy_{input}}$

Momentum: $\mathbf{p} = m\mathbf{v}$

Impulse-momentum theorem: $\mathbf{J} = \triangle \mathbf{p} = \mathbf{F}\triangle t$

Conservation of Total Momentum: total $\mathbf{p}_i$ = total $\mathbf{p}_f$

$$m_1\mathbf{v}_1 + m_2\mathbf{v}_2... = m_1\mathbf{v}'_1 + m_2\mathbf{v}'_2...$$

Collisions always conserve momentum

–Elastic collisions also conserve *KE*

–Inelastic collisions do NOT conserve *KE* (lose *KE*)

–Perfectly inelastic collisions lose the most *KE* (objects stick together after collision)

Angular Momentum: $L = I\omega$

Conservation of Total Angular Momentum: total L_i = total L_f

($I_i\omega_i = I_f\omega_f$ for a single object)

CHAPTER 6 FREESTANDING PRACTICE QUESTIONS

1. How much work is needed to lift a box of mass 2 kg up a height of 3 m using a pulley system with 75% efficiency?

A) 4 J
B) 8 J
C) 45 J
D) 80 J

2. An automobile with a certain shape experiences a drag force due to air resistance that is, in Newtons, equal to one-third the square of the car's speed, in meters per second. How much power would the engine have to supply to the wheels to balance this drag force when the car is moving at a constant speed of 30 m/s?

A) 10 W
B) 300 W
C) 9 kW
D) 27 kW

3. A young child is sliding down a hill at an incline of 30° on a sled with total combined mass of 10 kg. If the coefficient of friction between the hill and the sled is 0.3 and the length of the hill is 50 m, how much work has been done by gravity when the child reaches the bottom of the hill?

A) 1000 J
B) 2500 J
C) 3535 J
D) 4330 J

4. An experiment is conducted where a cue ball (mass 0.25 kg) moves at 10 m/s towards an adjacent numbered ball (mass 0.25 kg) at rest. In Trial 1, the collision is elastic. In Trial 2, the collision is perfectly inelastic. What is the speed of the cue ball immediately after the collision in Trial 1 and Trial 2 respectively?

A) 0 m/s and 5 m/s
B) 0 m/s and 10 m/s
C) 5 m/s and 0 m/s
D) 5 m/s and 5 m/s

5. A 200 kg roller coaster starts from rest 50 m above the ground. It falls toward the ground without any friction, then once it reaches ground level, the brakes are applied over 30 m in order to bring the coaster to a complete stop. How much work is done by the brakes?

A) 10×10^4 J
B) 10×10^5 J
C) -10×10^4 J
D) -10×10^5 J

6. A 7 kg ball is dropped from 20 m. If the speed just before it hits the ground is 18 m/s, what is the work done by air resistance?

A) 266 J
B) 13 J
C) −13 J
D) −266 J

CHAPTER 6 PRACTICE PASSAGE

Alice is playing with her little brother Jeff at an ice-skating rink that is entirely flat except for a ramp at one end that is at an upward incline of 30 degrees. Alice is pushing Jeff on a little toboggan that has blades on the bottom, so it glides along the surface of the ice without the effects of friction. Alice has a mass of 60 kg, Jeff has a mass of 28 kg and the mass of the toboggan is 2 kg.

Alice is pushing Jeff around the rink and decides that she wants to push him right up until the incline, then let go and see how far up the incline he goes. They start from rest 10 meters from the incline and she pushes him with a force that varies with the distance (Figure 1). Jeff goes speeding up the incline with a velocity of 2 m/s, travels a certain distance and then comes speeding down. At the bottom of the incline, Jeff's toboggan collides with Alice and the two of them travel across the ice.

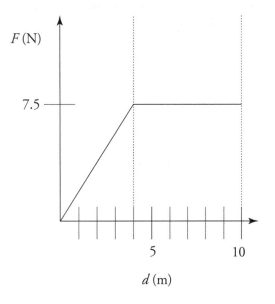

Figure 1 Graph of force vs. distance

Alice and Jeff keep sliding on the ice until the toboggan crashes into the end of the rink. One of the blades on the bottom of the toboggan has come loose in the crash and it no longer glides effortlessly on the ice. Alice once again pushes Jeff with a force given by Figure 1 and lets go just as they reach the incline. This time Jeff travels 10 centimeters less up the incline than he did before the toboggan broke.

1. How much work does Alice do from the moment she begins to push Jeff 10 m from the incline until she lets go just before the incline?

A) 60 J
B) 75 J
C) 0 J
D) There is not enough information to answer the question.

2. The first time Jeff goes up the incline, what distance along the incline does the toboggan travel before it comes to rest?

A) 0.2 m
B) 0.3 m
C) 0.4 m
D) 0.5 m

3. Assuming that the collision between Jeff and Alice at the bottom of the incline is perfectly inelastic, this tells us that:

    I. kinetic energy is conserved.
    II. momentum is conserved.
    III. the sum of the velocities before and after the collision is the same.

A) I only
B) II only
C) I and II only
D) I, II, and III

4. Imagine that instead of Alice jumping on the toboggan during the collision, they "bounce" off of one another in a perfectly elastic collision and they both speed off in different directions. If Jeff heads back up the incline with a speed of 2/3 m/s, with what speed is Alice moving away from the incline?

A) 1/3 m/s
B) 2/3 m/s
C) 1 m/s
D) 4/3 m/s

5. Once the toboggan has broken, if Jeff goes up the incline with the same initial velocity v as he did the first time, how much energy has been lost?

A) 1.0 J
B) 1.5 J
C) 10 J
D) 15 J

6. If Alice did 10 J of work while pushing Jeff in 5 seconds, and the force of friction due to the broken toboggan did −2 J of work, how much power did Alice exert?

A) 50 W
B) 2 W
C) 1.6 W
D) 1.5 W

7. If Jeff brought his friend Jeremy out to play with him and Alice pushes both of them from rest on the toboggan with the same force as given in Figure 1, how would the distance they travel up the incline and their initial velocity change from when just Jeff was being pushed (ignoring friction)?

A) The velocity would be greater and they would go further.
B) The velocity would be greater and they would go less far.
C) The velocity would be less and they would go further.
D) The velocity would be less and they would go less far.

SOLUTIONS TO CHAPTER 6 FREESTANDING QUESTIONS

1. **D**   Without the pulley system, lifting this box would require doing the work to increase the potential energy by *mgh*, which is (2)(10)(3) = 60 J. With a pulley system that has less than 100% efficiency, it will require more work, so the answer has to be greater than 60 J. Choice D is the only answer large enough. As a quick check, a 75% efficiency means that 75% of the work done would need to be put in to complete the task regardless, and 25% of the work goes to overcoming friction and other inefficiencies in the system. In this case, 75% of 80 J is 60 J, and this matches that the task would require 60 J without the pulleys. Be careful not to multiply the work required by 75% and choose C! That would be the right answer if the question told us that the pulley system required 60 J of work and asked how much work would be needed without the pulley system.

2. **C**   The word-equation given in the first sentence of the question stem can be expressed as $F_{\text{drag}} = \frac{1}{3}v^2$. (Neglect the dimensional incorrectness of the equation; the stem indicates that speed units of m/s will give force units of N here.) The question asks for power, and the relationship between force and power is $P = Fv$, so $P = (\frac{1}{3}v^2)(v) = \frac{1}{3}v^3$. Plug in the number given: $P = \frac{1}{3}(30)^3 = 9000$. Thus, the answer is 9 kW.

3. **B**   There are a couple of ways to approach this problem:

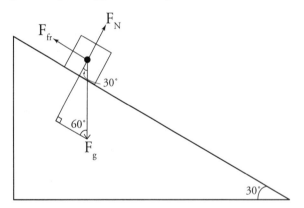

Number 1:

The formula for work is $W = Fd \cos \theta$, where *W* is the work, *F* is the force, *d* is the displacement and θ is the angle between the force and displacement vectors. To determine the work done by gravity, we use gravitational force and the length of the hill to get: $W = (mg)(d) \cos 60°$, where 60° is from the direction of gravitational force vertically down and *d* is along the ramp. Thus, $W = (10)(10)(50)(0.5) = 2500$ J.

Number 2:

We can resolve the F and d to be in the same direction, that is, take the component of the force acting in the same direction as the child's movement down the hill, eliminating the $\cos \theta$ (since $\cos 0° = 1$) from the equation. Then, we have, $F = mg \sin \theta$, where $\theta = 30°$. Thus, $W = Fd = (mg \sin \theta)d = (10)(10)(0.5)(50) = 2500$ J.

4.   A   In a perfectly inelastic collision, recall that total momentum is conserved but not total kinetic energy and that the balls all stick together. Initial momentum must be equal to final momentum. $p_{\text{initial}} = p_{\text{final}} = m_1 v_1 = (m_1 + m_2)v' \rightarrow v' = m_1 v_1 / (m_1 + m_2) = (0.25)(10) / (0.25 + 0.25)$ $= 5$ m/s. This is the value for Trial 2, eliminating choices B and C. For the elastic collision, kinetic energy must be conserved in addition to total momentum, and both objects can move at different velocities after the collision. Since momentum is conserved, $p_{\text{initial}} = p_{\text{final}} = m_1 v_1 = m_1 v_{1f} + m_2 v_{2f}$. Since $m_1 = m_2$, we have that $v_{2f} = v_1 - v_{1f}$. Similarly, if kinetic energy is conserved, then $KE_{\text{initial}} = KE_{\text{final}} = \frac{1}{2} m_1 v_1^2 = \frac{1}{2} m_1 v_{2f}^2 + \frac{1}{2} m_2 v_{2f}^2$. Therefore, $v_{2f}^2 = v_1^2 - v_{1f}^2$. In order for these two equations to hold true, v_{1f} must equal either 0 m/s or 10 m/s. Since 10 m/s would indicate the two balls did not collide at all (and 10 m/s for Trial 1 is not an option), the cue ball must have velocity of 0 m/s immediately following the elastic collision, transferring all kinetic energy to the numbered ball.

5.   C   This question requires you to use the work-kinetic energy theorem, which states that $W = \Delta KE$. The kinetic energy at the bottom is equal to the potential energy at the top, by conservation of energy, which is $mgh = (200)(10)(50) = 10^5$ J. The change in kinetic energy is the final kinetic energy minus the initial. Therefore, the work done by friction to bring the roller coaster to a stop is equal to $\Delta KE = -10^5$ J $= -10 \times 10^4$ J.

6.   D   The initial energy is $mgh = (7)(10)(20) = 1400$ J. The final energy is completely kinetic, $1/2(mv^2) = 1134$ J. The equation for conservation of energy with friction is $E_i + W_{\text{by friction}} = E_f$. Thus, the work done by friction is negative and equal to $1134 - 1400 = -266$ J.

SOLUTIONS TO CHAPTER 6 PRACTICE PASSAGE

1. **A** There are two methods of solving this problem. First, the work done by Alice is equal to the area under the graph given in Figure 1. This can be calculated in two steps. From $d = 0$ m to $d = 4$ m the work done is the area of the triangle: $\dfrac{(7.5 \text{ N})(4 \text{ m})}{2} = 15$ J. From $d = 4$ m to $d = 10$ m the work done is the area of the rectangle: $(7.5 \text{ N})(6 \text{ m}) = 45$ J. Therefore the total work is 60 J. The second method involves understanding that the work done by Alice is equal to the kinetic energy gained by the sled. This is equal to $(1/2)mv^2 = (1/2)(30 \text{ kg})(2 \text{ m/s})^2 = 60$ J.

2. **C** Jeff's initial kinetic energy can be computed by using the mass and velocity given and it is equal to $\dfrac{1}{2}(30 \text{ kg})(2 \text{ m/s})^2 = 60$ J. All of this energy is converted to potential energy at the top of the incline, therefore 60 J $= mgh$. This tells us that the height above the ground is 0.2 m. However, the question asks for the ground the toboggan covers, which is along the incline. So the correct answer is $\dfrac{(0.2 \text{ m})}{\sin(30°)} = 0.4$ m.

3. **B** The collision is perfectly inelastic, so momentum is conserved but kinetic energy is not. The sum of the velocities is not the same before and after the collision, which is a consequence of momentum being conserved.

4. **D** In a completely elastic collision you can conserve energy and momentum, so this question can be solved by conserving either. Using momentum, and taking the direction of Jeff's velocity before the collision as positive, the momentum before is $(30 \text{ kg})(2 \text{ m/s})$ and the momentum after is $(60 \text{ kg})(v) + (30 \text{ kg})(-\dfrac{2}{3} \text{ m/s})$. Setting these equal gives a velocity of $v = \dfrac{4}{3}$ m/s.

5. **D** The initial kinetic energy remains the same in both cases, therefore the potential energy at the top of the hill is the initial kinetic energy minus the energy lost. The change in potential energy, $mg\Delta h$, is equal to the energy lost. The difference in height is sin 30° multiplied by the change in distance traveled, which is $(\sin 30°)(0.1 \text{ m}) = 0.05$ m. The energy lost is then $(30 \text{ kg})(10 \text{ m/s}^2)(0.05) = 15$ J.

6. **B** The amount of work done by friction does not matter in this question. The power exerted by Alice is the work she does divided by the time it takes her. $\dfrac{(10 \text{ J})}{5 \text{ s}} = 2 \text{ J/s} = 2 \text{ W}$.

7. **D** This is a two-by-two question, meaning that two pieces of information are required in order to reach the correct answer. The work done is the same in both cases, so by the work-energy theorem, the kinetic energy is the same in both cases, and since the mass is larger in the second case, the velocity must be smaller. This eliminates choices A and B. All the kinetic energy is being converted to potential energy at the top of the hill, so the potential energy at the top of the hill is also the same in both cases. Again, since the mass is greater in the second case, the resulting height is less and that eliminates choice C.

Chapter 7
Thermodynamics

7.1 SYSTEMS, THERMAL PHYSICS, AND THERMODYNAMICS

As we've seen so far, work can be done on or by a physical system—a box on a ramp, a car's engine block hooked to several loops of rope attached to two pulleys, or a satellite launched into orbit are just a few examples—thereby increasing or decreasing the energy in that system. Broadly speaking, work is a *transfer of mechanical energy into or out of a system, from or to the environment.*

We ought to be careful here with our terms. In physics, as in chemistry and biology, you will hear a lot about *systems.* For our purposes, it is enough to define a system as the object or objects under examination, e.g., the things you want to answer questions about to do well on the MCAT. The *environment* is just the other objects and external forces outside the system. The environment may or may not be able to interact with the system. If the system is *closed,* then the environment cannot contribute matter to it; if the system is *isolated,* then the environment cannot contribute either matter or energy to it. If the system is *open,* then it is free to interact with the environment. This leads to a crucial point: systems obey conservation laws. Within the system, different forms of energy can *transform from one type to another but cannot spontaneously appear or cease to exist.* In other words, the only way the total energy in a system can change is if energy is *transferred* into or out of the system.

Consider a tennis ball in your hand. If you want to focus exclusively on the ball itself, you might call the ball "the system" and everything else "the environment." This is an open system; if you drop the ball, an external force in the environment (gravity) will do work on the ball, contributing to its increase in kinetic energy as it falls. Alternatively, you might want to look at the ball + the earth + gravity (the interaction between those two objects) as the system. In that case, when you drop the ball, one form of energy (gravitational potential energy) is transformed into another (kinetic energy).

But what about some other factors? For one thing, you could choose to throw the ball up in the air instead of just letting it idly drop to the ground. If we counted you as part of the environment, then we would say that the work you did on the ball in throwing it upward increased its kinetic energy: you transferred energy into the system. If we counted you as part of the system, we would have to explain the energy transformation in terms of the ATP turning to ADP and then AMP as your muscles contracted to allow you to throw the ball, and thus chemical potential energy was transformed into kinetic energy (for more on that, consult the *MCAT Biology Review!*). What about the air resistance the ball experiences as it falls through the air? As a frictional force, air resistance does what we have previously called "nonconservative" work on the ball, as it causes the ball to move more slowly (i.e., to have less kinetic energy) than it would if there were no air. Is this a violation of what we have said so far about energy conservation or transferring to and from the environment?

It is not. The problem is that so far we have considered only a limited number of kinds of energy, and we have neglected an important mode of energy transfer. Consider the tennis ball a bit more closely. Even as it sits apparently still in your hand, on the molecular level there is a tremendous amount of random motion. This is another form of energy internal to the system, which we'll call *thermal energy* (or sometimes just *internal energy,* though as you know from chemistry, there are other forms of internal energy such as chemical or nuclear energies). **Temperature** (T) is the macroscopic measure of this thermal energy per molecule. As the tennis ball falls, the frictional effects of air resistance do negative work on the ball, slowing it down, but they also cause the temperature of the ball to increase, because all of those tiny collisions between the air molecules and the molecules in the ball increase the thermal energy of the ball's molecules (as well as that of the air molecules that interact with the ball directly). That is to say, the individual molecules of the surface of the ball are moving faster than before, but in random directions (in addition to all moving toward the ground while the ball is falling). If you were to catch and hold the now slightly warmer ball in your hand, over time it would cool back to the temperature of the surrounding air. Its thermal energy would decrease, but it would be sitting perfectly still, so clearly it wasn't doing any work. It transferred energy to the environment by means of heat. **Heat** (Q) is the transfer of thermal energy between a system and its environment: $Q > 0$ when heat transfers *into* the system, $Q < 0$ when heat transfers *out* of the system. Please note this important distinction between *temperature* and *heat*, words that we use everyday in ways that can make them seem interchangeable. When we say *"it's hot* outside today," we're referring to the temperature, an indicator of the relatively high thermal energy per molecule of the local atmospheric system. When we then say "this weather *is making me hot* and sweaty," we're talking about heat, the transfer of the thermal energy from the atmosphere into our bodies. Note the difference in units as well: heat, as with energy, is measured in joules, whereas absolute temperature is measured in kelvins. Another important difference between temperature and thermal energy contained within a system (and transferrable as heat) is that temperature is an *intensive* property whereas thermal energy is an *extensive* one. That is to say, temperature (like density, for example) does not depend on the amount of a material present, but thermal energy (like mass) does. Imagine a block of stone at a temperature of 300 kelvins and containing 20,000 joules of thermal energy. If you split it in half, each half would still be 300 kelvins (not 150), but each would contain only 10,000 joules of thermal energy.

Thermodynamics concerns how macroscopic systems transfer and transform energy. As such, it is perhaps the broadest subject you'll study in preparation for physics on the MCAT, taking into account not only everything we've looked at so far in this text, but also extending into all the other science topics on the exam.

7.2 THE ZEROTH LAW OF THERMODYNAMICS

Thermal physics depends upon the quantity *temperature* being well defined in such a way that, if we stick thermometers on two different objects and get the same reading, we know there is something fundamentally similar about those two objects. This is unlike, say, length: a 2 m long metal rod does not have anything fundamentally in common with a 2 m long wooden plank. The **zeroth law of thermodynamics** provides this definition. It states that if one object is in thermal equilibrium with a second object, and that second object is in thermal equilibrium with a third object, then the first and third objects are in thermal equilibrium with each other. By *thermal equilibrium* we mean that, though the two bodies are in contact in such a way that heat is free to pass between them, no heat actually does so (or, more precisely, the same amount of heat passes each way). Practically, what this means is that Objects 1 and 3 are the same temperature. Technically, this *defines* temperature as a fundamental property, or *state variable,* of a system. It tells us that if we measured the temperatures of two objects (like our metal rod and wooden plank) to be the same, we would know that when we put the two in contact with each other, no net heat would be transferred between them.

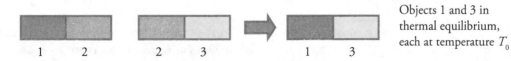

Objects 1 and 3 in thermal equilibrium, each at temperature T_0

The other *state variables* include pressure, volume, moles, and entropy. On the MCAT as in your college coursework, discussion of these variables crosses over between physics and chemistry (and possibly other disciplines), and the connections among those discussions can be confusing. One unifying idea you should keep in mind in all applications is that these variables define a *state function* for a system, which means they are macroscopic properties that reflect the microscopic conditions of that system and predict the future behavior of the system. The specific relation between the microscopic average kinetic energy per atom of a monatomic ideal gas (wherein kinetic energy is the only form of energy) is given by the following equation, sometimes called the equipartition of energy equation for ideal gases (k_B is the Boltzmann constant and is equal to 1.38×10^{-23} J/K).

$$\frac{1}{2}mv_{avg}^2 = \frac{3}{2}k_B T$$

Heat Transfer

In stating the zeroth law of thermodynamics, we relied upon the idea that bodies can achieve thermal equilibrium by heat transfer, the movement of thermal energy from one point to another. There are three mechanisms by which this is achieved.

Conduction

An iron skillet is sitting on a hot stove, and you accidentally touch the handle. You notice right away that there's been a transfer of thermal energy to your hand. The process by which this happens is known as **conduction**. The highly agitated atoms in the handle of the hot skillet bump into the atoms of your hand, making them vibrate more rapidly, thus heating up your hand.

Example 7-1: The rate at which materials conduct heat varies widely. Metals conduct heat well, meaning that heat moves through them rapidly. Materials like fiberglass, which is often used to provide thermal insulation in buildings, conduct heat very poorly. The *conduction rate* is described by the equation

$$P_{cond} = \frac{\Delta Q}{\Delta t} = -kA\frac{\Delta T}{\Delta x} = kA\frac{T_i - T_f}{L}$$

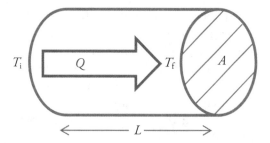

where k is a thermal conductivity constant dependent upon the material and the power P indicates the rate of thermal energy transfer. This energy is measured in joules as usual. (This is not an equation the

MCAT would expect you to have memorized.) Window glass typically has a thermal conductivity of $k = 1$ watt per meter per kelvin (recall that kelvins are a measure of absolute temperature with a scale equal to that of degrees Celsius). How many joules per second of heat are transferred out of a room at 25°C to an outside environment of at 0°C if there are two 2 × 1 meter single-paned windows in the room with a thickness of half a centimeter? Assume the walls are perfectly insulated.

Solution: Find the total area A by multiplying the dimensions of the windows and their total number: $A = 2 \times 2 \times 1 = 4 \text{ m}^2$. Applying the given equation then yields

$$\frac{\Delta Q}{\Delta t} = kA\frac{T_i - T_f}{L} = (1)(4)\frac{25 - 0}{0.5 \times 10^{-2}} = 200 \times 10^2 = 2 \times 10^4 \text{ J/s}$$

This is quite a bit of power, which is why it is a good idea to use double-paned or otherwise insulated windows in climates where it gets cold outside!

Convection

As the air around a candle flame warms, it expands, becomes less dense than the surrounding cooler air, and thus rises due to buoyancy. (We'll study buoyancy in the next chapter.) As a result, heat is transferred away from the flame by the large-scale (from the atoms' point of view anyway) motion of a fluid (in this case, air). This is (natural) **convection**.

Example 7-2: During circulation, the relatively warm blood moves from the heart to the extremities, where it cools slightly before returning to the heart. What best describes this process?

A. This is a natural convection process, as warm blood rises to the head while relatively cold blood sinks to the feet.
B. This is a natural convection process, as the expansion of the warm blood in the heart pushes blood out to the extremities via the arteries, whereas cooler blood at the extremities condenses and sinks toward the heart via the veins.
C. This is a forced convection process where the pumping action of the heart forces blood heated by the body's metabolic processes out to the extremities, which in turn forces the cooler blood back toward the heart (during which time it is heated).
D. This is a forced convection process where the pumping action of the heart compresses and thereby heats the blood. Its motion to the extremities is a result of this pressurization.

Solution: The heart is a pump: you should know that blood's motion through the body is caused by the heart, not by some passive physical process. Choices A and B are eliminated for not making sense: don't ignore your biology knowledge when answering physics questions if it's pertinent! Along that line of thought, the heart is not a pressure cooker: the heat of our bodies is produced by metabolic processes, the conversion of chemical energy to other forms (such as kinetic energy in the contraction of muscles throughout the body, which is why you feel hotter when exercising vigorously). Choice D doesn't adequately explain this and is therefore eliminated. Choice C is correct: the movement of the warm fluid and displacement of the cooler fluid is convection, but it is *forced convection* due to the pumping action. The process by which a convection oven works is analogous: the forced movement of the fluid (air) in the oven due to a fan results in faster heat transfer than in a normal oven that relies on natural convection and conduction.

Radiation

Sunlight on your face warms your skin. Radiant energy from the sun's fusion reactions is transferred across millions of kilometers of essentially empty space via electromagnetic waves. Absorption of the energy carried by these light waves defines heat transfer by **radiation**.

Thermal Expansion

Another response of materials to temperature difference is to change their physical dimensions, i.e., length and volume. Most materials expand as their temperature increases: this is why, for example, bridges have expansion slots, the metal grates you drive over every 10 meters or so. If the bridge got longer in response to an increase in temperature but had no room to expand, it would buckle and crack. The formula for linear thermal expansion is $\Delta L = \alpha L_0 \Delta T$, where ΔL is the change in length of the object, L_0 is its original length, and α is the coefficient of linear expansion of the material the object is made of. This is not typically an equation the MCAT expects you to have memorized.

7.3 THE FIRST LAW OF THERMODYNAMICS

Having defined two ways in which energy can transfer between the environment and a system (heat and work), as well as a way to measure the energy internal to the system (temperature), we are now ready to make a broader statement about conservation of energy than the ones we made in the preceding chapter. The first law of thermodynamics is just this statement: it says that *the total energy of the universe is constant.* Energy may be transformed from one form to another, but it cannot be created or destroyed.

The first law of thermodynamics can be expressed both tangibly and mathematically. To do this, consider the physical aspects of transferring energy to an object. Since energy cannot be created or destroyed, it must be transferred into some other form such as heat (Q) or work (W). Thus, we have the following mathematical statement of the first law:

First Law of Thermodynamics

$$\Delta E = Q - W$$

Pay close attention to the sign conventions we're using. Q is considered positive when heat is moving into the system, negative when it is coming out of the system. W is considered positive when the work is *being done by the system on the environment.* W is considered negative when the work is *being done by the environment on the system.* Unfortunately, this convention for work is opposite what is typically used in chemistry books, so you may remember the formula as $\Delta E = Q + W$, or with U in place of E, or with lower case letters. As long as you remember how the variables are being defined, when they are positive and negative, you shouldn't have any problems.

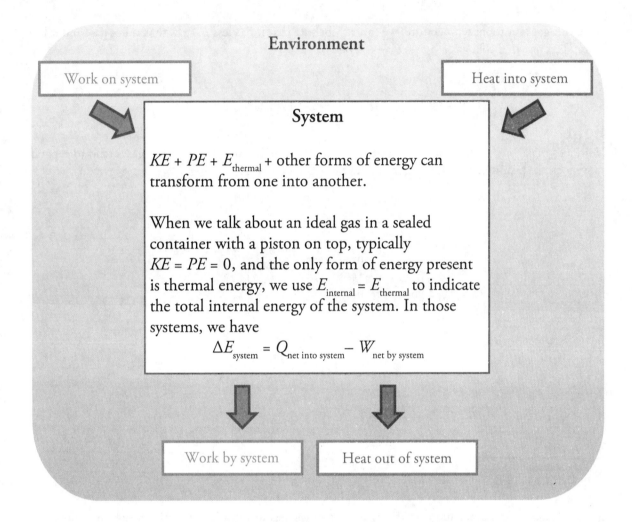

To analyze the First Law equation, let's take a sample of ideal gas at room temperature and put it into a container to make a closed (but not isolated) system. Let's use a metal cylinder that's welded shut at one end and sealed on the other end with a piston.

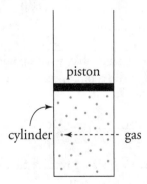

Starting with the energy component of the equation, we can consider the internal energy of the system. Again recall that for an ideal gas, the only form of internal energy is the kinetic energy of the atoms or molecules. The internal energy, $E_{internal}$, is proportional to the object's absolute temperature, T:

$$E_{internal} \propto T$$

Since this gas is at room temperature, we can say for sure that it has less $E_{internal}$ than a hot gas, and it has more $E_{internal}$ than a cold gas.

Heat

Now, let's make our gas hot. But before we do that, we learned somewhere that hot gases tend to expand, so we lock the piston in a fixed position to prevent it from moving:

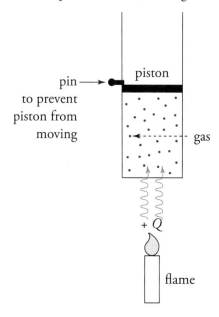

We gently apply the flame, and heat the cylinder and the gas inside. Since the piston does not move, no work is done, but energy is transferred as heat. We can sum up what's happening as

$$\Delta E_{internal} = Q, \, Q > 0$$

where we know that $E_{internal}$ has to increase because we feel that the gas and cylinder are getting hotter, and the additional energy is added to our system in the form of heat, Q.

If we let the hot gas and hot cylinder just sit on a table, what's going to happen over time? The hot cylinder and gas will cool down as they lose heat to the room, until they're at room temperature again. So, for this cooling down process, we'll have

$$\Delta E_{internal} = Q, \, Q < 0$$

where we know that $E_{internal}$ has to decrease because we feel that the gas and cylinder are cooling down, and energy is lost from our system in the form of heat, Q.

Work

Let's make the gas hot again. This time, let's remove the lock on the piston and allow it to move.

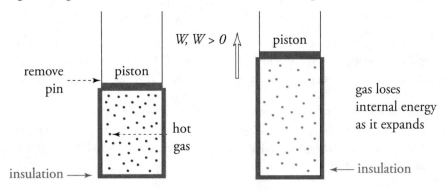

The hot gas pushes the piston up. Our gas is doing work, W, because it's applying a *force* and moving the piston a certain *distance*. As the piston moves, the volume of the gas increases since gases expand to fill their containers. Therefore, the ΔV in this example is positive. To quantify the work in a system, we not only need to know how much the volume of the system changes, but we also need to know how much pressure the gas exerts upward on the piston. Therefore, work can be defined as

$$W = P\Delta V$$

Due to an increase in volume, the work described in the case above has a positive value. A positive W is defined as work done *by* the system. When the weight on our piston moves up, it gains potential energy (the h in mgh is getting larger). Conservation of energy states that energy cannot be created or destroyed, but is simply moved around. Therefore, the energy gained by the weight must come from something else (the hot gas!). As long as the piston is well insulated, such that no heat (Q) can go in or out, we have

$$\Delta E_{internal} = -W, \; W > 0$$

where $E_{internal}$ of our gas has to decrease because energy is lost from our system in the form of doing work, W. Because the gas is losing energy as it expands and raises the piston, and we learned earlier that $\Delta E_{internal}$ is proportional to temperature, the *gas cools as it expands*.

Now, if after our gas has expanded and cooled as far as it's going to, we add more weight on the piston so that the piston and weights move down and compress the gas,

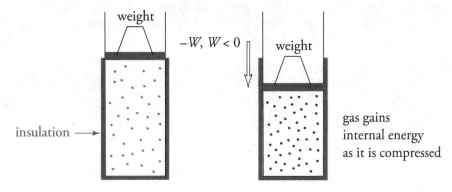

we have the situation for which

$$\Delta E_{internal} = +W, \ W < 0$$

Now, because ΔV is a negative value (because our gas has been compressed), this will lead to negative work being done *by the gas* (which is the same as *positive* work being done *on the gas*). In this situation, $E_{internal}$ has to increase because energy is gained by our system. Here, we'd see that our *gas warms as it is compressed*.

Thus, for processes in which no heat is exchanged between the gas and the environment, in general expanding gases cool and compressed gases warm. This is the principle behind how a steam engine, refrigerator, and air conditioner work.

Case 1: An Isobaric Process

An **isobaric** process is one that occurs at constant pressure. Consider heating our cylinder such that the volume of gas expands, pushing the piston upward, but the pressure remains constant because the weight on the piston is held constant, and that force divided by the area of the piston remains constant. If we plot pressure vs. volume for this process, the graph would look like this:

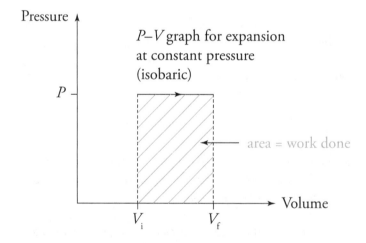

and the area under the curve would be equal to the work done by the gas on the piston. This means we can easily calculate W, without the use of calculus, since $W = P\Delta V$. Note that this is positive because ΔV is positive; when the arrow goes backward in the graph indicating $\Delta V < 0$, the area should be considered negative.

Case 2: An Isochoric Process

An **isochoric** process maintains a constant volume. Heating the gas with a locked piston would result in increasing pressure but no change in volume:

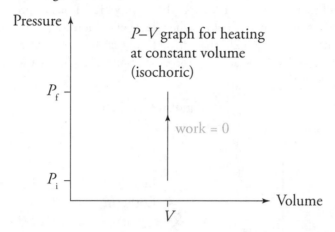

Therefore, no work is done. You can see this either by noticing that the area under the P-V graph is zero (since the graph is just a vertical line), or by realizing that if the volume didn't change, then the piston didn't move, and if there's no displacement of the piston, then there was no work done on the piston. Because $W = 0$, we know that $\Delta E = Q$.

Case 3: An Isothermal Process

When heat is allowed to pass freely between a system and its environment, an **isothermal** process can occur, where the temperature of the system remains constant. For example, for our gas to expand at constant temperature, the pressure must decrease (as governed by Boyle's law).

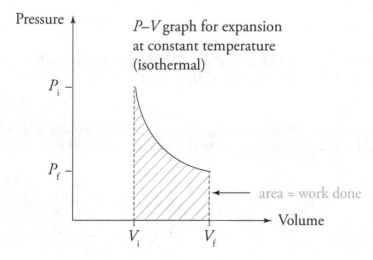

Again, the work done by the gas on the piston will be equal to the area under the curve. Since we know that E is directly proportional to T, we can say that in an isothermal process, $\Delta E = 0$ and $Q = W$.

Case 4: An Adiabatic Process

An **adiabatic** process occurs when no heat is transferred between the system and the environment, and all energy is transferred as work: the previous example with the insulated container is one instance. Another imperfect but real-world example is a rapidly expanding gas, which drops its pressure precipitously and simultaneously cools. This is the principle behind the release of compressed water vapor in a snow-making machine. The process happens so quickly that theoretically no heat is transferred; since $Q = 0$, we get $\Delta E_{internal} = -W$ (here the positive work done by the expanding gas is simply the pushing of the surrounding atmosphere out of the way).

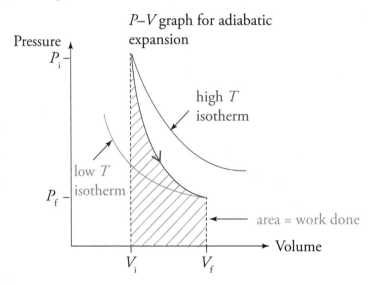

Example 7-3: For a perfectly insulated system, what are the values of $\Delta E_{internal}$ and Q if $W = +100$ J?

    A. $\Delta E_{internal} = -100$ J and $Q = 0$
    B. $\Delta E_{internal} = 0$ and $Q = -100$ J
    C. $\Delta E_{internal} = +100$ J and $Q = 0$
    D. $\Delta E_{internal} = 0$ and $Q = +100$ J

Solution: A perfectly insulated system allows no heat transfer (adiabatic), so $Q = 0$; this eliminates choices B and D. Now, by the first law of thermodynamics, $\Delta E_{internal} = Q - W = 0 - (+100$ J$) = -100$ J, so the answer is A.

Example 7-4: Suppose you want to raise the temperature of an ideal gas while adding the lowest possible amount of heat and doing no work on the gas. Which process should you use?

    A.   Isobaric
    B.   Isochoric
    C.   Isothermal
    D.   Adiabatic

Solution: An isothermal process will not raise the temperature of the gas at all by definition, so choice C is eliminated. An adiabatic process will not allow the transfer of heat into the gas, so choice D is eliminated. If you add heat during an isochoric process, the change in internal energy of the gas (which is directly proportional to the change in temperature) will be $\Delta E = Q$, whereas during an isobaric process it will be $\Delta E = Q - P\Delta V$, because the gas will expand as it increases in temperature; rearranging gives

$Q = \Delta E + P\Delta V$. Thus the isochoric process will require less heat to increase E and therefore T by some arbitrary amount. The correct choice is B.

This example illustrates the difference between two ideal gas heating processes. This distinction is quantified by the difference between *molar specific heats*. An ideal gas at constant volume will increase in temperature according to $Q = nC_V\Delta T$, where n is the number of moles and C_V is called the constant volume molar specific heat. An ideal gas at constant pressure, on the other hand, will increase in temperature according to $Q = nC_P\Delta T$, where C_P is called the constant pressure molar specific heat. The units of molar specific heat are $[C] = [Q] / [n][T] = $ J/mol-K. The exact values of the molar specific heats depend upon the type of gas (monatomic, diatomic, polyatomic), and you are unlikely to need to know them. However, as you already know from the preceding example that a constant pressure process requires more heat for an equal change in temperature than a constant volume process, it is worth noting that, in general, $C_P = C_V + R$, where R is the gas constant.

Example 7-5: The PV curve below represents a thermodynamic *cycle*, a series of reversible processes through which an ideal gas passes that return it to its initial state function. What area represents the net work done by the gas from steps 1 to 2 to 3 to 4 back to 1?

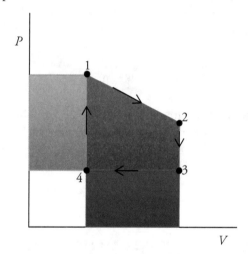

A. The blue trapezoid
B. The red rectangle
C. The blue trapezoid and the red rectangle
D. The blue trapezoid and both the red and green rectangles

Solution: The isochores 2→3 and 4→1 do no work, so we can ignore them. The process 1→2 does positive work $W_{1\to2} = P\Delta V$, which is the sum of the blue and red areas. The process 3→4 does negative work, because the volume decreases (this would correspond to the piston moving down, compressing the gas), $W_{3\to4} = P\Delta V$, which is the negative of the red area. Thus the sum of the four processes yields (blue + red) + 0 + (−red) + 0 = blue. The correct choice is A.

This example illustrates a couple of important facts about *thermodynamic cycles,* sequences of processes that lead a gas back to its original state function. This means that $\Delta E = 0$ for the overall cycle, and thus $Q = W$. During a cycle, the system either converts heat to work (for a clockwise cycle, like the one shown) or work to heat (for a counterclockwise cycle). Thermodynamic cycles are important as models of ideal heat engines. Indeed, many of the breakthroughs in the science of thermodynamics were made by engineers attempting to understand how to make more efficient engines.

Example 7-6: An ideal gas is held under pressure in an isolated container behind a thin membrane opposite which is vacuum, like an inflated balloon in a large evacuated room. The membrane is suddenly ruptured, like popping the balloon. What happens next?

A. Nothing: the membrane ruptures but the gas is unaffected.
B. The pressure and temperature both decrease rapidly.
C. The temperature decreases rapidly but the pressure stays constant.
D. The pressure decreases rapidly, but the temperature remains constant, since no heat is exchanged and no work is done.

Solution: If a gas is held under pressure and the source of the pressure is released, like suddenly removing the piston from the canister in the examples discussed previously, the pressure will spontaneously decrease to match that of the surroundings (this will be discussed in more detail in the next chapter on fluids). This eliminates choice A. The phenomenon described in this question is a special type of adiabatic process called a *free expansion:* it is nearly instantaneous, so there is no time for heat transfer, but because the membrane ruptures and there is nothing to push against, no work is done either. Applying the First Law equation thus yields

$$\Delta E = Q - W = 0 - 0 = 0.$$

Therefore there is no change in temperature either, and the correct choice is D. It might seem to you counterintuitive that something like popping a balloon could have such small apparent effect on the thermodynamic state of the system. You'd be right: something *does* increase, namely the *entropy* of the system.

7.4 THE SECOND LAW OF THERMODYNAMICS

As we have seen, the first law of thermodynamics is an expanded statement of conservation of energy, a principle we're familiar with from the realm of balls rolling down hills and blocks sliding across tables, as well as (now) gases being heated and expanding, doing work in the process. However, now that we have expanded our view of what counts as energy, it becomes apparent that many situations we would never expect to see do not in fact violate the principle of energy conservation. Imagine, for example, that you are looking at a wooden block resting on a normal horizontal table. All of the sudden, it begins sliding to the right. You'd be pretty surprised, and you'd probably start looking for the string (or the camera), because you would think that would violate the conservation of energy. However, suppose the block had a thermometer attached to it, and you noticed that as the block began to slide, its temperature began to lower. In that case, conservation of energy might not be violated: thermal energy was just transforming into kinetic energy. You would likely continue to object; it's one thing for a sliding block to slow down and stop due to friction, heating up in the process, but this doesn't typically work in reverse. Why *don't* things go backward? What directs the *arrow of time*? One answer is **entropy** and the **second law of thermodynamics.**

Entropy is a measure of the *disorder* of a system. What does this mean? Imagine the Great Pyramid of Giza, built so carefully of stacked stones that it has stood for over 4500 years. Now imagine those same six billion kilograms of stone scattered around hundreds of square kilometers of desert. The pyramid is ordered, the scattered stone is disordered. A microscopic analogy would be a diamond crystal, with its extremely regular and predictable organization of carbon atoms, versus the carbon atoms in pencil shavings scattered on a desk. The carbon atoms in the pencil shavings have much greater entropy than those in the crystal.

Without stating any equations you won't need to know, we can say qualitatively that *predictability* is one measure of order. If I tell you the first five cards in a deck are the ace, 2, 3, 4, and 5 of spades, you will probably feel pretty comfortable guessing the next card will be the 6 of spades, a lot more comfortable than if I shuffled the deck and asked you to predict the sixth card (technically, this is a function of information entropy and not physical entropy, but the details aren't important). By analogy, the entropy will be lower whenever there's a higher likelihood that, given you know the locations and velocities of some particles, you can deduce the same of other particles. Under this criterion, solids, with their regular arrays of atoms, have greater order and therefore less entropy than liquids, which have in turn less entropy than gases. Entropy is another *state variable*, one whose value corresponds to the microscopic order of the particles making up the system, just as temperature corresponds to the microscopic kinetic energy of those particles. The MCAT doesn't care about the mathematical details of this correspondence, and you are really likely to see quantitative entropy problems only in chemistry or biochemistry, not in physics.

The second law of thermodynamics states that the *entropy of an isolated system either stays the same or increases during any thermodynamic process*. If the system is closed, its entropy can decrease, but not without a corresponding greater increase in the entropy of the surrounding environment. Over a thermodynamic cycle, the rules are slightly different. If the entropy stays the same over a thermodynamic cycle, the cycle is said to be reversible, meaning that you could return from each state to the previous state by the same path in reverse (think of these paths as the curves on a *PV* graph), and that on returning there would be no indication of any change.

This means also that it is impossible for a system to convert all of the input heat (disordered energy) into work (ordered energy) during a thermodynamic cycle: it must always output some heat as well. Similarly, it is impossible to move heat from a colder system to a hotter one without inputting some work (work which, we've just discovered, must itself involve some output of heat). If the entropy increases over a series of processes (thereby making it not a true cycle), this indicates the process is *irreversible*. In the real world, all macroscopic processes are irreversible due to friction and other "loss" effects. A wooden block sliding on a horizontal table comes to a stop due to friction. Energy is conserved, converted from kinetic to thermal, but entropy increases, which is why you will never see the block spontaneously accelerate backward from whence it came. Things really can't go back to just the way they were.

Summary of Formulas

Energy flow into a system has a positive sign. Energy flow out of a system has a negative sign.

Temperature is defined by $\frac{1}{2}mv_{avg}^2 = \frac{3}{2}k_B T$ for a monatomic ideal gas.

The first law of thermodynamics states that energy cannot be created or destroyed. Based on this, $\Delta E = Q - W$.

The internal energy of an object is proportional to its temperature: $\Delta E \propto T$.

Work done by a gas: $W = P\Delta V$.

For an adiabatic process, $Q = 0$.

An isobaric process occurs at constant P, isothermal at constant T, and isochoric at constant V.

The change in absolute temperature of an ideal gas when heated is given by $Q = nC_V \cdot T$ or $Q = nC_P \cdot T$, depending upon whether the gas is heated at constant volume or constant pressure. $C_P = C_V + R$.

The second law of thermodynamics states that all processes tend toward maximum disorder, or entropy (S). It further states that heat cannot flow from a colder to a warmer object unless some work is done on the system to make it do so. Equivalently, the law says that heat cannot be converted totally to work by any cycle.

CHAPTER 7 FREESTANDING PRACTICE QUESTIONS

1. The linear thermal expansion of a metal rod is given by $\Delta L = \alpha L_0 \Delta T$. By how many degrees Celsius would the temperature of a rod have to increase for the rod's length to increase by 20%?

A) $\alpha L_0 / 5$
B) $1/5\alpha$
C) It depends on the original length of the rod.
D) Cannot be determined because kelvins must be used for ΔT.

2. An amount of heat Q is added to a system. Which of the following can result?

    I. Its temperature increases.
    II. Its phase changes.
    III. It undergoes isothermal expansion.

A) I only
B) I or II only
C) I or III only
D) I, II, or III

3. An expanding spring pushes a rigid cylinder of gas across a horizontal frictionless table. Consider the system to be the gas inside the cylinder. Which of the following sets of relations best describes what happens?

A) $W_{\text{on system}} > 0, Q > 0, \Delta KE > 0$
B) $W_{\text{on system}} = 0, Q = 0, \Delta KE = 0$
C) $W_{\text{on system}} > 0, Q = 0, \Delta KE > 0$
D) $W_{\text{on system}} > 0, Q < 0, \Delta KE > 0$

4. During adiabatic compression of a gas the temperature:

A) increases because no heat is transferred.
B) remains constant because heat is transferred.
C) remains constant because no heat is transferred.
D) decreases because heat is transferred.

5. A closed system consisting of a balloon expands by 5×10^{-2} L at constant temperature in an environment with a pressure of 1.0×10^5 Pa. What is the value of heat transfer in this process?

A) -5.0 J
B) -5.0 kJ
C) 5.0 J
D) 5.0 kJ

6. In the thermodynamic cycle shown below, the processes connecting points 2 and 3 and points 1 and 4 are adiabatic. What statement below is true?

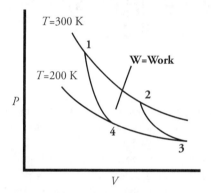

A) Work is done on or by the gas at every step.
B) Heat is exchanged only on processes 1-2 and 3-4.
C) The internal energy of the system returns to the same value after completing a cycle.
D) All of the above

CHAPTER 7 PRACTICE PASSAGE

Figure 1 shows a thin-walled, cylindrical metal container fitted with a tight-fitting but freely movable lightweight plastic piston and containing 0.25 mol of helium at 0°C and a pressure of 1 atm.

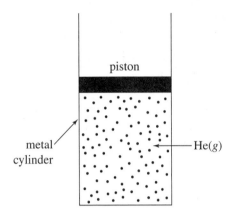

Figure 1

The volume, pressure, and temperature of the gas can be changed by various processes, such as by adding weights to the top of the piston or by heating the cylinder with a flame. The heat exchanged between the confined helium gas and the surroundings will be denoted by Q, where a positive value of Q indicates that the heat has been transferred *into* the gas; if Q is negative, heat has been transferred *out* of the gas. The work done on the gas will be denoted by W, where a positive value of W indicates that the gas does work on its surroundings; if W is negative, this means that the surroundings do work on the gas. The change in the internal energy of the gas is given by the equation.

$$\Delta E = Q - W$$

Equation 1

A student conducts the following series of experiments in a chemistry lab.

Experiment 1

The student measures the volume of the gas in the cylinder, places a known mass m on top of the piston, and then increases the temperature of the gas at constant pressure to 273°C.

Experiment 2

After the gas is allowed to cool back to 0°C at 1 atm pressure, the student locks the piston in place, and then increases the temperature of the gas to 273°C.

Experiment 3

After Experiment 2 is completed, the student unlocks the piston and a computer-controlled heat source maintains the temperature at a constant 273°C.

Experiment 4

After Experiment 2 is completed, the cylinder is completely wrapped in insulation before the piston is unlocked.

1. Experiment 4 is an example of an adiabatic process. Which of the following will always be true of an adiabatic process?

   A) The temperature will remain constant.
   B) $Q = W$
   C) $Q = -W$
   D) $Q = 0$

2. How do the pressure and volume of the gas change as a result of the procedures in Experiment 2?

   A) The pressure doubles, but the volume remains the same.
   B) The pressure stays the same, but the volume doubles.
   C) The pressure and volume both double.
   D) The pressure and volume both remain the same.

3. Which of the following best describes how the pressure and volume of the gas change as a result of Experiment 3?

   A) The pressure decreases, but the volume increases.
   B) The pressure increases, but the volume decreases.
   C) The pressure and volume both decrease.
   D) The pressure and volume both increase.

4. The student repeats Experiment 1 with a different cylinder and piston and finds that the volume increases from 0.025 m³ to 0.1 m³ at a constant pressure of 40 kPa. What is the value of W?

   A) −3000 J
   B) −300 J
   C) +300 J
   D) +3000 J

5. Let Q_3 and Q_4 denote the value of the heat transferred in Experiments 3 and 4, respectively, and let ΔE_3 and ΔE_4 represent the change in the internal energy of the gas in Experiments 3 and 4, respectively. Which one of the following statements is true?

A) $Q_3 < Q_4$ and $\Delta E_3 < \Delta E_4$
B) $Q_3 < Q_4$ and $\Delta E_3 > \Delta E_4$
C) $Q_3 > Q_4$ and $\Delta E_3 < \Delta E_4$
D) $Q_3 > Q_4$ and $\Delta E_3 > \Delta E_4$

6. After Experiment 4 is completed, the student places a 200-gram block on top of the piston, which pushes it down by 5 cm. As a result, the student should find that the internal energy of the gas:

A) decreases by 1 J.
B) decreases by 0.1 J.
C) increases by 0.1 J.
D) increases by 1 J.

SOLUTIONS TO CHAPTER 7 FREESTANDING QUESTIONS

1. **B** An increase of 20% in length is the same as saying $\Delta L/L_0 = 0.20$. This eliminates choice C. Substituting into the given equation yields

   $$\alpha \Delta T = \Delta L/L_0 = 0.2 \rightarrow \Delta T = 0.2/\alpha = 1/5\alpha.$$

   Choice D is eliminated because the scale of degrees Celsius and kelvins is the same, they just have different zeros ($-273°C = 0$ K).

2. **D** Obviously heat can raise the temperature of a system, and Item I is true (which doesn't eliminate anything). Heat can also melt a solid or boil a liquid without raising its temperature, so Item II is true, eliminating choices A and C. Heat additionally can expand a gas while it maintains constant temperature, so Item III is true, eliminating choice B. The point of the question is to reinforce that heat is a form of energy, not just something that makes other things "hot."

3. **C** An expanding spring exerts a force that causes a mass (the gas and its container, but even the gas has mass on its own) to displace, so it does positive work on the system, eliminating B. This work done on the system is mechanical, and because the gas is neither expanded nor compressed, simply translated, its kinetic energy increases. There is no friction and no mention of a temperature differential that would move heat into or out of the system, so $Q = 0$, eliminating choices A and D.

4. **A** During an adiabatic process, no heat is exchanged between the system and its surroundings ($Q = 0$). This eliminates choices B and D. For adiabatic processes, the change in internal energy of the system is equivalent to the negative work done by or positive work done on the system. When a gas is compressed, work is done on the gas. The temperature of the gas increases as a result.

5. **C** For a closed system at constant pressure, the magnitude of work can be calculated as $W = P\Delta V$. In this problem liters must be converted to m^3 as shown here:

   $$W = (1.0 \times 10^5 \text{ Pa})(5 \times 10^{-2} \text{ L})$$

   $$W = (1.0 \times 10^5 \text{ J/m}^3)(5 \times 10^{-2} \text{ L} \times 10^{-3} \text{ m}^3/\text{L})$$

   $$W = (1.0 \times 10^5 \text{ J/m}^3)(5 \times 10^{-5} \text{ m}^3) = 5.0 \text{ J}$$

   The balloon is expanding at constant temperature so work is being done by the balloon on the surroundings, so $W > 0$. Since the question asks for the heat transferred when $\Delta T = 0$, in an isothermal system $Q = W$. Therefore, $Q = +5.0$ J.

6.   **D**   Because every curve has a nonzero area beneath it, the statement in choice A is true; only vertical isochores describe processes in which $W = 0$. By definition, no heat is exchanged during adiabatic processes, but heat is exchanged in all other processes, so the statement in choice B is true. That's enough to make choice D correct, but it's also worth noting that the statement in choice C is true: a cycle that returns a gas to the same point on the PV diagram must return all state variables to the same value.

SOLUTIONS TO CHAPTER 7 PRACTICE PASSAGE

1.   **D**   If no heat is exchanged between the system and the surroundings, then $Q = 0$. Choice A is a trap: A process in which the temperature remains constant is called *isothermal*; do not confuse adiabatic with isothermal. The internal energy of the gas can be increased either by an exchange of heat or by work being performed on or by the gas. If Q is 0 but W is not, then ΔE will not be zero; as a result, the temperature of the gas will change.

2.   **A**   Since the piston is locked in place, the volume of the gas cannot change; this eliminates choices B and C. From the Ideal-Gas law, $PV = nRT$, we see that P is proportional to T. Since the absolute temperature doubles (from 0°C = 273 K to 273°C = 546 K), so does the pressure.

3.   **A**   Once the piston is unlocked, the hot gas can expand. Since a constant temperature is maintained, the gas expands isothermally. In an isothermal expansion of a gas, the pressure decreases while the volume increases.

4.   **D**   Because the volume of the gas increases, the gas does positive work against the piston, pushing it upwards. Because the gas does work on its surroundings, the value of W must be positive; this eliminates choices A and B. Since the pressure is constant, the force exerted by the gas is constant, so the expression $P\Delta V$ gives the magnitude of the work (it's just the area of a rectangle of base ΔV and height P). In this case, we have $W = P\Delta V = (40 \times 10^3 \text{ Pa})(0.075 \text{ m}^3) = 3000 \text{ J}$.

5.   **D**   In Experiment 3, T is constant, so E is constant (because the internal energy of a gas is directly proportional to its absolute temperature); thus, $\Delta E_3 = 0$. Since the gas does work pushing the piston upwards, W_3 is positive; as a result, $Q_3 = \Delta E_3 + W_3$ is positive. Experiment 4 describes an adiabatic process, so $Q_4 = 0$. Since the gas does work pushing the piston upwards, W_4 is positive, so $\Delta E_4 = Q_4 - W_4$ is negative. Therefore, $Q_3 > Q_4$ and $\Delta E_3 > \Delta E_4$.

6.   **C**   The weight on the piston pushes it down, and thus does work on the gas. The force is equal to the weight, $F = mg = (0.2 \text{ kg}) \times (10 \text{ N/kg}) = 2 \text{ N}$. Multiplying this by the distance, $d = 0.05 \text{ m}$, we find that the work done on the gas is $W = Fd = 0.1 \text{ J}$. Remember that $-W_{\text{on gas}} = W_{\text{by gas}} = -0.1 \text{ J}$. Because no heat is exchanged in Experiment 4, we have $\Delta E = Q - W = 0 - (-0.1 \text{ J}) = +0.1 \text{ J}$, so the internal energy of the gas increases by 0.1 J.

Chapter 8
Fluids and Elasticity
of Solids

8.1 HYDROSTATICS: FLUIDS AT REST

In this section and the next, we'll discuss some of the fundamental concepts dealing with substances that can flow, which are known as **fluids**. *Both liquids and gases are fluids*, but there are distinctions between them. At the molecular level, a substance in the liquid phase is similar to one in the solid phase in that the molecules are close to, and interact with, one another. The molecules in a liquid are able to move around a little more freely than those in a solid, in which the molecules typically only vibrate around relatively fixed positions. By contrast, the molecules of a gas are not constrained and fly around in a chaotic swarm, with hardly any interaction. On a macroscopic level, there is another distinction between liquids and gases. If you pour a certain volume of a liquid into a container of a greater volume, the liquid will occupy its original volume, whatever the shape and size of the container. However, if you introduce a sample of gas into a container, the molecules will fly around and fill the *entire* container.

Density and Specific Gravity

The **density** of a substance is the amount of mass contained in a unit of volume. In SI units, density is usually expressed in kg/m³ or g/cm³.

$$\text{density} = \frac{\text{mass}}{\text{volume}}$$

$$\rho = \frac{m}{V}$$

There is one substance whose density you should memorize: The density of liquid water is taken to be 1000 kg/m³ or 1 g/cm³. (Another useful version of the same value: 1 kg/L, where L stands for a liter; a liter is 1000 cm³.)

Sometimes the MCAT mentions **specific gravity**. This (poorly named) unitless number tells us how dense something is compared to water:

$$\text{specific gravity} = \frac{\text{density of substance}}{\text{density of water}}$$

$$\text{sp. gr.} = \frac{\rho}{\rho_{H_2O}}$$

For solids, density doesn't change much with surrounding pressure or temperature. For example, the density of marble is pretty close to 2700 kg/m^3 under most conditions. Liquids behave the same way: the density of water is pretty close to 1000 kg/m^3 under all conditions at which it's a liquid. However, the density of a gas changes markedly with pressure and temperature. (The ideal gas law tells us that $PV = nRT$, so the density of a sample of an ideal gas is given by the equation $\rho_{gas} = m/V = mP/nRT$, which depends on P and T.)

Example 8-1: Turpentine has a specific gravity of 0.9. What is the density of this liquid?

Solution: By definition, we have

$$\rho_{turpentine} = (\text{sp. gr.}_{turpentine})(\rho_{H_2O}) = (0.9)(1000\tfrac{kg}{m^3}) = 900\tfrac{kg}{m^3}$$

Example 8-2: A 2 cm^3 sample of osmium, one of the densest substances on Earth, has a mass of 45 g. What's the specific gravity of this metal?

Solution: The density of osmium is

$$\rho = \frac{m}{V} = \frac{45\text{ g}}{2\text{ cm}^3} = 22.5\tfrac{g}{cm^3}$$

Since this is 22.5 times the density of water (which is 1 g/cm^3), the specific gravity of osmium is 22.5.

Example 8-3: A cork has volume of 4 cm^3 and weighs 0.01 N. What is its density? What is its specific gravity?

Solution: Because the cork weighs 10^{-2} N, its mass is

$$m = \frac{w}{g} = \frac{10^{-2}\text{ N}}{10\,\tfrac{N}{kg}} = 10^{-3}\text{ kg}$$

Therefore, its density is

$$\rho_{cork} = \frac{m}{V} = \frac{10^{-3}\text{ kg}}{4\text{ cm}^3} \times \left(\frac{10^2\text{ cm}}{1\text{ m}}\right)^3 = \tfrac{1}{4} \times 10^3\,\tfrac{kg}{m^3} = 2.5 \times 10^2\,\tfrac{kg}{m^3}$$

and its specific gravity is

$$\text{sp. gr.}_{cork} = \frac{\rho_{cork}}{\rho_{H_2O}} = \frac{\tfrac{1}{4} \times 10^3\,\tfrac{kg}{m^3}}{10^3\,\tfrac{kg}{m^3}} = \tfrac{1}{4} = 0.25$$

Force of Gravity for Fluids

When solving questions involving fluids, it is often handy to know how to find the force of gravity acting on the fluid itself or objects that are immersed in the fluid. In previous chapters, we have used $F_{grav} = mg$ without too much difficulty. However, with fluids, it is more difficult to remove a portion of fluid from a tank, place it on a scale, and find its mass. Using the relationship between mass, volume, and density, we can redefine the magnitude of F_{grav} for fluids questions:

$$\rho = \frac{m}{V} \quad \rightarrow \quad m = \rho V \quad \rightarrow \quad \therefore F_{grav} = mg = \rho V g$$

With this new formula $F_{grav} = \rho V g$, it is important to make sure that the density (ρ) and the volume (V) describe the properties of the correct object or fluid.

Pressure

If we place an object in a fluid, the fluid exerts a contact force on the object. If we look at how that force is *distributed* over any small area of the object's surface, we have the concept of **pressure**:

Pressure

$$P = \frac{\text{force}_\perp}{\text{area}} = \frac{F_\perp}{A}$$

The subscript $\perp$ (which means "perpendicular") indicates that pressure is defined as the magnitude of the force acting *perpendicular* to the surface, divided by the area. We don't need to worry very much about this, because (for MCAT purposes) at any given point in a fluid the pressure is the same in all directions, which means that the force does not depend on the orientation of the force.

Although the formula for pressure involves "force," pressure is actually a *scalar* quantity, because the perpendicular force is the same for all orientations of surface. The unit of pressure is the N/m^2, which is called a **pascal** (abbreviated **Pa**). Because 1 N is a pretty small force and 1 m^2 is a pretty big area, 1 Pa is very small. Often, you'll see pressure expressed in kPa (or even in MPa). For example, at sea level, normal atmospheric pressure is about 100 kPa.

Let's imagine we have a tank of water with a lid on top. Suspended from the lid is a string attached to a thin metal sheet. The figures on the following page show you two views of this.

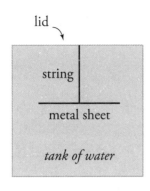

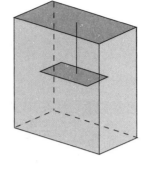

front view   side corner view

The weight of the water above the metal sheet produces a force that pushes down on the sheet. If we divide this force by the area of the sheet, w/A, we get the pressure, due to the water, on the sheet. The formula for calculating this pressure depends on the density of the fluid in the tank (ρ_{fluid}), the depth of the sheet (D), and the acceleration due to gravity (g).

$$P = \frac{w_{\text{fluid}}}{A} = \frac{m_{\text{fluid}}g}{A} = \frac{\rho_{\text{fluid}}V_{\text{fluid}}g}{A} = \frac{\rho_{\text{fluid}}ADg}{A} = \rho_{\text{fluid}}Dg$$

Hydrostatic Gauge Pressure

$$P_{\text{gauge}} = \rho_{\text{fluid}}gD$$

This formula gives the pressure due only to the fluid (in this case, the water) in the tank. This is called **hydrostatic gauge pressure**. It's called hydro*static*, because the fluid is at rest, and *gauge* pressure means that we don't take the pressure due to the atmosphere into account. If there were no lid on the water tank, then the water would be exposed to the atmosphere, and the *total* pressure at any point in the water would be equal to the atmospheric pressure pushing down on the surface *plus* the pressure due to the water (that is, the gauge pressure). So, below the surface, we'd have

$$P_{\text{total}} = P_{\text{atm}} + P_{\text{gauge}}$$

If the tank were closed to the atmosphere, but there were a layer of gas above the surface of the water, then the total pressure at a point below the surface would be the pressure of the gas pushing down at the surface plus the gauge pressure: $P_{\text{total}} = P_{\text{gas}} + P_{\text{gauge}}$. In general, we'll have

$$P_{\text{total}} = P_{\text{at surface}} + P_{\text{gauge}}$$

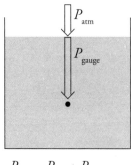

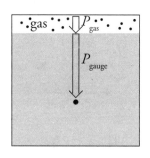

$$P_{total} = P_{atm} + P_{gauge} \qquad\qquad P_{total} = P_{gas} + P_{gauge}$$

in either case:

$$P_{total} = P_{at\ surface} + P_{gauge}$$

Notice that hydrostatic gauge pressure, $P_{gauge} = \rho_{fluid}gD$, is proportional to both the depth and the density of the fluid. *Total* pressure, however, is *not* proportional to either of these quantities if $P_{on\ surface}$ isn't zero.

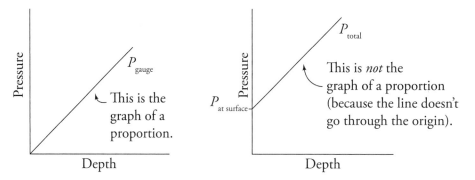

The lines in these graphs will be straight as long as the density of the liquid remains constant as the depth increases. Actually, ρ increases as the depth increases, but the effect is small enough that we generally consider liquids to be **incompressible**; that is, that the density of a liquid remains constant (so, in particular, the density doesn't increase with depth).

Example 8-4: The density of seawater is 1025 kg/m³. Consider a point X that's 10 m below the surface of the ocean.

a) What's the gauge pressure at X?
b) If the atmospheric pressure is 1.015×10^5 Pa, what is the total pressure at X?
c) Consider a point Y that's 50 m below the surface. How does the gauge pressure at Y compare to the gauge pressure at X? How does the total pressure at Y compare to the total pressure at X?

Solution:

a) The gauge pressure at X is

$$P_{\text{gauge}} = \rho_{\text{fluid}} gD = (1025 \tfrac{\text{kg}}{\text{m}^3})(10 \tfrac{\text{N}}{\text{kg}})(10 \text{ m}) = 1.025 \times 10^5 \text{ Pa}$$

b) The total pressure at X is the atmospheric pressure plus the gauge pressure:

$$P_{\text{total at X}} = P_{\text{atm}} + P_{\text{gauge}} = (1.015 \times 10^5 \text{ Pa}) + (1.025 \times 10^5 \text{ Pa}) = 2.04 \times 10^5 \text{ Pa}$$

c) Since P_{gauge} is proportional to D, an increase in D by a factor of 5 will mean the gauge pressure will also increase by a factor of 5. Therefore, the gauge pressure at Y will be $5(P_{\text{gauge at X}}) = 5.125 \times 10^5$ Pa. The total pressure at Y is equal to the atmospheric pressure plus the gauge pressure at Y, so

$$P_{\text{total at Y}} = P_{\text{atm}} + P_{\text{gauge}} = (1.015 \times 10^5 \text{ Pa}) + (5.125 \times 10^5 \text{ Pa}) = 6.14 \times 10^5 \text{ Pa}$$

Notice that $P_{\text{total at Y}}$ is not 5 times $P_{\text{total at X}}$. *Total* pressure is *not* proportional to depth.

Example 8-5: A large storage tank fitted with a tight lid holds a liquid. The space between the surface of the liquid and the lid of the tank is filled with molecules of the stored liquid in the gaseous phase. At a depth of 40 m, the total pressure is 520 kPa, while at a depth of 50 m, the total pressure is 600 kPa. What's the pressure of the gas above the surface of the liquid?

Solution: Let P_{gas} be the pressure that the gas exerts on the surface of the liquid. Then we have

$$P_{\text{total at } D_1 = 40 \text{ m}} = P_{\text{gas}} + \rho_{\text{fluid}} gD_1 = P_{\text{gas}} + \rho_{\text{fluid}} g(40 \text{ m}) = 520 \text{ kPa}$$
$$P_{\text{total at } D_1 = 50 \text{ m}} = P_{\text{gas}} + \rho_{\text{fluid}} gD_2 = P_{\text{gas}} + \rho_{\text{fluid}} g(50 \text{ m}) = 600 \text{ kPa}$$

We have two equations and two unknowns (P_{gas} and ρ_{fluid}). If we subtract the first equation from the second, we get $\rho_{\text{fluid}} g(10 \text{ m}) = 80$ kPa, which tells us that $\rho_{\text{fluid}} g = 8 \dfrac{\text{kPa}}{\text{m}}$. Plugging this back into either one of the equations will give us P_{gas}. Choosing, say, the first one, we find that

$$P_{\text{gas}} + \left(8 \frac{\text{kPa}}{\text{m}}\right)(40 \text{ m}) = 520 \text{ kPa} \rightarrow P_{\text{gas}} = 200 \text{ kPa}$$

Example 8-6: The containers shown below are all filled with the same liquid. At which point (A, B, C, D, E, or F) is the gauge pressure the lowest?

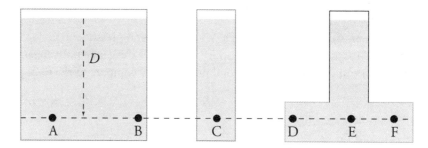

Solution: It's important to remember that the formula $P_{gauge} = \rho_{fluid}gD$ applies regardless of the shape of the container in which the fluid is held. If all the containers are filled with the same fluid, then the pressure is the *same* everywhere along the horizontal dashed line. This is because every point on this line (and within one of the containers) is at the same depth, D, below the surface of the fluid. The fact that the first container is wide, the second container is narrow, and the third container is wide at the base but has a narrow neck makes no difference. Even the fact that Points D and F (in the third container) aren't *directly* underneath a column of fluid of height D makes no difference either.

Pressure is the magnitude of the force per area, so pressure is a *scalar*. Pressure has no direction. The force *due to the pressure* is a vector, however, and the direction of this force on any small surface is always perpendicular to that surface. For example, in the figure below, the pressure at Point A is the same as the pressure at Point B, because they're at the same depth. But, as you can see, the direction of the force due to the pressure varies depending on the orientation of the surface (and even which side of the surface) the force is pushing on.

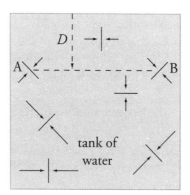

Buoyancy and Archimedes' Principle

Let's place a wooden block in our tank of water. Since the pressure on each side of the block depends on its average depth, we see that there's more pressure on the bottom of the block than there is on the top of it. Therefore, there's a greater force pushing up on the bottom of the block than there is pushing down on the top. The forces due to the pressure on the other four sides (left and right, front and back) cancel out, so the net fluid force on the block is upward. This net upward fluid force is called the **buoyant** force (or just **buoyancy** for short), which we'll denote by F_{Buoy} (or F_B).

We can calculate the magnitude of the buoyant force using Archimedes' principle:

Archimedes' Principle

The magnitude of the buoyant force
is equal to
the weight of the fluid displaced by the object.

When an object is partially or completely submerged in a fluid, the volume of the object that's submerged, which we call V_{sub}, is the volume of the fluid displaced.

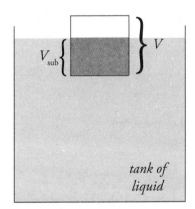

By multiplying V_{sub} by the density of the fluid, we get the *mass* of the fluid displaced; then, multiplying this mass by g gives us the weight of the fluid displaced. So, here's Archimedes' principle as a mathematical equation:

Archimedes' Principle

$$F_{\text{Buoy}} = \rho_{\text{fluid}} V_{\text{sub}} g$$

When an object floats, its submerged volume is just enough to make the buoyant force it feels balance its weight. That is, for a floating object, we always have $w_{\text{object}} = F_{\text{Buoy}}$. If an object's density is ρ_{object} and its volume is V, its weight will be $\rho_{\text{object}} V_{\text{object}} g$. The buoyant force it feels is $\rho_{\text{fluid}} V_{\text{sub}} g$. Setting these equal to each other, we find that

Floating Object in Equilibrium on Surface

$$w_{object} = F_{Buoy}$$

$$\frac{V_{sub}}{V} = \frac{\rho_{object}}{\rho_{fluid}}$$

So, if $\rho_{object} < \rho_{fluid}$, then the object will float; and the fraction of its volume that's submerged is the same as the ratio of its density to the fluid's density. *This is a very helpful fact to know for the MCAT.* For example, if the object's density is 3/4 the density of the fluid, then 3/4 of the object will be submerged (and vice versa).

If an object is denser than the fluid, then the object will sink. In this case, even if the entire object is submerged (in an attempt to maximize the buoyant force), the object's weight is still greater than the buoyant force. This leaves a net force in the downwards direction, causing the object to sink by accelerating downwards. If an object just happens to have the same density as the fluid, it will be happy hovering (in static equilibrium) underneath the fluid.

For an object that is completely submerged in the surrounding fluid, the actual weight of the object ($w_{object} = \rho_{object}Vg$) remains unchanged. However, the object's "apparent" weight is less due to the buoyant force "buoying" the object upwards. This corresponds to the measurement of a scale placed at the bottom of a tank of liquid in order to measure the apparent weight of the submerged object, or the normal force acting on the object.

Since the volume of the object is equal to the submerged volume ($V = V_{sub}$), the buoyant force F_{Buoy} on the object is equal to $\rho_{fluid}Vg$. Therefore,

$$\frac{w_{object}}{F_{Buoy}} = \frac{\rho_{object}Vg}{\rho_{fluid}Vg} = \frac{\rho_{object}}{\rho_{fluid}}$$

If the fluid in which the object is submerged is water, the ratio of the object weight to the buoyant force is equal to the specific gravity of the object.

Example 8-7: Ethyl alcohol has a specific gravity of 0.8. If a cork of specific gravity 0.25 floats in a beaker of ethyl alcohol, what fraction of the cork's volume is submerged?

    A.   4/25
    B.   1/5
    C.   1/4
    D.   5/16

Solution: Because the cork has a lower density than the ethyl alcohol, we know that the cork will float. Furthermore, the fraction of the cork's volume that will be submerged is

$$\frac{V_{sub}}{V} = \frac{\rho_{object}}{\rho_{fluid}} = \frac{(0.25)\rho_{H_2O}}{(0.8)\rho_{H_2O}} = \frac{0.25}{0.8} = \frac{\frac{1}{4}}{\frac{4}{5}} = \frac{5}{16}$$

Therefore, the answer is D.

Example 8-8: The density of ice is 920 kg/m³, and the density of seawater is 1025 kg/m³. Approximately what percent of an iceberg floats above the surface of the ocean (in other words, how much is "the tip of the iceberg")?

A. 5%
B. 10%
C. 90%
D. 95%

Solution: Because the ice has a lower density than the seawater, we know that the iceberg will float. Furthermore, the fraction of the iceberg's volume that will be submerged is

$$\frac{V_{sub}}{V} = \frac{\rho_{object}}{\rho_{fluid}} = \frac{920\ \frac{kg}{m^3}}{1025\ \frac{kg}{m^3}} \approx \frac{900}{1000} = 90\%$$

However, the answer is not C. The question asked what percent of the iceberg floats *above* the surface. So, if 90% is submerged, then 10% is above the surface, and the answer is B. Watch for this kind of tricky wording; it is a common MCAT tactic.

Example 8-9: A glass sphere of specific gravity 2.5 and volume 10^{-3} m³ is completely submerged in a large container of water. What is the apparent weight of the sphere while immersed?

Solution: Because the buoyant force pushes up on the object, the object's *apparent weight*, $w_{apparent} = w - F_{Buoy}$, is less than its true weight, w. Because the sphere is completely submerged, we have $V_{sub} = V$, so the buoyant force on the sphere is

$$F_{Buoy} = \rho_{fluid} V_{sub} g$$
$$= \rho_{H_2O} V g$$
$$= (1000\ \tfrac{kg}{m^3})(10^{-3}\ m^3)(10\ \tfrac{N}{kg})$$
$$= 10\ N$$

The true weight of the glass sphere is

$$w = \rho_{glass}Vg$$
$$= (\text{sp. gr.}_{glass} \times \rho_{H_2O})Vg$$
$$= (2.5 \times 1000 \ \tfrac{kg}{m^3})(10^{-3} \ m^3)(10 \ \tfrac{N}{kg})$$
$$= 25 \ N$$

Therefore, the apparent weight of the sphere while immersed is

$$w_{apparent} = w - F_{Buoy} = 25 \ N - 10 \ N = 15 \ N$$

Example 8-10: One way of measuring a person's body fat percentage is by comparing his weight in air to his weight while completely submerged in water. The principle is that fat is less dense than water (sp. gr. = 0.94) whereas bone and other tissues (average sp. gr. = 1.1) are more dense than water. If someone weighs 1050 N when weighed in air and 50 N when weighed fully submerged (with as little air in the lungs as possible), approximately what is his body fat percentage?

If the person has an apparent weight of 50 N when submerged, the buoyant force acting on him must be $w_{apparent} = w - F_B \rightarrow F_B = w - w_{apparent} = 1{,}050 \ N - 50 \ N = 1{,}000 \ N$. According to Archimedes' principle, the ratio of the man's weight to the buoyant force while completely submerged yields the ratio of his density to that of the fluid (in this case, water).

$$\frac{w}{F_B} = \frac{\rho_{man}}{1{,}000 \ kg/m^3} \rightarrow \frac{1{,}050 \ N}{1{,}000 \ N} = 1.05 = \frac{\rho_{man}}{1{,}000 \ kg/m^3} \rightarrow \rho_{man} = 1{,}050 \ kg/m^3$$

To achieve this density, the man must be some fraction of lean mass and the rest fat (note that we convert the given specific gravities of lean mass and fat to densities by multiplying by 1,000). Calling X the fraction of lean mass and omitting units for clarity:

$$1{,}100X + 940(1 - X) = 1{,}050 \rightarrow 1{,}100X - 940X = 160X = 110 \rightarrow X = \frac{110}{160} \approx \frac{2}{3}$$

Thus the man is about 70% lean mass and is 30% body fat mass.

Example 8-11: A balloon that weighs 0.18 N is then filled with helium so that its volume becomes 0.03 m³. (Note: The density of helium is 0.2 kg/m³.)

a) What is the net force on the balloon if it's surrounded by air? (Note: The density of air is 1.2 kg/m³.)

b) What will be the initial upward acceleration of the balloon if it's released from rest?

Solution:

a) Remember that gases are fluids, so they also exert buoyant forces. If an object is immersed in a gas, the object experiences a buoyant force equal to the weight of the gas it displaces. In this case, the balloon is completely immersed in a "sea" of air (so $V_{sub} = V$), and Archimedes' principle tells us that the buoyant force on the balloon due to the surrounding air is

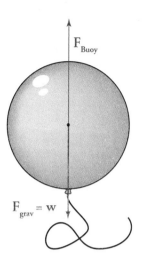

$$F_{Buoy} = \rho_{fluid} V_{sub} g$$
$$= \rho_{air} V g$$
$$= (1.2 \ \tfrac{kg}{m^3})(0.03 \ m^3)(10 \ \tfrac{N}{kg})$$
$$= 0.36 \ N$$

The weight of the inflated balloon is equal to the weight of the balloon material (0.18 N) plus the weight of the helium:

$$w_{total} = w_{material} + w_{helium}$$
$$= w_{material} + \rho_{helium} V g$$
$$= 0.18 \ N + (0.2 \ \tfrac{kg}{m^3})(0.03 \ m^3)(10 \ \tfrac{N}{kg})$$
$$= 0.18 \ N + 0.06 \ N$$
$$= 0.24 \ N$$

Because $F_{Buoy} > w_{total}$, the net force on the balloon is upward and has magnitude
$$F_{net} = F_{Buoy} - w_{total} = (0.36 \ N) - (0.24 \ N) = 0.12 \ N$$

b) Using Newton's second law, $a = F_{net} / m$ we find that

$$a = \frac{F_{net}}{m} = \frac{F_{net}}{\frac{w}{g}} = \frac{0.12 \ N}{\left(\frac{0.24 \ N}{10 \ m/s^2}\right)} = \frac{(0.12 \ N) \cdot (10 \ m/s^2)}{0.24 \ N} = \frac{10 \ m/s^2}{2} = 5 \ m/s^2$$

Pascal's Law

Pascal's law is a statement about fluid pressure. It says that a confined fluid will transmit an externally applied pressure change to all parts of the fluid and the walls of the container without loss of magnitude. In less formal language, if you squeeze a container of fluid, the fluid will transmit your squeeze perfectly throughout the container. The most important application of Pascal's law is to hydraulics.

Consider a simple hydraulic jack consisting of two pistons resting above two cylindrical vessels of fluid that are connected by a pipe. If you push down on one piston, the other one will rise. Let's make this more precise. Let F_1 be the magnitude of the force you exert down on one piston (whose cross-sectional area is A_1) and let F_2 be the magnitude of the force that the other piston (cross-sectional area A_2) exerts upward as a result.

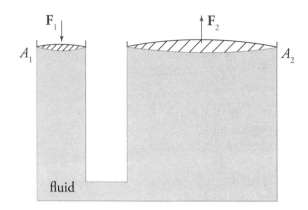

Pushing down on the left-hand piston with a force F_1 introduces a pressure increase of F_1 / A_1. Pascal's law tells us that this pressure change is transmitted, without loss of magnitude, by the fluid to the other end. Since the pressure change at the other piston is F_1 / A_1, we have, by Pascal's law,

$$\frac{F_1}{A_1} = \frac{F_2}{A_2}$$

Solving this equation for F_2, we get

$$F_2 = \frac{A_2}{A_1} F_1$$

So, if A_2 is greater than A_1 (as it is in the figure), then the ratio of the areas, A_2 / A_1, will be greater than 1, so F_2 will be greater than F_1; that is, *the output force, F_2, is greater than your input force, F_1*. This is why hydraulic jacks are useful; we end up lifting something very heavy (a car, for example) by exerting a much smaller force (one that would be insufficient to lift the car if it were just applied directly to the car).

This seems too good to be true; doesn't this violate some conservation law? No, since there's no such thing as a "Conservation of Force" law. However, there *is* a price to be paid for the magnification of the force. Let's say you push the left-hand piston down by a distance d_1, and that the distance the right-hand piston moves upward is d_2. Assuming the fluid is incompressible, whatever fluid you push out of the left-hand cylinder must appear in the right-hand cylinder. Since volume is equal to cross-sectional area times distance, the volume of the fluid you push out of the left-hand cylinder is $A_1 d_1$, and the extra volume of fluid that appears in the right-hand cylinder is $A_2 d_2$.

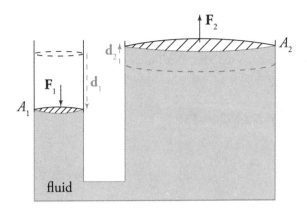

But these volumes have to be the same, so $A_1 d_1 = A_2 d_2$. Solving this equation for d_2, we get

$$d_2 = \frac{A_1}{A_2} d_1$$

If the area of the right-hand piston (A_2) is greater than the area of the left-hand piston (A_1), the ratio A_1 / A_2 will be *less* than 1, so d_2 will be less than d_1. In fact, the decrease in d is the same as the increase in F. For example, if A_2 is five times larger than A_1, then F_2 will be five times greater than F_1, but d_2 will only be *one-fifth* of d_1. We can now see that the product of F and d will be the same for both pistons:

$$F_2 d_2 = \left(\frac{A_2}{A_1} F_1 \right) \cdot \left(\frac{A_1}{A_2} d_1 \right) = F_1 d_1$$

Recall that the product of F and d is the amount of work done. What we have shown is that the work you do pushing the left-hand piston down is equal to the work done by the right-hand piston as it pushes upward. Just as when we discussed simple machines and mechanical advantage in Chapter 6, we can't cheat when it comes to work. True, we can do the same job with less force, but we will always pay for that by having to exert that smaller force through a greater distance. This is the whole idea behind all simple machines, not just a hydraulic jack.

Surface Tension

To complete our section on fluids at rest, we introduce the phenomenon of **surface tension**. We have all seen long-legged bugs that can walk on the surface of a pond or have watched a slowly-leaking faucet form a drop of water that grows until it finally drops into the sink. Both of these are illustrations of surface tension. The surface of a fluid can behave like an elastic membrane or thin sheet of rubber. A liquid will form a drop because the surface tends to contract into a sphere (to minimize surface area); however, when you see a drop hanging precariously from a faucet, its spherical shape is distorted by the pull of gravity. In fact, the reason it eventually falls into the sink is that the force due to surface tension causing the drop to cling to the head of the faucet is overwhelmed by the increasing weight of the drop. It can't hang on, and away it goes.

A standard way to define the surface tension is as follows. Imagine a rectangular loop of thin wire with one side able to slide up and down freely, thereby changing the enclosed area. If this apparatus is dipped into a fluid, a thin film will form in the enclosed area. Both the front face and the back face of the film are pulling upward on the free horizontal wire with a total upward force **F** against the wire's weight.

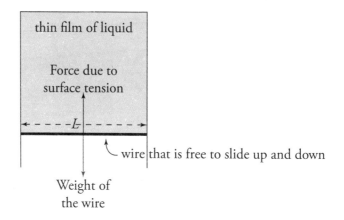

The strength of the surface tension force depends on the particular liquid and is determined by the *coefficient of surface tension*, γ, which is the force per unit length. Since there are *two* surfaces here (the front and the back), each of which acts along a length L, the force F due to surface tension acts along a total length of $2L$. The coefficient of surface tension is defined to be $\gamma = F/2L$, so $F_{\text{surf tension}} = 2\gamma L$. To give you an idea of the values of γ, the surface tension coefficient of water is 0.07 N/m at room temperature (and decreases as the temperature increases). A fluid with one of the highest surface tension coefficients is mercury. Its surface tension coefficient is nearly seven times greater than that of water: $\gamma_{\text{Hg}} = 0.46$ N/m at room temperature. Note that these values are really quite small. The surface of a pond of water can support the weight of a bug, but a frog isn't about to walk across the pond supported by surface tension.

8.2 HYDRODYNAMICS: FLUIDS IN MOTION

Flow Rate and the Continuity Equation

Consider a pipe through which fluid is flowing. The **flow rate**, f, is the volume of fluid that passes a particular point per unit time, like how many liters of water per minute are coming out of a faucet. In SI units, flow rate is expressed in m^3/s. To find the flow rate, all we need to do is multiply the cross-sectional area of the pipe at any point, A, by the average speed of the flow, v, at that point:

Flow Rate

$$f = Av$$

Be careful not to confuse flow rate with flow speed; flow rate tells us how *much* fluid flows per unit time; flow speed tells us how *fast* the fluid moves. There's a difference between saying that a hose ejects 4 liters of water every second (that's flow rate) and saying that the water leaves the hose at a speed of 4 m/s (that's flow speed).

If a pipe is carrying a liquid, which we assume is **incompressible** (that is, its density remains constant), then the flow rate must be the same everywhere along the pipe. Choose any two points in a flow tube carrying a liquid, Point 1 and Point 2. If there aren't any sources or sinks between these points (i.e., no leaks and no additional liquid), then the liquid that flows by Point 1 must also flow by Point 2, and vice versa. In other words, $f_1 = f_2$, or, since $f = Av$, we get $A_1 v_1 = A_2 v_2$; this is called the

Continuity Equation

$$A_1 v_1 = A_2 v_2$$

This tells us that when the tube narrows, the flow speed will increase; and if the tube widens, the flow speed will decrease. In fact, we can say that the flow speed is inversely proportional to the cross-sectional area (or to the square of the radius) of the pipe.

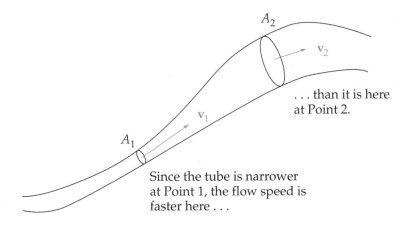

A_2

v_2

. . . than it is here
at Point 2.

v_1

A_1

Since the tube is narrower
at Point 1, the flow speed is
faster here . . .

Example 8-12: In the pipe shown above, if $A_2 = 9A_1$, then which of the following will be true?

A. $v_1 = 9v_2$
B. $v_1 = 3v_2$
C. $v_2 = 9v_1$
D. $v_2 = 3v_1$

Solution: If the cross-sectional area at Point 2 is 9 times the cross-sectional area at Point 1, then the flow speed at Point 2 will be 1/9 the flow speed at Point 1. That is, $v_2 = v_1 / 9$, or, solving for v_1, we get $v_1 = 9v_2$ (choice A).

Example 8-13: Before using a hypodermic needle to inject medication into a patient, a nurse tests the needle by shooting a small amount of the liquid into the air. The barrel of the needle is 1 cm in diameter, and the tip is 1 mm in diameter. If the nurse pushes the piston with a speed of 2 cm/s, how fast does the liquid come out the tip?

- A. 4 cm/s
- B. 20 cm/s
- C. 40 cm/s
- D. 200 cm/s

Solution: Cross-sectional area is proportional to the square of the diameter of the flow tube. In this case, the diameter decreases by a factor of 10 (from 1 cm to 1 mm), so the cross-sectional area decreases by a factor of $10^2 = 100$. Now, according to the continuity equation, if A decreases by a factor of 100, then v increases by a factor of 100. Therefore, the speed of the liquid coming out of the tip is $100 \times (2 \text{ cm/s}) = 200$ cm/s, choice D.

Example 8-14: A pipe of nonuniform diameter carries water. At one point in the pipe, the radius is 2 cm and the flow speed is 6 m/s.

a) What's the flow rate?

b) What's the flow speed at a point where the pipe constricts to a radius of 1 cm?

Solution:

a) At any point, the flow rate, f, is equal to the cross-sectional area of the pipe multiplied by the flow speed; therefore,

$$f = Av = \pi r^2 v = \pi (2 \times 10^{-2} \text{ m})^2 (6 \text{ m/s}) \approx 75 \times 10^{-4} \text{ m}^3/\text{s} = 7.5 \times 10^{-3} \text{ m}^3/\text{s}$$

b) By the continuity equation, we know that v, the flow speed, is inversely proportional to A, the cross-sectional area of the pipe. If the pipe's radius decreases by a factor of 2 (from 2 cm to 1 cm), A decreases by a factor of 4 because A is proportional to r^2. If A decreases by a factor of 4, then v will increase by a factor of 4. So, the flow speed at a point where the pipe's radius is 1 cm will be $4 \times (6 \text{ m/s}) = 24$ m/s.

Bernoulli's Equation

The most important equation in fluid dynamics is Bernoulli's equation, but before we state it, it's important to know under what conditions it applies. Bernoulli's equation applies to **ideal fluid** flow. A fluid must satisfy the following four requirements in order to be considered an ideal fluid:

- *The fluid is incompressible.*
  This works very well for liquids; gases are quite compressible, but it turns out that we can use the Bernoulli equation for gases provided the pressure changes are small.
- *There is negligible viscosity.*
  Viscosity is the force of cohesion between molecules in a fluid; think of it as internal friction for fluids. For example, maple syrup is more viscous than water, and there's more resistance to a flow of maple syrup than to a flow of water. (While Bernoulli's equation gives good results when applied to a flow of water, it would not give good results if it were applied to a flow of maple syrup.)
- *The flow is laminar.*
  In a tube carrying a flowing fluid, a *streamline* is just what it sounds like: a "line" in the stream. If we were to inject a drop of dye into a clear glass pipe carrying, say, water, we'd see a streak of dye in the pipe, indicating a streamline. The entire flow is called streamline (as an adjective) or laminar if the individual streamlines don't cross. When the flow is laminar, the fluid flows *smoothly* through the tube.

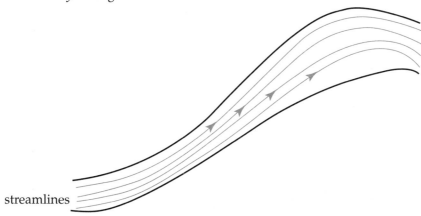

streamlines

The opposite of streamline flow is called **turbulent flow**. In this case, the flow is not smooth; it is chaotic (unpredictable). Turbulence is characterized by whirlpools and swirls (vortexes). At high enough speeds, all real fluids experience turbulent flow, and no simple equation can be applied to such a flow.

- *The flow rate is steady.*
  That is, the value of f is constant. If we're analyzing the water flowing through a garden hose connected to a faucet sticking out of the side of the house, turn the faucet handle to a particular setting and then leave it there. The flow rate through the hose must be steady while we're taking our measurements.

If these conditions hold—(1) the fluid is incompressible, (2) the flow is smooth (laminar), (3) there's no friction (viscosity), and (4) the flow rate is steady—then total mechanical energy will be conserved. *Bernoulli's equation is the statement of conservation of total mechanical energy for ideal fluid flow.* On the MCAT, you will often be told to consider a fluid to be ideal, allowing you to use Bernoulli's equation.

Bernoulli's Equation

$$P_1 + \tfrac{1}{2}\rho v_1^2 + \rho g y_1 = P_2 + \tfrac{1}{2}\rho v_2^2 + \rho g y_2$$

In this equation, ρ is the density of the flowing fluid, P_1 and P_2 give the pressures at any two points along a streamline within the flow, v_1 and v_2 give the flow speeds at these points, and y_1 and y_2 give the heights of these points above some chosen horizontal reference level.

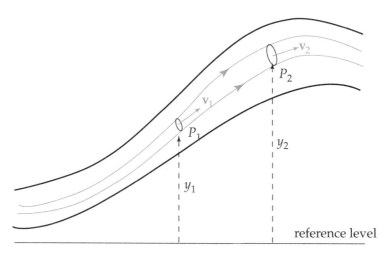

Although the equation may look complicated, notice that the two sides are the same, except all the subscripts on the left-hand side are 1's while all the subscripts on the right-hand side are 2's. Also, each $\frac{1}{2}\rho v_1^2$ term looks very much like the kinetic energy (sometimes it's referred to as kinetic energy density), and each term $\rho g y$ looks very much like gravitational potential energy. So, just take the equation you already know for conservation of total mechanical energy, $KE_1 + PE_1 = KE_2 + PE_2$, change the m's to ρ's, add P to both sides, and you've got Bernoulli's equation.

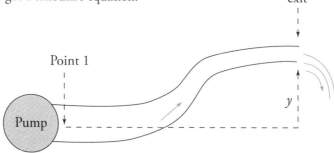

Example 8-15: In the figure above, a pump forces water at a constant flow rate through a pipe whose cross-sectional area, A, gradually decreases. At the exit point, A has decreased to 1/3 its value at the beginning of the pipe. If y = 60 cm and the flow speed of the water just after it leaves the pump (Point 1 in the figure) is 1 m/s, what is the gauge pressure at Point 1?

Solution: We'll apply Bernoulli's equation to Point 1 and the exit point, which we'll call Point 2. We'll choose the level of Point 1 as our horizontal reference level; this makes $y_1 = 0$. Now, because the cross-sectional area of the pipe decreases by a factor of 3 between Points 1 and 2, the flow speed must increase by a factor of 3; that is, $v_2 = 3v_1$. Since the pressure at Point 2 is P_{atm}, Bernoulli's equation becomes

$$P_1 + \tfrac{1}{2}\rho v_1^2 = P_{atm} + \tfrac{1}{2}\rho v_2^2 + \rho g y_2$$

This tells us that

$$
\begin{aligned}
P_1 - P_{atm} &= \rho g y_2 + \tfrac{1}{2}\rho v_2^2 - \tfrac{1}{2}\rho v_1^2 \\
&= \rho g y_2 + \tfrac{1}{2}\rho (3v_1)^2 - \tfrac{1}{2}\rho v_1^2 \\
&= \rho (g y_2 + 4v_1^2) \\
&= (1000 \ \tfrac{\text{kg}}{\text{m}^3})[(10 \ \text{m/s}^2)(0.6 \ \text{m}) + 4(1 \ \text{m/s})^2]
\end{aligned}
$$

$$\therefore P_{gauge\ at\ 1} = 10^4 \ \text{Pa}$$

Imagine that we punch a small hole in the side of a tank of liquid. We can use Bernoulli's equation to figure out the *efflux speed,* that is, how fast the liquid will flow out of the hole.

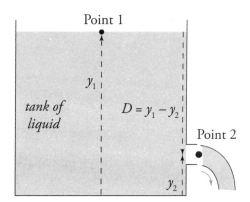

Let the bottom of the tank be our horizontal reference level, and choose Point 1 to be at the surface of the liquid and Point 2 to be at the hole where the water shoots out. First, the pressure at Point 1 is at atmospheric pressure; and the emerging stream at Point 2 is open to the air, so it's at atmospheric pressure, too. Therefore, $P_1 = P_2$, and these terms cancel out of Bernoulli's equation. Next, since the area at Point 1 is so much greater than at Point 2, we can assume that v_1, the speed at which the water level in the tank drops, is much lower than v_2, the speed at which the water shoots out of the hole. (Remember that by the continuity equation, $A_1 v_1 = A_2 v_2$; since $A_1 \gg A_2$, we'll have $v_1 \ll v_2$.) Because $v_1 \ll v_2$, we can say that $v_1 \approx 0$ and ignore v_1 in this case. So, Bernoulli's equation becomes

$$\rho g y_1 = \tfrac{1}{2}\rho v_2^2 + \rho g y_2$$

Crossing out the ρ's, and rearranging, we get

$$\tfrac{1}{2}v_2^2 = g(y_1 - y_2)$$
$$= gD$$
$$v_2 = \sqrt{2gD}$$

That is, $v_{efflux} = \sqrt{2gD}$, where D is the distance from the surface of the liquid down to the hole. This is called **Torricelli's result**. This equation should look familiar; it's basically the same formula that tells us how fast an object is going after it has fallen a distance h from rest.

Example 8-16: The side of an above-ground pool is punctured, and water gushes out through the hole. If the total depth of the pool is 2.5 m, and the puncture is 1 m above ground level, what is the efflux speed of the water?

Solution: We apply Torricelli's result, $v = \sqrt{2gD}$, where D is the distance from the surface of the pool down to the hole. If the puncture is 1 m above ground level, then it's 2.5 – 1 = 1.5 m below the surface of the water (because the pool is 2.5 m deep). Therefore, the efflux speed will be

$$v = \sqrt{2gD} = \sqrt{2(10 \text{ m/s}^2)(1.5 \text{ m})} = \sqrt{30 \text{ m/s}^2} \approx 5.5 \text{ m/s}$$

Example 8-17: A hole is opened at the bottom of a full barrel of liquid. When the efflux speed has decreased to 1/2 the initial efflux speed, the barrel is:

    A.   1/4 full
    B. $1/\sqrt{2}$ full
    C.   1/2 full
    D.   3/4 full

Solution: Torricelli's result tells us that the efflux speed is proportional to the square root of the height to the surface of the liquid in the barrel: $v \propto \sqrt{D}$. So, if v decreases by a factor of 2, then D has decreased by a factor of 4, and the answer is A.

Example 8-18: What does Bernoulli's equation tell us about a fluid at rest in a container open to the atmosphere?

Solution: Consider the figure below:

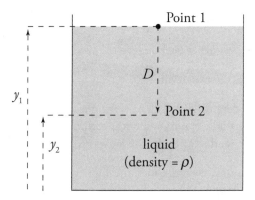

Because the fluid in the tank is at rest, both v_1 and v_2 are zero, and Bernoulli's equation becomes

$$P_1 + \rho g y_1 = P_2 + \rho g y_2$$

Since $P_1 = P_{atm}$, if we solve this equation for P_2, we get

$$P_2 = P_{atm} + \rho g(y_1 - y_2) = P_{atm} + \rho g D$$

which is the same formula we found earlier for hydrostatic pressure.

The Bernoulli Effect

Consider the two points labeled in the pipe shown below:

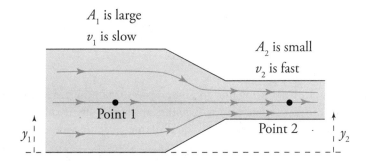

Since the heights y_1 and y_2 are equal in this case, the terms in Bernoulli's equation that involve the heights will cancel, leaving us with

$$P_1 + \tfrac{1}{2}\rho v_1^2 = P_2 + \tfrac{1}{2}\rho v_2^2$$

We already know from the continuity equation ($f = Av$) that the speed increases as the cross-sectional area of the pipe decreases. Since $A_2 < A_1$, we know that $v_2 > v_1$, and the equation above then tells us that $P_2 < P_1$. That is,

The pressure is lower where the flow speed is greater.

This is known as the **Bernoulli** (or **Venturi**) **effect**.

You may have seen a skydiver or motorcycle rider wearing a jacket that seems to puff out as they move rapidly through the air. The essentially stagnant air trapped inside the jacket is at a much higher pressure than the air whizzing by outside, and as a result, the jacket expands outward.

The drastic drop in air pressure that accompanies the high winds in a hurricane or tornado is another example. In fact, if high winds streak across the roof of a home, the outside air pressure is reduced so much that the air pressure inside the house (where the air speed is essentially zero) can be great enough to blow the roof off.

Example 8-19: A pipe of constant cross-sectional area carries water at a constant flow rate from the hot-water tank in the basement of a house up to the second floor. Which of the following will be true?

    A. The speed at which the water arrives at the second floor must be lower than the speed at which it left the water tank.

    B. The speed at which the water arrives at the second floor must be greater than the speed at which it left the water tank.

    C. The water pressure at the second floor must be lower than the water pressure at the tank.

    D. The water pressure at the second floor must be greater than the water pressure at the tank.

Solution: Because the flow rate is constant and the cross-sectional area of the pipe is constant, the flow speed will be constant (this follows from the continuity equation, $f = Av =$ constant). This eliminates choices A and B. Now, if the flow speeds v_1 and v_2 are the same, Bernoulli's equation becomes

$$P_1 + \rho g y_1 = P_2 + \rho g y_2$$

Because $y_2 > y_1$, it must be true that $P_2 < P_1$ (choice C).

Example 8-20: In a healthy adult standing upright, blood pressure in the arms and legs should be roughly equal. Suppose the height difference between elbow and ankle is 1 m. If one assumes that blood is an ideal fluid flowing through smooth rigid pipes of equal diameter, what would be the pressure difference between the arm and leg (the density of blood is about 1,025 kg/m³)?

Solution: According to Bernoulli's equation,

$$P_{arm} + \rho g y_{arm} + \tfrac{1}{2}\rho v_{arm}^2 = P_{leg} + \rho g y_{leg} + \tfrac{1}{2}\rho v_{leg}^2$$

The question stem states that the diameter of the pipes (the arteries and veins) should be assumed constant, so according to the continuity equation, $v_{arm} = v_{leg}$. Thus we have

$$\Delta P = P_{leg} - P_{arm} = \rho g y_{arm} - \rho g y_{leg} = \rho g (y_{arm} - y_{leg})(1{,}025 \text{ kg/m}^3)(10 \text{ m/s}^2)(1 \text{ m}) = 10{,}250 \text{ Pa}$$

For reference, this is about 80 torr, a huge pressure difference compared to typical healthy values of 120/80 torr. Clearly this result is suspicious. There are several reasons why one cannot validly apply Bernoulli's equation to blood flow, including that the heart is a pump (the flow is not under a constant pressure), the flexibility of the venous system, and the presence of valves in the circulatory system. However, one extremely important reason having to do with blood is its viscosity: blood is about 4 times more viscous than water (though the viscosity of blood varies depending upon several factors). This viscosity contributes to a resistance to flow, which leads to a pressure drop effect as blood gets further from the heart. One statement of *Poiseuille's law* for viscous fluid flow gives this pressure drop per unit length as

$$\frac{\Delta P}{L} = \frac{8\eta f}{\pi r^4}$$

where η is the viscosity coefficient of the fluid, f is flow rate, and r is the radius of the pipe.

8.3 THE ELASTICITY OF SOLIDS

Support beams for a building are compressed slightly under the heavy load they support; thick steel cables may be stretched in the construction of a bridge; and the ends of a connecting rod in a structure can be pushed or pulled in opposite directions, causing the rod to bend. These are some examples of the type of problem we'll look at in this section: the relationship between the forces applied to a solid object and the resulting change in the object's shape.

Stress

We'll look at three ways forces can be applied to an object: **tension** (stretching) forces, **compression** (squeezing) forces, and **shear** (bending) forces:

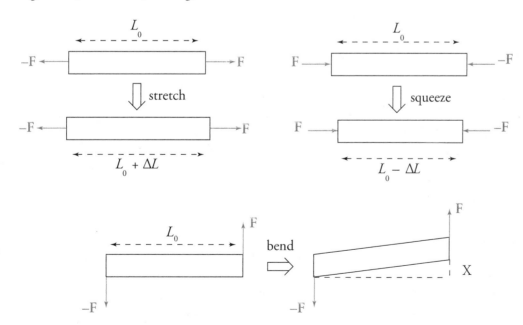

8.3

The magnitude of the force at either end, F, divided by the area over which it acts is called the **stress**:

Stress

$$\text{stress} = \frac{\text{force}}{\text{area}} = \frac{F}{A}$$

Stress is much like pressure, but they're not the same, because the force in the stress equation doesn't have to be perpendicular to the area over which it acts. For example, a shear force acts *parallel*, not perpendicular, to the areas at the ends. Nevertheless, we're still dividing a force by an area, so the unit of stress is the N/m^2, or pascal (Pa). It's *very important* to notice that stress is inversely proportional to the cross-sectional area, or, for an object with circular cross sections, inversely proportional to the *square* of the cross-sectional radius or diameter.

Strain

As a result of these forces, the object's shape will change. The ratio of the appropriate change in the length to the object's original length (see the figure above) is called the **strain**:

Strain

Tensile or Compressive	**Shear Strain**
$\text{strain} = \dfrac{\text{change in length}}{\text{original length}} = \dfrac{\Delta L}{L_0}$	$\text{strain} = \dfrac{\text{distance of shear}}{\text{original length}} = \dfrac{X}{L_0}$

The following mnemonic (though imprecise) may be helpful:

Stress is pressure. Strain is change.

Hooke's Law

The idea is simple: *Stress causes strain.* As long as the stress isn't too large—so that we don't permanently deform the object once the stress is removed (that is, allowing the object to display some *elasticity*)—then *stress and strain are proportional*. This is known as **Hooke's law**. For a tensile or compressive stress, the constant of proportionality is called **Young's modulus**; for a shear stress, it's called (what else?) the **shear**

modulus. The modulus depends on the type of material the object is made of; generally, the stronger the intermolecular bonds, the greater the modulus. A material's modulus can also depend on the type of stress the material is subjected to. For example, for the kind of steel used in building construction, the shear modulus is less than half its Young's modulus; this tells us that structural steel is weaker when subjected to shear forces than to tension or compression forces (that is, it's easier to bend steel than it is to stretch or compress it). It's even possible to have a Young's modulus for tension and a different one for compression. For example, human bone has two Young's moduli: The value of the modulus for compact bone under a tensile stress is about twice the value of the modulus for a compressive stress. Bone is more resistant to tension than to compression.

Hooke's Law

$$\text{stress} = \text{modulus} \times \text{strain}$$

Young's modulus is denoted by the letter Y or by E, while shear modulus is denoted by S or by G. Using E for Young's modulus (for tension and compression) and G for shear modulus, Hooke's law yields the following easy-to-remember formulas for tension/compression and for shear:

Tension/Compression

$$\frac{F}{A} = E\frac{\Delta L}{L_0}$$

$$\therefore \Delta L = \frac{FL_0}{EA}$$

Shear

$$\frac{F}{A} = G\frac{X}{L_0}$$

$$\therefore X = \frac{FL_0}{AG}$$

We call these the *Flea* and *Flag* formulas.

Example 8-21: A piece of rubber, originally 18 cm long, is stretched to a length of 20 cm. What strain has it undergone?

Solution: The change in length is $\Delta L = 20 \text{ cm} - 18 \text{ cm} = 2 \text{ cm}$. Therefore, the strain is

$$\frac{\Delta L}{L_0} = \frac{2 \text{ cm}}{18 \text{ cm}} = \frac{1}{9}$$

Example 8-22: What are the units of Young's modulus and the shear modulus?

Solution: Hooke's law says that stress = modulus × strain. Because strain has no units (we're dividing a length by a length), the units of the modulus must be the same as the units of stress: pascals.

Example 8-23: Two cylindrical rods with circular cross sections are identical except for the fact that Rod 2 has four times the diameter of Rod 1. If these two rods are subjected to identical compressive forces, how will the compression of Rod 2 compare to that of Rod 1?

Solution: First, the fact that Rod 2 has 4 times the diameter of Rod 1 means that Rod 2 has $4^2 = 16$ times the cross-sectional area. Therefore, if both rods experience identical compressive forces, the stress on Rod 2 will be 1/16 the stress on Rod 1 (because stress = force/area). Since the rods are made of the same material, their Young's moduli are the same, so, by Hooke's law, the strain on Rod 2 will be 1/16 the strain on Rod 1. Finally, because the rods had the same original length, the change in length of Rod 2 will be 1/16 of the change in length of Rod 1.

Example 8-24: Two objects are subjected to identical tensile stresses. The object with the greater value of Young's modulus will undergo:

- A. a smaller change in length.
- B. a greater change in length.
- C. less strain.
- D. greater strain.

Solution: Hooke's law says that stress = modulus × strain. If stress is a constant, then the strain is inversely proportional to the modulus. Therefore, the object with the greater value of Young's modulus will experience less strain (choice C). Notice that we can't say that choice A is correct, since we don't know the original lengths of the objects.

Example 8-25: Which material has the greater Young's modulus: rubber or glass?

Solution: Hooke's law says that stress = modulus × strain. Or, using the *Flea* formula, $\Delta L = FL_0 / EA$, and solving for E, we get $E = FL_0 / A\Delta L$. Now let's say we had a piece of glass and an identical piece of rubber: same original length, width, and height. If we apply the same force to both the glass and the rubber, which one will experience the greater change in length? The rubber, of course. Since E is *inversely* proportional to ΔL, we'd expect that E for rubber will be lower than E for glass. Or, equivalently, the value of E is greater for glass than for rubber. (In fact, the value of E for glass is nearly ten thousand times the value of E for rubber.) In general, the greater the value of E, the more difficult it is to stretch or compress the material; similarly, the greater the value of G (the shear modulus), the more difficult it is to bend the material.

Example 8-26: Two metal beams have the same length and cross-sectional area, but Beam X has twice the shear modulus of Beam Y. If each beam is subjected to the same shear forces, which beam will bend more and by what factor?

    A.   Beam X, by a factor of 2
    B.   Beam X, by a factor of 4
    C.   Beam Y, by a factor of 2
    D.   Beam Y, by a factor of 4

Solution: If the beams have the same cross-sectional area and are subjected to the same shear forces, the shear stress on the beams will be the same (since stress = force/area). By Hooke's law, then, the strain is inversely proportional to the modulus. If Beam X has twice the shear modulus, it will undergo 1/2 the strain. Since the beams had the same original length, Beam Y will bend more, by a factor of 2 (choice C).

Example 8-27: Hooke's law for a spring says that the magnitude of the force required to stretch or compress the spring from its natural length is given by the simple formula $F = kx$, where k is a constant (which depends on the spring) and x is the amount by which the spring is stretched or compressed. Is this formula for Hooke's law the same as the one given in this section?

Solution: Yes. Some of the letters may be different, but the idea is exactly the same: The force of tension or compression is proportional to the amount of stretch or compression. Let's take Hooke's law as given in this section, express it in the form of the *Flea* formula, $\Delta L = FL_0 / EA$, and rewrite it like this: $F = (EA / L_0) \cdot \Delta L$. Now, notice that this equation has exactly the same form as the equation $F = kx$:

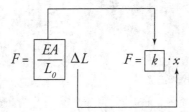

Summary of Formulas

HYDROSTATICS

Assume liquids are incompressible unless otherwise stated

Standard atmospheric pressure = 1 atm = 760 mmHg = 760 torr ≈ 100 kPa

Density: $\rho = \dfrac{m}{V}$

Specific gravity: $\text{sp.gr.} = \dfrac{\rho}{\rho_{H_2O}}$

$$\left(\rho_{H_2O} = 1000\,\tfrac{kg}{m^3} \text{ or } 1\,\tfrac{g}{cm^3} \text{ or } 1\,\tfrac{kg}{L} \right)$$

Force of gravity: $mg = \rho V g$

Pressure: $P = \dfrac{F_\perp}{A}$

Hydrostatic gauge pressure: $P_{gauge} = \rho_{fluid} g D$

> Hydrostatic gauge pressure is proportional to depth. Total hydrostatic pressure increases with increasing depth but is NOT proportional to depth.

Total hydrostatic pressure: $P_{total} = P_{at\ surface} + P_{gauge}$

Archimedes' principle: $F_{Buoy} = \rho_{fluid} V_{sub} g$

> Buoyant force is equal to the weight of the displaced fluid.

Floating object: $\rho_{object} < \rho_{fluid} \rightarrow w_{object} = F_{Buoy}$

$$\frac{V_{sub}}{V} = \frac{\rho_{object}}{\rho_{fluid}}$$

Apparent weight of submerged object: $w_{apparent} = w_{object} - F_{Buoy}$

Pascal's law: $\dfrac{F_1}{A_1} = \dfrac{F_2}{A_2}$

HYDRODYNAMICS

Conditions for ideal fluid:

- incompressible

- negligible viscosity

- laminar (non-turbulent)

- steady flow (satisfies continuity equation)

Flow rate: $f = Av$

Continuity equation: $A_1 v_1 = A_2 v_2$

Bernoulli's equation (ideal fluid):

- total energy (density) within all parts of an ideal fluid is the same

$$P_1 + \tfrac{1}{2}\rho v_1^2 + \rho g y_1 = P_2 + \tfrac{1}{2}\rho v_2^2 + \rho g y_2$$

Bernoulli principle ($y_1 = y_2$)

$$P_1 + \tfrac{1}{2}\rho v_1^2 = P_2 + \tfrac{1}{2}\rho v_2^2$$

- Fast flowing fluids have low pressure.

- Slow flowing fluids have high pressure.

Toricelli's result: $v_{efflux} = \sqrt{2gD}$

Poiseuille's law for flow rate of a viscous fluid: $\dfrac{\Delta P}{L} = \dfrac{8\eta f}{\pi r^4}$.

ELASTICITY OF SOLIDS

Stress: $\text{stress} = \dfrac{F}{A}$

Strain: $\text{strain} = \dfrac{\Delta L}{L_0}$

Hooke's law: $\text{stress} = \text{modulus} \times \text{strain}$

Tension or compression: $\Delta L = \dfrac{FL_0}{EA}$

Shear: $X = \dfrac{FL_0}{AG}$

CHAPTER 8 FREESTANDING PRACTICE QUESTIONS

1. Which of the following is true?

A) Compression in length increases with an increased area of applied force.
B) Compression in length increases with a decreased area of applied force.
C) Compression in length is larger with a smaller original length.
D) Compression in length is larger with a smaller Young's modulus.

2. A person is leaning on his elbow on a table. If the amount of force the table must exert to keep the person upright is F, the area of contact between the person and the table is A, and the angle that the person's arm makes with the table's surface is θ, how much pressure is exerted by the person on the table?

A) $\dfrac{F}{A}$

B) $\dfrac{F\sin\theta}{A}$

C) $\dfrac{F\cos\theta}{A}$

D) Since the force exerted by the person on the table is not given, the pressure exerted by the person on the table cannot be determined.

3. What is the maximum weight of an object that a 50 kg person could lift by standing on one piston of a hydraulic jack, if the jack's pistons are circular and have radii of 5 m and 10 m?

A) 500 N
B) 1000 N
C) 2000 N
D) 4000 N

4. If the blood in the body is taken to be an ideal fluid, which of the following is true of blood flow in arteries?

A) The flow speed of blood is the same through the complete peripheral vascular system at any given moment, but it varies over time.
B) The flow speed of blood is the same through the complete peripheral vascular system and does not vary over time.
C) The flow rate of blood is the same through the complete peripheral vascular system at any given moment, but it varies over time.
D) The flow rate of blood is the same through the complete peripheral vascular system and does not vary over time.

5. If the density of a person is approximately the density of water and the density of air is approximately 1 kg/m³, how many times greater is the weight of the person than the buoyant force from the air on the person?

A) 10
B) 100
C) 1000
D) 10000

6. Will an object with more mass but the same volume as another object sink faster in a non-viscous fluid?

A) No, because acceleration due to gravity is independent of the mass of the object being accelerated.
B) No, because the buoyant force is greater on an object with more mass.
C) Yes, because it weighs more, and the weight itself induces greater acceleration for the heavier object than for the lighter one.
D) Yes, because the buoyant force impedes the downward acceleration of a greater mass less than it does a lesser mass.

7. A particular eucalyptus tree has a density of 667 kg/m³ and a mass of 6000 kg. What volume of the tree would float above the surface of water?

A) 3 m³
B) 5 m³
C) 6 m³
D) 9 m³

CHAPTER 8 PRACTICE PASSAGE

Students are performing experiments in the laboratory using their knowledge of hydrostatics and hydrodynamics.

Experiment 1

Students are given five liquid substances and they are asked to find their densities. They also have a test block that they measure to have a mass of 50 g and a volume of 100 cm³. They place the test block into each liquid and measure how much of the test block is submerged in the water. Table 1 summarizes their results.

Liquid	Volume submerged	Float?
1	80 cm³	Yes
2	75 cm³	Yes
3	100 cm³	No
4	50 cm³	Yes
5	100 cm³	Yes

Table 1 Test block placed in different liquids

Experiment 2

The students are given four different complex objects that all have the same density. They place each object in a test liquid that has a specific gravity of 2. They record the submerged volume of the object by the measuring the displacement of the liquid. Their results are summarized in Table 2.

Object	Volume of displaced liquid
A	150 cm³
B	90 cm³
C	75 cm³
D	110 cm³

Table 2 Complex objects in a test liquid

Experiment 3

Students must create an irrigation system that takes water from a reservoir 80 cm deep to a wave pool across the room. A perfectly leveled, horizontal tube with constant circumference takes water from the bottom of the reservoir to the wave pool.

1. From Experiment 1, which liquid has the smallest density?

A) Liquid 4
B) Liquid 3
C) Liquid 5
D) Liquids 3 and 5

2. What is the specific gravity of Liquid 1?

A) 7/2
B) 5/8
C) 8/5
D) 2/7

3. What is the buoyant force acting on the test block in Liquid 5?

A) 2500 N
B) 500 N
C) 5 N
D) 0.5 N

4. Which object from Experiment 2 has the largest mass?

A) Object A
B) Object B
C) Object C
D) Object D

5. If the tubing used in Experiment 3 has a cross-sectional area of 0.02 m², what is the velocity of the water as it enters the wave pool? Assume the tubing is soft so that the pressure at the aperture from the reservoir is P_{atm}.

A) 2 m/s
B) 3 m/s
C) 4 m/s
D) 5 m/s

6. During Experiment 3, one student lowers the wave pool to the floor, 1.5 meters below the aperture in the reservoir. The water then flows through the tubing to the wave pool. As it flows, how does the flow speed at the reservoir aperture compare to the flow speed leaving the tubing into the wave pool?

A) $v_{\text{wave pool}} = \sqrt{v_{\text{reservoir}}^2 + 3g}$

B) $v_{\text{wave pool}} = \sqrt{v_{\text{reservoir}}^2 - 3g}$

C) $v_{\text{wave pool}} = v_{\text{reservoir}}$

D) Cannot be determined without knowing the instantaneous depth of the water in the reservoir and the wave pool.

7. Two objects made from the same material with the same mass are placed in a liquid, base first. The base of Object 2 is three times that of Object 1. What best describes the buoyant force on the objects?

A) Object 1 has a greater buoyant force acting on it because it has a larger volume submerged.

B) Object 2 has a greater buoyant force acting on it because it has a larger volume submerged.

C) Object 2 has a greater buoyant force acting on it because it has a larger area at its base.

D) The buoyant force acting on both objects is the same.

SOLUTIONS TO CHAPTER 8 FREESTANDING QUESTIONS

1. **D** The formula for change in length is $\Delta L = FL_0 / EA$, where ΔL is the change in length, F is the applied force, L_0 is the original length, E is the Young's modulus and A is the area of applied force. Choice B could be eliminated first because from our everyday knowledge, the more force is applied, the more compressed an object is. Of the remaining choices, only choice D fits the relationship described by the above formula.

2. **B** First, eliminate D because the force exerted by the table on the person, given as F, is equal in magnitude to the force exerted by the person on the table, according to Newton's third law. Next, the way that pressure, force, and area are related is $P = \dfrac{F_\perp}{A}$. Since the given angle is between the arm and the table, the vertical component of the force will be related to the sine of that angle. Thus, $P = \dfrac{F \sin \theta}{A}$. Choice A is wrong because it would be the pressure if the force were not at an angle, and choice C is wrong because it would be the pressure if the angle given were between the arm and a line perpendicular to the table's surface.

3. **C** Pascal's law states that $\dfrac{F_1}{A_1} = \dfrac{F_2}{A_2}$. Thus, $F_2 = \dfrac{F_1 A_2}{A_1}$. For the greatest force, A_1 should be small and A_2 should be large (that is, the person should stand on the smaller piston and put the object on the larger). If the person is standing on the piston, then the force applied is the person's weight, and the area of the circular pistons is πr^2, so $F_2 = \dfrac{(mg)(\pi r_2^{\,2})}{\pi r_1^{\,2}}$. Cancel π and plug in: $F_2 = \dfrac{(50 \times 10)(10^2)}{5^2}$. This comes out to 2000 N. Choice A is wrong because it is just the person's weight, and choice B is wrong because the force is proportional to the area, not to the radius. Choice D is wrong because volume (which would involve cubing the radius and gives this result) is not relevant here.

4. **C** This is a two-by-two question: determining whether the flow speed or flow rate is the relevant quantity will eliminate two answers, and determining whether the flow varies over time or not will eliminate the final wrong answer. The continuity equation states that flow rate is the same in a pipe, and arteries are enough like pipes that the same applies to them. The only assumption in the continuity equation is that the fluid is incompressible, and the question stem states that this fluid is an ideal liquid. Thus, eliminate choices A and B, because it is flow rate, not flow speed, that is the same through the complete peripheral vascular system. The difference between choices C and D is time variation, and the heart's pumping definitely is not steady. Between heartbeats, blood experiences much less pumping than it does during heartbeats. Therefore, the flow rate should vary over time, which eliminates choice D.

5. **C** The weight of a person, in terms of density, is $w_p = \rho_p V g$, where V is the volume of the person. The buoyant force from air on the person is $F_B = \rho_{air} V g$, where V is again the volume of the person because the whole person is submerged in air. This means that the only difference is the density of the person as compared to the density of air, and since we are told that the density of the person is approximately the density of water (1000 kg/m^3) and air has a density of approximately 1 kg/m^3, the relevant factor is 1000.

6. **D** Begin by setting up the forces and finding the acceleration. $F_{net} = ma$, as always, so (defining the sinking direction as positive) $w - F_B = ma$. Next, specify weight and the buoyant force: $mg - \rho_f V_{sub} g = ma$. Divide by m, which yields $a = g - \frac{\rho_f V_{sub} g}{m}$. For a larger mass, the subtracted buoyant force will be less, and subtracting less means ending up with a greater number, so yes, the acceleration is greater for an object with greater mass, provided that the compared objects are sinking in the same fluid on the same planet (that is, ρ_f and g are the same for the two objects) and they have the same volume (as the stem indicates they do). Notice that it is the buoyant force term that makes the difference here: mass canceled in the weight term. Objects fall at the same rate in a vacuum, so it can't be the weight itself that is causing this effect, which is the reason that choice C is wrong. It is the buoyant force that is responsible for the difference in accelerations. Choices A and B are wrong for their "No" answers; choice A gives a true justification (acceleration due to gravity is independent of the mass of the object being accelerated), but it neglects the effect of the buoyant force, and choice B gives an incorrect reason, since equal volumes mean that the magnitude of the buoyant force on each object is the same.

7. **A** Recall that for floating objects $\frac{\rho_o}{\rho_f} = \frac{V_{sub}}{V}$. Since the density of the object is 667 kg/m^3 and the density of water is 1000 kg/m^3, two-thirds of the object will be submerged and one-third will be above the surface of the water. Since $\rho = \frac{m}{V}$, then $V = \frac{m}{\rho} = \frac{6000}{667} = 9$ m^3. The total volume of the object is 9 m^3, and one-third of that is 3 m^3.

SOLUTIONS TO CHAPTER 8 PRACTICE PASSAGE

1. **B**   An object will only sink if its density is greater than the density of the liquid. Since the test object is the same for all liquids, and only sank in Liquid 3, then Liquid 3 has the smallest density.

2. **B**   The specific gravity is equal to ρ_{fl}/ρ_{water}, and the density of water is 1 g/cm^3. The density of the fluid is $\rho_{obj}V/V_{sub} = m_{obj}/V_{sub}$, therefore, the density of Liquid 1 is (50 g)/(80 cm^3), and the specific gravity is 5/8.

3. **D**   The buoyant force is equal to $\rho_{fl}{}'V_{sub}{}'g$. The density of Liquid 5 is given by $m_{obj}/V_{sub} = 0.5$ g/cm^3. Thus the buoyant force is equal to (50 g)(10 m/s^2) = (0.05 kg)(10 m/s^2) = 0.5 N.

4. **A**   Using the equation for objects floating on the surface $V_{sub}/V_{obj} = \rho_{obj}/\rho_{fluid}$, we know that V_{sub} is proportional to $V_{obj}{}'\rho_{obj} = m_{obj}$. Since V_{sub} is the only variable, we know that the object with the largest submerged volume has the largest mass, which is Object A.

5. **C**   The velocity of the water entering the tube is given by $v = (2gD)^{0.5} = 4$ m/s. The flow rate is constant, and the cross-sectional area of the tubing does not change, so the velocity at the wave pool is equal to the velocity as it exits the reservoir.

6. **C**   Don't make the mistake of applying the Bernoulli equation in cases when it would contradict the continuity principle! The passage states that the tubing has a constant circumference, from which you can deduce that it has a constant cross-sectional area (if the tubing were to become pinched, that would change the area, but the MCAT would never ask you to deduce that behavior). Because the flow rate remains constant and the area remains constant, so must the flow speed, by $f = Av$.

7. **D**   The buoyant force is given by $\rho_{fl}V_{sub}g$. Since the blocks have the same density, they will have the same volume submerged, and thus, they will have the same buoyant force acting on them.

Chapter 9
Electrostatics

9.1   ELECTRIC CHARGE

An atom is composed of a central nucleus (which is itself composed of protons and neutrons) surrounded by a cloud of one or more electrons. The fact that an atom is held together as a single unit is due to the fact that protons and electrons have a special property: They carry **electric charge**, which gives rise to an attractive force between them.

Electric charge exists in two varieties, which are called **positive** and **negative**. By convention, we say that protons carry positive charge and electrons carry negative charge. (Neutrons are well-named: They're neutral, because they have no electric charge.) The charge of a proton is $+e$, where e is called the **elementary charge**, and the charge of an electron is $-e$. Notice that the proton and the electron carry exactly the same amount of charge; the only difference in their charges is that one is positive and the other is negative.

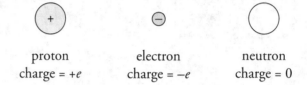

proton   electron   neutron

charge = $+e$ charge = $-e$ charge = 0

In SI units, electric charge is measured in **coulombs** (abbreviated **C**), and the value of the elementary charge, e, is 1.6×10^{-19} C.

Elementary Charge

$$e = 1.6 \times 10^{-19} \text{ C}$$

When an atom (or any other object) contains the same number of electrons as protons, its total charge is zero because the individual positive and negative charges add up and cancel. So, when the number of electrons (#e) equals the number of protons (#p), the object is *electrically neutral*. We say that an object is **charged** when there's an imbalance between the number of electrons and the number of protons. When an object has one or more extra electrons (#e > #p), the object is *negatively charged*, and when an object has a deficit of electrons (#e < #p), the object is *positively charged*. If a neutral atom has electrons removed or added, we say that it has been **ionized**, and the resulting electrically charged atom is called an **ion**. A positively charged ion is called a **cation**, and a negatively charged ion is called an **anion**. (An object can also become charged by gaining or losing protons, but these are usually locked up tight within the nuclei of the atoms. In virtually all cases, objects become charged by the transfer of *electrons*.)

Because an object can become charged only by losing or gaining electrons or protons, which can't be "sliced" into smaller pieces with fractional amounts of charge, the charge on an object can only be a whole number of $\pm e$'s; that is, charge is **quantized**. So, for any object, its charge is always equal to $n(\pm e)$, where n is a whole number. To remind us that charge is *quantized*, electric charge is usually denoted by the letter q (or Q).

> ### Charge is Quantized
>
> $$q = n(\pm e)$$
>
> where $n = 0, 1, 2...$

It is interesting to note that this quantization of charge applies to all fundamental particles either found in nature or created in the laboratory (e.g., muons, pions, etc.).

In chemistry, it's common to talk about the charge of an atom in terms of whole numbers like +1 or –2, etc. For example, we say that the charge of the fluoride ion, F^-, is –1, and the charge of the calcium ion, Ca^{+2}, is +2. This is just a convenient way of saying that the charge of the fluoride ion is –1 elementary unit (in other words, $-1e$), and the charge of the calcium ion is +2 elementary units, $+2e$. When we want to find the electric force between ions, we will express their charges in the proper unit (coulombs), and say, for example, that the charge of the fluoride ion is $-1e = -1.6 \times 10^{-19}$ C and the charge of the calcium ion is $+2e = +3.2 \times 10^{-19}$ C.

Finally, total electric charge is always conserved; that is, the total amount of charge before any process must always be equal to the total amount of charge afterward.[1]

Example 9-1: When you pet a cat, you rub electrons off the cat's fur, which are transferred to your hand. Assuming that you transfer 5×10^{10} electrons to your hand, what is the electric charge on your hand? What's the charge on the cat?

Solution: Because each electron carries a charge of $-e = -1.6 \times 10^{-19}$ C, and you've gained 5×10^{10} of them, the charge on your hand will be

$$(5 \times 10^{10})(-e) = (5 \times 10^{10})(-1.6 \times 10^{-19} \text{ C}) = -8 \times 10^{-9} \text{ C}$$

Since the cat has lost 5×10^{10} electrons, the charge on the cat will be

$$(5 \times 10^{10})(+e) = (5 \times 10^{10})(-1.6 \times 10^{-19} \text{ C}) = +8 \times 10^{-9} \text{ C}$$

Notice that the *net* charge before and after petting the cat was zero; all you've done is transfer charge.

---

[1] This does not mean that electric charge cannot be created or destroyed, which happens all the time. For example, in the reaction $e^- + e^+ \rightarrow \gamma + \gamma$ an electron (e^-) and its antiparticle (the positron, e^+, which is, in effect, a positively charged electron) meet and annihilate each other, producing energy in the form of two gamma-ray photons (γ), which carry no charge. Charge has been destroyed, but the total charge (zero, in this case) has been conserved. Conversely, charge can be created in the opposite process, when energy is converted to mass and charge (but always with zero total charge).

Example 9-2: How much positive charge is contained in 1 mole of carbon atoms? How much negative charge? What is the total charge?

Solution: Every atom of carbon contains 6 protons, so the amount of positive charge in one carbon atom is $q_+ = +6e$. Therefore, if N_A denotes Avogadro's number, the total amount of positive charge in 1 mole of carbon atoms is

$$Q_+ = N_A \times q_+ = N_A \times (+6e) = (6.02 \times 10^{23}) \times (6)(+1.6 \times 10^{-19} \text{ C}) = +6 \times 10^5 \text{ C}$$

Because every neutral carbon atom also contains 6 electrons, the amount of negative charge in a carbon atom is $q_- = 6(-e) = -6e = -q_+$, so the total amount of negative charge in 1 mole of carbon atoms is $Q_- = N_A \times q_- = -Q_+ \approx -6 \times 10^5 \text{ C}$. The total charge on the carbon atoms, $Q_+ + Q_-$, is zero.

9.2 ELECTRIC FORCE AND COULOMB'S LAW

If two charged particles are a distance r apart,

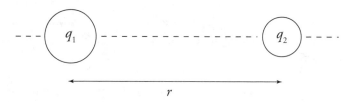

then the electric force between them, $\mathbf{F}_E$, is directed along the line joining them. The magnitude of this force is proportional to the charges (q_1 and q_2) and inversely proportional to r^2, as given by

---

Coulomb's Law

$$F_E = k \frac{|q_1 q_2|}{r^2}$$

The proportionality constant is k, and in general, its value depends on the material between the particles. However, in the usual case where the particles are separated by empty space (or by air, for all practical purposes), the proportionality constant is denoted by k_0 and called **Coulomb's constant**. This is a fundamental constant of nature (equal in magnitude, by definition, to 10^{-7} times the speed of light squared), and its value is $k_0 = 9 \times 10^9$ N·m²/C²:

Coulomb's Constant

$$k_0 = 9 \times 10^9 \ \tfrac{\text{N·m}^2}{\text{C}^2}$$

This is the value of k you should use unless you're specifically given another value (which would happen only if the charges were embedded in some insulating material that weakens the electric force).

The absolute value sign in the formula gives the magnitude of the force, whether repulsive or attractive. If direction (e.g., + or −) needs to be assigned, it should be done based on the fact that like charges (two positives or two negatives) repel each other, and opposite charges (one positive and one negative) attract. Note that the two electric forces in each of the following diagrams form an action–reaction pair.

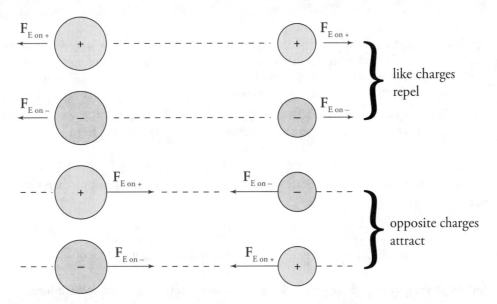

Example 9-3: Two charges, $q_1 = -2 \times 10^{-6} \, \text{C}$ and $q_2 = +5 \times 10^{-6} \, \text{C}$, are separated by a distance of 10 cm. Describe the electric force between these particles.

Solution: Using Coulomb's law, we find that

$$F_E = k_0 \frac{|q_1| q_2}{r^2} = (9 \times 10^9 \ \tfrac{\text{N·m}^2}{\text{C}^2}) \frac{(2 \times 10^{-6} \, \text{C})(+5 \times 10^{-6} \, \text{C})}{(10^{-1} \, \text{m})^2} = 9 \, \text{N}$$

Since one charge is positive and one is negative, the force is attractive, and each charge feels a 9 N force toward the other.

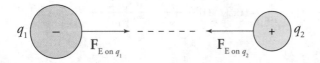

Example 9-4: A coulomb is a *lot* of charge. To get some idea just how much, imagine that we had two objects, each with a charge of 1 C, separated by a distance of 1 m. What would be the electric force between them?

Solution: Using Coulomb's law, we'd find that

$$F_E = k_0 \frac{q_1 q_2}{r^2} = (9 \times 10^9 \, \tfrac{\text{N} \cdot \text{m}^2}{\text{C}^2}) \frac{(1 \, \text{C})(1 \, \text{C})}{(1 \, \text{m})^2} = 9 \times 10^9 \, \text{N}$$

To write this answer in terms of a more familiar unit, let's use the fact that 1 pound (1 lb) is about 4.5 N, and 1 ton is 2000 lb:

$$F_E = (9 \times 10^9 \, \tfrac{\text{N} \cdot \text{m}^2}{\text{C}^2}) \cdot \frac{1 \, \text{lb}}{4.5 \, \text{N}} \cdot \frac{1 \, \text{ton}}{2000 \, \text{lb}} = \text{one million tons}$$

That's roughly equivalent to the weight of the Golden Gate Bridge! It's now easy to understand why most real-life situations deal with charges that are very tiny fractions of a coulomb; the *microcoulomb* (1 μC = 10^{-6} C) and the *nanocoulomb* (1 nC = 10^{-9} C) are more common "practical" units of charge.

Example 9-5: Consider a charge, +q, initially at rest near another charge, −Q. How would the magnitude of the electric force on +q change if −Q were moved away, doubling its distance from +q?

Solution: Coulomb's law is an inverse-square law, $F_E \propto 1 / r^2$, so if r increases by a factor of 2, then F_E will *decrease* by a factor of 4 (because $2^2 = 4$).

Example 9-6: Consider two plastic spheres, 1 meter apart: a little sphere with a mass of 1 kg and an electric charge of +1 nC, and a big sphere with a mass of 11 kg and an electric charge of +11 μC.

a) Find the electric force and the gravitational force between these spheres. Which force is stronger?
b) If the big sphere is fixed in position, and the little sphere is free to move, describe the resulting motion of the little sphere if it's released from rest.

Solution:

a) Using Coulomb's law, we find that the electric force between the spheres is

$$F_E = k_0 \frac{Qq}{r^2} = (9 \times 10^9 \, \tfrac{\text{N} \cdot \text{m}^2}{\text{C}^2}) \frac{(11 \times 10^{-6} \, \text{C})(1 \times 10^{-9} \, \text{C})}{(1 \, \text{m})^2} = 9.9 \times 10^{-5} \, \text{N} \approx 10^{-4} \, \text{N}$$

Using Newton's law of gravitation, the gravitational force between them is

$$F_G = G \frac{Mm}{r^2} = (6.7 \times 10^{-11} \, \tfrac{\text{N} \cdot \text{m}^2}{\text{kg}^2}) \frac{(1 \, \text{kg})(11 \, \text{kg})}{1 \, \text{m}^2} \approx 7.4 \times 10^{-10} \, \text{N}$$

Which force is stronger? It's no contest: The electric force is *much* stronger than the gravitational force. So, even though the spheres experience an attraction due to gravity, it is many orders of magnitude weaker than their electrical repulsion and can therefore be ignored.

b)   The net force on the little sphere is essentially equal to the electrical repulsion it feels from the big sphere (since the gravitational force is *so* much smaller, it can be ignored). Therefore, the initial acceleration of the little sphere is

$$a = \frac{F_E}{m} = \frac{10^{-4} \text{ N}}{1 \text{ kg}} = 10^{-4} \text{ m/s}^2$$

directed away from the big sphere. Notice that as the little sphere moves away, its acceleration does not remain constant. Because the electric force is inversely proportional to the square of the distance between the charges, as the little sphere moves away, the repulsive force it feels weakens, so its acceleration decreases. Therefore, the little sphere moves directly away from the big sphere with decreasing acceleration.

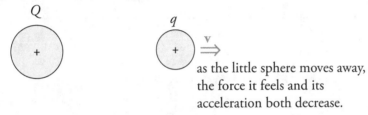

as the little sphere moves away, the force it feels and its acceleration both decrease.

Nevertheless, because the acceleration of the little sphere always points in the same direction (namely, away from the big sphere), the speed of the little sphere is always increasing, although the rate of increase of speed gets smaller as the little sphere gets farther away.

The Principle of Superposition for Electric Forces

Coulomb's law tells us how to calculate the force that one charge exerts on another one. What if two (or more) charges affect a third one? For example, what is the electric force on q_3 in the following figure?

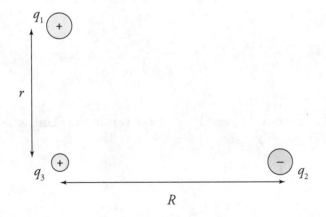

Here's the answer: If $\mathbf{F}_{1\text{-on-3}}$ is the force that q_1 *alone* exerts on q_3 (ignoring the presence of q_2) and if $\mathbf{F}_{2\text{-on-3}}$ is the force that q_2 *alone* exerts on q_3 (ignoring the presence of q_1), then the total force that q_3 feels is simply the vector sum $\mathbf{F}_{1\text{-on-3}} + \mathbf{F}_{2\text{-on-3}}$. The fact that we can calculate the effect of several charges by considering them individually and then just adding the resulting forces is known as the **principle of superposition**. (This important property will also be used when we study electric field vectors, electric potential, magnetic fields, and magnetic forces.)

The Principle of Superposition

The net electric force on a charge (q) due to a collection of other charges (Q's)

is equal to

the sum of the individual forces that each of the Q's alone exerts on q.

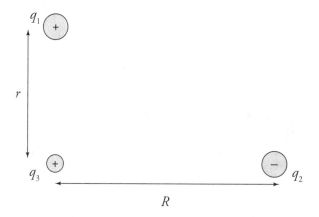

Example 9-7: In the figure above, assume that $q_1 = 2$ C, $q_2 = -8$ C, and $q_3 = 1$ nC. If $r = 1$ m and $R = 2$ m, which one of the following vectors best illustrates the direction of the net electric force on q_3?

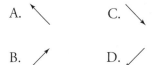

Solution: The individual forces $\mathbf{F}_{1\text{-on-3}}$ and $\mathbf{F}_{2\text{-on-3}}$ are shown in the figure below. Adding these vectors gives $\mathbf{F}_{\text{on 3}}$, which points down to the right, so the answer is C.

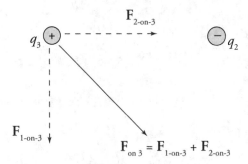

$$F_{1\text{-}on\text{-}3} = k_0 \frac{q_1 q_3}{r^2} = \left(9 \times 10^9 \frac{N \cdot m^2}{C^2}\right) \frac{(2\ C)(1 \times 10^{-9}\ C)}{(1\ m)^2} = 18\,N$$

(repulsive; away from q_1)

$$F_{2\text{-}on\text{-}3} = k_0 \frac{|q_2| q_3}{R^2} = \left(9 \times 10^9 \frac{N \cdot m^2}{C^2}\right) \frac{(8\ C)(1 \times 10^{-9}\ C)}{(2\ m)^2} = 18\,N$$

(attractive; toward q_2)

If the question had asked for the magnitude of the net electric force on q_3, then we'd use the Pythagorean theorem to find the length of the vector $\mathbf{F}_{on\,3}$. The vector $\mathbf{F}_{on\,3}$ is the hypotenuse of the right triangle whose legs are $\mathbf{F}_{1\text{-}on\text{-}3}$ and $\mathbf{F}_{2\text{-}on\text{-}3}$, so the magnitude of $\mathbf{F}_{on\,3}$ is found like this:

$$(\mathbf{F}_{on\,3})^2 = (\mathbf{F}_{1\text{-}on\text{-}3})^2 + (\mathbf{F}_{2\text{-}on\text{-}3})^2$$
$$= 18^2 + 18^2$$
$$= (18^2)(2)$$

$$\therefore \mathbf{F}_{on\,3} = 18\sqrt{2} \approx 25\,N$$

Example 9-8: In the figure below, assume that $q_1 = 1\ C$, $q_2 = -1\ nC$, and $q_3 = 8\ C$. If q_4 is a negative charge, what must its value be in order for the net electric force on q_2 to be zero?

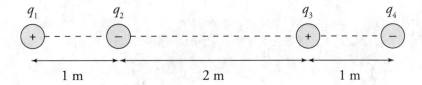

Solution: The individual forces $\mathbf{F}_{1\text{-on-2}}$, $\mathbf{F}_{3\text{-on-2}}$, and $\mathbf{F}_{4\text{-on-2}}$ are shown in the figure below. Notice that $\mathbf{F}_{1\text{-on-2}}$ and $\mathbf{F}_{4\text{-on-2}}$ point to the left, while $\mathbf{F}_{3\text{-on-2}}$ points to the right.

If we let $q_4 = -x$ C, then the magnitudes of the individual forces on q_2 are

$$F_{1\text{-on-2}} = k_0 \frac{q_1 |q_2|}{(r_{1-2})^2} = (9 \times 10^9 \ \tfrac{\text{N·m}^2}{\text{C}^2}) \frac{(1 \ \text{C})(1 \ \text{nC})}{(1 \ \text{m})^2} = 9 \ \text{N}$$

$$F_{3\text{-on-2}} = k_0 \frac{|q_2||q_3|}{(r_{2-3})^2} = (9 \times 10^9 \ \tfrac{\text{N·m}^2}{\text{C}^2}) \frac{(1 \ \text{nC})(8 \ \text{C})}{(2 \ \text{m})^2} = 18 \ \text{N}$$

$$F_{4\text{-on-2}} = k_0 \frac{|q_2||q_4|}{(r_{2-4})^2} = (9 \times 10^9 \ \tfrac{\text{N·m}^2}{\text{C}^2}) \frac{(1 \ \text{nC})(x \ \text{C})}{(3 \ \text{m})^2} = x \ \text{N}$$

In order for the net electric force on q_2 to be zero, the sum of the magnitudes of $\mathbf{F}_{1\text{-on-2}}$ and $\mathbf{F}_{4\text{-on-2}}$ must

be equal to the magnitude of $\mathbf{F}_{3\text{-on-2}}$. That is, $9 \ \text{N} + x \ \text{N} = 18 \ \text{N}$ so $x = 9$. Therefore, $q_4 = -x$ C $= -9$ C.

9.3 ELECTRIC FIELDS

There are several advantages to regarding electrical interactions in a slightly different way from the simple "charge Q exerts a force on charge q" mode of thinking. In this more sophisticated interpretation, the very existence of a charge (or a more general distribution of charge) alters the space around it, creating what we call an **electric field** in its vicinity. If a second charge happens to be there or to roam by, it will feel the effect of the field created by the original charge. That is, we think of the electric force on a second charge q as exerted *by the field*, rather than directly by the original charge(s). Qualitatively, we can represent electrical interactions as follows:

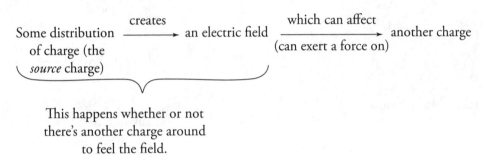

The charge(s) creating the electric field is/are called the **source charge(s)**; they're the source of the electric field. You may like to think of a source charge as a spider and its electric field as the spider's web. After a spider creates a web, when a small insect roams by, it is the web that ensnares the unfortunate bug, not the spider directly.

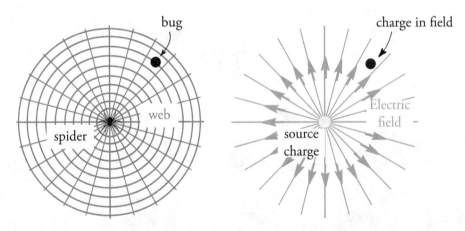

The figure on the right above illustrates one way to picture an electric field, but a few words of explanation are needed. First: An electric field is a **vector field**, which means that at each point in space surrounding the source charge, we associate a specific vector. The length of this vector will tell us the magnitude, or strength, of the field at that point, and the direction of the vector will tell us the direction of the resulting electric force that a *positive* test charge would feel if it were placed at that point. That's the convention: Although the charge that finds itself in an electric field can of course be positive or negative, for purposes of *illustrating* the field, we always think of a *positive* test charge. Because of this convention, *electric field vectors always point away from positive source charges and toward negative ones*. Also, the closer we are to the source charge, the stronger the resulting electric force a test charge would feel (because Coulomb's law is an *inverse*-square law). So, we expect the electric field vectors to be long at points close to the source charge and shorter at points farther away. The following figures illustrate the electric field due to a positive source charge and the electric field due to a negative source charge.

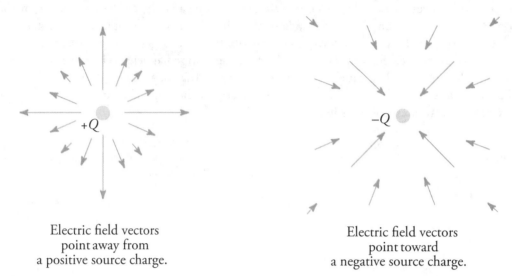

Electric field vectors
point away from
a positive source charge.

Electric field vectors
point toward
a negative source charge.

We can use Coulomb's law to find a formula for the strength of the electric field due to a point charge. Remember that a source charge creates an electric field whether or not there's another charge in the field to feel it. It takes *two* charges to create an electric *force*, but it takes only *one* (the source charge) to create an electric *field*. So, let's imagine we have a single source charge, Q, and another charge, q, at a distance r from Q.

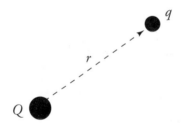

The force by Q, on the charge q, is, by Coulomb's law,

$$F_{\text{by } Q} = k\frac{|Q||q|}{r^2}$$

Now we ask, "What if q weren't there? Do we still have something?" The answer is *yes*, we have the electric field created by the source charge, Q. "So, if q weren't there, what if we removed q from the formula for the force exerted on it by Q? Would we still have something?" The answer is *yes*, we'd have the formula for the electric field, **E**, created by the single source charge Q.

Electric Field

$$E_{\text{by } Q} = k\frac{|Q|}{r^2}$$

In the formula for the force by Q on q, the variable r represents the distance from Q to q. However, if q is not there, what does r mean now? Answer: It's simply the distance from Q to the point in space where we want to know the electric field vector.

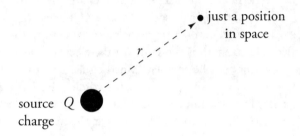

Example 9-9: Let $Q = +4$ nC be a charge that is fixed in position at the origin of an x-y coordinate system. What is the magnitude and direction of the electric field at the point (10 cm, 0)? At the point (–20 cm, 0)?

Solution: In the figure below, the point A is (10 cm, 0), which is 10 cm directly to the right of Q, and B is the point (–20 cm, 0), which is 20 cm directly to the left of Q.

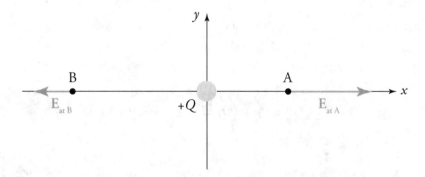

The electric field at point A is

$$E_{\text{at A}} = k_0\frac{Q}{(r_{\text{to A}})^2} = (9\times10^9 \ \tfrac{\text{N·m}^2}{\text{C}^2})\frac{(4\times10^{-9} \ \text{C})}{(10^{-1} \ \text{m})^2} = 3600 \ \tfrac{\text{N}}{\text{C}}$$

Since Q is positive, this means the electric field vector, $\mathbf{E}_{\text{at A}}$, points away from the source charge. Therefore, $\mathbf{E}_{\text{at A}}$ points in the positive x direction, which is usually written as the direction $\mathbf{i}$. So, if we wanted to write the complete electric field vector at point A, we'd write $\mathbf{E}_{\text{at A}} = (3600 \ \text{N/C})\mathbf{i}$.

The electric field at point B is

$$E_{\text{at B}} = k_0 \frac{Q}{(r_{\text{to B}})^2} = (9 \times 10^9 \, \tfrac{\text{N·m}^2}{\text{C}^2}) \frac{(4 \times 10^{-9} \, \text{C})}{(2 \times 10^{-1} \, \text{m})^2} = 900 \, \tfrac{\text{N}}{\text{C}}$$

Once again, $\mathbf{E}_{\text{at B}}$ points away from the source charge. Therefore, $\mathbf{E}_{\text{at B}}$ points in the negative x direction, which is usually written as the direction $-\mathbf{i}$. So, if we wanted to write the complete electric field vector at point B, we'd write $\mathbf{E}_{\text{at B}} = (900 \text{ N/C})(-\mathbf{i})$ or $-(900 \text{ N/C})\mathbf{i}$.

Notice from the formula $E = k|Q|/r^2$ that the electric field obeys an inverse-square law, like the electric force. So the strength of an electric field from a single source charge decreases as we get farther from the source; in particular, $E \propto 1/r^2$. Also, for a given source charge Q, the electric field strength depends only on r, the distance from Q. So at every point on a circle (or more generally a sphere) of radius r centered on the source charge, the electric field strength is the same. In the electric field vector diagram below on the left, all the field vectors at the points on the smaller dashed circle have the same length, indicating that the electric field magnitude is the same at all points on this circle. Similarly, all the field vectors at the points on the larger dashed circle have the same length, indicating that the electric field magnitude is the same at all points on *this* circle. (Note that the field vectors at the points on the larger circle are shorter than those at the points on the smaller circle.) However, notice that the magnitude may be the same at every point on each circle (because they're all the same distance r from the source charge) but the directions of the electric field vectors are all different on each circle. Therefore, we're forced to say that the electric field isn't the same at every point a distance r from Q because the directions are all different.

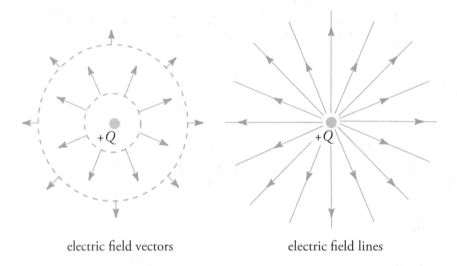

electric field vectors   electric field lines

The diagram on the left above and the two given earlier for the electric field produced by a positive source charge and by a negative source charge show the field represented by individual vectors. However, this is not the easiest way to draw an electric field.

Instead of drawing a bunch of separate vectors, we instead draw *lines* through them, like in the diagram on the right above. This drawing depicts the electric field using **field lines**. The direction of the field is indicated as usual; remember that, by convention, the electric field points away from positive source charges and toward negative ones and indicates the direction of the electric force that a positive test charge would feel if it were placed in the field.

Now that we've eliminated the separate vectors, it seems as though we've lost some information, namely, where the field is strong and where it's weak because we got this information from the lengths of the individual vectors. (Where the vectors were long, the field was strong, and where the vectors were shorter, the field was weaker.) However, we can still get a general idea of where the field is strong and where it's weak by looking at the *density* of the field lines: Where the field lines are cramped close together, the field is stronger; where the field lines are more spread out, the field is weaker.

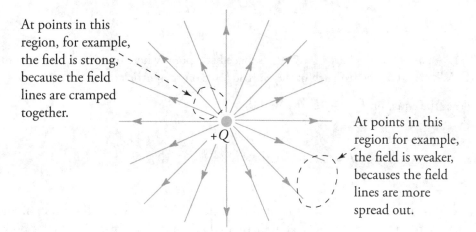

At points in this region, for example, the field is strong, because the field lines are cramped together.

+Q

At points in this region for example, the field is weaker, becauses the field lines are more spread out.

Now, let's imagine that we have a source charge Q creating an electric field, and another charge, q, roams in to the field. What force will q feel? We want to find an equation for the force on q due to the electric field. Recall the formulas above: $F_{on\,q} = k|Qq|\,/\,r^2$ and $E_{by\,Q} = k|Q|\,/\,r^2$. What would we need to do to E to get F? Just multiply it by q! That is, $F_{on\,q} = |q|\,E_{by\,q}$. It turns out that this very important formula works not just for the electric field created by a single source charge; it works for *any* electric field:

Electric Force and Field

$$\mathbf{F}_{on\,q} = q\mathbf{E}$$

Note that the absolute value symbol is useful when solving for the magnitude of force and electric field. The vector equation, $\mathbf{F}_E = q\mathbf{E}$, contains directional information and therefore does not need absolute values. Notice also from this formula that $E = F\,/\,|q|$, so the units of E are N/C, which you saw in Example 7-9. The equation $\mathbf{E} = \mathbf{F}\,/\,q$ also gives us the definition of the electric field: It's the force per unit charge.

Finally, before we get to some more examples, realize that we've had two important (boxed) formulas in this section on the electric field: $E = k|Q|\,/\,r^2$ and $\mathbf{F} = q\mathbf{E}$. In the first formula, Q is the charge that *makes* the field, while in the second formula, q is the charge that *feels* the field.

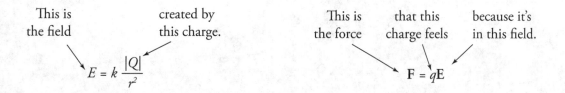

This is the field · · · created by this charge.

$E = k\dfrac{|Q|}{r^2}$

This is the force · · · that this charge feels · · · because it's in this field.

$\mathbf{F} = q\mathbf{E}$

Example 9-10: The magnitude of the electric field at a distance r from a source charge $+Q$ is equal to E. What will be the magnitude of the electric field at a distance $4r$ from a source charge $+2Q$?

Solution: The first sentence tells us that $kQ/r^2 = E$. Now, if we change Q to $2Q$ and r to $4r$, we find that E decreases by a factor of 8, because

$$E' = k\frac{Q'}{(r')^2} = k\frac{2Q}{(4r)^2} = \frac{2}{16} \cdot k\frac{Q}{r^2} = \frac{1}{8}E$$

Example 9-11: A particle with charge $q = 2\ \mu C$ is placed at a point where the electric field has magnitude 4×10^4 N/C. What will be the strength of the electric force on the particle?

Solution: From the equation $F_{on\ q} = qE$, we find that

$$F = (2 \times 10^{-6}\ C)(4 \times 10^4\ \tfrac{N}{C}) = 8 \times 10^{-2}\ N$$

Notice that we didn't need to know what created the field. If E is given, and the question asks for the force that some charge q feels in this field, all we have to do is multiply, $F = qE$, and we're done.

Example 9-12: In the diagram on the left below, the electric field at Point A points in the positive y direction and has magnitude 5×10^6 N/C. (The source charge is not shown.) If a particle with charge $q = -3$ nC is placed at point A, what will be the electric force on the particle?

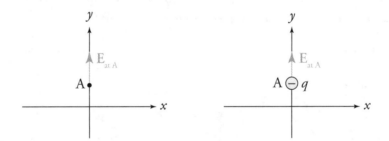

Solution: $\mathbf{E}_{at\ A}$ points in the positive y direction, which is usually written as the direction $\mathbf{j}$, so $\mathbf{E}_{at\ A} = (5 \times 10^6\ N/C)\mathbf{j}$. The equation $\mathbf{F}_{on\ q} = q\mathbf{E}$ then gives us

$$\mathbf{F} = (-3 \times 10^{-9})(5 \times 10^6\ \tfrac{N}{C})\mathbf{j} = (1.5 \times 10^{-2}\ N)(-\mathbf{j})$$

That is, the force will have magnitude 1.5×10^{-2} N and point in the negative y direction ($-\mathbf{j}$). Notice that whenever q is negative, the force $F_{\text{on } q}$ will always point in the direction *opposite* to the electric field.

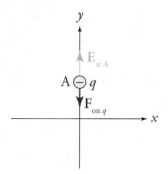

Example 9-13: A particle of mass m and charge q is placed at a point where the electric field is E. If the particle is released from rest, find its initial acceleration, **a**.

Solution: The acceleration of the particle is the force it feels divided by its mass: $\mathbf{a} = \mathbf{F}/m$. Because $\mathbf{F} = q\mathbf{E}$, we get

$$\mathbf{a} = \frac{\mathbf{F}}{m} = \frac{q\mathbf{E}}{m}$$

Notice that if q is negative, then **F** (and, consequently, **a**) will be directed *opposite* to the electric field **E**. Also, the question asked only for the *initial* acceleration, because once the particle starts moving, it will most likely move through locations where the electric field is different (in magnitude or direction or both), so the force on the particle will change; and if the force on the particle changes, so will the acceleration.

If a region contains a *uniform* electric field (i.e., same magnitude and direction at all points within the region), then the electrostatic force and the particle's acceleration will likewise be uniform. The Big 5 kinematics equations can therefore be used to solve for final velocity, time, etc. In addition, the formula $W = Fd \cos\theta$ can also be used to calculate the work done by or against the electrostatic force to move a charge from one position to another. A large conducting plate that is charged (or a parallel plate capacitor, as detailed in the next chapter) creates an electric field that is approximately uniform.

Example 9-14: A uniform electric field of strength 4×10^6 N/C points to the left as shown in the figure on the next page. A particle with charge $q = -20$ nC and mass $m = 10$ g is initially placed at point B.

a) If the particle is released from rest, toward which point will it move and how fast will it be traveling when it arrives?

b)   If the particle is again placed at point B and is now moved to point D, how much work is done "by the field"? (Note: In reality, forces do work, not fields; work done "by the field" is a commonly used expression.)

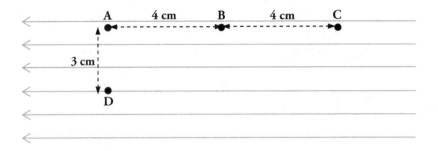

Solution:

a)   Negatively charged particles feel a force opposite the direction of the electric field, therefore the particle will move to point C. To find the final speed, the acceleration must first be calculated using Newton's Second Law:

$$|q|E = ma$$

$$a = |q|E \,/\, m = (20 \times 10^{-9}\ \text{C})(4 \times 10^{6}\ \text{N/C}) \,/\, (10 \times 10^{-3}\ \text{kg}) = 8\ \text{m/s}^2$$

Using Big 5 #5,

$$v^2 = v_0^2 + 2ad = 0 + 2(8\ \text{m/s}^2)(0.04\ \text{m}) = 0.64\ \text{m}^2/\text{s}^2$$

v is therefore 0.8 m/s.

b) $W = Fd\cos\theta = |q|Ed\cos\theta$. Since $\theta > 90°$ the work done by the field is negative. $\triangle BAD$ is a 3-4-5 triangle, so $d = 5$ cm. More importantly, $\cos\theta = -4/5$. Therefore,

$$W = (20 \times 10^{-9}\ \text{C})(4 \times 10^{6}\ \text{N/C})(0.05\ \text{m})(-4/5) = -3.2 \times 10^{-3}\ \text{J}$$

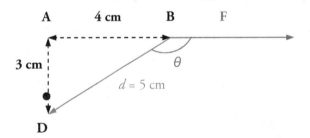

Notice that the work done by the field from point B to point D is the same as if the particle were moved from point B to point A. The field will only do work (whether positive or negative) if there is displacement in the direction of the electric field or opposite the field. This is similar to gravity, which only does work if there is displacement up or down. And as with gravity, the work done by the field is also path independent. This will be discussed in more depth later in the chapter.

The Principle of Superposition for Electric Fields

The pictures we've drawn so far have been of electric fields created by a single source charge. However, we can also have two or more charges whose electric fields overlap, creating one combined field. For example, let's consider an **electric dipole**, which, by definition, is a pair of equal but opposite charges:

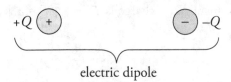

electric dipole

What if we regarded *both* of them as source charges; how would we find the electric field that they create together? By using the principle of superposition. If we wanted to find the electric field vector at, say, the point P in the diagram below,

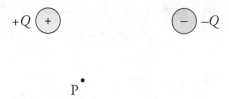

we'd first find the electric field vector, $\mathbf{E_+}$, at P due to the $+Q$ charge alone (ignoring the presence of the $-Q$ charge) and then we'd find the electric field vector, $\mathbf{E_-}$, at P due to the $-Q$ charge alone (ignoring the presence of the $+Q$ charge). The net electric field vector at P will then be the vector sum, $\mathbf{E_+} + \mathbf{E_-}$.

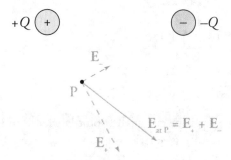

We can do this for as many points as we like and obtain a diagram of the electric field as a collection of vectors. The diagram in terms of electric field lines would look like this:

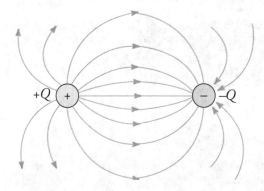

Notice that between the charges, where the field lines are dense, the field is strong; and as we move away from the charges, the field lines get more spread out, indicating that the field gets weaker.

9.3

Example 9-15: An electric dipole consists of two charges, $+Q$ and $-Q$, where $Q = 4$ μC, separated by a distance of $d = 20$ cm. Find the electric field at the point midway between the charges.

Solution: The electric field at P due to the positive charge is $E_+ = k_0 Q / \left(\frac{1}{2}d\right)^2$, pointing away from $+Q$, and the electric field at P due to the negative charge is $E_- = k_0 Q / \left(\frac{1}{2}d\right)^2$, pointing toward $-Q$ (which is in the same direction as $\mathbf{E}_+$).

$$+Q \;\bigoplus \qquad\qquad \mathrm{P} \bullet \overset{\mathrm{E_+}}{\underset{\mathrm{E_-}}{\longrightarrow}} \qquad\qquad \bigominus\; -Q$$

$$\overset{\longleftarrow\;\;\longrightarrow}{\tfrac{1}{2}d} \quad \overset{\longleftarrow\;\;\longrightarrow}{\tfrac{1}{2}d}$$

By the principle of superposition, the net electric field at P is the sum: $\mathbf{E} = \mathbf{E}_+ + \mathbf{E}_-$. The magnitude of $E_{\text{at P}}$ is $E_+ + E_- = k_0 Q / \left(\frac{1}{2}d\right)^2 + k_0 Q / \left(\frac{1}{2}d\right)^2 = 2 k_0 Q / \left(\frac{1}{2}d\right)^2$:

$$E = 2k_0 \frac{Q}{(\frac{1}{2}d)^2}$$

$$= 2(9 \times 10^9 \tfrac{\mathrm{N \cdot m^2}}{\mathrm{C^2}}) \frac{4 \times 10^{-6}\ \mathrm{C}}{(1 \times 10^{-1}\ \mathrm{m})^2}$$

$$= 7.2 \times 10^6 \tfrac{\mathrm{N}}{\mathrm{C}}$$

The direction of $\mathbf{E}_{\text{at P}}$ is away from $+Q$ and toward $-Q$:

$$+Q \;\bigoplus \qquad\qquad \underset{\mathrm{P}}{\bullet} \xrightarrow{\quad\mathrm{E}\quad} \qquad \bigominus\; -Q$$

Example 9-16: A positive charge, $+q$, is placed at the point labeled P in the field of the dipole shown below. Describe the direction of the resulting electric force on the charge. Do the same for a negative charge, $-q$, placed at the point labeled N.

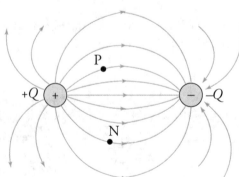

Solution: The electric field vector at any point is always *tangent* to the field line passing through that point and its direction is the same as that of the field line. Since $\mathbf{F} = q\mathbf{E}$, the force on a positive charge is in the same direction as $\mathbf{E}$ and the force on a negative charge is in the opposite direction from $\mathbf{E}$. The directions of $\mathbf{F}_{\text{on } q}$ and $\mathbf{F}_{\text{on } -q}$ are shown in the figure below.

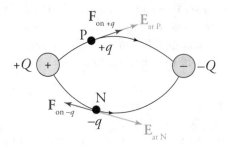

Conductors, Insulators, and Polarization

Most everyday materials can be classified into one of two major categories: *conductors* or *insulators* (also known as *dielectrics*). A material is a **conductor** if it contains charges that are free to roam throughout the material. Metals are the classic and most important conductors. In a metal, one or more valence electrons per atom are not strongly bound to any particular atom and are thus free to roam. If a metal is placed in an electric field, these free charges (called **conduction electrons**) will move in response to the field. Another example of a conductor would be a solution that contains lots of dissolved ions (such as saltwater).

Here's an interesting property of conductors: Imagine that we place a whole bunch of electrons on a piece of metal. It's now negatively charged. Since electrons repel each other, they'll want to get as far away from each other as possible. As a result, all this excess charge moves (rapidly) to the surface. Any net charge on a conductor resides on its surface. Since there's no excess charge within the body of the conductor, there cannot be an electrostatic field inside a conductor. You can block out external electric fields simply by surrounding yourself with metal; the free charges in the metal will move to the surface to shield the interior and keep $\mathbf{E} = 0$ inside.

By contrast, an **insulator (dielectric)** is a material that doesn't have free charges. Electrons are tightly bound to their atoms and thus are not free to roam throughout the material. Common insulators include rubber, glass, wood, paper, and plastic.

Now, let's study this situation: Start with a neutral metal sphere and bring a charge (a positive charge) Q nearby without touching the original metal sphere. What will happen? The positive charge will attract free electrons in the metal, leaving the far side of the sphere positively charged. Since the negative charge is closer to Q than the positive charge, there'll be a net attraction between Q and the sphere. So, even though the sphere as a whole is electrically neutral, the separation of charge induced by the presence of Q will create a force of electrical attraction between them.

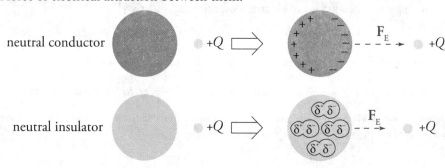

Now what if the sphere was made of glass (an insulator)? Although there aren't free electrons that can move to the near side of the sphere, the atoms that make up the sphere will become **polarized**. That is, their electrons will feel a tug toward Q, causing the atoms to develop a partial negative charge pointing toward Q (and a partial positive charge pointing away from Q). The effect isn't as dramatic as the mass movement of free electrons in the case of a metal sphere, but the polarization is still enough to cause an electrical attraction between the sphere and Q. For example, if you comb your hair, the comb will pick up extra electrons, making it negatively charged. If you place this electric field source near little bits of paper, the paper will become polarized and will then be attracted to the comb.[2]

9.4 ELECTRIC POTENTIAL AND POTENTIAL ENERGY

So far, we have viewed the electric field due to a source charge (or a more general charge distribution, such as a pair of charges or a plate) as a collection of vectors. This point of view allowed us to answer questions about other *vector* quantities, like force and acceleration. The basic equations for finding these quantities were $\mathbf{F} = q\mathbf{E}$ and $\mathbf{a} = \mathbf{F}/m = q\mathbf{E}/m$.

What if we wanted to answer questions about *scalar* quantities, like energy, work, or speed? It turns out that the easiest way to answer these questions is to view the electric field in a different way, in terms of a scalar field. First, it is useful to review a few facts about gravitational potential energy. As you'll recall, if an object of mass m is dropped from rest from a height h and hits the ground, $W_{\text{by grav}} = +mgh$ while $\Delta PE_{\text{grav}} = -mgh$. Similarly, if the object is lifted from the ground to a height h, $W_{\text{by grav}} = -mgh$, $W_{\text{against grav}} = +mgh$ and $\Delta PE_{\text{grav}} = +mgh$.

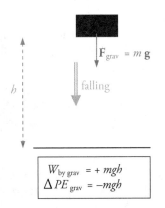

$$W_{\text{by grav}} = + mgh$$
$$\Delta PE_{\text{grav}} = -mgh$$

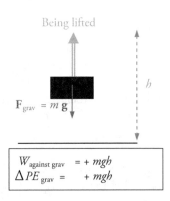

$$W_{\text{against grav}} = + mgh$$
$$\Delta PE_{\text{grav}} = + mgh$$

If an object moves "with nature" (i.e., in the direction that gravity points), then potential energy decreases. If an object moves "against nature", then potential energy increases. This is an important fact to remember going forward, as it will be applied to electric potential energy as well.

---

[2] The same phenomenon, in which the presence of a charge tends to cause polarization in a nearby collection of charges, is responsible for a kind of intermolecular force: Dipole-induced dipole forces are caused by a shifting of the electron cloud of a neutral molecule toward positively charged ions or away from a negatively charged ion; in each case, the resulting force between the ion and the atom is attractive.

The **London dispersion force**, in which electrically neutral molecules temporarily induce polarization in each other, is a much weaker version of the same phenomenon—again, electron clouds shift a little bit to create dipoles.

In the example below, a positively charged particle is fixed in place and a negatively charged particle is moved from point A to point B.

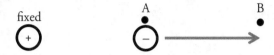

Without knowing the formula for electric potential energy, we can say that $\Delta PE_{elec} > 0$, since the particle is being moved "against nature".

Mathematically, we see that $W_{by\ grav} = -\Delta PE_{grav}$ and that $W_{against\ grav} = +\Delta PE_{grav}$. Similarly, we will be able to make an analogous statement about the relationship between the work done by or against the electric field and the change in electric potential energy. We will also be able to answer questions involving speed by using Conservation of Mechanical Energy.

To find the equation for electric potential energy, it is useful to first consider that charged particles not only create a vector field (i.e., the electric field), they also create a scalar field.

This scalar field has a name: it's called **electric potential** (or just **potential** for short).

Let Q be a point source charge. At any point P that's a distance r from Q, we say that the electric potential at P is the scalar given by this formula:

Electric Potential

$$\phi = k\frac{Q}{r}$$

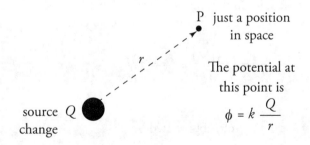

Notice the differences between this formula and the one for the electric field. First, the potential is kQ divided by r, while the electric field is kQ divided by r^2. Second, the electric field has a specific direction at each point (because it's a vector quantity); the potential, on the other hand, is not a vector, so it has no direction. For this reason, no absolute value symbol is needed. The sign of the potential is important in determining the behavior of nearby charges if they are placed in the field. While the electric field has the same magnitude at every point a distance r from Q, the field has a different direction at every point on the circle (or, more generally, the sphere) of radius r centered on Q. Therefore, we're forced to say that the electric field isn't the same at every point a distance r from Q because the directions are all different. The potential, however, is easier because it has no direction: The potential *is* the same at every point that's a distance r from Q.

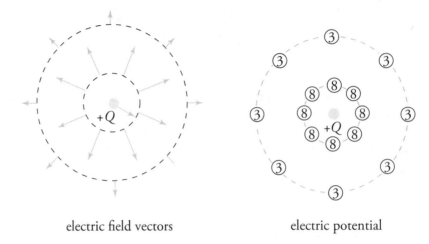

electric field vectors   electric potential

The dashed circles shown in the figure on the right above are called **equipotentials** ("equal potentials"), because the potential is the same at every point on them. For example, the potential is equal to 8 units everywhere on the inner dashed circle, and equal to 3 units everywhere on the outer dashed circle. As we move around on either dashed circle, the electric field changes (because the direction of **E** changes), but the potential doesn't change.

The formula given on the previous page for the potential, $\phi = kQ/r$, assumes that the potential decreases to 0 as we move far away from the source charges (that is, as $r \rightarrow \infty$); this is the standard, conventional assumption. With this formula, you can see that if Q is a positive charge, then the values of the potential due to this source charge are also positive (if Q is positive, then kQ/r is positive); on the other hand, the values of the potential due to a negative source charge are negative (if Q is negative, then kQ/r is negative). The sign of the potential (that is, whether it's positive or negative) is not an indication of a direction; remember, potential is a scalar, so it has no direction.

Before we get to some examples, it's important to mention that while there's no special name for the unit of electric field, there *is* a special name for the unit of electric potential:

$$[\phi] = [k]\frac{[Q]}{[r]} = \left(\tfrac{\mathrm{N \cdot m^2}}{\mathrm{C^2}}\right)\frac{\mathrm{C}}{\mathrm{m}} = \frac{\mathrm{N \cdot m}}{\mathrm{C}} = \frac{\mathrm{J}}{\mathrm{C}}$$

A joule per coulomb (J/C) is called a **volt**, abbreviated V.

Example 9-17: What is the electric potential at a distance of $r = 30$ cm from a source charge $Q = -20$ nC?

Solution: Using the formula $\phi = k_0 Q / r$, we find that

$$\phi = k_0 \frac{Q}{r} = (9 \times 10^9 \, \tfrac{\text{N} \cdot \text{m}^2}{\text{C}^2}) \frac{-20 \times 10^{-9} \, \text{C}}{30 \times 10^{-2} \, \text{m}} = -600 \text{ V}$$

Example 9-18: In the figure below, the potential at Point A is 1,000 V. What's the potential at Point B ?

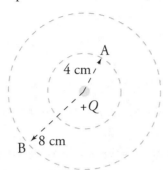

Solution: From the formula $\phi = k_0 Q / r$, we see that the potential is inversely proportional to r: Thus, $\phi \propto 1 / r$. Because the distance from Q to B is twice the distance from Q to A, the potential at B should be half the potential at A. Therefore, $\phi_{\text{at B}} = 500 \text{ V}$. (Notice that because the potential at A is 1,000 V, the potential at *every* point on the inner circle is 1,000 V; and since the potential at B is 500 V, the potential at *every* point on the outer circle is 500 V.)

Now that we know how to calculate electric potential, how do we use it to answer questions about the scalar quantities energy, work, and speed? The applications of electric potential all follow from this one fundamental equation:

Change in Electrical Potential Energy

$$\Delta PE = q\Delta\phi = qV$$

That is, the change in potential energy of a charge q that moves between two points whose potential difference is $\Delta\phi$ is just given by the product, $q\Delta\phi$; it also can be expressed as qV, where V is defined as the change in potential and is known as the *voltage*. For example, let's say a charge $q = +0.03$ C moves from a point on the inner circle to a point on the outer circle in the figure accompanying the preceding example:

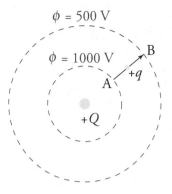

Then the change in the electrical potential energy of the charge q is

$$\Delta PE_{A \to B} = q\Delta\phi_{A \to B} = q(\phi_B - \phi_A) = (+0.03\,C)(500\,V - 1000\,V) = -15\,J$$

We expected that the change in potential energy would be negative (that is, the potential energy would decrease), because the positive charge is moving farther from the positive source charge (i.e., "with nature"). Because q moves in a way it naturally "wants" to move (since the positive charge q is naturally repelled by the positive charge Q), its potential energy should decrease.

If the charge q were instead pushed (by some outside force) from Point B to Point A (i.e., "against nature"), then its potential energy would increase:

$$\Delta PE_{B \to A} = q\Delta\phi_{B \to A} = q(\phi_A - \phi_B) = (+0.03\,C)(1000\,V - 500\,V) = +15\,J$$

What if the charge q were moved from one point on the outer circle (Point B, say) to another point on the outer circle, B'?

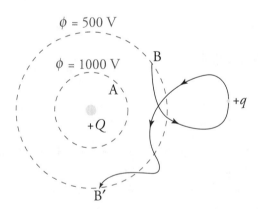

Its potential energy would not change. Because the potential is the same everywhere on the outer circle, the potential at B is the same as the potential at B', so the potential *difference* between Points B and B' is zero; and if $\Delta\phi = 0$, then $\Delta PE = 0$ as well. *A charge experiences no change in potential energy when its initial and final positions are at the same potential.*

The figure on the previous page also illustrates that the path taken by the charge is irrelevant. Like the gravitational force, the electric force is conservative; all that matters is where the charge began and where it ended; the specific path it takes doesn't matter.

Example 9-19: A charge $q = -8$ nC is moved from a position that's 10 cm from a charge $Q = +2$ µC to a position that's 20 cm away. What is the change in its electrical potential energy?

Solution: Let A be the initial point and B the final point; then the change in potential from Point A to Point B is

$$\Delta\phi = \phi_B - \phi_A = \frac{k_0 Q}{r_B} - \frac{k_0 Q}{r_A} = k_0 Q \left(\frac{1}{r_B} - \frac{1}{r_A} \right)$$

$$= (9 \times 10^9 \ \tfrac{\text{N·m}^2}{\text{C}^2})(2 \times 10^{-6} \ \text{C})\left(\tfrac{1}{0.2 \ \text{m}} - \tfrac{1}{0.1 \ \text{m}} \right)$$

$$= -9 \times 10^4 \ \text{V}$$

Therefore, the change in potential energy of the charge q is

$$\Delta PE = q \Delta\phi = (-8 \times 10^{-9} \ \text{C})(-9 \times 10^4 \ \text{V}) = 7.2 \times 10^{-4} \ \text{J}$$

We've seen that all charged particles naturally move to positions of lower potential energy. To accomplish this, notice in the preceding examples that *positively charged particles naturally tend toward lower potential and negatively charged particles tend toward higher potential.* To verify this mathematically, we have learned that $\Delta PE = q \Delta\phi$ or $\Delta\phi = \Delta PE / q$. Moving "with nature" means that ΔPE is negative. So if q is positive, then $\Delta\phi$ is (–)/(+) = (–), which means that potential decreases. If q is negative, then $\Delta\phi$ is (–)/(–) = (+), which means that potential increases.

A gravitational analogy may be useful. A positively charged particle can be thought of as any mass: it naturally "falls downward" when released from rest. Conversely, a negatively charged particle can be thought of as a helium balloon—it "rises upward." The electric field can be thought as **g**, which is a vector that points downward toward the center of the earth. Positively charged particles therefore naturally move in the direction of **E** and negatively charged particles naturally move opposite **E**. Finally, potential can be thought of as height above ground. Positives naturally move toward lower potential and negatives move toward higher potential. Note that negative potentials can be thought of as "heights" below ground. The rules above still apply.

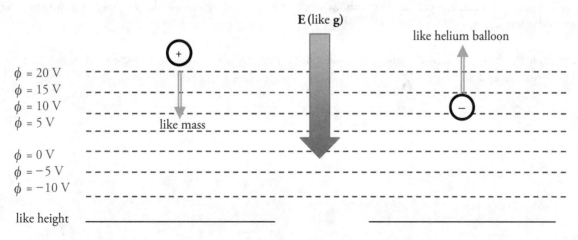

Now that we've seen examples of how to calculate changes in potential energy in an electric field by using the concept of electric potential, how do we answer questions about work or kinetic energy? By using equations we already know from mechanics.

What if we want to find the work done by the electric field as a charge moves? If we move objects around in a *gravitational* field, we remember that the change in gravitational potential energy is equal to the opposite of the work done by the gravitational field. That is, $\Delta PE_{grav} = -W_{by\,gravity}$, which is the same as $W_{by\,gravity} = -\Delta PE_{grav}$. Applying this same idea to an electric field, we can say that the work done by the electric field is equal to $-\Delta PE_{elec}$:

Work Done by Electric Field
$$W_{by\,electric\,field} = -\Delta PE_{elec}$$

Now what about kinetic energy? Well, if there's no friction (which will be the case for charges moving around in empty space) or other forces doing work as a charge moves, then mechanical energy is conserved; that is $KE + PE$ will remain constant. And if $KE + PE$ is constant, then $\Delta(KE + PE)$ will be zero. That is, ΔKE will be equal to $-\Delta PE$. Since we know how to calculate ΔPE, we can calculate ΔKE by just changing the sign of ΔPE:

$$\Delta KE = -\Delta PE$$

So, as long as you remember the fundamental formula for potential energy changes in an electric field, $\Delta PE = q\Delta\phi$, you can answer questions about work or kinetic energy in an electric field by just using the formulas above.

Example 9-20: In the figure below, a particle whose charge q is +4 nC moves in the electric field created by a negative source charge, $-Q$.

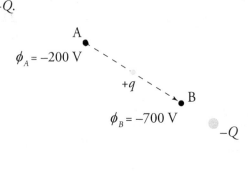

Find:

a) the change in potential energy,
b) the work done by the electric field, and
c) the change in kinetic energy of the particle as it moves from position A to position B.
d) If the mass of the particle is 10^{-8} kg and it started from rest at Point A, what will be its speed as it passes through Point B?

Solution:

a) $\Delta PE = q\Delta\phi = q\left(\phi_B - \phi_A\right) = \left(4\times 10^{-9}\,\text{C}\right)\left[\left(-700\,\text{V}\right)-\left(-200\,\text{V}\right)\right] = -2\times 10^{-6}\,\text{J}$

b) $W_{\text{by electric field}} = -\Delta PE_{\text{elec}} = -\left(-2\times 10^{-6}\,\text{J}\right) = 2\times 10^{-6}\,\text{J}$

c) $\Delta KE = \Delta PE_{\text{elec}} = -\left(-2\times 10^{-6}\,\text{J}\right) = +2\times 10^{-6}\,\text{J}$

d) If the particle started from rest at Point A, then $PE_{\text{at B}} = \Delta KE = +2\times 10^{-6}\,\text{J}$, so

$$\frac{1}{2}mv_B^2 = 2\times 10^{-6}\,\text{J} \;\rightarrow\; v_B^2 = \frac{2(2\times 10^{-6}\,\text{J})}{m} \;\rightarrow\; v_B = \sqrt{\frac{4\times 10^{-6}\,\text{J}}{10^{-8}\,\text{kg}}} = \sqrt{400\,\text{m}^2/\text{s}^2} = 20\,\text{m/s}$$

Example 9-21: An electric field pulls an electron from one position to another such that the change in potential is +1 V. By how much does the electron's kinetic energy change?

Solution: The change in potential energy is

$$\Delta PE = q\Delta\phi = (-1.6\times 10^{-19}\,\text{C})(+1\,\text{V}) = -1.6\times 10^{-19}\,\text{J}$$

so the change in kinetic energy is the opposite of this, $+1.6\times 10^{-19}$ C. This amount of energy is known as 1 **electron volt** (eV). In fact, the abbreviation for this unit makes the definition easy to remember: An electron (e^-) moving through a potential difference of 1 V experiences a kinetic energy change of $-q\Delta\phi = (e)(1\,\text{V}) = 1.6\times 10^{-19}\,\text{J} = 1$ eV. While the joule is the SI unit for energy, it's too big to be convenient when discussing atomic-sized systems. The electron volt is commonly used instead.

Example 9-22: An electric field pushes a proton from one position to another such that the change in potential is –500 V. By how much does the kinetic energy of the proton increase, in electron volts?

Solution: The change in potential energy is

$$\Delta PE = q\Delta\phi = (+e)(-500\,\text{V}) = -500\,\text{eV}$$

so the change in kinetic energy, ΔKE, is $-\Delta PE = -(-500\,\text{eV}) = +500$ eV.

9.4

The Principle of Superposition for Electric Potential

The formula $\phi = kQ/r$ tells us how to find the potential due to a single point source charge, Q. To find the potential in an electric field that's created by more than one charge, we use the principle of superposition. In fact, applying this principle is even easier here than for electric forces and fields because potential is a scalar. When we add up individual potentials, we're simply adding numbers; we're not adding vectors.

Let's illustrate with an example. In the figure below, the source charges $Q_1 = +10$ nC and $Q_2 = -5$ nC are fixed in the positions shown; the charges and the two points, A and B, form the vertices of a rectangle. What is the potential at Point A? at Point B?

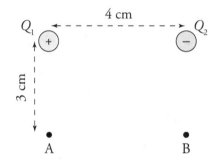

The potential at Point A due to Q_1 alone (ignoring the presence of Q_2) is

$$\phi_{A1} = k_0 \frac{Q_1}{r_{A1}} = (9 \times 10^9 \; \tfrac{\text{N} \cdot \text{m}^2}{\text{C}^2}) \frac{+10 \times 10^{-9} \; \text{C}}{3 \times 10^{-2} \; \text{m}} = 3000 \; \text{V}$$

Since Point A is 5 cm from Q_2 (it's the hypotenuse of a 3-4-5 right triangle), the potential at Point A due to Q_2 alone (ignoring the presence of Q_1) is

$$\phi_{A2} = k_0 \frac{Q_2}{r_{A2}} = (9 \times 10^9 \; \tfrac{\text{N} \cdot \text{m}^2}{\text{C}^2}) \frac{-5 \times 10^{-9} \; \text{C}}{5 \times 10^{-2} \; \text{m}} = -900 \; \text{V}$$

Therefore, the total electric potential at Point A, due to both source charges, is

$$\phi_A = \phi_{A1} + \phi_{A2} = (3000 \; \text{V}) + (-900 \; \text{V}) = 2100 \; \text{V}$$

Similarly, the total electric potential at Point B is

$$\phi_B = \phi_{B1} + \phi_{B2} = k_0 \frac{Q_1}{r_{B1}} + k_0 \frac{Q_2}{r_{B2}}$$

$$= (9 \times 10^9 \; \tfrac{\text{N} \cdot \text{m}^2}{\text{C}^2}) \frac{+10 \times 10^{-9} \; \text{C}}{5 \times 10^{-2} \; \text{m}} + (9 \times 10^9 \; \tfrac{\text{N} \cdot \text{m}^2}{\text{C}^2}) \frac{-5 \times 10^{-9} \; \text{C}}{3 \times 10^{-2} \; \text{m}}$$

$$= (1800 \; \text{V}) + (-1500 \; \text{V})$$

$$= 300 \; \text{V}$$

Example 9-23: A charge $q = 1$ nC is moved from position A to position B, along the path labeled a in the figure below. Find the work done by the electric field. How would your answer change if q had been moved from position A to position B, along the path labeled b?

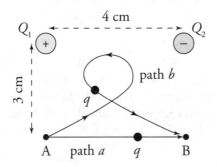

Solution: Path a begins at Point A, where $\phi_A = 2100\,\text{V}$, and ends at Point B, where $\phi_B = 300\,\text{V}$, so $\Delta\phi_{A\to B} = \phi_B - \phi_A = 300\,\text{V} - 2100\,\text{V} = -1800\,\text{V}$. Therefore, the change in potential energy of the charge q is

$$\Delta PE = q\Delta\phi = (1\times10^{-9}\text{ C})(-1800\text{ V}) = -1.8\times10^{-6}\text{ J}$$

This means that the work done by the electric field, $W_{by\,E}$, is equal to $-\Delta PE = 1.8\times10^{-6}$ J. If q had followed path b, the change in potential energy and the work done by the electric field would have been the same as for path a. The shape or length of the path is irrelevant; all that matters is the initial point and the ending point, and both paths begin at Point A and end at Point B.

We can't use the formula "work = force × distance" here, because the force is not constant during the object's displacement. To calculate work in an electric field, we use electric potential and the formula $W_{by\,E} = -\Delta PE_{elec}$.

Example 9-24: The figure below shows two source charges, $+2Q$ and $-Q$. What is the minimum amount of work that must be done by some outside force against the electric field to move a negative charge, $-q$, from position A to position B along the semicircular path shown?

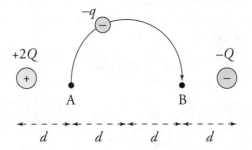

Solution: First, remember that neither the shape nor the length of the path matters; the fact that the path is a semicircle is irrelevant. All that matters is the initial point and the ending point of the path. Using the principle of superposition, the potentials at Points A and B are

$$\phi_A = \frac{k(+2Q)}{d} + \frac{k(-Q)}{3d} = \frac{5kQ}{3d} \quad\text{and}\quad \phi_B = \frac{k(+2Q)}{3d} + \frac{k(-Q)}{d} = -\frac{kQ}{3d}$$

9.4

Therefore, the change in potential energy of the charge $-q$ as it's moved from A to B is

$$\Delta PE = (-q)(\phi_B - \phi_A) = (-q)\left(\frac{-kQ}{3d} - \frac{5kQ}{3d}\right) = \frac{2kQq}{d}$$

Since the change in PE is positive, we know that the charge $-q$ is not moving as it would naturally on its own (after all, we can see from the figure that it's being moved from a point near a positive source charge, to which it's attracted, to a point near a negative charge, from which it's repelled). Therefore, some outside force is pushing this charge, doing work against the electric field. Since the work done *by* the electric field is $-\Delta PE = -2kQq/d$, the work done *against* the electric field by some outside force must be the opposite of this: $2kQq/d$.

Example 9-25: An electric dipole consists of a pair of equal but opposite charges, $+Q$ and $-Q$, separated by a distance d. What is the electric potential at the point (call it P) that's midway between these source charges?

Solution: The potential at P due to the positive charge alone is $k(+Q)/\left(\frac{1}{2}d\right)$, and the potential at P due to the negative charge alone is $k(-Q)/\left(\frac{1}{2}d\right)$. Adding these, we get zero, which is the potential at P due to both charges. (Notice that although the potential at P is zero, the electric field at P is *not* zero. We can have the "opposite" situation as well; that is, it's possible to have a point where the electric field is zero, but the potential is not. For example, if we had two equal source charges of the *same* sign, say $+Q$ and $+Q$, separated by a distance d, then the potential at the point that's midway between them would not be zero [it would be $2k(+Q)/\left(\frac{1}{2}d\right)$] but the electric field there *would* be zero.)

Example 9-26: An electric dipole consists of a pair of equal but opposite charges, $+Q$ and $-Q$, separated by a distance d. The dashed curves in the figure below are equipotentials. (Notice that the equipotentials are always perpendicular to the electric field lines, wherever they intersect. This is true for *any* electrostatic field, not just for the field created by a dipole.)

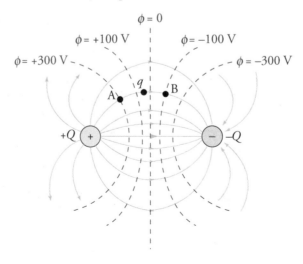

If a particle of mass $m = 1 \times 10^{-6}$ kg and charge $q = 5$ nC starts from rest at Point A and moves to Point B,

a) How much work is done by the electric field?
b) What is the speed of the particle when it reaches Point B?

Solution:

a) The work done by the electric field is equal to the opposite of the change in the particle's electrical potential energy $W_{\text{by E}} = -\Delta PE_{\text{elec}}$. Since the potential at Point A is $\phi_A = +300\,\text{V}$ (because A lies on the $\phi = +300\,\text{V}$ equipotential) and the potential at Point B is $\phi_B = -100\,\text{V}$ (because B lies on the $\phi = -100\,\text{V}$ equipotential), the change in potential from A to B is $\phi_B - \phi_A = (-100\ \text{V}) - (300\ \text{V}) = -400\ \text{V}$. Therefore,
$$W_{\text{by E}} = -\Delta PE_{\text{elec}} = -q\Delta\phi = -(5 \times 10^{-9}\ \text{C})(-400\ \text{V}) = 2 \times 10^{-6}\ \text{J}$$

b) Since the total work done on the particle is equal to its change in kinetic energy (the work-energy theorem), we have $\Delta KE = 2 \times 10^{-6}\,\text{J}$ Because the particle started from rest at Point A, we have $KE_{\text{at B}} = \Delta KE_{\text{A}\to\text{B}} = 2 \times 10^{-6}\,\text{J}$, so
$$\frac{1}{2}mv_B^2 = 2 \times 10^{-6}\,\text{J} \rightarrow v_B = \sqrt{\frac{2\left(2 \times 10^{-6}\,\text{J}\right)}{1 \times 10^{-6}\,\text{kg}}} = 2\,\tfrac{\text{m}}{\text{s}}$$

Example 9-27: The figure below shows several point source charges, $+Q_1$, $+Q_2$, $-Q_3$, and $-Q_4$, and the electric potential at various points (A, B, C, Z, Y, and Z) in the electric field they produce:

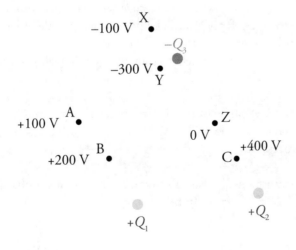

The difference in electric potential between two points is called the **voltage**, V. That is, $V = \Delta\phi$. For example, the voltage from Point A to Point B is $\phi_B - \phi_A = (+200\,\text{V}) - (+100\,\text{V}) = +100\,\text{V}$, and the voltage from X to Y is $V = (-300\,\text{V}) - (-100\,\text{V}) = -200\,\text{V}$.

9.4

a) How much work does the electric field do on a charge q = +2 μC as q is moved from Point X to Point C?

b) True or false? If the charge q is placed at Point Z, it will remain at this point because the electric potential is 0 V.

Solution:

a) The work done by the electric field is equal to the opposite of the change in the electrical potential energy $W_{by\,E} = -\Delta PE_{elec}$. Since $\Delta\phi = V$, the fundamental equation $\Delta PE = q\Delta\phi$ becomes simply

$$\Delta PE = qV$$

Since $V_{X \to C} = \phi_C - \phi_X = (+400\,\text{V}) - (-100\,\text{V}) = +500\,\text{V}$, we have

$$\Delta PE = qV = (2 \times 10^{-6}\,\text{C})(5 \times 10^{2}\,\text{V}) = 1 \times 10^{-3}\,\text{J}$$

Therefore, $W_{by\,E} = -1 \times 10^{-3}\,\text{J}$. (Does it make sense that ΔPE is positive and $W_{by\,E}$ is negative?

Yes, because a positive charge q would have to be pushed by some outside force from Point X (which is near a negative charge) to Point C (which is near a positive charge). When an external force has to do positive work against the electric field, the electrical potential energy increases and the work done by the electric field is negative.)

b) False. If q were placed at a point where the *electric field* was zero, *then* it would feel no force and remain there. However, if q is placed at a point where the electric potential is zero, it will be accelerated toward a point where the potential is lower (because q is positive; recall Example 7-21). In this case, q would be accelerated by the electric field toward the negative source charge $-Q_3$.

Example 9-28: During the active phase of the sodium-potassium pump, Na^+ ions are moved out of the cell against a potential difference of about 70 mV. How much work per sodium ion is done against the electric field during this process?

Solution: The work done against a field (or on a system, to use a more familiar phrasing for the same concept) is given by $W_{against\,E} = \Delta PE_{elec} = q\Delta\phi$. In this instance that yields $q\Delta\phi = (1.6 \times 10^{-19}\,\text{C})(7 \times 10^{-2}\,\text{V}) \approx 11 \times 10^{-21}\,\text{J} = 1.1 \times 10^{-20}\,\text{J}$.

Summary of Formulas

Elementary charge: $e = 1.6 \times 10^{-19}$ C

    charge of proton = $+e$; charge of electron = $-e$

Charge is quantized: $e = 1.6 \times 10^{-19}$ C

Coulomb's law: $F_{elec} = k \dfrac{|Q||q|}{r^2}$

    Opposite charges attract, like charges repel.

Coulomb's constant: $k_0 = 9 \times 10^9 \frac{Nm^2}{C^2}$

Principle of Superposition:

The net force, electric field, or electric potential on a charge q (for force) or point P (for electric field or electric potential) due to a collection of other charges (Qs) is equal to the sum of individual effects of each Q.

Electric field due to point charge Q: $E = k \dfrac{|Q|}{r^2}$

Direction of electric field:

    Positive charges want to move in the direction of the electric field (**E**).

    Negative charges want to move opposite the direction of the electric field (**E**).

Electric force and field: $\mathbf{F} = q\mathbf{E}$

Electric potential: $\phi = k\dfrac{Q}{r}$

(a scalar, not a vector)

    Positive charges want to move to regions of lower potential

    Negative charges want to move to regions of higher potential

Change in electrical *PE*: $\Delta PE_{elec} = q\Delta\phi = qV$

Work done by electric field: $W_{by\ E} = -\Delta PE_{elec}$

Change in *KE*: $\Delta KE = -\Delta PE$

For conductors, charge rests on the outer surface and the electric field inside is zero.

CHAPTER 9 FREESTANDING PRACTICE QUESTIONS

1. How far apart are two charges ($A = 10\ \mu C$ and $B = 12\ \mu C$) if the electric potential measured at point C midway between them is 10 V?

   A) 2×10^{-5} m
   B) 2×10^{5} m
   C) 4×10^{-4} m
   D) 4×10^{4} m

2. Two charges ($+q$ and $-q$) each with mass 9.11×10^{-31} kg are placed 0.5 m apart and the gravitational force (F_G) and electric force (F_E) are measured. If the ratio of F_G/F_E is 1.12×10^{-77}, what is the new ratio if the distance between the charges is halved?

   A) 2.24×10^{-77}
   B) 1.12×10^{-77}
   C) 5.6×10^{-78}
   D) 2.8×10^{-78}

3. Two equally positive charges are r distance apart. If the amount of charge on A is doubled and the distance between the charges is doubled, what is the ratio of new electric force to old electric force?

   A) 1/4
   B) 1/2
   C) 2
   D) 4

4. The amount of work required to move a charge in an electric field depends:

   A) only on the change in potential and not the path traveled.
   B) on both the change in potential and the path traveled.
   C) only on the path traveled and not the change in potential.
   D) on neither the path traveled nor the change in potential.

5. Which of the following pairs of electric forces form an action-reaction pair?

   I. Two positive charges, of different masses, placed at a distance d apart.
   II. Two negative charges, of equal masses, placed at a distance d apart.
   III. One positive charge and one negative charge, of equal masses, placed at a distance d apart.

   A) I and II only
   B) II and III only
   C) III only
   D) I, II and III

6. A hollow metal sphere of radius 0.5 m has a net charge of 2.0×10^{-6} C. A solid metal sphere of radius 0.5 m has a net charge of 4.0×10^{-6} C. The centers of the spheres are placed a distance 2 m apart and equilibrium is established. Compared to the electric field at the center of the hollow sphere, the electric field at the center of the solid sphere is:

   A) twice the magnitude.
   B) four times the magnitude.
   C) half the magnitude.
   D) equal in magnitude.

7. Starting from rest, a sphere of mass 2 kg and charge -0.1 C slides across a frictionless horizontal plane through a potential difference of 220 V. Determine the instantaneous velocity of the sphere the moment it has rolled through this potential.

   A) 4.7 m/s
   B) 5.1 m/s
   C) 5.5 m/s
   D) 6.1 m/s

CHAPTER 9 PRACTICE PASSAGE

In the Bohr model of the atom, electrons circle the point-like nucleus similar to the way planets orbit the Sun. Imagining that the atomic model is confined to motion in one plane, the orbit of the electrons can be drawn as circles with the nucleus in the center.

The atomic radius of an atom is defined as the length from the nucleus to the outermost electron and is generally within the tens to hundreds of picometers. The atomic radii of common atoms are as follows: hydrogen = 40 pm, helium = 30 pm, carbon = 80 pm. In the periodic table, atomic radius tends to increase as you go down each column of the table and decrease as you move from left to right across a period.

Current scientific thought suggests that the Bohr model is an oversimplification of atomic structure. Quantum mechanics states that the exact position of an electron at a given point in time cannot be known. Only the probability of electron existence in a region of space is known. However, the Bohr model of the atom wonderfully captures another aspect of quantum mechanics: the quantization of energy. The electrons can only have very specific energy values and the distinct orbits are a very good visual representation of this. Electrons can only move from one energy level to another if there is the exact energy configuration. When dropping from a higher energy to a lower energy, photons with the exact energy difference are emitted, and electrons can only move to a higher energy level if they absorb a photon of the exact energy difference.

1. What is the magnitude of the electric force a hydrogen nucleus exerts on its only orbiting electron in the Bohr model?

   A) 10^7 N
   B) 10 N
   C) 10^{-7} N
   D) 10^{-18} N

2. What is the electric potential a millimeter away from a carbon atom nucleus?

   A) 1.4×10^{-9} V
   B) 8.6×10^{-6} V
   C) 1.4×10^{-6} V
   D) 8.6×10^{-3} V

3. If the electric force between the nucleus and the outermost electron in ^{6}Li is F, what is the electric force between the nucleus and the outermost electron in ^{7}Li, given that the mass of a neutron is approximately 1/9th the mass of ^{6}Li?

   A) $F/9$
   B) $F/3$
   C) F
   D) $9F$

4. According to the Bohr model, the atomic radius decreases as you move from left to right in the periodic table. Which of the following helps to explain this phenomenon?

   I. The charge of the nucleus decreases as you move from left to right.
   II. The electric force between the electrons and the nucleus increases as you move from left to right.
   III. The work done by the electrons increases as you move from left to right.

   A) I only
   B) II only
   C) I and II only
   D) II and III only

5. An attractive force keeps the electron in ^{1}H orbiting the nucleus. Approximately what is the magnitude of the gravitational force, F_G, between the nucleus and the electron in terms of the magnitude of the electric force, F_E, between them? (Recall that $m_e = 9 \times 10^{-31}$ kg, $m_p = 2 \times 10^{-27}$ kg, and $G = 7 \times 10^{-11}$ m^{3}kg^{-1}s^{-2}.)

   A) $10^{-10}F_E$
   B) $10^{-20}F_E$
   C) $10^{-30}F_E$
   D) $10^{-40}F_E$

6. Imagine a lithium atom where the two electrons in the first energy level are at exact opposite sides of the nucleus and the electron in the second energy level is in line with the other electrons so that the three electrons and the nucleus all lie on a straight line. How much work would you need to apply to remove the outermost electron if the atomic radius is 100 pm and the distance between the first and second energy level is 50 pm?

A) $(ke/150) \times 10^{12}$ J
B) $(ke^2/150) \times 10^{12}$ J
C) $(ke/300) \times 10^{12}$ J
D) $(ke^2/300) \times 10^{12}$ J

7. Ionized hydrogen gas is placed in a region with a uniform electric field. All of the following are true EXCEPT:

A) The protons and the electrons will move in opposite directions.
B) The protons and the electrons will have the same magnitude of acceleration.
C) The protons will move in the direction of the electric field.
D) The electrons will move in the direction of higher potential.

SOLUTIONS TO CHAPTER 9 FREESTANDING PRACTICE QUESTIONS

1. **D**   This question requires us to remember the electric potential formula. The question stem tells us that C is the midway point between A and B, so if we can determine the distance between A and C (or B and C), we can double that distance to determine the distance between A and B. Since $\phi_{elec} = kQ/r$ is a scalar quantity, when we use the Principle of Superposition for Electric Potential, it is straight addition. Let C be the distance between A and C (note that it is also the distance between B and C since C is midway between A and B). Thus,

$$\phi_{elec} = \frac{kQ_A}{C} + \frac{kQ_B}{C}$$
$$C = (kQ_A + kQ_B)/\phi_{elec}$$
$$= [(9\times10^9)(10\times10^{-6}) + (9\times10^9)(12\times10^{-6})]/10$$
$$= [(90\times10^3) + (108\times10^3)]/10$$
$$= 1.98\times10^4 \text{ m} \approx 2\times10^4 \text{ m}$$

Now that we know how far apart A and C are (and also therefore how far apart B and C are), we double this distance to calculate how far apart A and B are (i.e., $2 \times (2 \times 10^4 \text{ m}) = 4 \times 10^4$ m).

2. **B**   To determine how the ratio changes, it is necessary to know the formulae for calculating F_G and F_E respectively ($F_G = GMm/r^2$ and $F_E = k|q_1||q_2|/r^2$). Both of gravitational force and electric force are inverse square laws with respect to r, the distance between the two charges. Therefore, G and E will vary in the same proportion so the ratio of G/E will be unchanged when the distance between the two charges or masses is varied.

3. **B**   The MCAT loves proportion questions, as they require us to remember the formulae for specific quantities. In this question, we need to recall the formula for electric force and how it varies with respect to the variable of distance. Given that $F_E = \dfrac{kq_1q_2}{r^2}$, the (original F_E) = $\dfrac{kq^2}{r^2}$ and the (new F_E) = $\dfrac{k(2q)(q)}{(2r)^2} = \dfrac{2kq^2}{4r^2} = \dfrac{kq^2}{2r^2} = \dfrac{1}{2}\left(\dfrac{kq^2}{r^2}\right) = \dfrac{1}{2}$ (original F_E). Therefore, the ratio of (new F_E)/(original F_E) = ($\dfrac{1}{2}$ original F_E)/(original F_E) = $\dfrac{1}{2}$.

4. **A**   The amount of work required to move a charge in an electric field depends only on the change in potential and is independent of the path traveled. Remember, like the gravitational field, the electric field is conservative.

5. **D** The electric force is a force in the same sense as gravity and friction are forces. In each of these three cases the pairs of forces are acting on the two separate objects, thereby satisfying Newton's third law. As such, each forms an action-reaction pair. Note that the mass in each case is irrelevant as the electric force is independent of the mass.

6. **D** The electric field inside of an electrostatic conductor is always zero. Therefore, the electric fields at the centers of the solid and hollow sphere are both equal in magnitude.

7. **A** Since $v_0 = 0$ (the sphere starts at rest), we need to calculate the kinetic energy gained by the sphere and use this to determine v_F. $\Delta PE = q\Delta\phi = -0.1$ C $(220$ V$) = -22$ J. Using $\Delta PE = -\Delta KE$, $\Delta KE = 22$ J. Finally, $\Delta KE = mv^2/2$, so $v = \sqrt{22}$. The MCAT does not expect you to have this square root memorized, but notice that it is less than $\sqrt{25}$, which is 5. We know that $\sqrt{22}$ is less than $\sqrt{25}$ so we can eliminate choices B, C and D.

SOLUTIONS TO CHAPTER 9 PRACTICE PASSAGE

1. **C** In this question we just can look at the powers of ten in each term separately from the specific numbers. The electric force is equal to $k|q_1||q_2|/r^2$, the powers of 10 give $(10^9)(10^{-19})$ $(10^{-19})/(10^{-12})(10^{-12}) = 10^{-5}$. Then, the other numbers are approximately $(9)(1.6)(1.6)/$ $(40)(40)$, which is approximately $25/1600$ which is on the order of 10^{-2}. Therefore, the magnitude of the electric force is 10^{-7}.

2. **B** A carbon nucleus contains six protons, and thus has a charge of $Q = 6e$. The electric potential one millimeter away from the nucleus is then $kQ/r = (9 \times 10^9)(6)(1.6 \times 10^{-19})/(10^{-3}) = 8.6 \times 10^{-6}$ V.

3. **C** The formula for electric force is $F = k|q_1||q_2|/r^2$, and does not depend on mass. Since an isotope does not change the charge of the nucleus, the electric force will not change.

4. **B** As you move from left to right in the periodic table there are more electrons added in the same shell and the nucleus has a greater positive charge. The added charges increase the electric force between the nucleus and the electrons, hence, attracting them closer together. Item I is not true (choices A and C can be eliminated); as you move from left to right the number of protons in the nucleus increases. Item III is false (choice D can be eliminated) since the electrons do no work as they orbit the nucleus because the electric potential does not change. Thus, Item II is the only correct answer.

5. **D** In this question you need to work with the powers of 10. The gravitational force is equal to Gm_1m_2/r^2, which is on the order of 10^{-45}, while the electric force is equal to $k|q_1||q_2|/r^2$, which is on the order of 10^{-5}. Thus, the gravitational force is approximately $10^{-40}F_E$. (To calculate it more precisely, the electric force is 1.4×10^{-7} N and the gravitational force is 7.88×10^{-47} N.)

6. **D** First, calculate the electric potential at the point of the outermost electron using the principle of superposition for electric potential:

$$\phi_2 = \phi_{\text{electron 1a}} + \phi_{\text{nucleus}} + \phi_{\text{electron 1b}}$$

$$= \frac{-ke}{50 \times 10^{-12}} + \frac{k(3e)}{100 \times 10^{-12}} + \frac{-ke}{150 \times 10^{-12}}$$

$$= \frac{ke}{50 \times 10^{-12}} \left(-1 + \frac{3}{2} - \frac{1}{3}\right)$$

$$= \frac{ke}{300 \times 10^{-12}}$$

Removing the electron requires that the final potential is equal to 0 (i.e., the electron is infinitely far away). Therefore, the work required to remove the electron is

$$W_{\text{against electric field}} = \Delta PE = q\Delta\phi = (-e)(0 - ke \,/\, 300 \times 10^{-12}) = ke^2 \,/\, 300 \times 10^{-12}.$$

7. **B** The direction of the electric field is defined as the direction of force a positive charge would experience. Likewise, negative charges feel a force opposite the direction of the electric field. Choices A and C are true statements, and therefore can be eliminated. Positive charges tend toward lower potential and negative charges tend toward higher potential. This eliminates choice D. The magnitude of the force experienced by a charge in an electric field is given by $F_E = |q|E$. Since protons and electrons have the same magnitude of charge, they will experience the same magnitude of force. Newton's Second Law tells us that $F_{\text{net}} = ma$. Since protons are more massive than electrons, they will experience a smaller acceleration.

Chapter 10
Electricity and Magnetism

10.1 ELECTRIC CIRCUITS

An electric circuit is a pathway for the movement of electric charge, consisting of a voltage source, connecting wires, and other components.

Current

Current can be defined as the movement of charge, but for the purposes of analyzing an electric circuit, we need a more precise definition. For example, imagine picking up a metal paper clip and untwisting it to make it relatively straight. If we could look inside this piece of metal wire at the individual atoms, we would see a lattice with about one electron per atom free to roam freely, unbound to any particular atom. These free electrons are known as **conduction electrons**. (Recall the discussion of metallic bonding in *MCAT General Chemistry*.) The conduction electrons in a metal are zooming around throughout the lattice at very high speeds. However, we only have a current when there is a *net* movement of charge. Let's look at this a little more closely.

The figure below shows an imagined magnified view inside a metal wire. The conduction electrons move at an average speed on the order of a million meters per second ($v \sim 10^6$ m/s). If we chose any cross-sectional slice of the wire, we would see that these conduction electrons cross from left to right as often as they cross from right to left. So, while there is movement of charge, there's no *net* movement of charge; that is, there's no current.

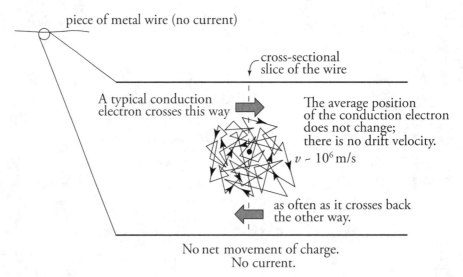

So how would this same piece of wire look if there *were* current in it? Superimposed on the conduction electrons' going-nowhere-fast zooming, we would see that there's a slight drift in one particular direction. This is known as the electrons' **drift velocity** (v_d). If we chose any cross-sectional slice of the wire, we'd see that these conduction electrons move across it from, say, left to right more often than they cross back. Thus, the average positions of the conduction electrons do change and there is a *net* movement of charge (in the case pictured below, negative charge to the right). This is **current**.

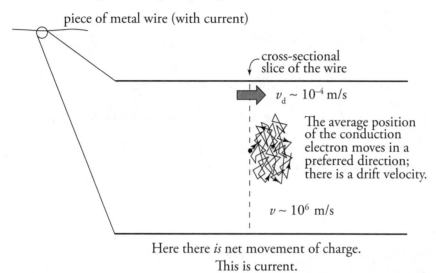

piece of metal wire (with current)

cross-sectional slice of the wire

$v_d \sim 10^{-4}$ m/s

The average position of the conduction electron moves in a preferred direction; there is a drift velocity.

$v \sim 10^6$ m/s

Here there *is* net movement of charge.
This is current.

In the first figure, there was no drift velocity and, therefore, no preferred direction for the movement of charge and no current. In the figure above, however, there is a drift velocity, so there is a flow of charge: a current.

Now, how do we measure current? Since current is the flow of charge, it makes sense to measure current as the amount of charge that moves past a certain point per unit time. Current is denoted by the letter I, and is equal to charge (Q) divided by time (t):

Current

$$I = \frac{Q}{t}$$

The unit of current is the coulomb per second (C/s), which has its own special name: the **ampère** (or just **amp**, for short), abbreviated **A**. Thus, 1 A = 1 C/s.[1] Since we know that one coulomb is a lot of charge (recall Example 9-4 in the preceding chapter), we would expect that one amp is a lot of current. The following table shows that even a small fraction of a coulomb is enough to kill you.

<u>Current</u>	<u>Physiological Effect</u>
~ 0.01 A	slight tingling
~ 0.02 A	painful; muscles may contract around source (can't let go)
~ 0.05 A	painful; can't let go; breathing difficult
~ 0.1 to 0.2 A	ventricular fibrillation (potentially fatal arrhythmia)
> 0.2 A	severe burning; breathing stops; heart stops (may be restarted)

Example 10-1: Within a metal wire, 5×10^{17} conduction electrons drift past a certain point in 4 seconds. What is the magnitude of the current?

Solution: The magnitude of charge that passes the point in $t = 4$ seconds is

$$Q = ne = (5 \times 10^{17})(1.6 \times 10^{-19} \text{ C}) = 8 \times 10^{-2} \text{ C}$$

Therefore, the value of the current is

$$I = \frac{Q}{t} = \frac{8 \times 10^{-2} \text{ C}}{4 \text{ s}} = 0.02 \text{ A}$$

Example 10-2: A typical ion channel in a cellular membrane might allow the passage of 10^7 sodium ions to flow through in one second. What is the magnitude and direction of this ionic current?

Solution:

$$I = \frac{Q}{t} = \frac{(10^7)1.6 \times 10^{-19} \text{ C}}{1 \text{ s}} = 1.6 \times 10^{-12} \text{ A}$$

Because sodium ions are positive, the direction of current flow is the same as the one in which the charges are moving. (It is interesting to note that this current of ions into and out of the cell does not obey Ohm's Law generally, so predicting the current based upon voltage difference across the membrane is impossible.)

---

[1] Notice that current is defined in about the same way that we defined *flow rate* in Chapter 8: amount of stuff per unit time. You can think of current as the flow rate of charge.

Voltage

Now that we know how to measure current, the next question is, *What causes it?* Look back at the picture of the wire in which there was a current. What would make an electron drift to the right? One answer is to say that there's an electric field inside the wire, and since negative charges move in the direction opposite to the electric field lines, electrons would be induced to drift to the right if the electric field pointed to the left:

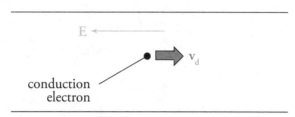

Another (equivalent) answer to the question, "What would make an electron drift to the right?" is that there's a potential difference (a voltage) between the ends of the wire. Because we know that negative charges naturally move toward regions of higher electric potential, electrons would be induced to drift to the right if the right end of the wire were maintained at a higher potential than the left end.

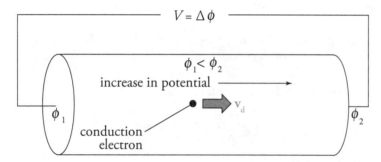

For our purposes in analyzing circuits, this second interpretation of the answer will be the one we use: that is, *it is a voltage that creates a current*. If there's no voltage (no potential difference), then the conduction electrons will just zoom around their original positions, going essentially nowhere; without a potential difference, they'd have no reason to do anything differently.

It is not uncommon to see the voltage that creates a current referred to as **electromotive force** (**emf**), since it is the cause that sets the charges into motion in a preferred direction. Notice, however, that calling it a "force" really isn't correct; it's a voltage.

Resistance

Now that we know what current is, how to measure it, and what causes it, the next question is, *How much do we get?* The answer is, *It depends*. If we took a paper-clip wire and touched its two ends to the terminals of a battery, we'd get a measurable current. Now imagine picking up a rubber band and cutting it, so that it becomes essentially a straightened out "wire" of rubber. If we took this rubber wire and touched its two ends to the terminals of the same battery, we'd get essentially zero current. What's the difference? The metal wire and the rubber wire have very different **resistances**. Metals are conductors and rubber is an insulator. That is, metals have a very low intrinsic resistance, while insulators (like rubber) have a very high intrinsic resistance to the flow of charge. Since insulators have very few free electrons, there's going to be virtually no current, even with an applied voltage, which is why we got essentially zero current with our rubber wire.

Let V be the voltage applied to the ends of an object, and let I be the resulting current. By definition, the resistance of the object, R, is given by this equation:

Resistance

$$R = \frac{V}{I}$$

The unit of resistance is the volt per amp (V/A), which has its own special name: the **ohm**, abbreviated Ω (the Greek letter capital *omega*—get it? "<u>ohm</u>ega"). Thus, $1\ \Omega = 1$ V/A. Notice from the definition that for a given voltage, a large I means a small R, and a small I means a big R; that is, for a fixed voltage, resistance and current are inversely proportional.

Example 10-3: When the potential difference between the ends of a wire is 12 V, the current is measured to be 0.06 A. What's the resistance of the wire?

Solution: Using the definition of resistance, we find that

$$R = \frac{V}{I} = \frac{12\ \text{V}}{0.06\ \text{A}} = 200\,\Omega$$

There's another way to calculate the resistance, using a formula that does not depend on V or I. Instead, it expresses the resistance in terms of the material's *intrinsic* resistance, which is known as its **resistivity** (and denoted by ρ, not to be confused with the material's density):

Resistance and Resistivity

$$R = \rho \frac{L}{A}$$

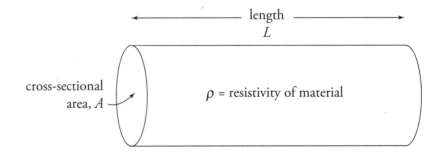

Notice that resistance and resistivity are not the same thing. Each material has its own resistivity; its *intrinsic* resistance. However, the resistance R depends on how we shape the material. For example, if we had two aluminum wires, one that was long and thin and another that was short and thick, both would have the same resistivity (because they're both made of the same material, aluminum), but the wires would have different resistances. The long, thin wire would have the greater resistance because R is proportional to L and inversely proportional to A.

Example 10-4: Consider two copper wires. Wire #1 has three times the length and twice the diameter of Wire #2. If R_1 is the resistance of Wire #1 and R_2 is the resistance of Wire #2, then which of the following is true?

  A. $R_2 = (2/3)R_1$
  B. $R_2 = (4/3)R_1$
  C. $R_2 = 6R_1$
  D. $R_2 = 12R_1$

Solution: We're told that $L_1 = 3L_2$, and since $d_1 = 2d_2$, we know that $A_1 = 4A_2$ (because area is proportional to the *square* of the diameter). Since both wires have the same resistivity (because they're both made of the same material), we find that

$$\frac{R^2}{R^1} = \frac{\rho L_2 / A_2}{\rho L_1 / A_1} = \frac{L_2}{L_1} \cdot \frac{A_1}{A_2} = \frac{1}{3} \cdot 4 = \frac{4}{3} \rightarrow R_2 = \frac{4}{3}R_1$$

Thus, the answer is B.

Example 10-5: The wire used for lighting systems is usually No. 12 wire, in the American Wire Gauge (AWG) system. The diameter of No. 12 wire is just over 2 mm (which means a cross-sectional area of 3.3×10^{-6} m^2). What would be the resistance of half a mile (800 m) of No. 12 copper wire, given that the resistivity of copper is 1.7×10^{-8} Ω·m?

Solution: Using the equation $R = \rho L / A$, we get

$$R = \rho \frac{L}{A} = (1.7 \times 10^{-8} \ \Omega \cdot m) \frac{8 \times 10^2 \ m}{3.3 \times 10^{-6} \ m^2} \approx 4 \ \Omega$$

If we wanted to give a more precise formula for the resistance in terms of resistivity, we would have to include the temperature dependence. The resistivity of conductors generally increases slightly with temperature. However, unless specifically mentioned otherwise, assume that the MCAT will treat resistivity as a constant.

Ohm's Law

The definition of resistance, $R = V/I$, is usually written more simply as $V = IR$, and known as **Ohm's law.**

> **Ohm's Law**
>
> $$V = IR$$

However, the actual statement of Ohm's law isn't $V = IR$; rather, it's a statement about the behavior of certain conductors, and it isn't true for all materials. A material is said to obey Ohm's law if its resistance, R, remains constant as the voltage is varied; another requirement is that the current must reverse direction if the polarity of the voltage is reversed.[2] On the MCAT, you can assume that materials are "ohmic" unless you are specifically told otherwise.

Resistors

A resistor is a component in an electric circuit that has a specific (and usually known) resistance. When we analyze a circuit, we generally ignore the resistance of the connecting metal wires and think of the resistance as being concentrated solely in the resistors placed in the circuit. We can do this because metal wires are such good conductors, i.e., their resistance is very low. Recall that in Example 8-4, we calculated that even half a mile of household wire has a resistance of only 4 Ω.

In the real world, a resistor is typically a little cylinder filled with an alloy (of carbon or of nickel and copper) and often encircled by colored bands to indicate the numerical value of its resistance, like this:

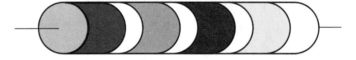

In circuit diagrams, however, a resistor is denoted by the following symbol:

Electric circuits on the MCAT may contain just one resistor, but it's more likely that they'll have two or more. There are two ways the MCAT will combine resistors: in series or in parallel. Two or more resistors are said to be in **series** if each follows the others along a single connection in a circuit. For example, these two resistors are in series, because R_2 directly follows R_1 along a single path.

---

2 Some materials don't behave this way, and the relationship between voltage and current is more complex; on the MCAT, however, it's safe to assume that $V = IR$ applies unless you're told otherwise.

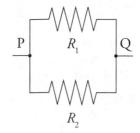

Resistors in Series

On the other hand, two or more resistors are said to be in **parallel** if they provide alternative routes from one point in a circuit to another. For example, the following two resistors are in parallel, because we get from Point P to Point Q in the circuit *either* by traveling through R_1 *or* by traveling through R_2; we don't go through both resistors like we would if they were in series.

Resistors in Parallel

Typically, we analyze a circuit by first transforming it into a simpler one, one that contains just a single resistor. Therefore, we need a way to turn combinations of resistors (series combinations and parallel combinations) into a single, equivalent resistor; that is, one resistor that provides the same overall resistance as the combination. Here are the formulas:

resistors in series

single
equivalent resistor

$$R_{eq} = R_1 + R_2$$

R_{eq}

resistors in parallel

$$R_{eq} = \frac{R_1 R_2}{R_1 + R_2}$$

R_{eq}

So, for resistors in series, we simply add the resistances. For example, if a 20 Ω resistor is in series with a 30 Ω resistor, this combination is equivalent to a single 50 Ω resistor, because 20 + 30 = 50. Notice that for a series combination, the equivalent resistance is always greater than the largest resistance in the combination; that's why the "R" is bigger in the figure above for the series combination.

For resistors in parallel, the formula is a little more complicated. If we have two resistors in parallel, we get the equivalent resistance by taking the product of the resistances (R_1R_2) and dividing this by their sum $(R_1 + R_2)$. For example, if a 3 Ω resistor is in parallel with a 6 Ω resistor, this combination is equivalent to a single 2 Ω resistor, because (3 × 6) divided by (3 + 6) is equal to 2. For a parallel combination, the equivalent resistance is always less than the smallest resistance in the combination; that's why the "R_{eq}" is smaller in the figure above for the parallel combination.

The "product over sum" formula for parallel resistors only works for *two* resistors. If you have three or more resistors in parallel, do them two at a time. Here's an example:

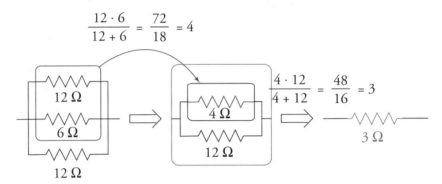

We could have also found the same answer this way:

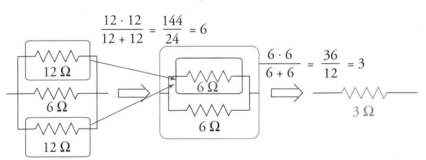

For resistors in series, we just add the individual resistances, no matter how many we have in a row. For example, if we have the following four resistors in series: 10 Ω, 20 Ω, 30 Ω, and 40 Ω, then we can reduce this combination of four series resistors to a single equivalent resistance of 100 Ω, because 10 + 20 + 30 + 40 = 100.

The formula for calculating the equivalent resistance, R, for a parallel combination of resistors R_1, R_2, ... is usually given as:

$$\frac{1}{R} = \frac{1}{R_1} + \frac{1}{R_2} + ...$$

This formula works for any number of resistors in parallel, not just two. If you prefer this formula, that's perfectly okay. However, you may find adding the fractions to be messier than the "product over sum" rule above. Also, be sure to avoid the common error of forgetting to take the reciprocal of the left-hand side to get your final answer.

Example 10-6: Show that the equivalent resistance of two identical resistors in series is twice the resistance of either resistor, but the equivalent resistance of two identical resistors in parallel is half the resistance of either resistor.

Solution: Let the resistance of each resistor be R. Then, if two such resistors are in series, the equivalent resistance is $R_{eq} = R + R = 2R$. However, if two such resistors are in parallel, then their equivalent resistance is

$$R_{eq} = \frac{R \cdot R}{R + R} = \frac{R^2}{2R} = \frac{R}{2}$$

Example 10-7: What is the equivalent or total resistance of the following combination of resistors?

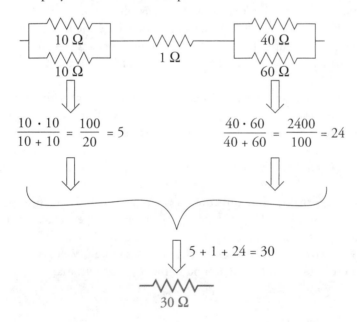

Solution: Here we have a mixture of parallel *and* series combinations. There's a parallel combination (the pair of 10 Ω resistors) that's in series with both a 1 Ω resistor and another parallel combination (the 40 Ω and 60 Ω resistors). To simplify this, we work in steps:

Therefore, the given combination of resistors is equivalent to a single 30 Ω resistor.

DC Circuits

Now that we know how to simplify series and parallel combinations of resistors, we're ready to analyze circuits. The simplest circuit consists of a voltage source (most commonly, it's a battery), a connecting wire between the terminals of the voltage source, and a resistor. As an example, imagine hooking up a light bulb to a typical flashlight battery; one wire connects the positive terminal of the battery to one of the "leads" on the light bulb, and another wire connects the other lead on the bulb to the negative terminal of the battery. This completes the circuit. The diagram on the right below shows the way this real-life circuit would be drawn schematically.

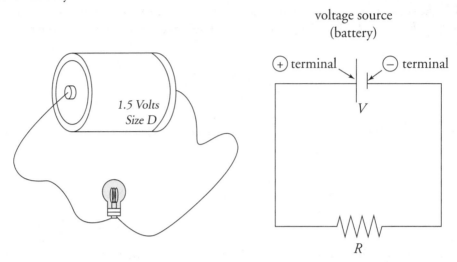

The pair of adjacent parallel lines denotes the voltage source. The job of the voltage source is to maintain a potential difference (a voltage) between its terminals; the value of this voltage is denoted by V or sometimes by ε, for emf (electromotive force). Remember that a voltage is needed to create a current. The terminal that's at the higher potential is denoted by the longer line and called the **positive terminal**; the terminal that's at the lower potential is denoted by the shorter line and called the **negative terminal**.

Once the circuit is set up, we know what will happen inside the metal wires: conduction electrons will drift toward the higher potential terminal; that is, they'll drift away from the negative terminal, toward the positive terminal. The direction of the flow of conduction electrons would be clockwise in the diagram as drawn. However, there is a convention that is followed when discussing the direction of the current. *The direction of the current is taken to be the direction that <u>positive</u> charge carriers would flow, even though the actual charge carriers that do flow might be negatively charged.* (Sounds like the convention for defining the direction of the electric field, doesn't it? "The direction of the electric field is taken to be the direction of the force that a positive charge would feel, even if the actual charge that gets placed in the field isn't positive." In fact, that's the reason for the convention about the direction of the current; to keep things consistent.) Even though we know electrons are drifting clockwise in this circuit, we'd say that the current, I, flows counterclockwise from the positive terminal around to the negative terminal.

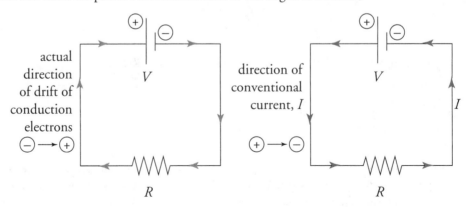

If we were asked for the value of the current in this circuit, this question would be easy to answer. We know V and R, and we want I. Using the equation $V = IR$, we'd say that

$$I = \frac{V}{R}$$

For example, if $V = 1.5$ V and $R = 150$ Ω, then $I = 0.01$ A. So, what made this problem so easy? The answer: There was only one resistor. This will usually be our goal: to simplify a circuit with multiple resistors into a circuit with just a single equivalent resistor. (We say "usually" because there are some question types that can be answered without changing the circuit into one with just a single resistor; we'll show you some examples of those, too.)

In order to simplify a circuit with multiple resistors, we first need a way to turn resistors in series and resistors in parallel into a single equivalent resistor; this we already know how to do. However, there are two other important quantities in circuits besides R; namely, I and V. We also need to know what happens to these other quantities when we convert a series or parallel combination of resistors into a single resistor. The following figure contains this needed information:

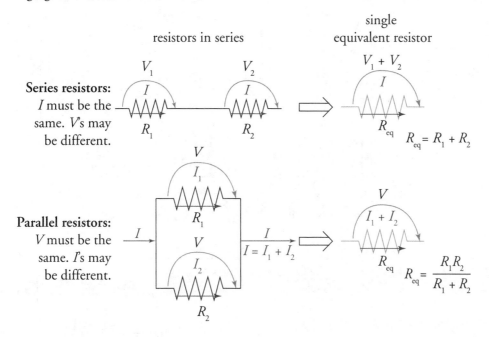

Resistors in series always share the same current, and resistors in parallel always share the same voltage drop. However, the voltage drops across series resistors will be different (and the currents through parallel resistors will be different) if the resistances are different.

With all this information at hand, we're ready to tackle an example. Consider the following circuit:

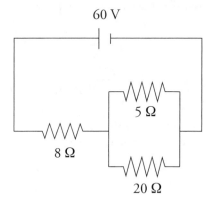

We'll find the current in the circuit, the current through each resistor, and the voltage across each resistor. The first stage of the solution involves simplifying this multiple-resistor circuit into a circuit with just a single equivalent resistor, like this:

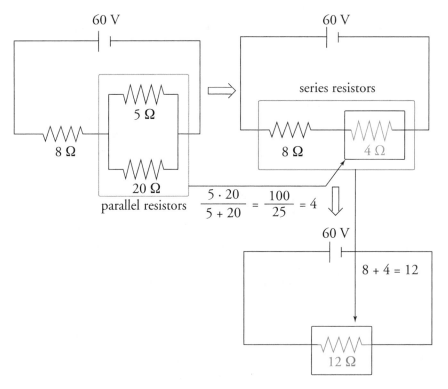

Now that we have an equivalent circuit with just one resistor, we can find the current:

$$I = \frac{V}{R} = \frac{60\text{ V}}{12\ \Omega} = 5\text{ A}$$

If we want to find the currents through (and the voltages across) the individual resistors in the original circuit, we have to work backward. The key to "working backward" is to ask at each stage: "What am I going back to?" If the answer is, "a *series* combination," then the value you bring back is the *current*, because series resistors share the same current. If the answer is, "a *parallel* combination," then the value you bring back is the *voltage*, because parallel resistors share the same voltage.

going back to series combination → bring *I*

going back to parallel combination → bring *V*

Let me illustrate this "working backward" technique with our circuit above. You should read this figure starting at the bottom, then up, then to the left... in other words, in the *reverse* order from what we did before because now we're working backward:

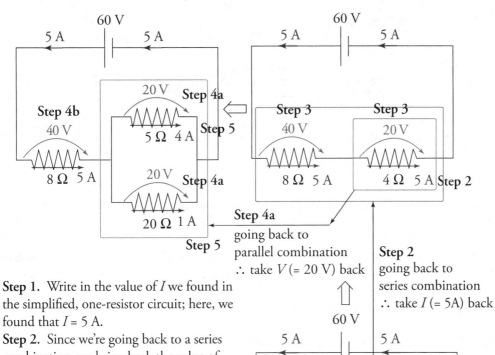

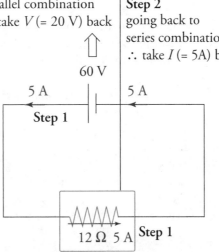

Step 1. Write in the value of *I* we found in the simplified, one-resistor circuit; here, we found that *I* = 5 A.

Step 2. Since we're going back to a series combination, we bring back the value of the current, *I* = 5 A.

Step 3. Use *V* = *IR* to find the voltage across each individual series resistor; here, we get *V* = (5 A)(8 Ω) = 40 V for the first resistor, and *V* = (5 A)(4 Ω) = 20 V for the second resistor.

Step 4a. Since we're going back to a parallel combination, we bring back the value of the voltage, *V* = 20 V.

Step 4b. Simply copy the information for the 8 Ω resistor, since that resistor doesn't change when we go back.

Step 5. Use *I* = *V/R* to find the current across each individual parallel resistor; here, we get *I* = (20 V)/(5 Ω) = 4 A for the top resistor, and *I* = (20 V)/(20 Ω) = 1 A for the bottom resistor.

Now that we have found all the information for the original circuit,

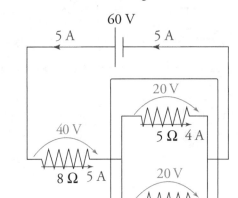

there are a couple of important things to notice, things that will hold true in any circuit. They are consequences of **Kirchhoff's laws** (pronounced "Keer-koff").

- *For a circuit containing one battery as the voltage source, the sum of the voltage drops across the resistors in any complete path starting at the (+) terminal and ending at the (–) terminal matches the voltage of the battery.*

For our circuit above, we have 40 V + 20 V = 60 V. (We don't add the 20 V twice, because these resistors are in parallel; each charge carrier moving through the circuit would go *either* across the 20 V voltage as it drifts through the top resistor in the parallel combination *or* across the 20 V voltage as it drifts through the bottom resistor; it doesn't go through both resistors.)

- *The amount of current entering the parallel combination is equal to the sum of the currents that pass through all the individual resistors in the combination.*

For our circuit above, we have 5 A = 4 A + 1 A.

Besides asking about resistance, current, and voltage, the MCAT can also ask about power. When current passes through a resistor, the resistor gets hot: it dissipates heat. The rate at which it dissipates heat energy is the **power dissipated by the resistor**. The formula used to calculate this power, P, is known as the **Joule heating law**.

Power Dissipated by a Resistor: Joule Heating Law
$$P = I^2 R$$

So, for our circuit above, we find that:

the power dissipated by the 8 Ω resistor is $I^2R = (5\text{ A})^2(8\ \Omega)$ $\quad$ = 200 W
the power dissipated by the 5 Ω resistor is $I^2R = (4\text{ A})^2(5\ \Omega)$ $\quad$ = 80 W
the power dissipated by the 20 Ω resistor is $I^2R = (1\text{ A})^2(20\ \Omega)$ $\quad$ = 20 W
the total power dissipated by all resistors is the sum: $\qquad$ 300 W

The power *supplied* to the circuit by the voltage source (like a battery) is given by this formula: $P = IV$. So, for our circuit above, we find that

power supplied by the 60 V battery is $P = IV = (5\text{ A})(60\text{ V}) = 300$ W

Notice that these answers match:

power dissipated by all resistors = 300 W = power supplied by the battery

This is simply a consequence of Conservation of Energy, so it will be true in general:

- *The total power dissipated by the resistors is equal to the power supplied by the battery.*

Sometimes, a circuit may contain more than one battery, and in some of these cases, the battery with the lower voltage will be *absorbing* power from the battery with the higher voltage (that is, from the "boss battery" that supplies the power to the circuit). The power *absorbed* by a battery is also given by the formula $P = IV$, and the italicized statement above should then read:

- *The total power dissipated by the resistors and absorbed by other voltage sources (i.e., the total power used by the circuit) is equal to the power supplied to the circuit by the highest-voltage power source.*

One more note: The Joule heating law, $P = I^2R$, can be written as $P = I(IR) = IV$, so, in fact, we need just one formula for the power dissipated or supplied by *any* component in a circuit:

> **Power**
>
> $$P = IV$$

However, if you use the formula $P = IV$ to find the power dissipated by a resistor, *be careful* that you only use the *V for that resistor*, and not the *V* for the entire circuit. So, for our circuit above, we'd find that:

the power dissipated by the 8 Ω resistor is $\quad IV = (5\text{ A})(40\text{ V}) = 200$ W
the power dissipated by the 5 Ω resistor is $\quad IV = (4\text{ A})(20\text{ V}) =$ 80 W
the power dissipated by the 20 Ω resistor is $\quad IV = (1\text{ A})(20\text{ V}) =$ 20 W

giving us the same answers we found before when we used the formula $P = I^2R$.

Along with questions about power, there could also be questions about energy. Simply remember the definition: power = energy/time, so

$$\text{energy} = \text{power} \times \text{time}$$

For example, how much energy is dissipated in 5 seconds by the 5-ohm resistor in the circuit above? We calculated that the power dissipated by this resistor is $P = 80$ W $= 80$ J/s; so the energy dissipated in $t = 5$ seconds is $Pt = (80$ J/s$)(5$ s$) = 400$ J.

In some circuits (in practice, most of them), one or more of the resistors are actually doing something useful besides just heating up. However, the circuit diagrams and the calculations we do will be the same. For example, a motor will be shown as a resistor in an MCAT circuit; so will a light bulb (which is really just a resistor that happens to get so hot that some of the energy dissipated is emitted as light rather than heat). In either case, the calculations for these components are the same as treating each as a regular resistor. Notice that if you want to calculate the work that can be done by a motor, you'll wind up multiplying power by time.

Finally, a common and useful model/analogy for an electric circuit is a stream of water traveling down a series of waterfalls, with a pump in the collecting pool at the bottom to take the water back up to the top again. The battery (voltage source) is like the pump, and the voltage of the battery is the height it lifts the water. The current is the water, and each resistor is a waterfall. Resistors in series share the same current, because however much water drops down one waterfall must drop down the next one in the line (it has nowhere else to go); the heights of these waterfalls can of course be different, which is why the voltage drops for series resistors may be different. Parallel resistors are parallel waterfalls: They provide different paths for the water to drop from one point in the stream to a lower point. Because such waterfalls connect the same higher point to the same lower point, their heights must be the same; this is why parallel resistors always share the same voltage drop. One waterfall in parallel might be very narrow and only allow a small amount of water to flow down, while another waterfall in the same parallel (side-by-side) combination might be wide and thus allow more water to flow down; this is why resistors in parallel may have different currents. However, the total amount of water entering the top of the parallel waterfall combination must go down all the waterfalls in that combination (again, the water has nowhere else to go); this illustrates why the amount of current entering the parallel combination is equal to the total amount of current that passes through all the resistors in the combination. Finally, the total height of the waterfalls must be the same as the height through which the pump lifts the water from the collecting pool at the bottom; this illustrates why the total voltage drop across the resistors matches the voltage of the battery.

circuit	stream of water flowing down waterfalls with pump at the bottom
current	the flow rate of the water
resistor	waterfall
series	one waterfall after another
parallel	side-by-side waterfalls
voltage	for resistor: height of waterfall (distance water falls)
	for battery: total height the pump lifts the water to start a new cycle
resistance	relative width of channel in the water circuit (narrower width = higher resistance; wider = lower resistance)

Here's a diagram of the water stream and waterfalls that would be analogous to the circuit we analyzed above.

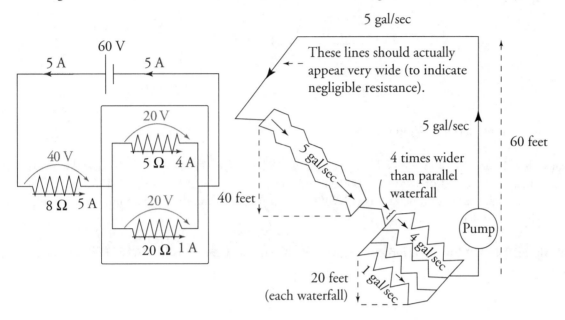

Example 10-8: Verify that the formulas $P = IV$ and $P = I^2R$ are dimensionally correct by showing that the product of current and voltage (IV) and the product of current squared and resistance (I^2R), both have the same units of power.

Solution: First, because $[I] = C/s$ and $[V] = J/C$, we have

$$[IV] = [I][V] = \frac{C}{s} \cdot \frac{J}{C} = \frac{J}{s} = W = \text{watt} = [P]$$

Next, because $[I] = C/s$ and $[R] = \Omega = V/A$, we have

$$[I^2R] = [I]^2[R] = \left(\frac{C}{s}\right)^2 \cdot \frac{V}{A} = \frac{C^2}{s^2} \cdot \frac{\frac{J}{C}}{\frac{C}{s}} = \frac{C^2}{s^2} \cdot \frac{J \cdot s}{C^2} = \frac{J}{s} = W = \text{watt} = [P]$$

Example 10-9: A portion of a circuit is shown below:

$$10\,\Omega \quad \overset{1A}{} \quad 40\,\Omega \quad 20\,\Omega$$

If the current through the 10-ohm resistor is 1 A, what is the current through the 20-ohm resistor?

A. 0.25 A
B. 0.5 A
C. 1 A
D. 2 A

Solution: Because these resistors are in series, they all share the same current. If the current in the first resistor is 1 A, then the current through each of the other resistors is also 1 A. The answer is C.

Example 10-10: A portion of a circuit is shown below:

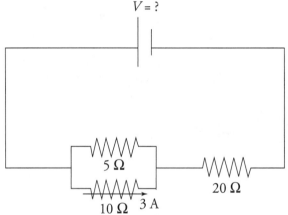

If the current through the 12-ohm resistor is 1 A, what is the value of the current I?

Solution: The voltage drop across the top resistor is $V = IR = (1 \text{ A})(12 \text{ }\Omega) = 12$ V. Because the resistors are in parallel, the voltage drop across the bottom resistor must also be 12 V. Using $I = V/R$, we find that the current through the bottom resistor is $(12 \text{ V})/(4 \text{ }\Omega) = 3$ A. Therefore, the total amount of current passing through the parallel combination is 1 A + 3 A = 4 A.

Example 10-11: With the information given in the circuit diagram below, what is the voltage of the battery?

A. 150 V
B. 210 V
C. 240 V
D. 300 V

Solution: The voltage drop across the bottom resistor in the parallel combination is $V = IR = (3 \text{ A})(10 \text{ }\Omega)$ = 30 V. Because the top and bottom resistors in this combination are in parallel, the voltage drop across the top resistor must also be 30 V. Using $I = V/R$, we find that the current through the top resistor is $(30 \text{ V})/(5 \text{ }\Omega) = 6$ A. Therefore, the total amount of current passing through the parallel combination is 6 A + 3 A = 9 A. Since this much current flows through the 20-ohm resistor, the voltage drop across the 20-ohm resistor is $V = IR = (9 \text{ A})(20 \text{ }\Omega) = 180$ V. Because the total voltage drop across the resistors must match the voltage of the battery, we have $V = 30$ V + 180 V = 210 V, so the answer is B. (Remember: We don't add the 30 V voltage drop twice here; choice C is a trap.)

Example 10-12: A portion of a circuit is shown below:

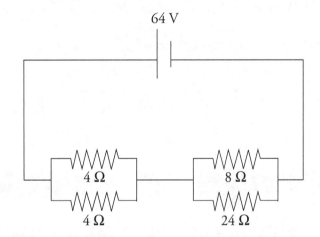

If the current entering the parallel combination is 12 A, how much current flows through the 120-ohm resistor?

Solution: Because the 60-ohm bottom resistor has half the resistance of the 120-ohm top resistor, twice as much current will flow through the bottom resistor as through the top one. So, if we let X stand for the current in the top resistor, then the current in the bottom resistor is $2X$. Because 12 A enters the parallel combination, we must have $X + 2X = 12$ A, so $X = 4$ A. Therefore, the current in the top resistor is 4 A (and the current in the bottom resistor is 8 A). Notice that the voltage drop across the top resistor is $V = IR = (4\text{ A})(120\text{ }\Omega) = 480$ V, and the voltage drop across the bottom resistor is $V = IR = (8\text{ A})(60\text{ }\Omega) = 480$ V. The fact that these voltages match (as they must for parallel resistors) verifies that our answer is correct.

Example 10-13: How much energy is dissipated in 10 seconds by the 24-ohm resistor in the following circuit?

A. 480 J
B. 640 J
C. 720 J
D. 960 J

Solution: The pair of parallel 4-ohm resistors is equivalent to a single 2-ohm resistor [because $(4 \times 4)/(4 + 4) = 2$], and the parallel 8-ohm and 24-ohm resistors are equivalent to a single 6-ohm resistor [because $(8 \times 24)/(8 + 24) = 192/32 = 6$]. These equivalent resistors are in series, so the overall equivalent resistance for the circuit is $2\text{ }\Omega + 6\text{ }\Omega = 8\text{ }\Omega$. This means the current in the circuit is $I = V/R_{eq} = 64/8 = 8$ A. When these 8 amps enter the second parallel combination (the one with the 8-ohm and 24-ohm resistors), it must split up in such a way that the current through the 8-ohm resistor is 3 times the current through the 24-ohm resistor. (Because the 8-ohm resistor has 1/3 the resistance of the 24-ohm resistor, it will get 3 times the current.) So, if we let X stand for the current in the 24-ohm resistor, then the current through the 8-ohm resistor is $3X$; this gives $X + 3X = 8$ A, so $X = 2$ A. Thus, the current in the 24-ohm resistor is 2 A. [The current in the 8-ohm resistor is $3X = 6$ A. The voltage drop across the 8-ohm resistor is $(6 \text{ A})(8 \text{ } \Omega) = 48$ V, and the voltage drop across the 24-ohm resistor is $(2 \text{ A})(24 \text{ } \Omega) = 48$ V; the fact that these match verifies that our calculation is correct.] Since the current in the 24-ohm resistor is 2 A, the power dissipated by this resistor is $P = I^2R = (2^2)(24) = 96$ W. Therefore, the energy dissipated by this resistor in 10 seconds is $(96 \text{ W})(10 \text{ s}) = 960$ J, and the answer is D.

Example 10-14: What is the current in the 100-ohm resistor shown below?

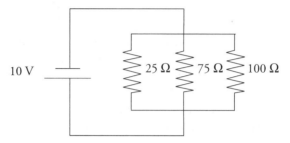

Solution: For this question, we don't need to begin by finding the single equivalent resistance of the given parallel combination, because we already know the voltage across the 100-ohm resistor. The parallel combination is attached directly to the terminals of the battery, so the voltage across each of the resistors must be 10 V. Because we know both V and R, we can find I in one step: $I = V/R = (10 \text{ V})/(100 \text{ } \Omega) = 0.1$ A.

Example 10-15: What is the current in the circuit below?

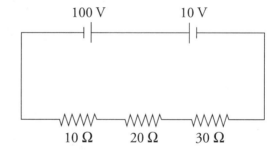

Solution: This circuit contains two batteries. The 100-volt battery wants to send current clockwise. (Remember: We consider current as the directed motion of positive charge, and positive charge carriers would move away from the positive terminal, around the circuit to the negative terminal.) However, the 10-volt battery would want to send current the opposite way: counterclockwise. Since the 100-volt battery has the higher voltage (or, equivalently, the greater emf), it's the "boss" battery. Therefore, current will flow clockwise, but the effective emf will be reduced to $100 - 10 = 90$ V, because the 10-volt battery is opposing the 100-volt boss battery. The equivalent resistance is $10 + 20 + 30 = 60 \text{ } \Omega$ (the resistors are in series), so the current in the circuit will be $I = V/R_{eq} = (90 \text{ V})/(60 \text{ } \Omega) = 1.5$ A. (Note: The 10-volt battery is being charged by the 100-volt boss battery.)

Example 10-16: A toaster oven is rated at 720 W. If it draws 6 A of current, what is its resistance?

Solution: Here, we're given P and I, and asked for R. Since $P = I^2R$, we find that

$$R = \frac{P}{I^2} = \frac{720\ \text{W}}{(6\ \text{A})^2} = 20\ \Omega$$

Example 10-17: Current passes through an insulated resistor of resistance R, mass m, and specific heat c. The voltage across this resistor is V. If the resistor absorbs all the heat it generates, find an expression for the increase in temperature of the resistor after a time t. (All values are expressed in SI units.)

Solution: The amount of heat energy generated (and absorbed) by the resistor is $Q = Pt$, where $P = IV = (V/R)V = V^2/R$. (Here, Q stands for heat not charge.) Now, using the fundamental equation $Q = mc\Delta T$ (from general chemistry), we have

$$\Delta T = \frac{Q}{mc} = \frac{Pt}{mc} = \frac{\frac{V^2}{R}t}{mc} = \frac{V^2 t}{Rmc}$$

All real batteries have **internal resistance**, which we denote by r. Let ε denote the emf of the battery; this is its "ideal" voltage (i.e., the voltage between its terminals when there's no current). Once a current is established, the internal resistance causes the voltage between the terminals to be different from ε. If the battery is supplying current I to the circuit, then the **terminal voltage**, V, is less than ε and given by $V = \varepsilon - Ir$. (On the other hand, if the circuit is *supplying* current to the battery [charging it up] then the terminal voltage is greater than ε and given by the equation $V = \varepsilon + Ir$.) The internal resistance is actually *between* the terminals in a real battery, but in circuit diagrams, the internal resistance is drawn next to the battery, like this:

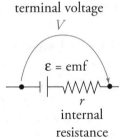

terminal voltage
V

$\varepsilon = $ emf

r
internal
resistance

However, unless you are told otherwise, you may assume that all batteries are ideal and have no internal resistance.

Example 10-18: The battery shown in the circuit below has an emf of 100 V and an internal resistance of 5 Ω. What is its terminal voltage in this circuit? (*Note:* It's not uncommon to see a dashed box drawn around the battery and its internal resistance; this emphasizes that *r* is actually inside the battery.)

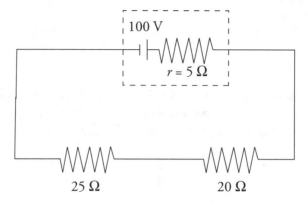

A. 80 V
B. 90 V
C. 100 V
D. 110 V

Solution: The three resistors in this circuit are in series, so the equivalent resistance for the circuit is 5 + 25 + 20 = 50 Ω. Because the emf is 100 V, the current in the circuit is

$$I = \varepsilon \,/\, R = (100 \text{ V})(50 \,\Omega) = 2 \text{ A}$$

The terminal voltage is therefore

$$V = \varepsilon - Ir = (100 \text{ V}) - (2 \text{ A})(5 \,\Omega) = 90 \text{ V}$$

The answer is B. (*Note:* You could eliminate choices C and D immediately; the terminal voltage must be *less* than the emf because the battery is supplying current to the circuit.)

Example 10-19: The diagram below shows a point X held at a potential of $\phi = 60$ V connected by a combination of resistors to a point (denoted by G) that is **grounded**. *The ground is considered to be at potential zero.* What is the current through the 100-ohm resistor?

60 V

X

60 Ω

30 Ω

100 Ω

G
ground

Solution: The parallel resistors are equivalent to a single 20 Ω resistor, which is then in series with the 100 Ω resistor, giving an overall equivalent resistance of 20 + 100 = 120 Ω. Since the potential difference between points X and G is $V = \phi_X - \phi_G = 60 - 0 = 60$ V, the current in the circuit (and through the 100-ohm resistor) is

$$I = V / R = (60 \text{ V})/(120 \,\Omega) = 0.5 \text{ A}$$

Example 10-20: The diagram below shows a battery with an emf of 100 V connected to a circuit equipped with a switch, S.

a)   What is the current in the circuit when the switch is open?

b)   What is the current in the circuit when the switch is closed?

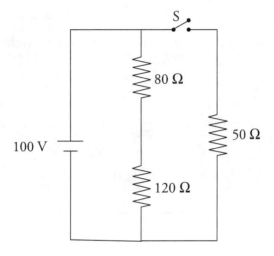

Solution:

a)   With the switch open (as pictured above) the 50 Ω resistor is effectively taken out of the circuit; no current will flow in that branch. Current will flow only in the part of the circuit shown below:

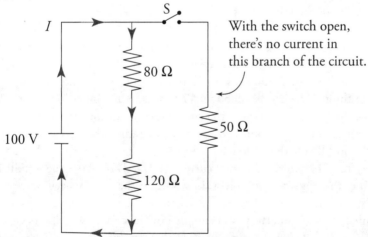

The two resistors that *are* in the circuit when the switch is open are in series, so the total equivalent resistance is 80 + 120 = 200 Ω; thus, the current is

$$I = V / R = (100 \text{ V})/(200 \text{ Ω}) = 0.5 \text{ A}$$

b)   With the switch closed, all the resistors are part of the circuit, and there will be current in all the branches. Let's find the equivalent resistance. The 80 Ω and 120 Ω resistors are in series, so they're equivalent to a single 80 + 120 = 200 Ω resistor, which is then in parallel with the 50 Ω resistor. This gives an overall equivalent resistance of 40 Ω because $(200 \times 50)/(200 + 50)$ is equal to 40. Therefore, the current supplied to the circuit in this case is $I = V/R_{eq}$ = (100 V)/(40 Ω) = 2.5 A.

Example 10-21: Three identical light bulbs are connected to a battery, as shown:

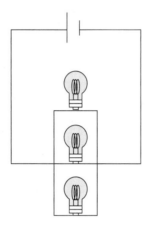

What will happen if the middle bulb burns out?

  A. The other two bulbs will go out.
  B. The light intensity of the other two bulbs will decrease, but they won't go out.
  C. The light intensity of the other two bulbs will increase.
  D. The light intensity of the other two bulbs will remain the same.

Solution: Let V be the voltage of the battery, and let R be the resistance of each light bulb. The current through each light bulb (that is, through each resistor) is $I = V/R$. If the middle bulb burns out, then the middle branch of the parallel combination is severed; but current can still flow through the top and bottom bulbs, and the current through each will still be $I = V/R$. Because the intensity of the light is directly related to the power each one dissipates, the fact that the current doesn't change means that $P = I^2R$ won't change, so the light intensity of the other two bulbs will remain the same. The answer is D. [What *will* change if the middle bulb burns out? Before the middle bulb burns out, the current through each of the three bulbs is $I = V/R$, so the battery must be providing a total current of $3I = 3V/R$. After the middle bulb burns out, the current through each of the other two bulbs is still $I = V/R$, so the battery need only provide a total current of $2I = 2V/R$. That is, the total current through the circuit will decrease (since, after all, there are only two bulbs to light, not three). In addition, the power supplied by the battery will also decrease, from $P = (3I)(V)$ = $3V^2/R$ to $P = (2I)(V) = 2V^2/R$, and the battery will last longer. Finally, notice that if the three bulbs were wired in *series* rather than in parallel, then if any one of the bulbs burned out, they'd all go out because the circuit would be broken.]

Measuring Circuit Values

To verify that a circuit is operating properly, or to troubleshoot one that is malfunctioning, we need to be able to measure the voltage and current in different parts of the circuit. **Voltmeters** are used to measure the potential difference between two points in a circuit, and **ammeters** are used to measure the current through a particular point in the circuit. At the core of each of these devices is a **galvanometer**.

A galvanometer on its own is an apparatus that sensitively measures current using the interaction between currents and magnetic fields (discussion of the particulars of this interaction is left to the final section of this chapter). Current enters the galvanometer and travels through a coil that is wound around the base of a needle. The coil is situated in an external magnetic field in such a way that whenever current runs through the coil, magnetic forces deflect the galvanometer needle. The degree of deflection indicates the amount of current running through the device.

To construct an ammeter, we need to have a small, known fraction of the current we are trying to measure running through the galvanometer (because the galvanometer is very sensitive, a large current will over-load it). For instance, let's take a look at the circuit we discussed earlier in this section. Say that we want to measure the current flowing through each of the resistors. To do so, all we need to do is connect the ammeter in series with the resistor of interest.

To measure the current through the 8 Ω resistor:

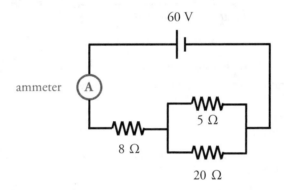

To measure the current through the 5 Ω resistor:

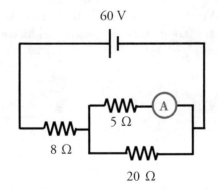

When we connect the ammeter to the circuit, we are adding an additional resistance to the circuit, known as the *internal resistance, r,* of the meter. In reality, this internal resistance is roughly equal to a small *shunt resistance, R_s,* connected in parallel with the ideal galvanometer (G) and its own much larger series resistance, R_g, used to ensure that only a small current actually passes through the galvanometer (the internal resistance of the galvanometer itself is approximated to be zero, a sound assumption given the large value of the R_g).

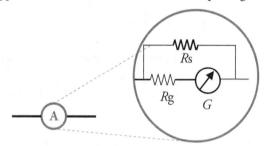

Since we don't want the ammeter to interfere with the circuit in the process of measuring it, we want our ammeter to have as low of an internal resistance as possible so that there is as little voltage dropped over this resistor as possible. The way to achieve this is for the shunt resistance to be very small, because the shunt resistance is very close to the total internal resistance of the ammeter:

$$r = \frac{R_s R_g}{R_s + R_g} = R_s \times \frac{R_g}{R_s + R_g} \xrightarrow{R_g \gg R_s} R_s \times 1 = R_s$$

Another way to think about this is that we want the equivalent resistance of the combination of the ammeter's internal resistance and the resistor of interest to be as close to the original resistance of the resistor as possible.

Example 10-22: A typical ammeter might have an internal resistance of $r = 0.1$ mΩ. If we are measuring the current through the 5 Ω resistor in the circuit above, what would be the equivalent resistance of the ammeter and resistor connected in series?

Solution: Just add the resistances: $R_{eq} = 5\ \Omega + 1 \times 10^{-4}\ \Omega \approx 5\ \Omega$.

Although a galvanometer is intrinsically a current-measuring device, it can also be used to measure voltage, since we know that current and voltage are proportional. To do this, we'll want to connect the voltmeter across the resistor of interest, so that it can measure the potential difference from one side of the resistor to the other.

To measure the voltage across the 8 Ω resistor:

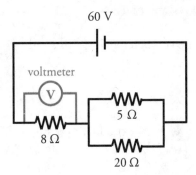

To measure the voltage across the 5 Ω resistor:

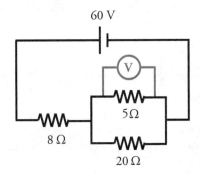

Just like an ammeter, a voltmeter also has an internal resistance. In this case, however, the internal resistance is connected in parallel to resistor of interest. Again, we want to minimize any impact to the original circuit, so for the voltmeter we'll want the internal resistance to be as large as possible to minimize any current going through the voltmeter. A typical voltmeter might have an internal resistance of 10 MΩ. This is achieved by using a large resistance R_g in series with the galvanometer, as shown below. If we again assume the resistance of G is negligible, then $r = R_g$.

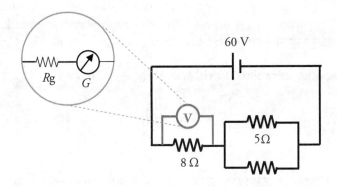

Example 10-23: When connecting a voltmeter to a circuit, we want the equivalent resistance of the combination to be as close to the original resistance as possible. In the circuit above, if $r = R_g = 10 \text{ M}\Omega$ when measuring the voltage across the 8 Ω resistor, find

a) the equivalent resistance of the voltmeter and resistor, and
b) the measured voltage.

Solution:

a) The equivalent resistance is given by the product over sum rule for resistors in parallel:
$R_{eq} = (10 \times 10^6 \ \Omega)(8 \ \Omega)/(10 \times 10^6 \ \Omega + 8 \ \Omega) \approx (10 \times 10^6 \ \Omega)(8 \ \Omega)/(10 \times 10^6 \ \Omega) = 8 \ \Omega$.

b) This is the same circuit we solved previously in the beginning of the subsection on DC circuits, when we found that the voltage across the 8 Ω resistor was 40V. (This would be a good time to confirm you remember how to solve for currents and resistances across circuit elements by solving for this result again). Because we have just confirmed that the voltmeter does not appreciably affect the resistance across this circuit element, the measured value will be the same as the calculated value.

10.2 CAPACITORS

A pair of conductors that can hold equal but opposite charges is known as a **capacitor**. The conductors can be of any shape, but the most common capacitor consists of a pair of parallel metal plates; it's known as a **parallel-plate capacitor**:

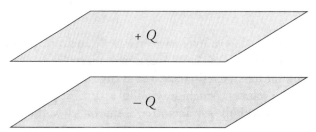

Notice that one plate carries a positive charge and the other plate carries an equal amount of negative charge. Therefore, the *net* charge on a capacitor is zero. However, whenever we talk about the "charge on a capacitor," we always mean the magnitude of charge on either plate, which is $+Q$.

In circuit diagrams, a capacitor is denoted by either of these two symbols:

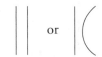

The first question we'll answer is, "How do we create a charged capacitor?" Take an uncharged parallel-plate capacitor, and hook the plates to the terminals of a battery. Conduction electrons in the connecting wires will be repelled from the negative terminal and flow to one plate, while electrons from the other plate will be attracted toward the positive terminal of the battery. The current rises quickly at first, but it gradually dies out as the plates acquire charge. The plate that's connected to the positive terminal becomes positively charged, and the plate that's connected to the negative terminal becomes negatively charged. Since the positive plate has a higher potential than the negative plate, the potential difference between the plates opposes the potential difference of the battery. Charge will stop flowing when the potential difference between the plates matches the voltage of the battery because at that point the circuit will look like one that has two opposing voltage sources.

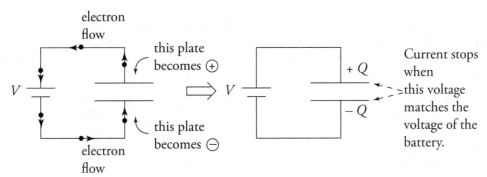

If V is the potential difference between the plates of a charged capacitor, and Q is the charge on the capacitor, then Q and V are proportional. The proportionality constant, C, is called the **capacitance**:

Charge on a Capacitor

$$Q = CV$$

From this equation we can see that the unit of capacitance is coulomb per volt (C/V), which has its own name: the **farad**, abbreviated F. Therefore, 1 C/V = 1 F. Because a coulomb is a lot of charge, we'd expect a farad to be a lot of capacitance. Most real-life capacitors have capacitances that are on the order of a few microfarads.

The capacitance is determined only by the sizes of the plates and how far apart they are (and, as we'll see a little later, whether there's anything between the plates). For a parallel-plate capacitor with empty space between the plates, C is given by the following equation:

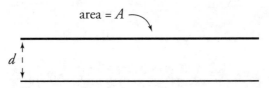

Capacitance of a Parallel Plate Capacitor

$$C = \varepsilon_0 \frac{A}{d}$$

where A is the area of each plate, d is their separation, and ε_0 is a fundamental constant of nature. (The constant ε_0 is known as the **permittivity of free space**; it's equal to $1/(4\pi k_0)$, where k_0 is Coulomb's constant, so the approximate numerical value of ε_0 is 8.85×10^{-12} F/m.)

The capacitance C depends only on A and d. Although $Q = CV$, the capacitance C does not depend on either Q or V; it only tells us how Q and V will be related. If you were given an uncharged capacitor, you could determine C without charging it up, by using the formula $C = \varepsilon_0 A/d$.

Intuitively, capacitance measures the plates' "capacity" for holding charge at a certain voltage. Let's say we had two capacitors with different capacitances, and we wanted to store as much charge as we could while keeping V low. We'd choose the capacitor with the greater capacitance because it would be able to hold more charge per volt.

Example 10-24: A capacitor has a capacitance of 2 nF. How much charge can it hold at a voltage of 150 V?

Solution: We're given C and V, and asked for Q. Using the equation $Q = CV$, we find that

$$Q = CV = (2 \times 10^{-9} \text{ F})(150 \text{ V}) = 3 \times 10^{-7} \text{ C}$$

(This means that the positive plate will have a charge of $+Q = 3 \times 10^{-7}$ C, and the negative plate will have a charge of $-Q = -3 \times 10^{-7}$ C.)

Example 10-25: A charged capacitor has charge Q, and the voltage between the plates is V. What will happen to C if Q is doubled?

Solution: Nothing. For a given capacitor, C is a constant. Because $Q = CV$, we see that Q is proportional to V. Doubling Q will not affect C; what *will* happen is that V will double.

Example 10-26: What will happen to the capacitance of a parallel-plate capacitor if the plates were moved closer together, halving the distance between them?

Solution: From the equation $C = \varepsilon_0 A/d$, we see that C is inversely proportional to d. Thus, if d is decreased by a factor of 2, then C will increase by a factor of 2.

Example 10-27: How big would the plates of a parallel-plate capacitor need to be in order to make the capacitance equal to 1 F, if $d = 8.85$ mm?

Solution: We'll start with the equation $C = \varepsilon_0 A/d$ and solve for A:

$$A = \frac{Cd}{\varepsilon_0} = \frac{(1 \text{ F})(8.85 \times 10^{-3} \text{ m})}{8.85 \times 10^{-12} \frac{\text{F}}{\text{m}}} = 10^9 \text{ m}^2$$

(If the plates were squares, they'd have to be nearly 20 miles on each side to make $A = 10^9$ square meters! Now you can see that 1 F is a *lot* of capacitance.)

Now that we know the basic equation for capacitance ($Q = CV$) and how to calculate it ($C = \varepsilon_0 A/d$), the next question is, "What's a capacitor used for?" For MCAT purposes, a parallel-plate capacitor has two main uses:

1. To create a uniform electric field, and
2. To store electrical potential energy.

Let's go over each one.

When we studied electric fields in the preceding chapter, we noticed that the electric field created by one or more point source charges varied, depending on the location. For example, as we move farther from the source charges, the field gets weaker. Even if we stay at the same distance from, say, a single source charge, the direction of the field changes as we move around. Therefore, we could never obtain an electric field that was constant in both magnitude and direction throughout some region of space from point-source charges. However, the electric field that's created between the plates of a charged parallel-plate capacitor *is* constant in both magnitude and direction throughout the region between the plates; in other words, a charged parallel-plate capacitor can create a *uniform* electric field. The electric field, **E**, always points from the positive plate toward the negative plate, and it's the same magnitude at every point between the plates, whether we choose a point closer to the positive plate, closer to the negative plate, or right in the middle between them.

Because **E** is so straightforward (it's the same everywhere between the plates), the equation for calculating it is equally straightforward. The strength of **E** depends on the voltage between the plates, *V*, and their separation distance, *d*. We call the equation "Ed's formula":

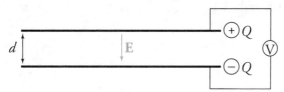

Ed's Formula

$$V = Ed$$

The equation $F = qE$ showed us that the units of E are N/C (because $E = F/q$). Ed's formula now tells us that the units of E are V/m (because $E = V/d$). You'll see both newtons-per-coulomb and volts-per-meter used as units for the electric field; it turns out that these units are exactly the same.

Example 10-28: The charge on a parallel-plate capacitor is 4×10^{-6} C. If the distance between the plates is 2 mm and the capacitance is 1 µF, what's the strength of the electric field between the plates?

Solution: Since $Q = CV$, we have $V = Q/C = (4 \times 10^{-6} \text{ C})/(10^{-6} \text{ F}) = 4$ V. Now, using the equation $V = Ed$, we find that

$$E = \frac{V}{d} = \frac{4 \text{ V}}{2 \times 10^{-3} \text{ m}} = 2000 \tfrac{\text{V}}{\text{m}}$$

Example 10-29: The plates of a parallel plate capacitor are separated by a distance of 2 mm. The device's capacitance is 1 μF. How much charge needs to be transferred from one plate to the other in order to create a uniform electric field whose strength is 10^4 V/m?

Solution: Because $Q = CV$ and $V = Ed$, we find that

$$Q = CEd = (1 \times 10^{-6} \text{ F})(10^4 \tfrac{\text{V}}{\text{m}})(2 \times 10^{-3} \text{ m}) = 2 \times 10^{-5} \text{ C}$$

Example 10-30: A proton (whose mass is m) is placed on top of the positively charged plate of a parallel-plate capacitor, as shown below.

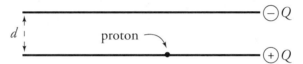

The charge on the capacitor is Q, and the capacitance is C. If the electric field in the region between the plates has magnitude E, which of the following expressions gives the time required for the proton to move up to the other plate?

A. $d\sqrt{\dfrac{eQ}{mC}}$

B. $d\sqrt{\dfrac{m}{eQC}}$

C. $d\sqrt{\dfrac{2eQ}{mC}}$

D. $d\sqrt{\dfrac{2mC}{eQ}}$

Solution: Once we find the acceleration of the proton, we can use Big Five #3, with $v_0 = 0$ (namely, $y = \tfrac{1}{2}at^2$) to find the time it will take for the proton to move the distance $y = d$. The acceleration of the proton is F/m, where $F = qE = eE$ is the force the proton feels; this gives $a = eE/m$. (We're ignoring the gravitational force on the proton because it is so much weaker than the electric force.) Now, since $E = V/d$ and $V = Q/C$, the expression for a becomes $a = eQ/mdC$. Substituting eQ/mdC for a, and d for y, Big Five #3 gives us

$$y = \frac{1}{2}at^2 \rightarrow d = \frac{1}{2} \cdot \frac{eQ}{mdC}t^2 \rightarrow t = d\sqrt{\frac{2mC}{eQ}}$$

The answer is D. Another way we could have attacked this question is to look at the answer choices and see if they make sense. If choice A were correct, then it would imply that a greater charge Q would *increase* the time required for the proton to move to the top plate. This doesn't make sense because a greater Q would create a greater force on the proton, giving it a greater acceleration, thus making it move faster, and causing t to decrease. We can also see that choice C can't be correct, for the same reason. Choice B could be eliminated because the units don't work out to be seconds, as shown below; therefore, the answer *had* to be D.

$$[d]\sqrt{\frac{[m]}{[e][Q][C]}} = m\sqrt{\frac{\text{kg}}{\text{C}\cdot\text{C}\cdot\frac{\text{C}}{\text{V}}}} = m\sqrt{\frac{\text{kg}}{\text{C}\cdot\text{C}\cdot\frac{\text{C}}{\text{J/C}}}} = \frac{\text{m}}{\text{C}^2}\sqrt{\text{kg}\cdot\text{J}} = \frac{\text{m}}{\text{C}^2}\sqrt{\text{kg}\cdot\frac{\text{kg}\cdot\text{m}^2}{\text{s}^2}} = \frac{\text{kg}\cdot\text{m}^2}{\text{C}^2\cdot\text{s}} \neq \text{s}$$

Example 10-31: An electron is projected horizontally into the space between the plates of a parallel-plate capacitor, as shown below, where the electric field has a magnitude of 56 V/m. The initial velocity of the electron is horizontal and has a magnitude of $v_0 = 5 \times 10^6$ m/s.

a) What is the force on the electron while it's in the region between the plates? (Neglect gravity.) What's the acceleration of the electron in this region? (Note: electron mass $\approx 9 \times 10^{-31}$ kg.)

b) How long would it take the electron to cover the horizontal distance L through the capacitor?

c) Describe the electron's trajectory through this region.

Solution:

a) Because the electric field $\mathbf{E}$ is constant between the plates, the force on the electron is also constant and given by $\mathbf{F} = q\mathbf{E} = -e\mathbf{E}$; this force points upward, in the direction opposite to the electric field (because q is negative), toward the positively charged top plate. Substituting in the numerical values gives $F = eE = (1.6 \times 10^{-19}$ C$) \times (56$ N/C$) = 9 \times 10^{-18}$ N. If the mass of the electron is m, then its acceleration, $\mathbf{a}$, is $\mathbf{F}/m$. Like $\mathbf{F}$, the acceleration is uniform and vertical, pointing upward, toward the top plate. The magnitude of $\mathbf{a}$ is $a = F/m = (9 \times 10^{-18}$ N$)/(9 \times 10^{-31}$ kg$) = 10^{13}$ m/s^2.

b) Because the acceleration of the electron is vertical, the electron's horizontal velocity will not change. Because v_{0x} is always equal to v_{0x}, the time required to traverse the 10 cm horizontal distance through the region between the plates is

$$x = v_x t \rightarrow t = \frac{x}{v_x} = \frac{x}{v_{0x}} = \frac{L}{v_{0x}} = \frac{10 \times 10^{-2} \text{ m}}{5 \times 10^6 \text{ m/s}} = 2 \times 10^{-8} \text{ s}$$

c) Because the acceleration is constant, we can use The Big Five to describe the motion of the electron. In fact, the motion of the electron between the plates is just like the motion of a projectile whose initial velocity is horizontal. The only difference is that while a projectile would curve downward in a half-parabola, the electron in the figure above will curve upward. Adapting Big Five #3 to vertical motion (in the y direction), we have $y = v_{0y}t + \frac{1}{2}a_y t^2$. Because

$v_{0y} = 0$, this equation simplifies to $y = \frac{1}{2}a_y t^2$. Now, in the time t that the electron moves through the region between the plates (which we found in part *b*) its vertical displacement will be $y = \frac{1}{2}\left(10^{13}\,\text{m/s}^2\right)\left(2 \times 10^{-8}\,\text{s}\right)^2 = 2 \times 10^{-3}\,\text{m} = 2\,\text{mm}$. Therefore, the electron will just hit the right edge of the top plate.

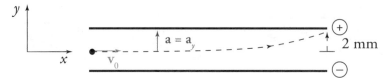

Now let's look at the second important use of a capacitor: as a storage device for electrical potential energy. We can think of the process of charging a capacitor as a transferal of electrons from one plate to the other. The plate that the electrons are taken from is left positively charged, and the plate the electrons are transferred to becomes negatively charged. Also, because we're simply transferring charge from one plate to the other, we are always assured at each moment that the plates carry equal but opposite charges.

During this charging process, an outside agent (the voltage source) must do work against the electric field that's created between the plates of the capacitor. Once we begin the process of transferring electrons from one plate to the other, it becomes increasingly difficult to transfer more. After all, it takes effort to remove more electrons from the plate that is left positively charged, *and* it takes effort to place them on the plate that is negatively charged. The fact that we have to "fight" against the system means we're storing potential energy.

This transferal is fighting against the electric field.

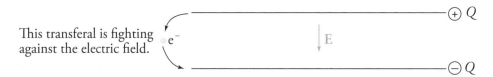

To increase the charge on the capacitor, work is required to remove extra electrons from the positive plate and move them to the negative plate. This work against the electric field is stored as electrical potential energy.

Because it requires more work to transfer more charge, we'd expect that the amount of potential energy stored should depend on Q, the final charge on the capacitor; that is, as Q increases, so should the *PE*. We'd also expect that the amount of stored *PE* should depend on the voltage between the plates. After all, we defined potential difference, V, by the equation $\Delta PE = qV$, where q was the charge that moved between the points whose potential difference was V. Hence, the higher voltage V leads to an increase in stored potential energy. If the final charge on the capacitor is Q and the final resulting voltage is V, then *PE* is proportional to both Q and V. Here's how we can intuitively find the formula for *PE* in this case: We transferred a total amount of charge equal to Q, fighting against the voltage that prevailed at each stage. If the final voltage is V, then the average voltage during the charging process is $\frac{1}{2}V$. Since ΔPE is equal to charge times voltage, we get $\Delta PE = Q \cdot \left(\dfrac{1}{2} V \right) = \dfrac{1}{2} QV$. At the beginning of the charging process, when there was no charge on the capacitor, we had $PE_i = 0$, so $\Delta PE = PE_f - PE_i = PE_f - 0 = PE_f$. Therefore, we have $PE_f = \dfrac{1}{2} QV$:

> **Electrical PE Stored in a Capacitor**
>
> $$PE = \tfrac{1}{2} QV$$

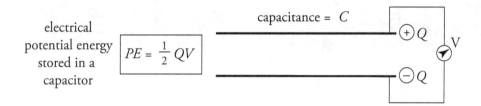

electrical potential energy stored in a capacitor

$$PE = \frac{1}{2} QV$$

capacitance = C

$\oplus Q$

V

$\ominus Q$

Using the fundamental equation $Q = CV$, we can rewrite this equation in terms of C and V, or in terms of Q and C:

$$PE = \frac{1}{2} QV = \frac{1}{2} CV^2 = \frac{Q^2}{2C}$$

If you lift a rock off the ground, you do work against the gravitational field of the earth, and, as a result, you store gravitational potential energy. To recapture this stored energy, you let the rock fall back to the ground, transferring the gravitational potential energy into mechanical kinetic energy. Similarly, if you transfer electrons from one plate of a capacitor to the other, you do work against the electric field of the capacitor, and, as a result, you store electrical potential energy. To recapture this stored electrical energy, you let the electrons go back to their original plate, effectively **discharging** the capacitor. The movement of electrons can be used in a productive manner by providing a path for them and placing some electrical devices along the way. As a result, the electrons that return to the plate end up passing through, say, a light bulb, and the current causes the bulb to light. We've been able to tap into the energy stored in the capacitor to do useful work. When we connect the charged capacitor plates by a wire with some resistor(s) along it, the charge drains off rapidly at first, but the rate at which the charge leaves gradually decreases as time goes on. The same is true of the resulting current; it too starts off high and then gradually drops to zero as the capacitor discharges.

Discharging a Capacitor

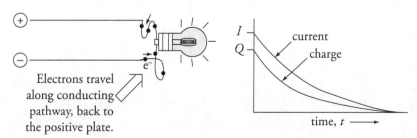

Electrons travel along conducting pathway, back to the positive plate.

I

Q

current

charge

time, t ⟶

Example 10-32: A defibrillator contains a circuit whose primary components are a battery, a capacitor, and a switch. When the heart is undergoing ventricular fibrillation, the normally ordered electrical signals that organize the heart's pumping behavior are out of sync. The strong current delivered by the conducting paddles of the defibrillator can depolarize the entirety of the heart and potentially reset its orderly pumping triggered by the SA node. The defibrillator circuit first charges the capacitor with the battery. During the application and discharging of the circuit, a switch is closed to allow the capacitor to discharge through the paddles and the patient's tissue. Which of the following graphs best illustrates the voltage between the capacitor plates during this latter process?

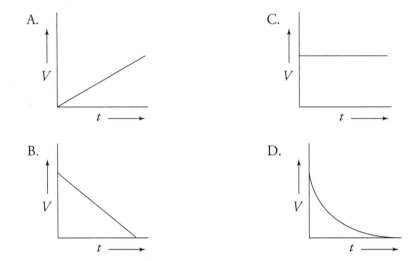

Solution: As the capacitor loses charge, Q decreases. Since $V = Q/C$, we know that V must decrease, too. This eliminates choices A and C. The charge drains off rapidly at first, but the rate at which the charge leaves gradually decreases as time goes on; therefore, the decrease in Q (and therefore in V also) is not linear. Thus, the best graph is the one in choice D. (The defibrillator circuit will also feature an *inductor* or *solenoid*, described later in this chapter. This has the effect of slowing the discharge of the capacitor and prolonging the application of current sufficiently to completely depolarize the heart.)

Dielectrics

If the plates of a capacitor were touching at the start of the charging process, then we'd effectively have a single conductor, not a pair, and no transferal of electrons from one plate to the other could begin; it wouldn't work as a capacitor. And if the plates were ever allowed to touch during the charging process, the capacitor would discharge almost immediately, since the transferred electrons would have a direct route back to the positive plate. All the electrical potential energy that had been stored would be lost in an instant, without any useful work being done by the stored energy. So for a capacitor to be useful, we need to keep the plates from touching.

Let's consider ways to do that. One way would be to mount them on separate insulating handles, like this:

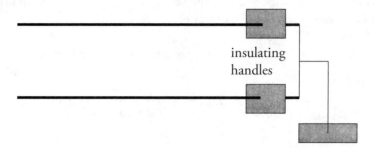

insulating
handles

That could work, but the way it's typically done is to sandwich a slab of insulating material between the plates. Such an insulator is known as a **dielectric**:

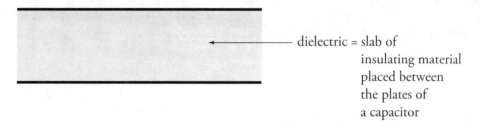

dielectric = slab of
insulating material
placed between
the plates of
a capacitor

Not only does a dielectric keep the plates from touching, but there's also a bonus: *The presence of a dielectric always increases the capacitance.* For the capacitor whose plates are mounted on insulating handles, with vacuum (or, for all practical purposes, air) between the plates, the capacitance is given by the equation we gave earlier: $C = \varepsilon_0 A/d$. However, if the capacitor is fitted with a dielectric, the capacitance is multiplied by a factor of K, where K is known as the **dielectric constant** of the insulating material. For example, wax paper is a dielectric, with a dielectric constant of about 3.5. If a parallel-plate capacitor were fitted with wax paper as a dielectric, the capacitance would be multiplied by 3.5. Other common dielectrics are teflon and certain plastics and ceramics.

Here's the formula for the capacitance of a parallel-plate capacitor with a dielectric:

Capacitance of a Parallel-Plate Capacitor with a Dielectric

$$C_{\substack{\text{with} \\ \text{dielectric}}} = K \cdot C_{\substack{\text{without} \\ \text{dielectric}}} = K\varepsilon_0 \frac{A}{d}$$

The value of K for vacuum is exactly 1, which makes sense since having empty space between the plates means there's *no* dielectric. The MCAT will assume that $K = 1$ for air as well because the actual value of K for air (~1.0005) is so close to 1. A capacitor with just air between its plates is known simply as an *air capacitor*. K is never less than 1, which is the reason dielectrics always increase capacitance.

Example 10-33: The area, A, of each plate of a parallel-plate capacitor satisfies the equation $\varepsilon_0 A = 10^{-10}$ F·m. If the plates are separated by a distance of 2 mm and this space is filled by a sheet of mica with a dielectric constant of 6, what is the capacitance of this capacitor?

Solution: The presence of the mica increases the capacitance by a factor of 6, so:

$$C_{\substack{\text{with}\\ \text{dielectric}}} = K \cdot C_{\substack{\text{without}\\ \text{dielectric}}} = K\varepsilon_0 \frac{A}{d} = 6 \cdot \frac{10^{-10} \text{ F·m}}{2 \times 10^{-3} \text{ m}} = 3 \times 10^{-7} \text{ F}$$

Example 10-34: The inner and outer surfaces of a cell membrane act as plates in a parallel-plate capacitor. Consider a 1 μm² section of an axon: The dielectric constant of the membrane is 8 and the membrane is 6 nm thick. If the voltage across the membrane is 70 mV, what is the approximate magnitude of charge that resides on each side of this 1 μm² section? (*Note:* $\varepsilon_0 = 8.85 \times 10^{-12}$ C²/N·m²)

Solution: The capacitance is $C_{\text{with dielectric}} = K\varepsilon_0 A / d$, with $K = 8$, so

$$Q = CV = K\varepsilon_0 \frac{A}{d} \cdot V = (8)(8.85 \times 10^{-12} \tfrac{\text{C}^2}{\text{N·m}^2}) \cdot \frac{1 \text{ μm}^2 \cdot \left(\frac{1 \text{ m}}{10^6 \text{ μm}}\right)^2}{6 \times 10^{-9} \text{ m}} \cdot (70 \times 10^{-3} \text{ V}) \approx 1 \times 10^{-15} \text{ C}$$

Example 10-35: The capacitance of a certain air capacitor whose plates are separated by a distance of 1 mm is 4 pF. If the plates are moved apart to a distance of 2.2 mm to accommodate a slab of porcelain of thickness 2.2 mm that is then inserted between them, the capacitance becomes 12 pF. What is the dielectric constant of porcelain?

Solution: The capacitance without the porcelain is $C_{\text{without dielectric}} = \varepsilon_0 A / d_1$, and the capacitance with the porcelain is $C_{\text{with dielectric}} = K\varepsilon_0 A / d_2$. The ratio of these values is

$$\frac{C_{\text{with dielectric}}}{C_{\text{without dielectric}}} = \frac{K\varepsilon_0 A / d_2}{\varepsilon_0 A / d_1} = K\frac{d_1}{d_2} = K\frac{1 \text{ mm}}{2.2 \text{ mm}} = \frac{K}{2.2}$$

Now, because the capacitance increased by a factor of 3, we have

$$\frac{K}{2.2} = 3 \rightarrow \quad \therefore K = 6.6$$

The presence of a dielectric can affect other properties of a capacitor besides capacitance. However, the ways a dielectric affects the charge, voltage, and electric field depend on whether the capacitor is connected or disconnected from the battery that charged it.

Let's begin by looking at the case in which a capacitor without a dielectric is charged by a battery and then disconnected from it. What happens if we then insert a dielectric between the plates? First, since the capacitor is disconnected from the battery, the charge that exists on the plates is trapped and cannot change. Therefore, Q remains constant. Because the capacitance C increases, the equation $Q = CV$ tells us that the voltage will decrease; in fact, because Q stays constant and C increases by a factor of K, we see that V will decrease by a factor of K. Next, using the equation $V = Ed$, we see that because V decreases by a factor of K, so does E. Finally, using the equation $PE = \frac{1}{2}QV$, we conclude that since Q stays constant and V decreases by a factor of K, the stored electrical potential energy decreases by a factor of K.

We can look at this a little more closely: First, why does the electric field strength, E, decrease in this case? The dielectric is an insulator, so although the field between the plates won't move any free electrons through the material, it will polarize the molecules. That is, the electric field will create tiny dipole moments in the molecules of the insulator, with the negative (δ^-) ends closer to the positive plate and the positive (δ^+) ends closer to the negative plate. As a result, we'll have a layer of negative charge at the surface of the dielectric that's near the positive plate and a layer of positive charge at the surface of the dielectric that's near the negative plate. These layers of induced charge on the opposite surfaces of the dielectric are the source of a new electric field through the dielectric, $\mathbf{E}_{induced}$, a field that points in the opposite direction from the electric field created by the charged capacitor plates themselves (because electric fields always point from positive and toward negative source charges).

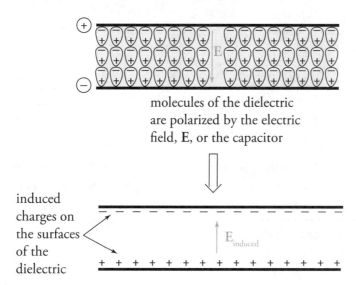

molecules of the dielectric
are polarized by the electric
field, **E**, or the capacitor

induced
charges on
the surfaces
of the
dielectric

$\mathbf{E}_{induced}$

The total electric field between the plates is then the sum of the field created by the plates, **E**, and the field created by the layers of induced charge on the surfaces of the dielectric, $\mathbf{E}_{induced}$. Because $\mathbf{E}_{induced}$ points in the direction *opposite* to **E**, the *net* field strength is reduced to $E - E_{induced}$. This is the physical reason why the electric field magnitude is reduced in this case.

We also found that the potential energy would be reduced if we inserted a dielectric after disconnecting the capacitor from the charging battery. Where did this energy go? Most of it is stored as electrical potential energy inside those induced dipoles in the dielectric. (Unfortunately, that stored energy is hard to recapture in a useful way.) You would notice that as you began to place the dielectric between the plates, the electric field would actually pull it in; thus, some of the stored potential energy turns into kinetic energy of the dielectric as it was pulled into the space between the capacitor plates. Finally, there would be some heat production (the usual MCAT answer to "Where did the energy go?").

Now let's examine the case in which a capacitor without a dielectric is first charged up and then while it's still connected to its voltage source, we insert a dielectric between its plates. First, since the capacitor is still connected to the battery, the voltage between the plates must match the voltage of the battery.

Therefore, V will not change.[3] Because the capacitance C increases, the equation $Q = CV$ tells us that the charge Q must increase; in fact, because V doesn't change and C increases by a factor of K, we see that Q will increase by a factor of K. Next, using the equation $V = Ed$, we see that because V doesn't change, neither will E. Finally, using the equation $PE = \frac{1}{2}QV$, we conclude that since V doesn't change and Q increases by a factor of K, the stored electrical potential energy increases by a factor of K. An important point to notice is that V doesn't change because the battery will transfer additional charge to the capacitor plates. This increase in Q offsets any momentary decrease in the electric field strength when the dielectric is inserted (because the molecules of the dielectric are polarized, as above) and brings the electric field strength back to its original value. Furthermore, as more charge is transferred to the plates, more electrical potential energy is stored.

The following figure summarizes the effects on the properties of a capacitor with the insertion of a dielectric in the two cases:

charge capacitor to voltage V charge capacitor to voltage V

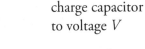

then disconnect battery and insert dielectric   keep battery connected and insert dielectric

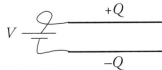

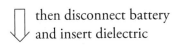

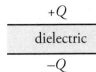

- C increases by factor of K
- Q stays the same
- V decreases by a factor of K
- E decreases by a factor of K

- C increases by factor of K
- Q increases by a factor of K
- V stays the same
- E stays the same

[3] This analysis assumes that the circuit has no resistance, so the newly increased capacitance can be "filled up" instantaneously. In practice, voltage in the capacitor would drop at first but then rise quickly until it was again equal to the battery's voltage.

Example 10-36: An air capacitor is charged and disconnected from the battery. The electric field between the plates is **E**. Now, a dielectric with dielectric constant $K = 4$ is inserted between the plates. What is the electric field created by the layers of induced charges on the surfaces of the dielectric?

    A. $3E/4$ opposite the direction of **E**
    B. $E/4$ opposite the direction of **E**
    C. $E/4$ in the same direction of **E**
    D. $3E/4$ in the same direction of **E**

Solution: The question is asking for $\mathbf{E}_{induced}$. First, $\mathbf{E}_{induced}$ points in the *opposite* direction from **E**, so the answer must be either A or B. To find the magnitude of $\mathbf{E}_{induced}$, we use the fact that $E - E_{induced} = E/K$; since $K = 4$, we see that $E_{induced} = 3E/4$. Thus, the answer is A.

Example 10-37: A parallel-plate capacitor, with air between the plates, is charged to a voltage of $V = 1000$ V by a battery. The values of Q, E, and PE are also measured. The battery is then disconnected from the capacitor and a dielectric with dielectric constant $K = 4$ is inserted between the plates. The values of V, Q, E, and PE are measured again. Which of these values did *not* change?

    A. V
    B. Q
    C. E
    D. PE

Solution: Since the battery was disconnected from the capacitor after charging, the value of Q does not change: there's nowhere for charges to go and no source of new charges. The values of V, E, and PE will all decrease by a factor of K. The answer is B.

Example 10-38: Cell membranes have a dielectric number of about 9. If the internal potential of the cell is about 70 mV lower than the external potential, how much charge could accumulate on a square micrometer of phospholipid layer with a thickness of 8 nanometers ($\varepsilon_0 \approx 9 \times 10^{-12}$ F/m)?

Solution:

$$C = \frac{K\varepsilon_0 A}{d} = \frac{9(9 \times 10^{-12} \text{ F/m})(10^{-6} \text{ m})^2}{8 \times 10^{-9}} \approx 10^{-14} \text{ F}$$

Now the charge this cell membrane capacitor can hold at the given voltage is $Q = CV = (10^{-8}$ F$)$ $(70 \times 10^{-3}$ V$) = 7 \times 10^{-16}$ C. This may not seem like much, but considering that the charge of one sodium or potassium ion is 1.6×10^{-19} C, this amounts to about 4 billion ions. This is NOT what actually happens to a living cell, mind you, because a living cell is not a passive participant in its local environment (and there are chemical considerations in addition to electrical ones).

Dielectric Breakdown

Dielectrics have another purpose besides keeping the plates apart and increasing the capacitance. The illustration earlier for a discharging capacitor showed the plates connected by a conducting wire; the electrons on the negative plate used this pathway to travel back to the positive plate. This type of controlled discharge is necessary if we are to tap into the motion of these electrons to do useful work (like lighting a light bulb). But why don't the extra electrons on the negative plate just jump across the gap to the positive plate, without traveling through a conducting wire pathway? They can, but only under extreme circumstances.

For an air capacitor, the maximum electric field strength is about 3 million volts per meter. If the value of E were to exceed this maximum value, the air would no longer act as an insulator. Electrons would be pulled out of the molecules, ionizing the air, and the electrons on the negative plate would then have a conducting pathway through the air; we'd see a spark as the capacitor discharged very rapidly. When the electric field strength between the plates becomes so strong that the dielectric (which is supposed to act as an insulator) is ionized, providing a route for the electrons on the negative plate to return to the positive plate, we say that the dielectric has suffered **dielectric breakdown**. This is essentially what causes lightning. The bottom region of a thundercloud is negatively charged and the surface of the earth below the cloud is positively charged; these surfaces act as the oppositely charged plates in a huge parallel-plate capacitor. When the voltage V becomes so great that $E = V/d$ exceeds 3 million volts per meter, the air is ionized, and charge is transferred in a spectacular bolt of lightning.

The presence of a dielectric increases this maximum electric field strength. As a result, capacitors with dielectrics can hold more charge (and thus store more potential energy) without the threat of dielectric breakdown. For example, wax paper has a **dielectric strength** that's about 5 times greater than that of air; in other words, the maximum electric field that a piece of wax paper can withstand is about 15 million volts per meter, 5 times what air could withstand. If the maximum E is increased by a factor of 5, the maximum V that the plates can support is increased by a factor of 5 (since V is proportional to E). Because $PE = \frac{1}{2}CV^2$, a capacitor with wax paper as a dielectric not only has a capacitance 3.5 times greater than an air capacitor (because $K = 3.5$ for wax paper), but its maximum V is increased by 5. Therefore, a capacitor with a wax paper dielectric can store $(3.5) \times 5^2 = 87.5$ times more potential energy than the same capacitor with just air between the plates.

Except for enjoying a great lightning display or causing a spark to jump across the gap in your car's spark plugs, dielectric breakdown is something that you typically want to avoid. In electrical devices that contain capacitors, if any of the capacitors suffer dielectric breakdown this generally means that a hole is burned through the dielectric, and the capacitor must then be replaced.

Example 10-39: An air capacitor has a capacitance of 1 μF. If its plates are separated by a distance $d = 1$ mm, what is the maximum amount of charge the capacitor could hold before dielectric breakdown occurs? (Dielectric strength of air = 3 million volts per meter)

Solution: Because $V = Ed$, we can find the maximum voltage that the capacitor can withstand:

$$V_{max} = E_{max}d = \left(3 \times 10^6 \tfrac{v}{m}\right)\left(10^{-3}\,m\right) = 3000\,V.$$ Now, because $Q = CV$, we find that

$$Q_{max} = CV_{max} = (1 \times 10^{-6}\,F)(3000\,V) = 3 \times 10^{-3}\,C$$

Combinations of Capacitors

Like resistors, capacitors can also be placed in series and in parallel within a circuit. In this section, we'll see how to find the equivalent capacitance for each of these cases.

Capacitors in **parallel** all have the same voltage (like *resistors* in parallel), but the equivalent capacitance is the sum of the individual capacitances (like resistors in *series*):

$$\text{equivalent capacitance} \atop \text{for capacitors in parallel} \qquad \boxed{C_{eq} = C_1 + C_2 + C_3 + \ldots}$$

For example, in the figure below, the equivalent capacitance, C_{eq}, is 2 μF + 3 μF + 4 μF = 9 μF:

capacitors in parallel

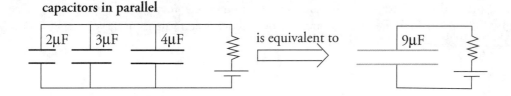

Capacitors in **series** all have the same charge (similar to *resistors* in series all having the same current), but the equivalent capacitance is found from the same formula that we used for resistors in *parallel*:

$$\text{equivalent capacitance} \atop \text{for capacitors in series} \qquad \boxed{\frac{1}{C_{eq}} = \frac{1}{C_1} + \frac{1}{C_2} + \frac{1}{C_3} + \ldots}$$

Equivalently, we could simplify the capacitors two at a time using the expression *product/sum*. For example, in the figure below, the equivalent capacitance, C_{eq}, is 2 μF, because 1/12 + 1/6 + 1/4 = 1/2. (We could also calculate it as (12 × 6)/(12 + 6) = 4 and (4 × 4)/(4 + 4) = 2.)

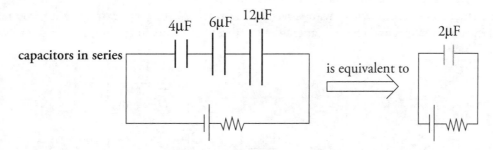

Example 10-40: Three uncharged capacitors are arranged in a circuit as shown.

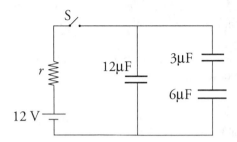

After the switch S has been closed for a long time and electrostatic equilibrium is reached, how much charge is on the 6 μF capacitor?

Solution: The 3 μF and 6 μF capacitors are in series, so they're equivalent to a single 2 μF capacitor, because (3 × 6)/(3 + 6) = 2. Therefore, the circuit shown above is equivalent to

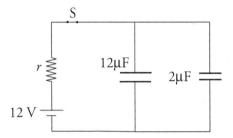

These two capacitors are in parallel, so both will have the same voltage: 12 V, since the plates of each are connected to the terminals of a 12 V battery. Now, using the equation $Q = CV$, we see that the charge on the 2 μF capacitor will be

$$Q = (2 \ \mu F)(12 \ V) = 24 \ \mu C$$

Since the 2 μF capacitor is equivalent to the series combination consisting of the 3 μF and 6 μF capacitors, the charge on each of these capacitors must be the same, 24 μC. (For extra practice, you may wish to verify the final voltages and charges on each of the three capacitors in the original circuit; the answers are shown below.)

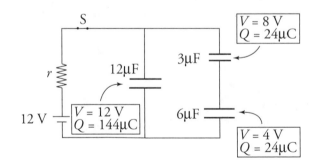

10.3 ALTERNATING CURRENT

In Section 8.1, we discussed circuits in which the current flowed in one direction only; such current is called **direct current** (DC). However, the electrical current that we use in our homes and offices every day is **alternating current** (AC), because the direction of the current changes: first one way, then the opposite way, then back again, and so on. The electrons that drift in the wires (and whose flow constitutes the current) are constantly forced to shuttle back and forth. While this may seem a little silly, producing an alternating voltage (and thus an alternating current) on a scale that supplies electricity to entire cities is far easier than producing a steady, direct voltage.

An AC generator creates a sinusoidally varying voltage. The voltage starts at, say, zero, and climbs to a peak value (called the amplitude), then falls back to zero; at this point, the polarity reverses, and the voltage again rises to its peak value then falls back to zero, and the cycle starts again. When we graph this time-varying voltage, we show the first half of the cycle as positive and the second half as negative; the negative voltage simply means that it "points" in the opposite direction from the voltage in the first half of the cycle. Thus, when the voltage is positive, the current flows in one direction. When the voltage is negative, the current flows in the opposite direction. In cases where the circuit contains only a source of alternating voltage and resistors, the current is in phase with the voltage, and we also consider Ohm's law to hold: That is, the voltage and current are related by $v = iR_{eq}$, where R_{eq} is the equivalent resistance of the circuit.

Note: It's customary when discussing time-varying voltages and currents to use lower-case letters; v and i, rather than V and I. The capital letters then denote the *maximum* values of v and i.

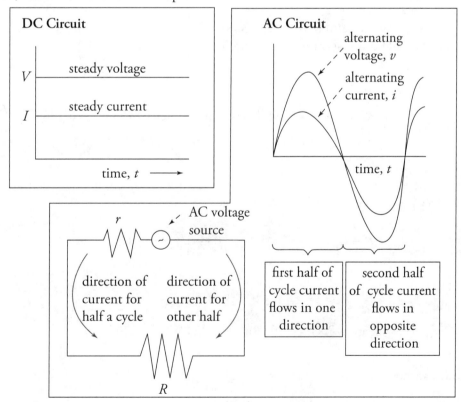

Notice that since v and i are constantly changing in an AC circuit, we can't talk about *the* voltage or *the* current. Instead, we talk about a kind of average voltage and average current. The particular average that is most useful is known as the **root-mean-square**, abbreviated **rms**. To form the rms of a quantity, we square it, average it over a cycle (that is, find the mean), then take the square root; it's the *root* of the *mean* of the *square* (hence root-mean-square). Fortunately, what all this boils down to is that the rms of a quantity is equal to its maximum divided by $\sqrt{2}$.

RMS Voltage and RMS Current

$$V_{rms} = \frac{v_{max}}{\sqrt{2}} = \frac{V}{\sqrt{2}} \quad \text{and} \quad I_{rms} = \frac{i_{max}}{\sqrt{2}} = \frac{I}{\sqrt{2}}$$

Recall that the power dissipated by a resistor in a DC circuit is given by the equation $P = I^2R$ and the power supplied by a voltage source is given by $P = IV$. For an AC circuit, we say that the average power dissipated by a resistor is $\bar{P} = I_{rms}^2 R$ and the average power supplied by the voltage source is $\bar{P} = I_{rms}V_{rms}$. This is why the rms average is one we use; it keeps the formulas the same as they were for DC circuits.

Example 10-41: Homes are typically supplied with 110 V rms.

    a)   What's the maximum voltage?

    b)   How much energy (in kWh) is used in 2 hours by a device whose resistance is 110 ohms?

    c)   How much would this cost if the electric company charges you 8¢ per kWh?

Solution:

    a)   Since 110 V is the rms voltage, we find the maximum voltage by multiplying V_{rms} by $\sqrt{2}$:

$$v_{max} = \sqrt{2} \cdot V_{rms} \approx (1.4)(110 \text{ V}) = 154 \text{ V}$$

    b)   Energy is power × time, so we can find the energy consumed by this device by multiplying the average power it consumes by the time. Since

$$\bar{P} = I_{rms}^2 R = \left(\frac{V_{rms}}{R}\right)^2 R = \frac{V_{rms}^2}{R} = \frac{(110 \text{ V})^2}{110 \text{ }\Omega} = 110 \text{ W}$$

    we have

$$\text{energy} = \bar{P} \times t = (110 \text{ W})(2 \text{ h}) = 220 \text{ Wh} = 0.220 \text{ kWh}$$

    c)   To calculate how much this would cost, we multiply this by 8¢/kWh:

$$\text{cost} = 0.220 \text{ kWh} \times \frac{\$0.08}{\text{kWh}} = \$0.0175 = 1\tfrac{3}{4} \text{ cents}$$

10.4 MAGNETIC FIELDS AND FORCES

Electric fields are created by electric charges; **magnetic fields** are created by *moving* electric charges. If a charge is at rest, it produces an electric field in the surrounding space. If this charge were to move, it would create an additional force field, a magnetic field, in the surrounding space. Since charge in motion constitutes a current, we can also say that magnetic fields are produced by electric currents. A permanent bar magnet is a source of a magnetic field because of the multitude of microscopic currents due to motions of the orbiting electrons within the metal; therefore, even a bar magnet's magnetic field is ultimately due to charges in motion.

If we place a charge q in a given electric field, $\mathbf{E}$, the force that the field will exert on this charge is given by the equation $\mathbf{F}_E = q\mathbf{E}$. We now need a similar formula to tell us the force that a magnetic field would exert on a charge q. First, a magnetic field can only exert a force on a charge that is *moving* through the field. A magnetic field is produced by moving charges and it exerts a force only on other moving charges. A magnetic field will exert no force on a charge that's at rest. The letter $\mathbf{B}$ is used to denote a magnetic field. The formula for the force that a magnetic field exerts on a charge q is as follows:

Magnetic Force

$$\mathbf{F}_B = q(\mathbf{v} \times \mathbf{B})$$

---

where $\mathbf{v}$ is the velocity of the charge q. Notice that if $\mathbf{v} = 0$ (that is, if the charge is at rest), then $\mathbf{F}_B$ will also be 0.

The formula $\mathbf{F}_B = q(\mathbf{v} \times \mathbf{B})$ involves the *cross product* of $\mathbf{v}$ and $\mathbf{B}$. You don't need to worry about calculating the vector components of the cross product; there is a much simpler way of finding $\mathbf{F}_B$ that is more than adequate for the MCAT. First, the magnitude of $\mathbf{F}_B$ is given by this equation:

Magnitude of Magnetic Force

$$F_B = |q|vB\sin\theta$$

---

where θ is the angle between $\mathbf{v}$ and $\mathbf{B}$. Notice that if $\mathbf{v}$ is parallel to $\mathbf{B}$, then $\theta = 0°$, and, since $\sin 0° = 0$, we get $\mathbf{F}_B = 0$. So, a charge could be moving through a magnetic field and yet feel no force if its direction of motion is parallel to the magnetic field lines. The same will be true if $\mathbf{v}$ is anti-parallel to $\mathbf{B}$ (that is, if the direction of $\mathbf{v}$ is exactly opposite to the direction of $\mathbf{B}$), since in this case, we have $\theta = 180°$ and $\sin 180° = 0$, so again we get $\mathbf{F}_B = 0$. If $\mathbf{v} \perp \mathbf{B}$, then $\theta = 90°$, and since $\sin 90° = 1$, the magnitude of $\mathbf{F}_B$ becomes simply $F_B = |q|vB$. From this equation, we can find the SI unit for magnetic field strength:

$$[B] = \frac{[F_B]}{[q][v]} = \frac{N}{C \cdot m/s} = \frac{N}{\frac{C}{s} \cdot m} = \frac{N}{A \cdot m}$$

One newton per amp-meter (1 N/A·m) is renamed one **tesla**, abbreviated $\mathbf{T}$. That is, B is measured in teslas.

10.4

Now that we know how to find the magnitude of F_B, all we need is a way to find the direction. The direction of F_B will depend on whether the charge q that moves through the field is positive or negative. Just like the force due to an electric field, the force due to a magnetic field also depends on the sign of the charge: If **B** exerts a force in a particular direction on a charge $+q$ moving with velocity **v**, then it would exert a force in the opposite direction on $-q$ moving with velocity **v**. In addition, magnetic forces have the following strange property: *The direction of F_B is always perpendicular to both* **v** *and* **B**. For example, if we had a magnetic field whose field lines pointed across this page (say, from left to right), and a positive charge q travels down the page, then the direction of the force F_B that q feels would be out of the plane of the page. The direction of F_B will always be perpendicular to the plane containing the vectors **v** and **B**. Since we're now dealing with a situation in which we'll have vectors in *three* dimensions, we need a notation to indicate when a vector points into, or out of, the plane of the page. Here are the symbols:

Now let's learn how to find the direction of the magnetic force, F_B, acting on a particle of charge q moving with velocity **v** through a magnetic field **B**. It involves the **right-hand rule** and the **left-hand rule**. You use the right-hand rule if the charge q moving through the field is positive, and the left-hand rule if q is negative.[4] Here's how the rules work.

First, determine whether the charge moving through the magnetic field is positive or negative.

If q is *positive*, use your *right* hand and the *right*-hand rule.

If q is *negative*, use your *left* hand and the *left*-hand rule.

Whether you use the right-hand rule or the left-hand rule, you will always follow these steps:

1. Orient your hand so that your thumb points in the direction of the velocity **v**.
2. Point your fingers in the direction of **B**.
3. The direction of F_B will then be perpendicular to your palm.

---

[4] Another method which many people prefer is always to use the right-hand rule, and then reverse the result (in other words, solve for the direction of the force on a positive charge, and then realize that the force on a negative charge is in exactly the opposite direction).

Think of your palm pushing with the force $\mathbf{F}_B$; the direction it pushes is the direction of $\mathbf{F}_B$.

Right-Hand Rule:

For determining the direction of
the magnetic force, $\mathbf{F}_B$,
on a *positive* charge

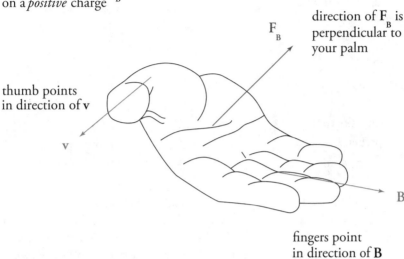

direction of $\mathbf{F}_B$ is
perpendicular to
your palm

F_B

thumb points
in direction of $\mathbf{v}$

v

B

fingers point
in direction of $\mathbf{B}$

Left-Hand Rule:

For determining the direction of
the magnetic force, $\mathbf{F}_B$,
on a *negative* charge

direction of $\mathbf{F}_B$ is
perpendicular to
your palm

F_B

v

thumb points
in direction of $\mathbf{v}$

fingers point
in direction of $\mathbf{B}$

B

For example, let's say we have a positive charge q moving with velocity $\mathbf{v}$ to the right across the plane of this page through a magnetic field $\mathbf{B}$ directed toward the top of the page. How would you find the direction of the resulting magnetic force on this moving charge? Since q is positive, use your right hand, and lay it flat on this page with your palm facing up; notice that in this orientation, your thumb points to the right (as it should since your thumb always points in the direction of the particle's velocity, $\mathbf{v}$) and your fingers point up toward the top of the page (as they should since your fingers always point in the direction

10.4

10.4

of the magnetic field, **B**). The direction of $\mathbf{F}_B$ is perpendicular to your palm, pointing out of the plane of the page, and so we symbolize the direction of $\mathbf{F}_B$ by ◉. In this case, the charged particle would start curling out of the plane of the page as a result of the magnetic force it feels.

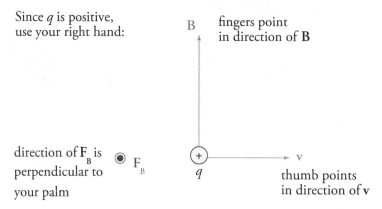

Now let's examine what would happen in the previous example if the charged particle had been *negative*. That is, we have a *negative* charge q moving with velocity **v** to the right across the plane of this page through a magnetic field **B** directed toward the top of the page. How would you find the direction of the resulting magnetic force on this moving charge? Since q is negative, use your *left* hand, and lay it flat on this page with your palm facing *down*; notice that in this orientation, your thumb points to the right (as it should since your thumb always points in the direction of the particle's velocity, **v**) and your fingers point up toward the top of the page (as they should since your fingers always point in the direction of the magnetic field, **B**). The direction of $\mathbf{F}_B$ is perpendicular to your palm, pointing *into* the plane of the page, and so we symbolize the direction of $\mathbf{F}_B$ by ⊗. In this case, the charged particle would start curling into the plane of the page as a result of the magnetic force it feels.

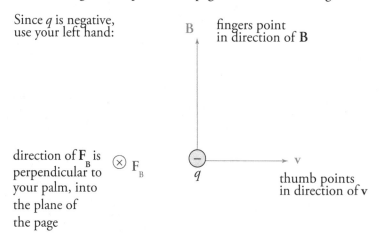

Practice the right- and left-hand rules and verify each of the following:

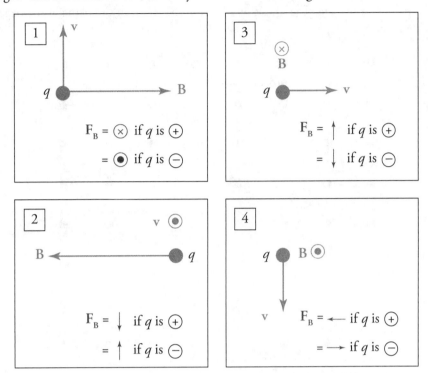

Because the magnetic force a charge feels is always perpendicular to the velocity of the charge, *magnetic forces do no work*. Recall that if a force **F** is perpendicular to the displacement **d** of an object, then this force **F** does zero work, because $W = Fd \cos \theta$ and $\theta = 90°$; since $\cos 90° = 0$, we get $W = 0$. Since magnetic forces never do work, they can never change the kinetic energy of a particle, meaning that *KE* is constant. (This follows from the work-energy theorem, $W = \Delta KE$.) Since magnetic forces cannot change the kinetic energy of a particle, they can't change the speed of a particle. All magnetic forces can do is make charged particles change their direction; they can't make them speed up or slow down.

The formula given earlier for the magnitude of the magnetic force is $|q| vB \sin\theta$, where θ is the angle between **v** and **B**. On the MCAT, it's most common to have a constant magnetic field and $\mathbf{v} \perp \mathbf{B}$; in this case, $\theta = 90°$, and because $\sin 90° = 1$, the magnitude of F_B becomes $F_B = |q| vB$. Further, if $\mathbf{v} \perp \mathbf{B}$, the subsequent motion of the charged particle will be uniform circular motion, with the magnetic force providing the centripetal force. Recall that in uniform circular motion, the centripetal force is always perpendicular to the particle's velocity and the particle's speed is constant; all the particle does is continuously change direction as it moves in a circular path. This is consistent with what we said in the previous paragraph about magnetic forces: they don't change the speed of a particle, only its direction. The case of a charged particle executing uniform circular motion in a constant magnetic field is so important for the MCAT, that we'll do the following example in detail.

Example 10-42: A proton is injected with velocity **v** into a region of constant magnetic field **B** that points out of the plane of the page. The direction of **v** is to the right, in the plane of the page, as shown in the diagram below:

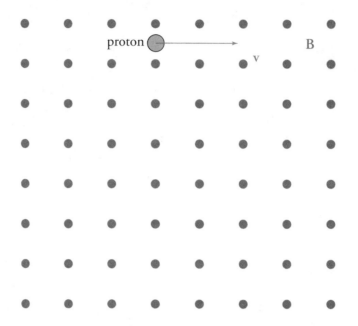

a)   Describe the subsequent motion of the proton.
b)   Find the radius of the circular trajectory it follows.

Solution:

a)   Because the proton is a positive charge, we use the *right*-hand rule to find the direction of the magnetic force it feels. With **v** to the right and **B** out of the page, we find that $\mathbf{F}_B$ points downward in the plane of the page:

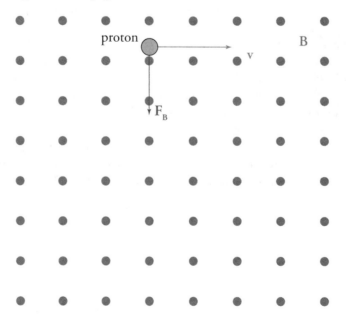

As a result, the proton will curve downward, and as it does, it is still continuously acted on by the magnetic force, but because the direction of **v** changes, so will the direction of $\mathbf{F_B}$. For example, when the proton is at the position shown in the following figure, the direction of $\mathbf{F_B}$ will be to the left:

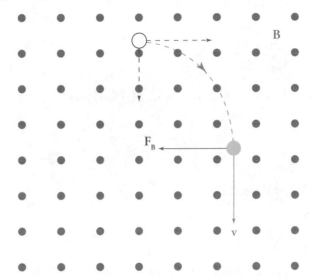

We can now see that the proton will continue to curve in a circular path, traveling clockwise:

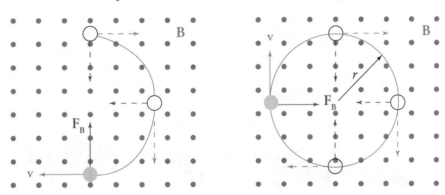

b) To find the radius of the circular path, we use the fact that the magnetic force provides the centripetal force to write

$$qvB = \frac{mv^2}{r}$$

where m is the mass of the proton. (We can drop the absolute value signs on the charge q because q is positive here.) Substituting $q = e$ (remember, it's a proton), then canceling one v from the right-hand side and solving for r, we get

$$r = \frac{mv}{eB}$$

Example 10-43: A particle with positive charge q and mass m moving with speed v undergoes uniform circular motion in a constant magnetic field **B**. If the radius of the particle's path is r, which one of the following expressions gives the magnitude of the momentum of the particle?

   A. qB/r
   B. r/qB
   C. rB/q
   D. qBr

Solution: Since the magnetic force provides the centripetal force, we have

$$qvB = \frac{mv^2}{r}$$

Canceling one v from the right-hand side, we get $qB = mv/r$, so $mv = qBr$. The answer is D.

Example 10-44: A particle with positive charge q and mass m moving with speed v undergoes uniform circular motion in a constant magnetic field **B**. If the radius of the particle's path is r, which of the following expressions gives the particle's orbit period (in other words, the time required for the particle to complete one revolution)?

   A. $2\pi/qvB$
   B. $2\pi m/qB$
   C. $qvB/2\pi m$
   D. $qB/2\pi m$

Solution: Since the magnetic force provides the centripetal force, we have

$$qvB = \frac{mv^2}{r}$$

Canceling one v from the right-hand side and solving for r, we get $r = mv/qB$. The time required for the particle to complete one revolution is equal to the total distance traveled by the particle in one revolution (the circumference, $2\pi r$) divided by the particle's speed, v. This gives

$$T = \frac{2\pi r}{v} = \frac{2\pi \cdot \dfrac{mv}{qB}}{v} = \frac{2\pi m}{qB}$$

Therefore, the answer is B. (*Note:* T is called the *cyclotron period*. Notice that it does *not* depend on r or v. Whether the particle moves rapidly in a large circle or more slowly in a smaller circle, it doesn't matter: the orbit period is determined solely by the mass and charge of the particle, and the magnitude of the magnetic field.)

Example 10-45: A sulfide ion, S^{2-}, moving with speed v_0 enters a region containing a uniform magnetic field **B**. If the vector $\mathbf{v}_0$ makes an angle of 30° with **B**, what is the magnitude of the initial magnetic force on this ion?

A. $ev_0B/4$
B. $ev_0B/2$
C. ev_0B
D. $2ev_0B$

Solution: The charge on this ion is $-2e$, so the initial magnetic force the ion feels has magnitude

$$F_B = |q|vB\sin\theta = |-2e| \cdot v_0 B \sin 30° = 2e \cdot v_0 B \cdot \tfrac{1}{2} = ev_0 B$$

The answer is C.

Example 10-46: A particle with negative charge $-q$ moving with speed v_0 enters a region containing a uniform magnetic field **B**. If the vector $\mathbf{v}_0$ makes an angle of 30° with **B**, what is the particle's speed 8 seconds after entering the field?

A. $v_0/4$
B. v_0
C. $2v_0$
D. $4v_0$

Solution: Since magnetic forces do no work, the kinetic energy (and thus the speed) of the particle will be unchanged. The answer is B.

Example 10-47: A particle with charge q moves with velocity **v** through a region of space containing a uniform electric field, **E**, *and* a uniform magnetic field, **B**. Which of the following expressions gives the total electromagnetic force on the particle?

A. $q(\mathbf{E} + \mathbf{B})$
B. $q(\mathbf{v} \times \mathbf{E} + \mathbf{B})$
C. $q\mathbf{v} \times (\mathbf{E} + \mathbf{B})$
D. $q(\mathbf{E} + \mathbf{v} \times \mathbf{B})$

Solution: The electric force on the particle is $\mathbf{F}_E = q\mathbf{E}$, and the magnetic force is $\mathbf{F}_B = q(\mathbf{v} \times \mathbf{B})$. Therefore, the *total* electromagnetic force is

$$\mathbf{F}_E + \mathbf{F}_B = q\mathbf{E} + q(\mathbf{v} \times \mathbf{B}) = q(\mathbf{E} + \mathbf{v} \times \mathbf{B})$$

The answer is D.

Note: The total electromagnetic force is known as the **Lorentz force**.

Example 10-48: The figure below shows a charged parallel-plate capacitor with a uniform electric field, **E**, in the space between its plates. A uniform magnetic field, **B**, is also produced in the space between the capacitor plates by another device.

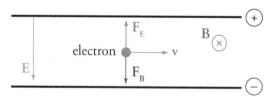

At what speed would an electron need to travel between the plates in order to pass through undeflected? (Ignore gravity.)

    A. E/B
    B. B/E
    C. EB
    D. EB^2

Solution: In between the plates, the direction of the electric force, F_E, on the electron is upward. Using the left-hand rule (because the particle carries a negative charge), we find that the direction of the magnetic force, F_B, is downward.

Therefore, these two forces point in opposite directions. They'll cancel (giving $F_{net} = 0$) and allow the particle to pass through undeflected if these forces have the same magnitude. The magnitude of the electric force is $F_E = |q|E = |-e|E = eE$, and the magnitude of the magnetic force is $F_B = |q|vB = |-e|vB = evB$. Therefore, we'll have $F_B = F_E$ when $evB = eE$. Solving this equation for v, we find that $v = E/B$, choice A.

Example 10-49: A uniform magnetic field **B** exerts a force F_B on a particle with charge q moving with velocity **v** through the field. Which of the following gives the magnetic force that the same field would exert on a particle of charge $2q$ moving with velocity $-2v$?

    A. $-8F_B$
    B. $-4F_B$
    C. $4F_B$
    D. $8F_B$

Solution: If **B** exerts a force of F_B on a charge q moving with velocity **v**, then it would exert a force of $-F_B$ on a charge q moving with velocity $-v$. Now, because F_B is proportional to q and to v, if q and v both double, then F_B will be multiplied by a factor of $2 \cdot 2 = 4$. Therefore, the force that **B** would exert on a particle of charge $2q$ moving with velocity $-2v$ is $-4F_B$, choice B.

Example 10-50: The figure below shows a simple mass spectrometer. It consists of a source of ions that are accelerated from rest through a potential difference V and then enter a region containing a uniform magnetic field **B** that points out of the plane of the page and is perpendicular to the initial velocity, **v**, of the ion as it enters. Once an ion enters the magnetic field, it travels in a semicircular path until it strikes the detector, which records its arrival and the distance, d, from the opening.

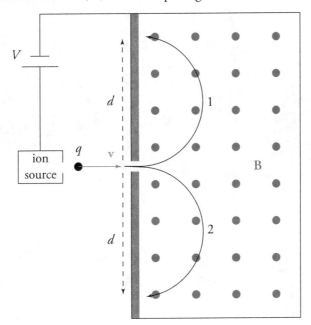

a) An ion of charge $+q$ and mass m will enter the magnetic field with what speed? Write v in terms of q, m, and V.

b) Which semicircular path would a cation follow: 1 or 2?

c) If you were using this device in a lab to analyze a sample containing various isotopes of an element, how would you find the mass of a cation striking the detector if all you knew were q, V, B, and d?

Solution:

a) The ion loses electrical potential energy in the amount qV, and as a result, gains kinetic energy, $\frac{1}{2}mv^2$. Therefore, $\frac{1}{2}mv^2 = qV$, so $v = \sqrt{2qV/m}$.

b) The right-hand rule (for a positive charge) tells us that if **v** points to the right and **B** points out of the plane of the page, then $\mathbf{F}_B$ points downward:

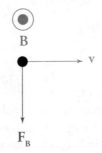

Since $\mathbf{F}_B$ points downward when the particle is at the opening, a cation would follow path 2, because $\mathbf{F}_B$ provides the centripetal force and thus points toward the center of the path. The following diagram illustrates this:

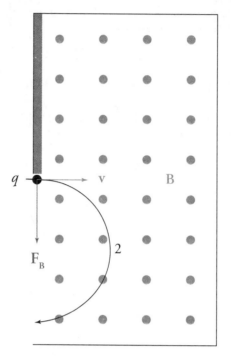

c) Since the magnetic force provides the centripetal force, we have

$$qvB = \frac{mv^2}{r}$$

Canceling one v from the right-hand side and solving for m (the mass of the cation) gives

$$m = \frac{qBr}{v}$$

From the diagram, we see that $r = \frac{1}{2}d$, and from part (a), $v = \sqrt{2qV/m}$, so we get

$$m = \frac{qB \cdot \frac{1}{2}d}{\sqrt{2qV/m}}$$

Squaring both sides and solving for m, we find that the mass of the cation is

$$m = \frac{qB^2 d^2}{8V}$$

Sources of Magnetic Fields

Now that we know how a given magnetic field affects a charged particle, we'll now look at how the magnetic field was created in the first place. Recall that charges *in motion* produce a magnetic field. A current is charge in motion, so electric currents produce magnetic fields. Let's take the simplest possible case: An electric current moving in a straight line. The magnetic field lines created by the current wrap around the current, forming closed loops. To find the direction of these magnetic field loops, we use the right-hand rule because by convention we consider a current I to be the direction that positive charges would move.[5] Imagine grabbing the wire in your right hand in such a way that your thumb points in the direction of the velocity of the charges (that is, in the direction of I). The way that your fingers wrap around the wire gives the direction of the magnetic field. Verify the directions of the **B**-field loops for the wires shown below; remember, magnetic field "lines" are actually circles that wrap around the wire. (That's the end of the right-hand rule in this situation. We are not trying to figure out the direction of the magnetic force that a given magnetic field exerts on a charged particle; we're now finding the magnetic field. Your thumb and fingers mean the same thing now as they did before: Your thumb points in the direction of the motion of the relevant charge (the charge making the field) and your fingers point in the direction of the magnetic field, **B**.)

current-carrying wire perpendicular to page with current coming *out* of the plane of the page

current-carrying wire perpendicular to page with current going *into* the plane of the page

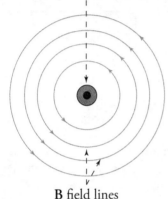

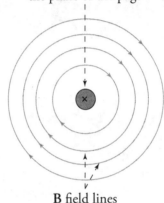

B field lines

B field lines

In these next two diagrams, the **B**-field circles look like ellipses because of perspective; here the current-carrying wires lie in the plane of the page, and the **B**-field circles are perpendicular to the page, going into (or out of) the page above the wire and out of (or into) the page below the wire.

With the current pointing to the left, the **B** field lines go into the page above the wire . . .

With the current pointing to the right, the B field lines come out of the page above the wire . . .

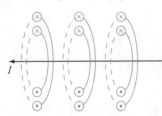

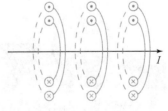

and come out of the page below the wire.

and go into the page below the wire.

[5] Though it's uncommon on the MCAT, it's possible you'll be asked about the field produced by a single moving charge, not a current. If the charge is positive you simply use the method given here; if the charge is negative you could use the left-hand rule, or use the right-hand rule and then reverse the direction of the answer; in other words, the field lines created by a negative charge circle in the opposite direction from those created by a positive charge.

The magnitude of the magnetic field created by a straight wire carrying a current I is proportional to I and inversely proportional to the distance r from the wire:

$$B \propto \frac{I}{r}$$

Hence, the magnetic field will be stronger if the current is increased or if we are positioned closer to the wire.

Circular wire loops that carry current also create magnetic fields. In the figure below, notice that the field lines are nearly vertical near the center of the circular wire loop that lies along the central axis. At the center of the loop, the magnitude of **B** is proportional to the current, I, and inversely proportional to the radius of the wire loop ($B \propto I/r_{loop}$). If the current in the wire loop had been traveling in the opposite direction (that is, clockwise), then each of the arrows on the **B**-field lines would point in the opposite direction.

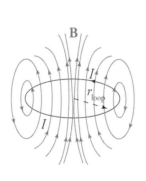
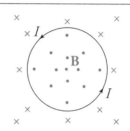

counterclockwise current:
B field points out of
page inside the loop
and points into the page
outside the loop

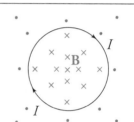

clockwise current:
B field points into page
inside the loop
and points out of the
page outside the loop

Imagine taking a long wire and wrapping it tightly around a cylinder, like a paper-towel tube. The result will look like a spring; we can also consider it to be like a lot of circular loops close together. Such a helical coil of wire is called a **solenoid**. The magnetic field it produces inside the cylinder is parallel to the central axis and achieves its maximum magnitude *on* the central axis, getting weaker as we move away from the center, closer to the coils:

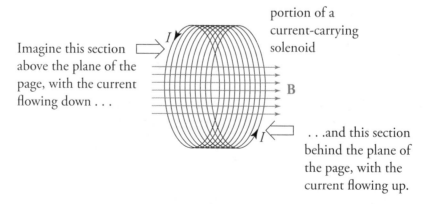

Imagine this section
above the plane of the
page, with the current
flowing down . . .

portion of a
current-carrying
solenoid

. . .and this section
behind the plane of
the page, with the
current flowing up.

If the solenoid has many windings and if the length is much greater than its diameter, then the magnetic field in the interior is nearly uniform and is proportional to the current (I) and to the number of turns per unit length (N/L): $B \propto I(N/L)$. Hence, the magnetic field will be stronger if the current is increased or if the solenoid wire loops are tightly packed.

Example 10-51: The figure below shows a long straight wire carrying a current, I. An electron is projected above the wire and initially parallel to it.

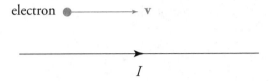

Which of the following best illustrates the direction of the magnetic force on the electron at the position shown?

A. $\downarrow$ C. $\otimes$

B. $\odot$ D. $\uparrow$

Solution: Since the current in the wire points to the right, the direction of the magnetic field **B** above the wire is out of the plane of the page. Using the left-hand rule (since the electron is a negative charge),

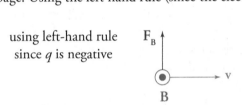

we find that the direction of the magnetic force $\mathbf{F}_B$ is upward, away from the wire, so choice D is correct.

Example 10-52: The figure below shows two long, straight wires carrying current. The top wire carries a current $I_1 = I$ to the left, while the bottom wire carries a current $I_2 = 2I$ to the right.

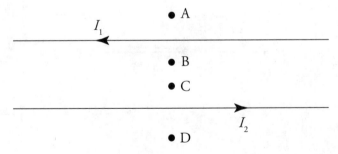

Points A and B are equidistant from the top wire, and Points C and D are equidistant from the bottom wire. Furthermore, the distance between Points B and C is the same as the distance between B and the top wire, which is also the same as the distance between C and the bottom wire. Of these four points, where is the total magnetic field the weakest?

Solution: First, we notice that the magnetic field created by the top wire, $\mathbf{B}_1$, encircles the wire, with the magnetic field circles centered on the top wire and pointing into the plane of the page above the wire and out of the page below it. Similarly, the magnetic field created by the bottom wire, $\mathbf{B}_2$, also encircles the wire, with the magnetic field circles centered on the bottom wire and pointing out of the plane of the page above the wire and into the page below it:

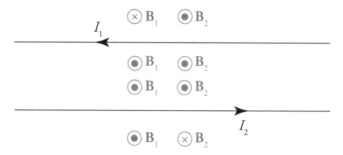

So, we can immediately rule out choices B and C; between the wires, the individual magnetic fields point in the same direction, so their magnitudes add, giving a strong field in this region. However, above the top wire and below the bottom wire, the individual magnetic fields point in opposite directions, so their magnitudes subtract; therefore, of the choices given, the field is weakest at either Point A or Point D. Because $I_2 = 2I$, Point D is closer to the higher-current wire, so to calculate the net $\mathbf{B}$ field at Point D, we'd subtract a small quantity (the contribution from the weaker-current, which is also farther away) from a large quantity (the contribution from the close higher-current). By contrast, to calculate the net $\mathbf{B}$ field at Point A, the quantity we'd subtract is larger than the one we subtracted to find the field at Point D and the positive term here is smaller than the positive term in the calculation of the field at Point D. Therefore, we expect the field at Point A to be weaker than at Point D. If this "intuitive" argument is unconvincing, let's do some math to back it up:

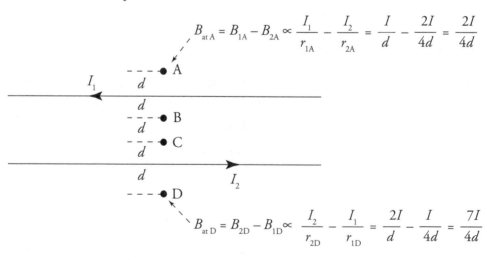

Example 10-53: The figure on the following page shows a circular loop of wire in the plane of the page, carrying a current I. A proton is projected with velocity $\mathbf{v}$, such that $\mathbf{v}$ lies in a plane slightly above and parallel to the plane of the loop, as shown:

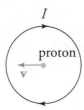

Which of the following best illustrates the direction of the magnetic force on the proton at the position shown?

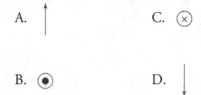

Solution: Since the current in the loop travels clockwise, the direction of the magnetic field **B** above the center of the loop points *into* the plane of the page. Using the right-hand rule (since the proton is a positive charge),

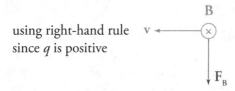

we find that the magnetic force $\mathbf{F}_B$ is in the plane above and parallel to the plane of the loop and with a direction as illustrated by choice D.

Example 10-54: The figure below shows a portion of a long narrow solenoid carrying a current, I. An alpha particle (α) is projected with velocity **v** down the central axis of the solenoid, as shown:

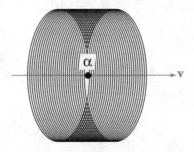

Which of the following best illustrates the direction of the magnetic force on the alpha particle?

D. None of the above

Solution: At the position of the alpha particle, the magnetic field **B** created by the current-carrying sole-noid is directed along the central axis; that is, either in the same direction as **v** or in the opposite direction from **v**, depending on the direction of the current in the wire loops. In either case, though, the magnetic force will be zero. (Remember that if **v** is parallel or anti-parallel to **B**, then $F_B = 0$.) The answer is D.

Magnets

A permanent bar magnet creates a magnetic field that closely resembles the magnetic field produced by a circular loop of current-carrying wire:

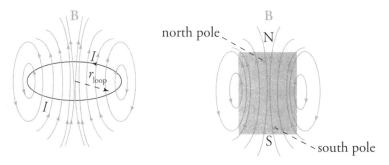

By convention, the magnetic field lines emanate from the end of the magnet designated the **north pole** (**N**) and then curl around and re-enter the magnet at the end designated the **south pole** (**S**). The magnetic field created by a permanent bar magnet is due to the electrons; they have an intrinsic spin (remember the spin quantum number, m_s, from general chemistry) and they orbit their nuclei; therefore, they are charges in motion, the ultimate source of all magnetic fields. If a piece of iron is placed in an external magnetic field (for example, the one created by a current-carrying solenoid) the individual magnetic dipole moments of the electrons will be forced to more or less line up. Because iron is *ferromagnetic*, these now-aligned magnetic dipole moments tend to retain this configuration, thus permanently magnetizing the bar and causing it to produce its own magnetic field.

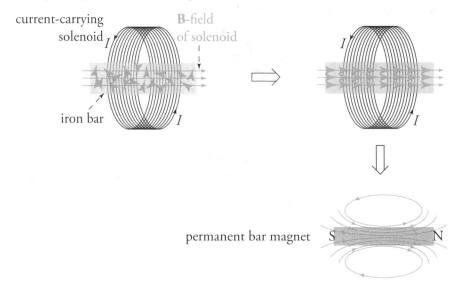

As with electric charges, like magnetic poles repel each other, while opposite magnetic poles attract each other:

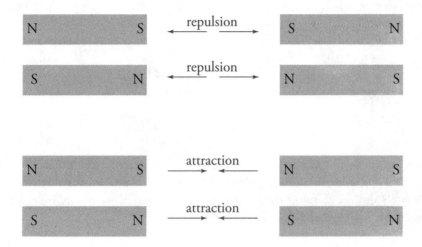

However, while you can have a positive electric charge all by itself, you can't have a single magnetic pole all by itself: the existence of a lone magnetic pole has never been confirmed. That is, there are no magnetic *monopoles*; magnetic poles always exist *in pairs*. If you cut a bar magnet into two pieces, you wouldn't get a piece with just an N and another piece with just an S; you'd get two separate and complete magnets, each with a N–S pair:

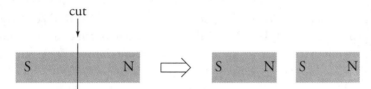

Example 10-55: An MRI scanner functions according to some subtle quantum mechanical principles, but at its most basic, it takes advantage of the fact that spinning protons (namely the two hydrogen nuclei in every water molecule in your body) function as tiny magnets. An extremely powerful, constant external magnetic field $\mathbf{B}_0$ is applied to the body, causing these proton magnets to align. Why? When a magnet is placed in a magnetic field, it tends to align with the field (or, slightly less likely, exactly opposite it), so that the vector from the S pole to the N pole of the magnet is parallel to the field lines.

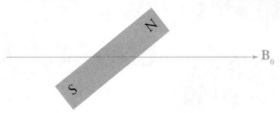

Given that the uniform magnetic field $\mathbf{B}_0$ in the figure above exerts the same magnitude of force on the N pole as it does on the S pole and the magnetic force on a pole is along the field line, what can you say about the net force and net torque on the magnet?

10.4

Solution: Because the $\mathbf{B}_0$ field will exert a force $\mathbf{F}_B$ on the N pole and a force of $-\mathbf{F}_B$ on the S pole, the net force on the magnet will be zero ($\mathbf{F}_B + -\mathbf{F}_B = 0$). However, the net torque will not be zero, since the magnetic force produces a clockwise torque on each pole, tending to align the magnet parallel to the field line.

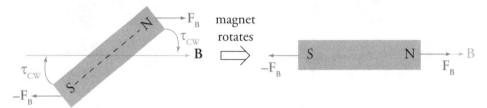

The tiny proton magnets don't actually align statically with the external field, but rather precess around that alignment, the way a teetering spinning top does before it falls over. It is the frequency of this precession that is ultimately utilized to make the protons emit radio waves, which are then detected and translated into images by the MRI machine.

The rotating Earth itself is the source of a (nonuniform) magnetic field, which surrounds the planet and traps electrons and protons emitted by the Sun, making them spiral throughout curved regions called the Van Allen belts. (Protons tend to be confined in Van Allen belts close to Earth's surface, while electrons spiral around in belts farther from the surface. These energetic trapped protons can ionize nitrogen and oxygen in the upper atmosphere, creating cations and electrons. When these cations and electrons recombine, energy is emitted. This is the source of the light that produces the aurora borealis [and, in the southern hemisphere, the aurora australis].) The magnetic poles are *near*, but not *at*, the geographic poles; also notice that it's the magnetic *south* pole that's near the geographic North Pole, and the magnetic *north* pole that's near the geographic South Pole. After all, the magnetic north pole of a compass needle points (roughly) toward geographic north, but we know that it's *opposite* magnetic poles that attract, so the compass needle must be attracted to the magnetic south pole.

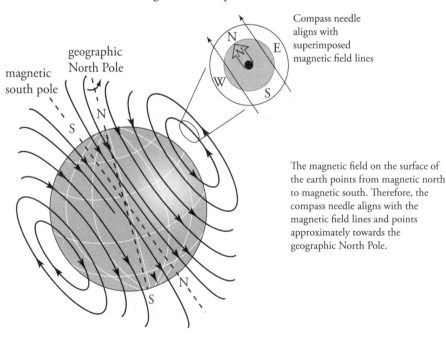

Compass needle aligns with superimposed magnetic field lines

The magnetic field on the surface of the earth points from magnetic north to magnetic south. Therefore, the compass needle aligns with the magnetic field lines and points approximately towards the geographic North Pole.

Example 10-56: The magnitude of Earth's magnetic field is roughly 1 gauss (1 G) at the surface; the **gauss** is a very common (non-SI) unit of magnetic field strength, with 1 G equal to 10^{-4} T. If a proton moving with speed $v = 5 \times 10^6$ m/s in the atmosphere experiences a magnetic field strength of 0.5 G, what force (magnetic or gravitational) has the greater effect? (*Note*: mass of proton $\approx 1.7 \times 10^{-27}$ kg.)

Solution: The gravitational force on the proton is

$$F_{\text{grav}} = mg = (1.7 \times 10^{-27} \text{ kg})(10 \tfrac{\text{N}}{\text{kg}}) = 1.7 \times 10^{-26} \text{ N}$$

The maximum magnetic force on the proton is

$$F_{\text{B}} = qvB = evB = (1.6 \times 10^{-19} \text{ C})(5 \times 10^6 \tfrac{\text{m}}{\text{s}})(0.5 \times 10^{-4} \text{ T}) = 4 \times 10^{-17} \text{ N}$$

Since $F_{\text{B}} \gg F_{\text{grav}}$, we see that it's the magnetic force that is chiefly responsible for the proton's motion through Earth's atmosphere.

Example 10-57: Two bar magnets are fixed in position, and a proton is projected with velocity **v** into the region between adjacent opposite poles, as shown below:

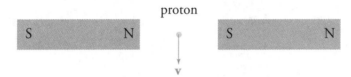

Which of the following best illustrates the direction of the magnetic force on the proton at the position shown?

A. ⟵   C. ⊗

B. ⊙   D. ⟶

Solution: On the outside of the magnet(s), **B** points from the N pole to the S pole.

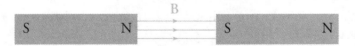

Using the right-hand rule (for a positive charge) where **B** points to the right and **v** is downward, then **F**$_B$ points out of the plane of the page:

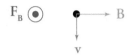

Therefore, the answer is B.

Example 10-58: An electron initially travels with velocity **v**, directed into the plane of the page, near a bar magnet, as illustrated below:

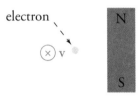

Which of the following arrows best illustrates the direction of the magnetic force on the electron at the position shown?

A. ⟵   C. ↑

B. ↓   D. ⟶

Solution: Because the **B** field points from the N pole to the S pole (*outside* the magnet), the direction of the **B** field at the position of the electron is downward:

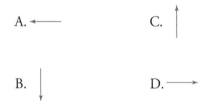

The left-hand rule (for a negative charge) tells us that if **B** points downward and **v** is directed into the plane of the page, then **F**$_B$ points to the right:

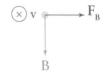

Therefore, the answer is D.

Example 10-59: The following figure shows an electromagnet with an iron core. Since iron is ferromagnetic, the magnetic field created by the current-carrying coil aligns the magnetic dipole moments of electrons in the iron, creating a magnetic field throughout the iron.

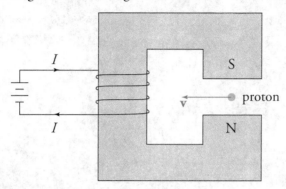

If a proton is projected with velocity **v** between the poles as shown, which of the following best illustrates the direction of the magnetic force on the proton at the position shown?

A. C.

B. D.

Solution: Because outside the magnet the B field always points from the N pole to the S pole, the direction of the **B** field at the position of the proton is upward:

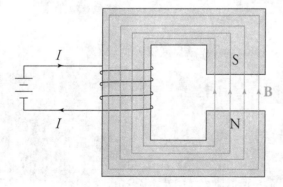

The right-hand rule (for a positive charge) tells us that if **B** points upward and **v** is directed to the left, then $\mathbf{F}_B$ points into the plane of the page:

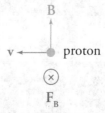

Therefore, the answer is C.

Summary Of Formulas

CIRCUITS

Current: $I = \dfrac{Q}{t}$

- in the direction of "flow of positive charge"

- actual flow of electrons is in the opposite direction

Resistance: $R = \rho \dfrac{L}{A}$ (ρ = resistivity, not density)

Ohm's law: $V = IR$ (where R is constant as V varies)

Resistors in series: $R_{eq} = R_1 + R_2 + ...$

Resistors in parallel: $\dfrac{1}{R_{eq}} = \dfrac{1}{R_1} + \dfrac{1}{R_2} + ...$ or $R_{eq} = \dfrac{R_1 R_2}{R_1 + R_2}$ (two at a time)

Current is the same for resistors in series; voltage is the same for resistors in parallel.

Kirchhoff's Rules:

- The sum of the voltage-drops across the resistors in any complete path is equal to the voltage of the battery.

- The amount of current entering a parallel combination of resistors is equal to the sum of the currents that pass through the individual resistors.

Power of circuit element: $P = IV = I^2 R = \dfrac{V^2}{R}$

Total power supplied by a battery equals the total power dissipated by the resistors.

The ground is at potential zero (potential = 0).

Root-mean-square quantities for AC circuit:

$$V_{rms} = \frac{V_{max}}{\sqrt{2}} \, , \, I_{rms} = \frac{I_{max}}{\sqrt{2}}$$

Average power of circuit element in AC circuit:

$$\bar{P} = \left(I_{rms} \right)^2 R = I_{rms} V_{rms}$$

PARALLEL PLATE CAPACITORS

Charge on a capacitor: $Q = CV$

- The capacitance does not depend on voltage or charge. It is determined by the formula below.

Capacitance:

no dielectric: $C = \varepsilon_0 \dfrac{A}{d}$

with dielectric: $C_{with\ dielectric} = KC_{without\ dielectric} = K\varepsilon_0 \dfrac{A}{d}$ [K = dielectric constant]

- Inserting a dielectric always increases the capacitance. If the battery remains attached, V is constant; if the battery is taken away Q is constant.

Electric field in parallel-plate capacitor:

$$V = Ed$$

Stored potential energy in capacitor:

$$PE = \frac{1}{2}QV = \frac{1}{2}CV^2 = \frac{Q^2}{2C}$$

- The work done by the battery to charge the capacitor = PE.

Capacitors in series: $\dfrac{1}{C_{eq}} = \dfrac{1}{C_1} + \dfrac{1}{C_2} + ...$ or $C_{eq} = \dfrac{C_1 C_2}{C_1 + C_2}$ [two at a time]

Capacitors in parallel: $C_{eq} = C_1 + C_2 + ...$

MAGNETIC FORCE AND FIELD

Magnetic force on moving charge q:

$$\mathbf{F}_B - q(\mathbf{v} \times \mathbf{B})$$

$$F_B = |q| vB \sin\theta \quad (\theta = \text{angle between } \mathbf{v} \text{ and } \mathbf{B})$$

Direction of $\mathbf{F}_B$: use right-hand rule if q is positive; use left-hand rule if q is negative (or use right-hand rule and reverse the answer)

$\mathbf{F}_B$ is always perpendicular to both $\mathbf{v}$ and $\mathbf{B}$

$\mathbf{B}$ created by long, straight current-carrying wire: $B \propto I / r$

$\mathbf{B}$ created by a solenoid: $B \propto I \dfrac{N}{L}$ (L = length of solenoid, N = number of coils)

The magnetic force never changes the speed of a particle, and does NO work on the particle.

Magnetic field lines created by a magnet will point north to south.

The north pole of a magnet wants to line up with the direction of an external magnetic field; the south pole wants to line up opposite the field.

CHAPTER 10 FREESTANDING PRACTICE QUESTIONS

1. A helium nucleus traveling at speed v feels a magnetic force of magnitude F_B due to a solenoid that produces a magnetic field. If the number of turns per unit length in the solenoid is doubled while the current is kept constant, what is the magnitude of the force that the helium nucleus feels if it is traveling with the same speed in the same direction?

A) $0.5F_B$
B) $1F_B$
C) $2F_B$
D) $4F_B$

2. Capacitor C_1 has a capacitance of 5 F and holds an initial charge $Q_{1,i} = 40$ C. Capacitor C_2 has a capacitance of 15 F and holds an initial charge $Q_{2,i} = 60$ C. The two capacitors are in a circuit with an open switch S between them, as shown in the figure below. When the switch closes, the charges on the capacitors will redistribute. What is the quantity of charge, $Q_{1,f}$ and $Q_{2,f}$, on each capacitor a long time after the switch closes?

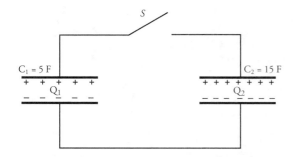

A) $Q_{1,f} = 25$ C, $Q_{2,f} = 75$ C
B) $Q_{1,f} = 75$ C, $Q_{2,f} = 25$ C
C) $Q_{1,f} = 50$ C, $Q_{2,f} = 50$ C
D) $Q_{1,f} = 40$ C, $Q_{2,f} = 60$ C

3. An air capacitor stores potential energy. If you wanted the potential energy to double by adding a dielectric between the plates while keeping the voltage constant, what would have to be the value of the dielectric constant?

A) 0.5
B) 2
C) 4
D) 8

4. Determine the total power dissipated through the circuit shown below in terms of V, R_1, R_2, and R_3.

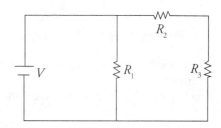

A) $\dfrac{V^2}{R_1 + R_2 + R_3}$

B) $\dfrac{R_1 + R_2 + R_3}{V^2}$

C) $\dfrac{R_1(R_2 + R_3)}{V^2(R_1 + R_2 + R_3)}$

D) $\dfrac{V^2(R_1 + R_2 + R_3)}{R_1(R_2 + R_3)}$

5. Lightning is an atmospheric discharge of electricity that can propagate at speeds of up to 60,000 m/s and can reach temperatures of up to 30,000°C. A single lightning strike lasts for approximately 250 ms and can transfer up to 500 MJ of energy across a potential difference of 2 10^7 volts. Estimate the total amount of charge transferred and average current of a single lightning strike.

A) 6.25×10^{-4} coulombs, 8×10^7 amps
B) 6.25×10^{-4} coulombs, 2.5×10^{-3} amps
C) 25 coulombs, 100 amps
D) 25 coulombs, 8×10^7 amps

6. Which of the following changes will increase the resistance of a closed circuit system?

   I. Replacing the wire with one made of the same metal that has a smaller cross sectional area
   II. Placing a voltmeter in series with the rest of the circuit
   III. Doubling the wire length in the closed circuit

A) III only
B) I and III only
C) II and III only
D) I, II and III

7. If the resistance of a wire in a household appliance becomes 4 times its original value, which of the following statements is/are correct?

   I. The voltage of the wire becomes quadrupled.
   II. The current through the wire becomes 1/4th the original value.
   III. The power consumed by the appliance becomes quadrupled.

A) I only
B) II only
C) I and III only
D) II and III only

CHAPTER 10 PRACTICE PASSAGE

A current-carrying wire will generate a magnetic field around the wire that varies with current in the wire, i, and the distance from the wire, r. The strength of the magnetic field generated can be calculated using the equation

$$B = \mu_0 i / 2\pi r$$

Equation 1

where B is the magnitude of the magnetic field generated and μ_0 is a constant known as the permeability of free space. The direction of the magnetic field generated will always be circular around the wire.

A physics student is conducting an experiment to test the effects on charged particles of the magnetic field created by wires. Two long wires are stretched parallel to each other a distance 20 cm apart. Each wire is connected to a voltage source and a grounded point so that a current will flow through the wire. Three separate test paths are established and marked in Figure 1. The wires are fixed in place, so any forces experienced by the wires will not cause them to move.

The charged particle used in the experiment is a lightweight (mass, m) negatively charged (charge, $-q$) metal marble. For each experiment, the marble is injected along the test path with a constant initial velocity, v, which is parallel to the wires. The magnetic field created by the wires exerts a magnetic force on the marble, causing the velocity to change direction from the initial velocity direction. Because the marble rolls without slipping, frictional effects are assumed to be negligible.

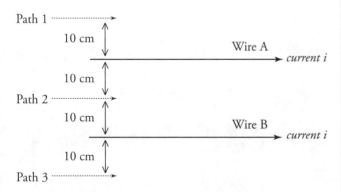

Figure 1 Complete setup for Trial 1 with the three test paths marked

In the first trial of the experiment, the student has the same voltage drop across both wires and the current, i, in both wires is going from left to right, as shown in Figure 1. The metal marble was injected along each test path, and its initial change in direction recorded in Table 1. In the second trial of the experiment, the current in Wire A remained the same, but the current in Wire B was doubled. Again, the metal marble was injected along each test path, and its initial change in direction recorded in Table 1.

Trial	Test Path	Initial Change in Direction of Marble
1	1	Up, away from Wire A ($\uparrow$)
1	2	No change in direction, marble passes straight along path 2 ($\rightarrow$)
1	3	Down, away from Wire B ($\downarrow$)
2	1	Up, away from Wire A ($\uparrow$)
2	2	Up, toward Wire A and away from Wire B ($\uparrow$)
2	3	Down, away from Wire B ($\downarrow$)

1. Which of the following best explains why the marble on Path 2 did not change direction in Trial 1 of the experiment?

A) The net magnetic force acting on the marble was zero because the net magnetic field was zero along Path 2 since the magnetic field created from Wire A was equal in magnitude and opposite in direction from the magnetic field created from Wire B.

B) The net magnetic force acting on the marble was zero because the magnetic fields created by the two wires along Path 2 resulted in forces that were an action-reaction pair.

C) The net magnetic force acting on the marble was not zero, but the magnetic fields created by the two wires resulted in forces on the marble that were parallel to the wires and kept the marble on Path 2.

D) The net magnetic force acting on the marble was not zero because the marble increased velocity as it traveled on Path 2.

2. What is the magnitude and direction of the magnetic field on Path 2 in Trial 2 if $i = 6$ A?

A) magnitude is 30 μ_0/π direction is into the page
B) magnitude is 30 μ_0/π direction is out of the page
C) magnitude is 60 μ_0/π direction is into the page
D) magnitude is 60 μ_0/π direction is out of the page

3. How much work is done by the magnetic force on the marble on Path 3 in Trial 2 in terms of the variables given in the passage?

A) $qv\mu_0 i/2\pi$
B) $qv\mu_0 i/2\pi r$
C) $qv\mu_0 ir/2\pi$
D) 0

4. Assuming the same voltage drop is used for both trials of the experiment, how might the student double the current in Wire B in Trial 2?

A) Increase the resistance by a factor of 2
B) Decrease the resistance by a factor of 2
C) Increase the resistance by a factor of 4
D) Decrease the resistance by a factor of 4

5. Which of the following best describes the negative charge on the metal marble?

A) The negative charge means the electric field inside the marble points in, toward the center of the marble.
B) The negative charge means the electric field inside the marble points out, away from the center of the marble.
C) There is no electric field inside the marble since the negative charge is spread evenly on the surface of the marble.
D) There is no electric field inside the marble since conductors absorb charge and neutralize it.

6. The student wanted to conduct a Trial 3 of the experiment where the current in Wire A is the same as in Trial 1, and the current in Wire B is the same magnitude as Wire A but in the opposite direction. Predict the results of Trial 3 of the experiment.

  I. The initial change in direction of the marble on Path 1 is up, away from Wire A ($\uparrow$)
  II. The initial change in direction of the marble on Path 2 is no change in direction ($\rightarrow$)
  III. The initial change in direction of the marble on Path 3 is up, toward Wire B ($\uparrow$)

A) I only
B) I and II only
C) I and III only
D) I, II, and III

SOLUTIONS TO CHAPTER 10 FREESTANDING QUESTIONS

1. **C** The magnetic field generated by a solenoid is proportional to IN/L, so doubling the number of turns per unit length will double the magnetic field. The magnitude of the force in a magnetic field is proportional to the magnetic field strength, therefore it will double if the magnetic field strength doubles.

2. **A** The sum of the charges, Q_{tot}, on the two capacitors is 100 C. After Switch S is closed, capacitors C_1 and C_2 are connected together and must have the same terminal voltage V. Q_{tot} remains 100 C. After a long time, the charge has become redistributed between the two capacitors. If the final charge on C_1 is $Q_{1,f}$ then the final charge on C_2 is $Q_{2,f} = Q_{tot} - Q_{1,f}$. Therefore $V = Q_{1,f}/C_1 = Q_{2,f}/C_2 = (Q_{tot} - Q_{1,f})/C_2$. Solving for $Q_{1,f}$ gives $Q_{1,f} = Q_{tot}/4 = 25$ C and $Q_{2,f} = 75$ C.

3. **B** The potential energy is equal to $1/2 \, QV = 1/2 \, (CV)V$. When you add a dielectric, the capacitance gets multiplied by the dielectric constant K, giving $1/2 \, KCV^2$. Therefore, in order to increase the potential energy by a factor of 2, K must be 2 if V is to stay constant.

4. **D** Power can be expressed as $P = V^2/R$. Therefore, begin by determining total resistance of the circuit, R_{TOT}. In this circuit, R_2 and R_3 are connected in series, and are connected in parallel to R_1. R_2 and R_3 can be reduced to $R_{EQ} = R_2 + R_3$. This equivalent resistor connects in parallel to R_1, and can be further reduced to $R_{TOT} = R_1 \, (R_2 + R_3)/(R_1 + R_2 + R_3)$. Use this equation for total resistance in the equation for power to yield $P = V^2/R_{TOT}$, or choice D.

5. **C** Change in electrical potential energy is given by the equation $\Delta PE = qV$. The problem states that there is an energy transfer of 500 megajoules across a potential difference of 20 megavolts. Solving for q yields a charge transfer of 500 MJ / 20 MV, or 25 coulombs. The problem states that the time over which the charge is transferred is 250 msec, or 0.25 seconds. Using the equation $I = Q/t$, the average current can be calculated as 25 coulombs / 0.25 seconds, or 100 amps.

6. **D** Item I is correct because the electrical resistance of a metal wire is inversely proportional to its cross sectional area (choices A and C can be eliminated). Note that since both remaining choices include Item III, Item III must be correct and we only need to evaluate Item II. Item II is also correct. The internal resistance of a voltmeter is very high, and thus adding a voltmeter will increase the resistance of the whole system (choice B can be eliminated and choice D is correct). Item III is in fact correct. According to the formula $R = \rho L/A$, the resistance of the wire is directly proportional to its length L. Therefore, as the length of the wire increases, so does the overall resistance of the system.

7. **B** Item I is false. The voltage is the electromotive force that drives the current through the wire. Therefore, it remains constant and unaffected by the increase in resistance (choices A and C can be eliminated). Note that the remaining choices both include Item II so Item II must be true: according to the equation $V = IR$, when V is constant, the current I is inversely proportional to the resistance R. Item III is false. The power P is expressed by the equation $P = IV$, where I is the current through the wire and V is the voltage that drives the current. Since V stays constant, and I becomes 1/4 of the original value, the power P would be $1/4 \, I \times V = 1/4 \, IV$, which is 1/4 the original power output (choice D is wrong and choice B is correct).

SOLUTIONS TO CHAPTER 10 PRACTICE PASSAGE

1. **A** In Trial 1 along Path 2, the magnitude of each magnetic field can be calculated using Equation 1. Since the current is the same in each wire, and along Path 2 the distance from each wire is the same, then the magnitude of the magnetic field created by each wire is the same. The direction of the magnetic field created by the wires can be found by using the right hand rule. Pointing the thumb of the right hand in the direction of the current (to the right) and curling the fingers around the wire shows the direction of the magnetic field created. Along Path 2, Wire A creates a magnetic field that is into the page. The magnetic field created by Wire B along Path 2 is out of the page. So the magnetic field created by Wire A is equal in magnitude and opposite in direction from the magnetic field created by Wire B, and the net magnetic field along Path 2 is zero. The magnetic force, F, exerted by a magnetic field, B, on a particle moving with velocity, v, and charge q, is calculated as $F = |q|vB \sin \theta$ where θ is the angle between v and B. Since $B = 0$ along Path 2, then $F = 0$. By Newton's second law, $F = ma$ where a is the acceleration. Since $F = 0$ then $a = 0$ and the velocity is constant in both magnitude and direction. Choices C and D are incorrect, since the net force on the marble is zero. Choice B is incorrect because there is no action-reaction pair since all forces are acting on the same object. The correct answer is choice A.

2. **B** In Trial 2 along Path 2, the magnitude of each magnetic field can be calculated using Equation 1. The magnetic field created by Wire A is $\mu_0 i/2\pi r = \mu_0 6/2\pi (0.1) = 30 \ \mu_0/\pi$ and the magnetic field created by Wire B is $\mu_0 i/2\pi r = \mu_0 6(2)/2\pi (0.1) = 60 \ \mu_0/\pi$. The direction of the magnetic field created by the wires can be found by using the right hand rule. Pointing the thumb of the right hand in the direction of the current (to the right) and curling the fingers around the wire shows the direction of the magnetic field created. Along Path 2, Wire A creates a magnetic field that is into the page. The magnetic field created by Wire B along Path 2 is out of the page. Since the magnetic fields created by each wire are in opposite directions, the net field is in the direction of the field with the larger magnitude. The field created by Wire B has the larger magnitude, so the net field is out of the page. This eliminates choices A and C. The magnitude of the net field is the difference in the two magnitudes. So $60 \ \mu_0/\pi - 30 \ \mu_0/\pi = 30 \ \mu_0/\pi$. The correct answer is choice B.

3. **D** The work done by magnetic forces is always zero. The magnetic force on an object is always perpendicular to the velocity of the object. The work done is always calculated by multiplying the force times the distance traveled times the cosine of the angle between them. Since the angle between the force and the distance will always be $90°$, then $\cos 90° = 0$, and the work will always be zero. The correct answer is choice D.

4. **B** The current in a wire can be calculated using $V = IR$ where V is the voltage, I is the current, and R is the resistance. Since the voltage is constant in this case, then the resistance needs to be decreased in order to increase the current. This eliminates choices A and C. In order to increase current by a factor of 2, then the resistance needs to be decreased by a factor of 2. The correct answer is choice B.

5. C   The metal marble is a spherical conductor, and the excess charge will be distributed evenly around the surface of the marble. (Since the metal is a conductor, the charges are free to move. Since the individual negative charges oppose each other, they move to be as far from each other as possible.) With the charges distributed evenly on the surface of the sphere, there is no electric field inside the sphere, eliminating choices A and B. Choice D is false. The correct answer is choice C.

6. C   The direction of the magnetic field created from Wire A is found using the right hand rule: the direction of the magnetic field created by Wire A is out of the page on Path 1, and into the page on Path 2 and Path 3. The direction of the magnetic field created from Wire B is also found using the right hand rule: the direction of the magnetic field created by Wire B is into the page on Path 1 and Path 2, and out of the page on Path 3. On both Path 1 and Path 3, the magnetic fields generated by each wire are in opposite directions from each other, so the net magnetic field direction is determined by the magnetic field with the largest magnitude. Since current is the same in both wires, then, using Equation 1, the magnetic field magnitude is largest where the distance from the wire is least. For Path 1, the magnetic field created from Wire A will have the least distance and so the largest magnitude, therefore the net magnetic field will be out of the page. For Path 3, the magnetic field created from Wire B will have the least distance and so the largest magnitude, therefore the net magnetic field will be out of the page. This information is summarized below.

Path	Direction of Magnetic Field Created by Wire A	Direction of Magnetic Field Created by Wire B	Direction of Net Magnetic Field
1	Out of Page	Into Page	Out of Page
2	Into Page	Into Page	Into Page
3	Into Page	Out of Page	Out of Page

The direction of the magnetic force from the magnetic field on the moving negatively charged marble can be found using the left hand rule (remember e"left"ron so negative charges use the left hand). For Path 1 and Path 3, the magnetic field is out of the page, so the force is up ($\uparrow$). So Items I and III are correct. This eliminates choices A and B. For Path 2, the magnetic field is into the page, so the force is down ($\downarrow$), and Item II is not correct. This eliminates choice D. The correct answer is choice C.

Chapter 11
Oscillations and Waves

11.1 OSCILLATIONS

Any motion that regularly repeats is referred to as **periodic** or **harmonic motion**. Common examples include an object undergoing uniform circular motion, a mass oscillating on a spring and a pendulum. This type of motion can be characterized by its **period** or **frequency**.

Period

The time it takes an object to move through one full cycle of motion is called the period. For an object undergoing uniform circular motion, the period is the time it takes to make one revolution. For a mass on a spring or a pendulum, it is the time it takes to make a round trip (i.e., the final position and velocity must be the same as the initial values). The period is denoted by T and is measured in seconds.

Example 11-1: The bob on a pendulum moves from point A to point B in 0.5 seconds. What is the period of oscillation?

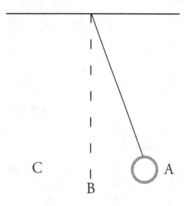

Solution: A to B represents one-quarter of a period. A full period is the time it takes for the bob to move from A to B to C to B and back to A. So $T = 4(0.5 \text{ s}) = 2 \text{ s}$.

Frequency

Rather than timing one cycle to find the period, we can instead count the number of cycles that occur in one second. This is known as the frequency, denoted by f. The units of f are cycles per second, or **hertz** (Hz).

Now the first thing we notice is that period and frequency are reciprocals. After all, the period is "the number of seconds per cycle," and the frequency is "the number of cycles per second." So, we have these fundamental relationships:

Period and Frequency

$$f = \frac{1}{T} \quad \text{and} \quad T = \frac{1}{f}$$

Every type of oscillation has a period and a frequency, but there is a special class of oscillations in which these quantities have a unique property. This "ideal" type of oscillatory motion is referred to as **simple harmonic motion** (often abbreviated SHM). A mass oscillating on a spring exhibits SHM.

The spring in the series of diagrams below is fixed at its left end and has a block attached to its right end. When the spring is neither stretched nor compressed (i.e., when it's at its natural length, as shown in Diagram 1 below) we say the spring is at its **equilibrium position**. In general, the point at which the net force on the block is zero, which in this case is when the spring is at its natural length, is called the equilibrium position, and we label it $x = 0$.

Now, imagine that we stretch the spring (Diagram 1 to Diagram 2), and let go. Once released, the spring pulls back to the left, going through its equilibrium position and then to the point of maximum compression. From here, the spring pushes back to the right, passing again through its equilibrium position, and returning to the point of maximum extension. If friction is negligible, this back-and-forth motion will continue indefinitely, and the time it takes for the block to go through one period, for example, from Diagram 2 to Diagram 6, is a constant.

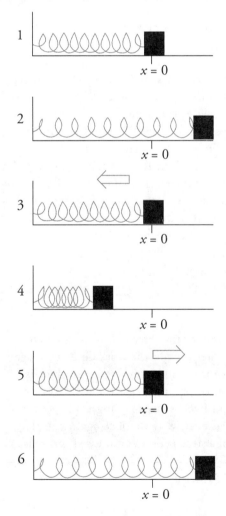

The Dynamics of SHM

Force

Let's first describe the motion of the block attached to the spring from the point of view of the force it feels. The spring exerts a force on the block that's proportional to its displacement. If we call the equilibrium position $x = 0$, then the force exerted by the spring is given by

> **Hooke's Law**
>
> $$\mathbf{F} = -k\mathbf{x}$$

The proportionality constant, k, called the **spring constant**, tells us how strong the spring is; the greater the value of k, the stiffer (and stronger) the spring.

As we can see from Hooke's Law, the units of k are newton/meter. Since a meter is a large distance to stretch or compression a spring, the values for k are often large.

What is the role of the minus sign in Hooke's law? Look back at the diagrams on the previous page. Since we're calling the equilibrium position $x = 0$, when the block is to the right of equilibrium, its position, x, is positive. At this point, the stretched spring wants to pull back to the left; because the direction of the force of the spring is to the left, we indicate this direction by calling it negative. Similarly, when the block is to the left of equilibrium, its position, x, is negative. At this point, the compressed spring wants to push back to the right; because the direction of the force of the spring is to the right, we indicate this direction by calling it positive. We see that the direction of the spring force is always directed opposite to its displacement from equilibrium, and for this reason, the minus sign is needed in Hooke's law. Furthermore, because the spring is always trying to restore the block to equilibrium, we say that spring provides the **restoring force**; it's this force that maintains the oscillations. The fact that the restoring force exerted by the spring obeys Hooke's Law (i.e., the force is directly proportional to the distance from equilibrium) is the reason why the block undergoes simple harmonic motion.

Energy

Unfortunately, knowing an equation for the force doesn't allow us to solve directly for other things, such as the speed of the block at some later time or the work done by or against the spring: The force changes as the block moves, so acceleration is not uniform. However, there is a way to figure out these quantities by using energy. When we pull on the spring to get the oscillations started, we're exerting a force over a distance; that is, we're doing work. Because we're doing work against the spring, the spring stores potential energy, called **elastic potential energy**. If we once again call the equilibrium position of the spring $x = 0$, then the potential energy of a stretched or compressed spring is given by this equation:

> **Elastic Potential Energy**
>
> $$PE_{\text{elastic}} = \tfrac{1}{2}kx^2$$

It follows that $W_{\text{by spring}} = -\Delta PE_{\text{elastic}}$ and $W_{\text{against spring}} = \Delta PE_{\text{elastic}}$. To justify this, imagine an external force is stretching a spring from $x = 0$ to $x = X$. The minimum force required to do this is opposite the spring force: $+kx$. From mechanics, we learned that the work done by a variable force is equal to the area under the force vs. position graph.

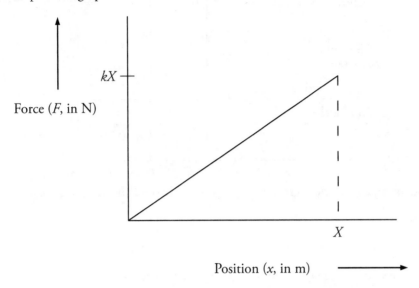

The area under curve is the area of a triangle with base equal to X and height equal to kX. So $PE = W_{\text{against spring}} = (1/2)bh = (1/2)(X)(kX) = (1/2)kX^2$.

We can also use conservation of energy to find the speed of a oscillating mass on a spring at any given position.

When we release the block from rest in Diagram 2 from page 383, the spring is stretched and the block isn't moving, so all the energy is in the form of elastic potential energy. This potential energy turns into kinetic energy, until at $x = 0$ (equilibrium), all the energy has been converted to kinetic energy. As the block rushes past equilibrium, this kinetic energy gradually turns back into elastic potential energy until the point where the spring is at maximum compression and it's all transformed back to potential energy. The compressed spring then pushes outward, converting its potential energy back to kinetic; the block rushes through equilibrium again, and kinetic energy is transformed back to potential energy, until it reaches its starting point (Diagram 6 from page 381) at maximum extension. At this instant, we're back to our full reserve of elastic potential energy (and no kinetic energy), and the process is ready to repeat.

As a result, we can look at the motion of the block from the point of view of the back-and-forth transfer between elastic potential energy and kinetic energy.

The maximum displacement of the block from equilibrium is called the **amplitude**, denoted by A. This positive number tells us how far to the left and right of equilibrium the block will travel. So, in the series of diagrams above, the block's position at maximum extension is $x = +A$, and its position at maximum compression is $x = -A$.

We can summarize the dynamics of the oscillations in this table:

	at $x = -A$	at $x = 0$	at $x = +A$
magnitude of restoring force	max	0	max
magnitude of acceleration	max	0	max
$PE_{elastic}$ of spring	max	0	max
KE of block	0	max	0
speed (v) of block	0	max	0

Because we're ignoring any frictional forces during the oscillations of the block, total mechanical energy will be conserved. That is, the sum of the block's kinetic energy, $\frac{1}{2}mv^2$, and the spring's potential energy, $\frac{1}{2}kx^2$, will be a constant. We can use this fact to figure out the maximum speed of the block. At the instant the block is passing through equilibrium, all the potential energy of the spring has been transformed into kinetic energy of the block. If the amplitude of the oscillations is A, then the maximum elastic potential energy, $\frac{1}{2}kA^2$ (the value of $\frac{1}{2}kx^2$ when $x = \pm A$), is completely converted to maximum kinetic energy at $x = 0$. This gives us:

$$PE_{elastic,\ max} \rightarrow KE_{max}$$

$$\tfrac{1}{2}kA^2 = \tfrac{1}{2}mv^2$$

$$\therefore v_{max} = A\sqrt{\frac{k}{m}}$$

Example 11-2: A block of mass m attached to a spring with constant k oscillates horizontally on a frictionless surface with amplitude A. In which case does the spring do more work, moving the mass from $x = A$ to $x = A/2$ or from $x = A/2$ to $x = 0$?

Solution: In both cases the spring does positive work, since the restoring force is in the same direction as the motion of the block. Since the force is not constant, we cannot use the formula $W = Fd\cos\theta$. Instead, the work done by the spring is given by $W = -\Delta PE_{elastic} = -(PE_{final} - PE_{initial})$.

From $x = A$ to x to $A/2$:

$$W = -(\frac{1}{2}k[A/2]^2 - \frac{1}{2}kA^2) = -(\frac{1}{8}kA^2 - \frac{1}{2}kA^2) = \frac{3}{8}kA^2$$

From $x = A/2$ to $x = 0$:

$$W = -(\frac{1}{2}k[0]^2 - \frac{1}{2}k[A/2]^2) = -(0 - \frac{1}{8}kA^2) = \frac{1}{8}kA^2$$

Notice that even though the distance travelled is the same in each case, the average force exerted by the spring is greater from $x = A$ to $x = A/2$ than it is from $x = A/2$ to $x = 0$, and therefore the work done by the spring is also greater.

Example 11-3: A block of mass 200 g is oscillating on the end of a horizontal spring of spring constant 100 N/m and natural length 12 cm. When the spring is stretched to a length of 14 cm, what is the acceleration of the block?

Solution: When the spring is stretched by 2 cm, Hooke's law tells us that the force exerted by the spring has a magnitude of $F = kx = (100$ N/m$)(0.02$ m$) = 2$ N. Therefore, by Newton's second law, the acceleration of the block will have a magnitude of $a = F/m = (2$ N$)/(0.2$ kg$) = 10$ m/s^2.

Example 11-4: If the block in Example 11-3 above were replaced with a block of mass 800 g, how would its maximum speed change?

Solution: The equation derived above, $v_{max} = A\sqrt{k/m}$, tells us that v_{max} is inversely proportional to the square root of the mass of the oscillator. Therefore, if m increases by a factor of 4, v_{max} will decrease by a factor of 2.

The Kinematics of SHM

Earlier it was mentioned that a mass oscillating on a spring exhibits "ideal" oscillatory motion, which is called simple harmonic motion, and that this motion is the result of Hooke's Law (i.e., the restoring force is directly proportional to the distance from equilibrium). But what makes this motion different than non-ideal oscillations? It turns out (using calculus) that the frequency and period only depend on the spring constant, k, and the mass of the block, m.

$$f = \frac{1}{2\pi}\sqrt{\frac{k}{m}} \quad \text{and} \quad T = 2\pi\sqrt{\frac{m}{k}}$$

Notice that neither f nor T depends on A, the amplitude. This is why we call the motion of the block on the spring *simple* harmonic motion. This is not an obvious statement. If a mass on a spring is pulled back 1 cm or pulled back 10 cm (assuming the spring is still within its elastic limit), the time it takes to complete one cycle is exactly the same. As an example of an oscillating system that does not exhibit simple harmonic motion, imaging a ball bouncing. Removing air resistance and assuming that the bounces are completely elastic, the ball will continue to bounce to the same height from which it was released. However, dropping the ball from 1 cm will take less time to fall and rise than dropping it from 10 cm (which can be proven with the Big 5 equations).

It's possible for a system to oscillate because of a restoring force that is not directly proportional to the displacement. If this were the case, the frequency and period would depend on the amplitude; we'd still call the motion *harmonic*, which just means back-and-forth, but we wouldn't call it *simple* harmonic.

Example 11-5: Suppose that the block shown in the series of diagrams on the first page of this chapter requires 0.25 sec to move from Diagram 4 to Diagram 6. What is the frequency of the oscillations?

Solution: The interval from Diagram 4 to Diagram 6 represents *half* a cycle, which requires *half* a period to complete. If half a period is 0.25 sec, then the period is 0.5 sec. Therefore, the frequency, f, is $1/T = 1/(0.5 \text{ s}) = 2$ Hz.

So far we have examined the simple harmonic motion of a mass on a horizontal spring, where the system is in equilibrium when the spring is at its rest length. If the spring is now rotated so that it is suspended vertically and a mass is attached, will the oscillations still be simple harmonic? The answer is yes. The formulas for period and frequency are exactly the same. The force of gravity, however, does affect the situation. The weight of the block will naturally stretch the spring so that equilibrium ($F_{net} = 0$) no longer occurs when the spring is at its rest length. The new equilibrium position is when the upward force of the spring exactly balances the weight: $kx = mg$. When the spring is stretched beyond this point and released, the mass will oscillate around the new equilibrium position. It is often convenient to rename the new equilibrium position $x = 0$. This enables us to "ignore gravity". In other words, measuring x from equilibrium instead of measuring from the rest length of the spring, it becomes exactly like a horizontal spring, but with a longer rest length. We can therefore still use the equations

$$-kx = ma \text{ and } v_{max} = A\sqrt{\frac{k}{m}}$$

Pendulums

Besides the spring-block simple harmonic oscillator, there's another oscillator that the MCAT will expect you to know about: the simple pendulum. If the connecting rod or string between the suspension point and the object at the end of a pendulum has negligible mass (so that all the mass is in the object at the end of the rod or string), and if there is no friction at the suspension point during oscillation, we say the pendulum is a **simple pendulum**.

The displacement of the mass is not taken as a distance from equilibrium (as in the spring-block case), but rather as the angle it makes with the vertical. The vertical (shown as a dashed line in the figure below) is the equilibrium position, $\theta = 0$. The restoring force here is gravity; specifically, it's equal to $mg \sin \theta$, which is the component of the object's weight in the direction toward equilibrium.

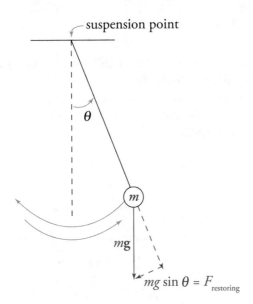

Strictly speaking, a pendulum does not undergo simple harmonic motion because the restoring force is not proportional to the displacement ($mg \sin \theta$ is not exactly proportional to θ). However, if the angle is small, then $\sin \theta \approx \theta$ (in radians), so the restoring force can be approximated as $mg\,\theta$, which is proportional to θ.[1] In this case, we can treat the motion as simple harmonic, and the frequency and period are given by the following equations:

$$f = \frac{1}{2\pi}\sqrt{\frac{g}{l}} \text{ and } T = 2\pi\sqrt{\frac{l}{g}}$$

where l is the length of the pendulum and g is the acceleration due to gravity. Observe that in the case of simple harmonic motion of a simple pendulum, the mass of the swinging object does not affect the frequency or period of oscillation.

Example 11-6: The bob (mass = m) of a simple pendulum is raised to a height h above its lowest point and released. Find an expression for the maximum speed of the pendulum.

Solution: When the bob is at height h above its lowest point, it has gravitational potential energy equal to mgh (relative to its lowest point). As it passes through the equilibrium position, all this potential energy is converted to kinetic energy. Therefore, $mgh = \frac{1}{2}mv_{max}^2$, and we get $v_{max} = \sqrt{2gh}$. This is the speed of the bob as it passes through equilibrium, which is where it attains its maximum speed.

---

[1] The conversion between degrees and radians is as follows: 180 degrees = π radians. If the angle is given in degrees, the restoring force is approximately $mg\,\theta(\pi/180°)$, which is still proportional to θ.

11.2 WAVES

A **mechanical wave** is a series of disturbances (i.e., oscillations) within a medium that transfers energy from one place to another. The medium itself is not transported, just the energy. Examples included a vibrating string or sound. Mechanical waves cannot exist without a medium. In a later chapter we will discuss **electromagnetic waves**, which do not need a medium. This is because the electric and magnetic fields oscillate rather than physical matter.

Transverse Waves

Perhaps the simplest example of wave is one we can create by wiggling one end of a long rope:

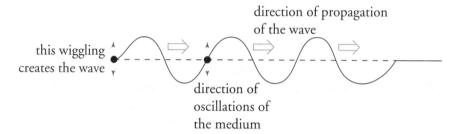

This wave uses the rope as the medium, traveling from one end to the other. Notice that the wave is moving horizontally, but the rope itself is moving up and down. That's why this is called a **transverse** wave: The wave travels (propagates) in a direction that's *perpendicular* to the direction in which the medium is vibrating.

Frequency and Period

The most fundamental characteristic of a wave is its frequency. If we pick a spot on the rope and count how many times it moves up and down (the number of round trips it makes) in one second, we've just measured the **frequency**, f, which we express in hertz (cycles per second).

The **period** of a wave, T, is the reciprocal of the frequency, and is the amount of time it takes any spot on the rope to complete one cycle (in this case, one up-and-down round trip).

These definitions for frequency and period are same as for a mass on a spring or a pendulum. Each particle of rope oscillates up and down with simple harmonic motion. However, we can also think of the frequency and period of a wave in a different way. Instead of focusing on the oscillations, we can observe "pulses" moving the right. Frequency can be thought as the number of pulses that pass a given point per unit time and period is the time it takes between pulses.

Wavelength and Amplitude

The figure below identifies the **crests** (**peaks**) and **troughs** of the wave. The distance from one crest to the next (i.e., the length of one cycle of the wave) is called the **wavelength**, denoted by λ, the Greek letter lambda. We can also measure the wavelength by measuring the distance from one trough to the next, or, in fact, between any two consecutive corresponding points along the wave.

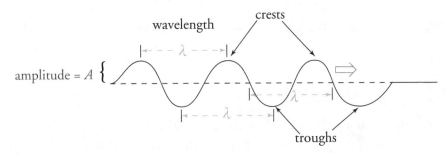

The **amplitude** of a wave, A, is the maximum displacement from equilibrium that any point in the medium makes as the wave goes by. In the case of a wave on a rope, the amplitude is the distance from the original horizontal position of the rope up to a crest; it's also the distance from the horizontal position down to a trough.

Wave Speed

To figure out how fast the wave travels, we just notice that the wave travels a distance of λ in time T; that is, λ is the length of one wave cycle, and T, the period, is the time required for one wave cycle to go by. Since distance = rate × time, we get $\lambda = vT$. Solving this for v gives us $\lambda(1/T) = v$ and since $f = 1/T$, the equation becomes $v = \lambda f$. *This is the most important equation for waves and one of the most important equations for the MCAT.*

> **Wave Equation**
> $$v = \lambda f$$

Two Big Rules for Waves

Notice that the second equation for the wave speed shows that v does not depend on f (or λ). While this may seem to contradict the first equation, $v = \lambda f$, it really doesn't. The speed of the wave depends on the characteristics of the rope: how tense it is, and what it's made of. We can wiggle the end at any frequency we want, and the speed of the wave we create will be a constant. However, because $\lambda f = v$ must always be true, a higher f will mean a shorter λ (and a lower f will mean a longer λ). Thus, changing f doesn't change v: It changes λ. This brings up our first big rule for waves:

> **Big Rule 1:** The speed of a wave is determined by the type of wave and the characteristics of the medium, *not* by the frequency.

For example, the speed of a transverse wave on a rope is given by:

$$v = \sqrt{\frac{\text{tension}}{\text{linear density}}}$$

The linear density of a rope is its mass per unit length. Notice that the tension and linear density are properties of the medium, and that this equation is independent of wave properties of frequency, wavelength, and amplitude.

Note that two different types of wave can move with different speeds through the same medium; for example, sound and light move through air with very different speeds. There are exceptions to Big Rule 1, but the only one the MCAT will expect you to know about is *dispersion*, which is discussed in Chapter 13, on Optics. Any other exception would be discussed in the passage; otherwise, you can assume the rule applies.

Our second big rule for waves concerns what happens when a wave passes from one medium into another. Because wave speed is determined by the characteristics of the medium, a change in the medium implies a change in wave speed, but the frequency won't change.

> **Big Rule 2:** When a wave passes into another medium, its speed changes, but its frequency does *not*.

The reasoning behind this makes sense if you focus on a wave as a series of pulses. Frequency is the number of pulses that pass by per unit time. It stands to reason that, if a certain number of pulses per second arrives at the boundary between two different media, then the same number of pulses per second must leave, passing into the new medium. In other words, rate in = rate out. This is similar to the Equation of Continuity in fluids and the rule for electric current passing through resistors in series.

Because f is constant, Rule 2 tells us that the wavelength is proportional to wave speed.

Notice that Rule 1 applies to different waves in one medium, while Rule 2 applies to a single wave in different media. Memorize these rules. The MCAT loves waves.

Example 11-7: A transverse wave of frequency 4 Hz travels at a speed of 6 m/s along a rope. What would be the speed of a 12 Hz wave along this same rope?

Solution: Big Rule 1 for waves says that the speed of a wave is determined by the type of wave and the characteristics of the medium, not by the frequency. If all we do is change the frequency, the wave speed will not change: The wave speed will still be 6 m/s. (What *will* change? The wavelength. Because $\lambda = v/f$, a change in f with no change in v will change λ.)

Example 11-8: Which one of the following statements is true concerning the amplitude of a wave?

   A. Amplitude increases with increasing frequency.
   B. Amplitude increases with increasing wavelength.
   C. Amplitude increases with increasing wave speed.
   D. None of the above.

Solution: The amplitude is determined by how much energy we put into the wave to get it started. If we wiggle the rope up and down through a large distance (a large amplitude), this takes more energy on our part, and as a result, the wave carries more energy. However, the amplitude doesn't depend on f, λ, or v. The answer is D.

Example 11-9: A wave of frequency 12 Hz has a wavelength of 3 m. What is the speed of this wave?

Solution: Using the equation $v = \lambda f$, we find that $v = (3 \text{ m})(12 \text{ Hz}) = 36 \text{ m/s}$.

Example 11-10: An electrocardiogram responds to changes in the electric potential of the heart from a number of different angles and distances, and represents a different pair combinations of these signals (voltages) as deflections of several needles under which runs graph paper moving horizontally at a constant speed. Suppose a patient has a resting heart rate of 60 beats per minute and the tape runs through the machine at 4 cm/s. What is the wavelength over which the pattern should repeat?

Solution: 60 beats/min = 1 beat/s, or a period of 1s and frequency of 1 Hz. The wave speed, v, is simply the speed at which the tape runs under the needle: $v = 4$ cm/s. Thus $\lambda = v/f = 4$ cm/s / 1 Hz = 4 cm.

Example 11-11: What happens when the wave shown below passes from the thick, heavy rope into the thinner, lighter rope?

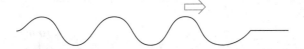

Solution: According to Big Rule 2 for waves, when a wave passes into another medium, its speed changes, but its frequency does not. How does the speed change? Because the rope is lighter (i.e., it has a lower linear density), the equation for wave speed on a string (given above) tells us that v will *increase*. So, if v increases but f doesn't change, then λ will also increase because $\lambda = v/f$.

Example 11-12: A certain rope transmits a 2 Hz transverse wave of amplitude 10 cm with a speed of 1 m/s. What would be the wavelength of a 5 Hz transverse wave of amplitude 8 cm on this same rope?

Solution: First, ignore the amplitudes; they're included in the question only to make things seem more complicated than they are. The amplitude of a wave indicates how much energy the wave transports, but it has nothing to do with wavelength, period, frequency, or wave speed (recall Example 11-8 above). Now, if a

2 Hz transverse wave has a speed of 1 m/s on this rope, then a transverse wave of *any* frequency will have a speed of 1 m/s on this rope; that's what Big Rule 1 for waves tells us. Thus, if f = 5 Hz and v = 1 m/s, then

$$\lambda = \frac{v}{f} = \frac{1 \, \text{m/s}}{5 \, \text{Hz}} = 0.2 \, \text{m}$$

Example 11-13: How long will it take a wave of wavelength λ and period T to travel a distance d?

A. $\lambda T d$

B. $\dfrac{\lambda d}{T}$

C. $\dfrac{T d}{\lambda}$

D. $\dfrac{\lambda T}{d}$

Solution: First, let's see if we can eliminate any choices because the units don't work out correctly. We're being asked for an amount of time, so the answer must have the dimension (and units) of time. Choice A can't be correct, since it has units of $[\lambda][T][d]$ = m·sec·m = m²·sec. Notice that both λ and d have units of meters, which we don't want in the answer, so these units must cancel. Therefore, B can't be correct either since λ and d are multiplied by each other, rather than being divided as they should to make their units cancel.

One difference between the two remaining choices is that in C, the distance d is in the numerator, while in D, the distance d is in the denominator. Now, let's think about this: More time will be required for the wave to travel a greater distance. In other words, the bigger d is, the greater the travel time should be. Therefore, we can eliminate D; after all, since d is in the denominator in choice D, a larger d will result in a smaller amount of time, which doesn't make sense. Thus, the answer must be C.

Here's an alternate solution using equations. Because *distance* = *speed* × *time* ($d = vt$), we know that $t = d/v$. We can find v using the wave equation $v = \lambda f$, and since $f = 1/T$, we find that

$$t = \frac{d}{v} = \frac{d}{\lambda f} = \frac{d}{\lambda} \cdot \frac{1}{f} = \frac{d}{\lambda} \cdot T = \frac{T d}{\lambda}$$

The answer is indeed C, just as we figured out by checking units and using logic.

11.3 INTERFERENCE OF WAVES

When two or more waves are superimposed on each other, they will combine to form a single resultant wave. This is called **interference**. The amplitude of the resultant wave will depend on the amplitudes of the combining waves *and* on how these waves travel relative to each other.

If crest meets crest, and trough meets trough, we say that the waves are **in phase** with each other. Their amplitudes will *add*, and we say the waves interfere **constructively**. However, if the crest of one wave coincides with the *trough* of the other (and vice versa), we say that the waves are exactly **out of phase** with each other. In this case, their amplitudes *subtract*, and we say that the waves interfere **destructively**.

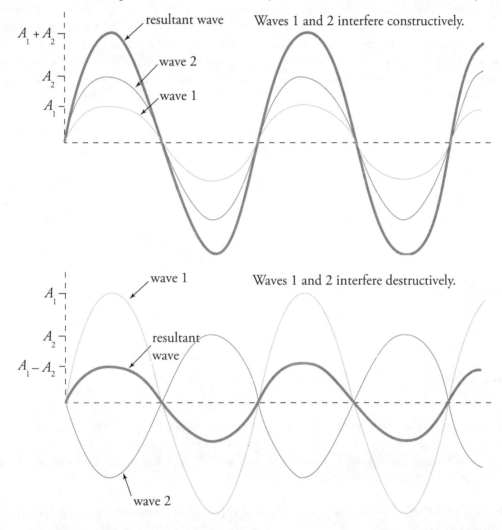

A passage might also say that waves that are directly opposite each other in amplitude are *180 degrees out of phase*, or *π radians out of phase*; it is common to refer to a whole cycle or wave as being 360 degrees or 2π radians, as if it were a circle. If the waves aren't exactly in phase (0°, 360°, or 2π radians) or exactly out of phase (180° or π radians), the amplitude of the resultant wave will be somewhere between the difference and the sum of the amplitudes of the interfering waves.

The interfering waves may also have different wavelengths. These waves will produce a more complicated-looking resultant wave, but we'd still say the waves interfere constructively where they reinforce each other, and destructively where they tend to cancel each other out.

The preceding pictures of waves that are in phase and out of phase can also be thought of graphs representing the displacement at a fixed location as a function of time. As example, imagine a cork floating in calm water. Source 1 creates a wave, which travels through the water, causing the cork to bob up and down. A graph of the cork's motion as a function of time would be sinusoidal (i.e., it looks like a Wave 1 in the picture except that the distance from maximum to maximum is the period rather than the wavelength).

Similarly, if Source 2 were acting alone, Wave 2 would cause the cork to bob up and down. The graph of this motion as a function of time would look similar to the picture of Wave 2. If Wave 1 and Wave 2 both arrive at the cork, they will interfere. If the waves are in phase when they arrive at the cork (i.e., crests arrive at the same time, troughs arrive at the same time, etc.) or if they are 180° out of phase when they arrive at the cork (i.e., the crest of one wave arrives simultaneously with the trough of the other), the graph of the cork's motion as a function of time would like the resultant waves in the picture. Note that if the waves have different frequencies (and wavelengths), then the graph of the cork's motion will not look like a sine or cosine, but will be more complicated. An example of this is **beats**, which are discussed in the next chapter.

Be careful on the MCAT. If you see a picture of a sine or cosine, make sure you can determine whether it is an actual wave (pictured at a fixed time), or a graph of one particle's motion as a function of time.

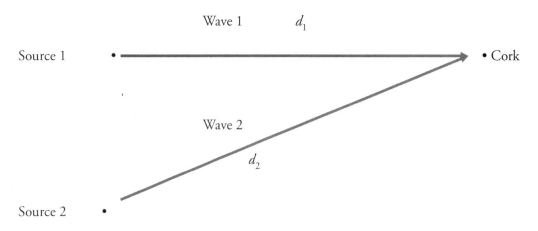

How can you determine whether two waves are in phase, 180° out of phase or something in between? One way is to look at *path difference*. In the above picture, imagine Source 1 and Source 2 emit identical waves that are exactly in phase. Just because they are initially in phase does not mean they will be in phase when they arrive at the cork. The reason is because Wave 2 had to travel a larger distance than Wave 1. The path difference = $d_2 - d_1$. The general rule is:

- If the path difference = $n\lambda$ and, ($n = 0, 1, 2, \ldots$), the waves will be in phase and will therefore constructively interfere.
- If the path difference = $(n + \frac{1}{2})\lambda$, the waves will be 180° out of phase and will therefore destructively interfere.

If Wave 2 travels an integer number of wavelengths farther than Wave 1, the crests from each will still arrive at the same time. If Wave 2 travels $\lambda/2$, $3\lambda/2$, $5\lambda/2$, etc. farther than Wave 1, the crest from one wave will arrive simultaneously with a trough from the other wave. Note that if the cork in the picture experiences constructive interference, it does not mean than neighboring corks will. The distance from the sources to the other corks would be different. An example of this is Young's Double-Slit experiment, where the two sources are small holes in a screen emitting light that is in phase. On the opposite wall is a screen that features alternating bright and dark fringes. Bright fringes are the result of constructive interference and dark fringes are the result of destructive interference. They alternate, since the path difference changes as you move up or down the screen.

11.4 STANDING WAVES

Let's say that we have a long rope with one end in our fingers and the other end attached to a wall. We wiggle the rope up and down at a certain frequency, f, and create waves of frequency f that travel down the length of the rope. When they hit the wall, they'll be reflected. We now have two waves on the same rope (the wave we continue to generate plus the reflected wave) with the same frequency and amplitude but traveling in opposite directions. These waves will interfere. If the frequency is just right, the resulting wave seems to stand still; the rope continues to vibrate up and down, but the resultant wave no longer travels. The combination of these traveling waves produces a **standing wave**, with the horizontal positions of the crests and troughs remaining fixed.

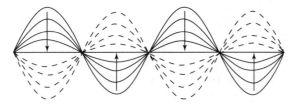

Notice that each point along the rope has its own amplitude. Some points don't vibrate up and down at all; these points are called **nodes** (points of <u>no</u> displacement). Halfway between any two consecutive nodes are points where the amplitude is maximized; these positions are called **antinodes**. Every other point has an amplitude that's smaller than the amplitude at the antinode positions.

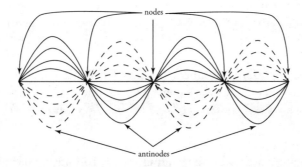

To figure out the conditions under which a standing wave will be formed, we'll look at the three simplest standing waves. In the figure at the top of the next page, we have a rope of length L. The first picture shows the simplest standing wave that can form if we have nodes at the two ends; the second and third pictures show the next simplest standing waves that the rope could support.

The distance between any two consecutive nodes is always one-half of the wavelength. The first picture shows us that one of these half-wavelengths is equal to L; in the second picture, two half-wavelengths are equal to L; and in the third picture, three half-wavelengths are equal to L.

11.4

Notice the pattern that emerges relating the length of the rope and the wavelength of the standing wave.

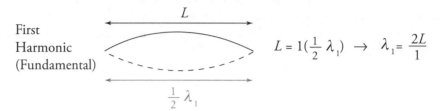

First
Harmonic
(Fundamental)

$$L = 1(\tfrac{1}{2}\lambda_1) \rightarrow \lambda_1 = \frac{2L}{1}$$

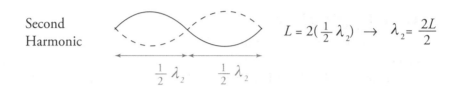

Second
Harmonic

$$L = 2(\tfrac{1}{2}\lambda_2) \rightarrow \lambda_2 = \frac{2L}{2}$$

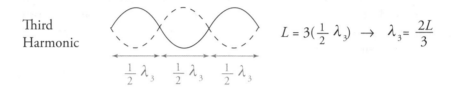

Third
Harmonic

$$L = 3(\tfrac{1}{2}\lambda_3) \rightarrow \lambda_3 = \frac{2L}{3}$$

Standing-Wave Wavelengths for Two Fixed Ends

$$\lambda_n = \frac{2L}{n} \quad \text{where} \quad n = 1, 2, 3\ldots$$

The only standing waves that can be supported are those for which the length of the rope is equal to a whole number of half-wavelengths, so the wavelength must be twice the length of the rope divided by a whole number:

The number n is called the **harmonic number**. The first harmonic is usually called the **fundamental** because once we know the **fundamental wavelength**, λ_1, we automatically know all the other harmonic wavelengths, because we can write λ_n in terms of λ_1, like this: $\lambda_n = \lambda_1/n$.

Because the equation $v = \lambda f$ must always be true, and only certain wavelengths are allowed for a standing wave, then only certain frequencies will give standing waves. To find the harmonic frequencies, we just write $\lambda_n f_n = v$, and solve for f_n:

Standing-Wave Frequencies for Two Fixed Ends

$$f_n = \frac{n}{2L}v \quad \text{where} \quad n = 1, 2, 3\ldots$$

In the same way that the fundamental wavelength can be used to figure out all the other harmonic wavelengths, the fundamental frequency can be used to figure out all the other harmonic frequencies: $f_n = nf_1$. Memorizing this equation is helpful for the MCAT.

It is possible to create standing waves with only one fixed end (node) and one non-fixed end (antinode), but the appropriate formulas to find frequency and wavelength for this situation are discussed in Chapter 12. Regardless of the type of standing wave, the formula to find the appropriate harmonic from the fundamental frequency still holds ($f_n = nf_1$).

Example 11-14: If a rope of length 6 m supports a standing wave with exactly four nodes (which includes the ends of the rope), what is the wavelength of the standing wave?

Solution: Draw the standing wave. It should look just like the third harmonic drawn on the previous page. Therefore, the wavelength is $\lambda_3 = 2L/3 = 2(6 \text{ m})/3 = 4$ m.

Example 11-15: The speed of a transverse traveling wave along a certain 4-meter-long rope is 24 m/s. Which of the following frequencies could cause a standing wave to form on this rope, assuming both ends of the rope are fixed?

- A. 32 Hz
- B. 33 Hz
- C. 34 Hz
- D. 35 Hz

Solution: The fundamental frequency for this rope is $f_1 = (1/2L)v = 3$ Hz. All harmonic frequencies are whole-number multiples of the fundamental, so any frequency that could cause a standing wave to form on the rope must be a multiple of 3 Hz. Of the choices given, only choice B, 33 Hz, is a multiple of 3 Hz.

Example 11-16: For a particular rope, it's found that the fundamental frequency is 6 Hz. What's the third-harmonic frequency?

Solution: From the equation $f_n = nf_1$, we get $f_3 = 3f_1 = 3(6 \text{ Hz}) = 18$ Hz.

Example 11-17: For a particular rope, it's found that the second-harmonic frequency is 8 Hz. What's the fifth-harmonic frequency?

Solution: The equation $f_n = nf_1$ gives us $f_2 = 2f_1$. This means that $f_1 = f_2/2 = (8 \text{ Hz})/2 = 4$ Hz. Therefore, $f_5 = 5f_1 = 5(4 \text{ Hz}) = 20$ Hz.

Example 11-18: The second-harmonic wavelength for a rope fixed at both ends is 0.5 m. How fast do transverse waves travel along this rope if the fundamental frequency is 4 Hz?

Solution: Using the equation $\lambda_n = \lambda_1/n$, we get $\lambda_2 = \lambda_1/2$. This means that $\lambda_1 = 2\lambda_2 = 2(0.5 \text{ m}) = 1$ m. Now, multiplying any harmonic wavelength by its corresponding harmonic frequency will give us the wave speed. In particular, we have $v = \lambda_1 f_1$, so $v = (1 \text{ m})(4 \text{ Hz}) = 4$ m/s.

Summary of Formulas

Simple Harmonic Motion (SHM) requires:

- dynamics condition: restoring force is directly proportional to displacement from equilibrium ($x = 0$) and points towards that equilibrium point

- kinematics condition: frequency and period are independent of the amplitude of oscillations

Hooke's law (spring): $F = -kx$

Elastic potential energy (spring): $PE_{elastic} = \frac{1}{2}kx^2$

Spring-block oscillator frequency: $f = \dfrac{1}{2\pi}\sqrt{\dfrac{k}{m}}$

Simple pendulum frequency (small oscillations): $f = \dfrac{1}{2\pi}\sqrt{\dfrac{g}{l}}$

Period/frequency
(all harmonic motion and waves): $T = 1/f$

Wave equation: $v = \lambda f$

Two Big Rules for Waves to be used with wave equation:

1) Wave speed v depends on wave type and the medium, not on frequency

2) A single wave passing between media maintains a constant frequency

Standing wave on a rope (both ends fixed nodes)

Standing-wave wavelengths: $\lambda_n = \dfrac{2L}{n}$ $(n = 1, 2, 3, \ldots)$

$\lambda_n = \dfrac{\lambda_1}{n}$

Standing-wave frequencies: $f_n = \dfrac{n}{2L}\,v$ $(n = 1, 2, 3, \ldots)$

$f_n = nf_1$

CHAPTER 11 FREESTANDING PRACTICE QUESTIONS

1. A 2 kg mass is attached to a massless, 0.5 m string and is used as a simple pendulum by extending it to an angle $\theta = 5°$ and allowing it to oscillate. Which of the following changes will increase the period of the pendulum?

A) Replacing the mass with a 1 kg mass
B) Changing the initial extension of the pendulum to a 10° angle
C) Replacing the string with a 0.25 m string
D) Moving the pendulum to the surface of the moon

2. A 100 kg bungee jumper attached to a bungee cord jumps off a bridge. The bungee cord stretches and the man reaches the lowest spot in his descent before beginning to rise. The force of the stretched bungee cord can be approximated using Hooke's law, where the value of the spring constant is replaced by an elasticity constant, in this case, 100 kg/s^2. If the cord is stretched by 30 m beyond its vertical equilibrium length at the lowest spot of the man's descent, then what his acceleration at the lowest spot?

A) 0 m/s^2
B) 10 m/s^2
C) 20 m/s^2
D) 30 m/s^2

3. A physics student is doing a wave experiment with a 1 m long cord stretched across the lab table. In the middle of the cord, a 1 cm section is painted red. A specially designed machine creates vibrations so that a sine wave will travel on the cord from the east side of the table to the west side of the table. The vibrations of the sine wave are parallel to the table and peak at the north side of the table and the south side of the table. Which of the following best describes the motion of the red spot?

A) The spot moves from east to west along the sine wave.
B) The spot moves from west to east along the sine wave.
C) The spot remains in a fixed location on the table.
D) The spot vibrates between the north side and south side of the table.

4. A parent is pushing a young child on a swing at the playground. When the parent stops pushing, the child's swinging motion continues without assistance. Assume the chain on the swing has negligible mass and any friction is negligible. Which of the following would need to be true in order for the child's motion on the swing to be considered simple harmonic motion?

I. The mass of the child is not too large
II. The child is not swinging too high, so the angle between the swing and the vertical is not too big
III. The tension in the chain of the swing is negligible

A) I only
B) II only
C) I and III
D) I, II, and III

5. Immediately before a performance, a musician breaks a guitar string. The only string available to repair the guitar is twice the linear density of the string normally used. How can the musician adjust the new string so that it will still have the correct frequency? (Note: $v = (\text{Tension}/\mu)^{0.5}$, where μ = linear mass density.)

A) The tension of the new string should be twice the tension of the old string.
B) The tension of the new string should be half the tension of the old string.
C) The amplitude of the new string should be twice the amplitude of the old string.
D) The amplitude of the new string should be half the amplitude of the old string.

6. The speed of a 2 kg mass on a spring is 4 m/s as it passes through its equilibrium position. What is its frequency if the amplitude is 2 m?

A) 1/5 Hz
B) 1/3 Hz
C) 3 Hz
D) 5 Hz

7. The distance from a trough to a crest is 20 cm on a 3 m rope of 1 kg. If the tension in the rope is 3 N, what is the period? (Note: $v = [\text{tension/linear density}]^{0.5}$)

A) 1/15 s
B) 2/15 s
C) 15/2 s
D) 15 s

CHAPTER 11 PRACTICE PASSAGE

A physics student conducts an experiment to study pendulums and momentum. Using an apparatus known as *Newton's cradle*, the student conducts two different trials. The Newton's cradle apparatus consists of five identical steel balls of equal size and mass. Each ball is suspended from two wires that connect it to a frame, so that the ball is in the air and can move side to side in a single plane. The balls are suspended so that they are touching each other and are free to move individually or as a group. Each ball can be considered a simple pendulum since the hanging wires have negligible mass. Assume there is no friction in the pendulum mechanism.

For the first trial, Ball A is raised at an angle, θ, from the vertical and let go. The ball swings down and hits Ball B. Momentum is transferred through Balls B, C, and D to Ball E, causing Ball E to swing up to a maximum angle, θ, from the vertical on the right while Balls A, B, C, and D are stationary. Then Ball E swings down and hits Ball D, transferring momentum through Balls D, C, and B to Ball A, causing Ball A to swing up again to the same maximum angle, θ, from the vertical while Balls E, D, C, and B are stationary. The period for this motion is measured to be 1.5 seconds.

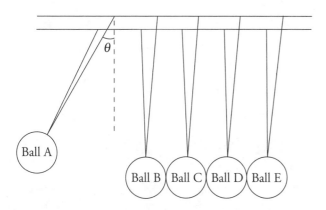

Figure 1 Newton's Cradle Apparatus with Ball A raised at the start of Trial 1

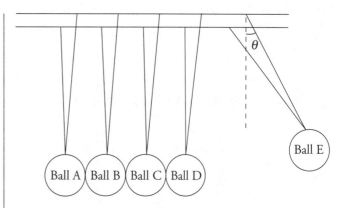

Figure 2 Newton's Cradle Apparatus after transfer of momentum to Ball E during Trial 1

For the second trial, both Ball A and Ball B are lifted together to the same angle, θ, as in the first trial. The result of the swing is that both Ball D and Ball E swing up on the right with the same displacement angle, θ. As in the first trial, momentum is conserved.

1. Which of the following is true during the experiment?

A) Kinetic energy is not conserved and the collisions are inelastic.
B) Kinetic energy is not conserved and the collisions are elastic.
C) Kinetic energy is conserved and the collisions are inelastic.
D) Kinetic energy is conserved and the collisions are elastic.

2. Which of the following is true when Ball E is at half of its maximum height as measured from its lowest point?

   I.   The kinetic energy is half of the total mechanical energy.
   II. The velocity is half of the maximum velocity of the ball.
   III. The time elapsed from the time Ball E started in motion to the time it reached half of its maximum height is half of the period.

A) I only
B) I and III
C) II and III
D) I, II, and III

3. What should be the measured period in Trial 2?

A) 1.0 seconds
B) 1.5 seconds
C) 2.0 seconds
D) 3.0 seconds

4. For Ball E, how does the maximum velocity in Trial 2, v_2, compare to the maximum velocity in Trial 1, v_1?

A) $v_2 = (1/2)v_1$
B) $v_2 = \left(1\sqrt{2}\right)v_1$
C) $v_2 = v_1$
D) $v_2 = 2v_1$

5. To help record results, the student attached pens of negligible mass to balls A and E and scrolled paper perpendicular to the axis of motion of the Newton's cradle. The paper scrolls at a rate of 20 cm/s underneath the pens during the trials. What is the wavelength of the resulting wave graphed in Trial 1 (assume the pens are rigged to align parallel to the paper when the cradle isn't in motion)?

A) 13 cm
B) 20 cm
C) 30 cm
D) 33 cm

6. If L is the length of each string, what is the maximum height of Ball E in Trial 1 above its lowest position?

A) $L - \cos \theta$
B) $L - L \cos \theta$
C) $L + L \cos \theta$
D) $L \cos \theta$

7. In both Trial 1 and Trial 2 of the experiment, the number of balls that moved on the right side was the same as the number of balls lifted on the left side to start the motion, while all the central balls remained stationary. Which of the following changes to the experiment would most likely result in not having the same number of balls swing on each side of the apparatus?

A) Raise three balls on the left side to start the motion.
B) Increase the length of the wires holding the balls.
C) Change the masses of the balls so that each mass is different from the others.
D) Add a small space between each of the balls as they hang on the apparatus.

SOLUTIONS TO CHAPTER 11 FREESTANDING QUESTIONS

1. **D** Based on the equation $T = 2\pi\sqrt{\frac{L}{g}}$, we know that the period does not depend on either the mass or the initial angle of extension, eliminating choices A and B. Furthermore, we know that decreasing the length of the string will decrease the period, eliminating choice C. Moving the pendulum to the surface of the moon will lower the gravitational acceleration, which would increase the period. Therefore, choice D is correct.

2. **C** A force diagram of the jumper at the lowest spot is shown below.

$$F_{bungee} = (100 \text{ kg/s}^2)(30 \text{ m}) = 3000 \text{ N}$$

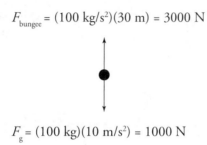

$$F_g = (100 \text{ kg})(10 \text{ m/s}^2) = 1000 \text{ N}$$

Since the force up is greater than the force down, there is a net upward force of 2000 N on the jumper and an upward acceleration. Acceleration = F/m = (2000 N)/(100 kg) = 20 m/s².

3. **D** A sine wave is a transverse wave, so the vibration direction is perpendicular to the direction of propagation. The question states that the wave vibrates between the north and south and propagates from east to west. The red spot is simply a part of the cord and will vibrate in the same direction the cord is vibrating (choice C is wrong), namely between the north and south. Since a wave only transports energy, not material, it would be impossible for the spot to propagate along the wave, eliminating choices A and B and leaving choice D as the correct answer.

4. **B** Simple harmonic motion is by definition when the restoring force is proportional to the displacement of the object. In this case, the swing is similar to a simple pendulum (a simple pendulum has no mass in the material connecting the end of the pendulum to the rotation point, and the question states the chain has negligible mass). For a simple pendulum to experience simple harmonic motion, the restoring force must be proportional to the displacement. In this case, the displacement is the angle, θ, between the swing and the vertical. The restoring force is the component of the weight directed toward the vertical. For a child of mass, m, the restoring force is $mg \sin \theta$. If the angle is small, then $\sin \theta$ approximates θ, so the motion is considered simple harmonic motion. Thus, Item II is true, eliminating choices A and C. Item I is false: The mass of the child will impact the magnitude of the restoring force, but will not indicate whether the motion is simple harmonic motion (choice D can be eliminated and choice B is correct). Item III is also false: The tension in the chain will have a variable value that depends upon the component of the weight directed along the chain, but it will have no impact on whether the motion is simple harmonic motion.

5. **A** The amplitude of the wave on the string will not impact the frequency of the wave or the wave speed, eliminating choices C and D. Since the frequency = wave speed / wavelength, in order to keep the frequency constant, the wave speed should be kept constant. Wave speed is proportional to the square root of tension / linear density ($v = (\text{Tension}/\mu)^{0.5}$) and since linear density is doubled, then tension should also be doubled in order to keep wave speed constant. The correct answer is choice A.

6. **B** The kinetic energy is at a maximum at the equilibrium position, and is equal to the potential energy at the amplitude: $\frac{1}{2}kA^2 = \frac{1}{2}mv_{max}^2$. This equation can be solved for the spring constant, $k = 8$ N/m. The spring constant and the mass are all you need to determine the frequency from $f = \frac{1}{2\pi}\sqrt{k/m}$, giving a frequency of approximately 0.33 Hz.

7. **B** The speed of the wave is $\sqrt{3/(\frac{1}{3})} = 3$ m/s. From $v = f\lambda$, and knowing that the wavelength is 40 cm = $\frac{2}{5}$ m, the frequency is 15/2 Hz, making the period $\frac{2}{15}$ s.

SOLUTIONS TO CHAPTER 11 PRACTICE PASSAGE

1. **D** By definition, if a collision is elastic then kinetic energy is conserved and if a collision is inelastic then energy is not conserved, eliminating choices B and C. Momentum is always conserved during a collision. Before the collision, all the momentum is with Ball A, so $p_{before} = mv_A$. After the collision, all the momentum is with Ball E, so $p_{after} = mv_E = p_{before}$ so $v_A = v_E$. Since the masses and velocities are the same for Ball A and Ball E, the kinetic energy of Ball A before the collision = the kinetic energy of Ball E after the collision, so kinetic energy is conserved and the collision is elastic. The correct answer is choice D.

2.　**A**　When Ball E is at its maximum height, all of its energy is potential energy and $E_{total} = PE_{max} = mgh_{max}$. When Ball E is at half of its maximum height, its potential energy is $mg(\frac{1}{2})h_{max} = (\frac{1}{2})PE_{max} = (\frac{1}{2})E_{total}$. Since the total mechanical energy is the sum of the potential energy and the kinetic energy, then the other half of the total energy must be kinetic energy. Item I is true (choice C can be eliminated). When the ball is at its lowest point, all of its mechanical energy will be kinetic energy and $E_{total} = KE_{max} = \frac{1}{2}mv^2_{max}$. As discussed above, at half the maximum height, half the total mechanical energy is kinetic energy. So $\frac{1}{2}E_{total} = \frac{1}{2}KE_{max} = \frac{1}{4}mv^2_{max} = KE_{half}$. The kinetic energy can also be calculated using the velocity at the half height, v_{half}. So $KE_{half} = \frac{1}{2}mv^2_{half} = \frac{1}{4}mv^2_{max}$ and $v_{half} = \frac{1}{\sqrt{2}}v_{max}$. Item II is false (choice D can be eliminated). The period is the time for one full cycle. This is the time from Ball A dropping, through Ball E rising, Ball E dropping, and Ball A rising again. The entire time Ball E is moving is half of the period. The time for it to rise half way is approximately 1/8 of the entire period. Item III is false (choice B can be eliminated). The correct answer is choice A.

3.　**B**　Period depends on the length of the wire and the acceleration due to gravity $T = 2\pi\sqrt{\frac{L}{g}}$. Neither of these changed between Trial 1 and Trial 2, so the period should be the same in Trial 2 as in Trial 1. The correct answer is choice B.

4.　**C**　For a pendulum, the maximum velocity is at the lowest point (when $\theta = 0$). For Ball E, this occurs after the collision of Ball A, and again after falling from its maximum height. For both trials, since the angle of displacement is the same for Ball E, then the height of the ball is the same, the maximum potential energy is the same, the maximum kinetic energy is the same, and the maximum velocity is the same. The correct answer is choice C. (Note: The total mechanical energy for the system will be doubled in Trial 2 compared to Trial 1, but the question is asking specifically about Ball E, not the whole system.)

5.　**C**　The rate of the paper is the rate of propagation of the wave. Since $v = f\lambda$, and $f = 1/T$, we have that $\lambda = vT$. Then, $\lambda = (20 \text{ cm/s})(1.5 \text{ s}) = 30 \text{ cm}$. The correct answer is choice C.

6. **B** The easiest way to solve this is to remember that at $\theta = 0°$ the height = 0. Plugging in $0°$ for the angle in each of the answer choices, only choice B gives the correct value of height = 0, eliminating choices A, C, and D. Another (longer) way solve the question is using a sketch like the one below.

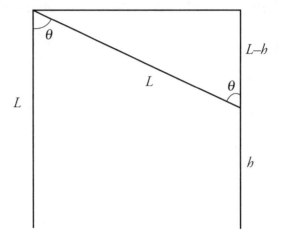

Using the sketch and basic trigonometry the equation is $\cos \theta = (L - h)/L$ and $h = L - L \cos \theta$. The correct answer is choice B.

7. **C** Momentum is always conserved, so the momentum before the collision must equal the momentum after the collision. Since the balls all have the same mass, momentum is conserved when the number of balls in motion before the collision equals the number in motion after the collision. It seems likely that raising three balls to start the motion would result in three balls moving on the right side to conserve momentum (in fact, this is what happens), which is the pattern the question seeks to avoid, eliminating choice A. Changing the length of the wires will change the period of motion, but will not affect the collisions and the number of balls in motion, eliminating choice B. A small space between the balls does not affect their momentum, momentum will still be conserved, and the same number of balls will still move on each side of the apparatus, eliminating choice D. Changing the masses of the balls so that each is different means that a different combination of balls needs to move at potentially different speeds in order to conserve momentum, and a different number of balls would move on each side of the apparatus. The correct answer is choice C.

Chapter 12
Sound

12.1 SOUND WAVES

Sound waves don't travel in the same way that waves on a rope do. The waves we've looked at so far are transverse waves: The direction in which the particles of the conducting medium oscillate is perpendicular to the direction in which the wave travels. If, however, the direction in which the particles of the conducting medium oscillate is *parallel* to the direction in which the wave travels, we call the wave **longitudinal**. Sound waves (also known as compression waves) are longitudinal waves in gas, liquid, or solid; when a compression wave's frequency is between 20 Hz and 20 kHz, humans can perceive it as what we commonly call sound.

Let's take a closer look at sound waves. As a stereo speaker, vocal fold, or tuning fork vibrates, it creates regions of high pressure (**compressions**) that alternate with regions of low pressure (**rarefactions**). These pressure waves are transmitted through the air (or some other medium) and can eventually reach our ears and brain, which translate the vibrations into sound.

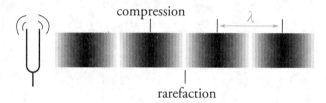

Like other waves, a longitudinal compression wave has a wavelength, a speed, a frequency, a period, and an amplitude. The equation $v = \lambda f$ holds, as do the two Big Rules for waves.

Sound can travel in any medium: gas, liquid, or solid. Its speed depends on two things: the medium's resistance to compression (quantified by its *bulk modulus B*) and its density, according to the equation $v_{sound} = \sqrt{\dfrac{B}{\rho}}$. On the MCAT, knowing the relationship is good enough—you won't have to calculate the speed of sound in a given medium. However, you should know that in general, *sound travels slowest through gases, faster through liquids, and fastest through solids.* The speed of sound in air is about 340 m/s (that's about 760 miles per hour), but it varies slightly with temperature, pressure, and humidity.

Example 12-1: A sound wave of frequency 440 Hz (this note is *concert A*, or the A above middle C) travels at a speed of 344 m/s through the air in a concert hall. How fast would a note one octave higher, 880 Hz, travel through the same concert hall?

  A. 172 m/s
  B. 344 m/s
  C. 516 m/s
  D. 688 m/s

Solution: Altering the frequency will not affect the wave speed. Remember Big Rule 1 for waves. Therefore, the answer is B.

Example 12-2: A siren produces sound waves in the air. If the frequency of the waves is gradually decreasing, which of the following changes to the waves is most likely also occurring?

A. The wavelength is increasing.
B. The wave speed is decreasing.
C. The amplitude is decreasing.
D. The period is decreasing.

Solution: Because the wave speed is set by the medium (the air, in this case), the wave speed is a constant. Since $v = \lambda f$, this means that λ and f are inversely proportional. So, if f is decreasing, then λ must be increasing, choice A.

Example 12-3: What is the wavelength of a sound wave of frequency 170 Hz if the wave speed is 340 m/s?

Solution: Using $v = \lambda f$ we find that $\lambda = v/f = (340 \text{ m/s})/(170 \text{ Hz}) = 2$ m.

Example 12-4: A typical medical ultrasound scan uses frequencies in the MHz range. What would happen to an ultrasound signal as it passed from air into body tissues?

A. Its wavelength and speed would both decrease.
B. Its wavelength and speed would both increase.
C. Its wavelength would decrease and its speed would increase.
D. Its wavelength would increase and its speed would decrease.

Solution: When a wave passes into a new medium, its frequency does not change (the specific frequency range is irrelevant). Therefore, when traveling through the body, the frequency of the sound wave will be the same as it was in the air. However, we know that sound waves generally travel faster through liquids and solids than they do through gases, so we'd expect the wave speed through the body to be faster. Because the equation $v = \lambda f$ is always true, the same f at a faster v means a greater wavelength. Therefore, the answer is B. (Note that almost all of the ultrasound wave would reflect off the skin if it were incident on it from air: this is why a gel is first applied to the skin before the emitter/detector is placed on the skin, so that no air interrupts the signal.)

Example 12-5: When a longitudinal compression wave of frequency 700 Hz travels through a brass rod, its wavelength is 5 m. How fast does sound travel through brass?

Solution: Using $v = \lambda f$, we find that $v = (5 \text{ m})(700 \text{ Hz}) = 3500$ m/s.

12.2   STANDING SOUND WAVES IN PIPES

Just as we can have standing waves on a rope caused by the interference of two oppositely directed transverse waves with equal amplitudes, standing sound waves in a pipe can be caused by the interference of two oppositely directed longitudinal waves of equal amplitude.

The analysis of these standing waves is similar to that of a string attached at each end. In that case, the ends correspond to nodes (because there is no motion). Since the distance between nodes is some whole number of half-wavelengths, this gave us formulas for the different frequencies and wavelengths that the standing waves can have. In the case of pipes, we also need to know what corresponds to each end. The ends of a pipe can either be open to the atmosphere or closed.

It turns out that the open end of a pipe (technically, just beyond it) corresponds to an antinode. To be more specific, these are often referred to as displacement antinodes (maximum displacement). They are also called pressure nodes (constant pressure). The closed end of a pipe corresponds to a displacement node (no motion) or a pressure antinode (maximum pressure fluctuations). The pressure varies most where there is no motion and the motion varies most where there is constant pressure.

Pipes are often classified as *open pipes* (open on each end) or *closed pipes* (open on one end and closed on the other).

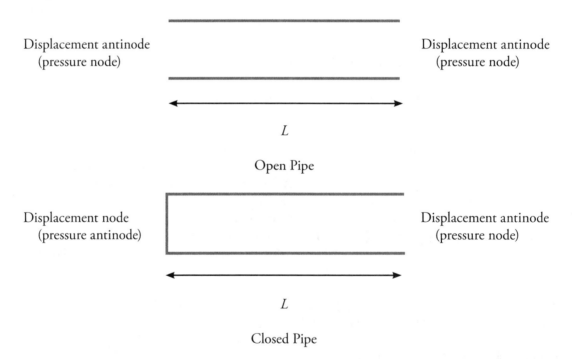

Displacement antinode
(pressure node)

Displacement antinode
(pressure node)

L

Open Pipe

Displacement node
(pressure antinode)

Displacement antinode
(pressure node)

L

Closed Pipe

In the case of the open pipe, the distance between displacement antinodes (or pressure nodes) is equal to a whole number of half-wavelengths. The formulas for wavelength and frequency are therefore the same as for the string attached at each end: $\lambda_n = 2L / n$ and $f_n = nv / 2L$, where the harmonic number, n, is any positive whole number, and v now refers to the speed of sound in air.

To visualize the harmonic modes, it is convenient to represent the standing waves as transverse.

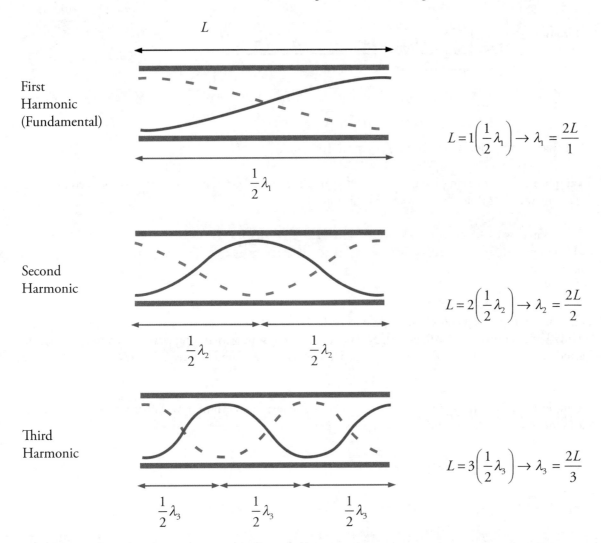

In the case of the closed pipe, the distance between a displacement antinode (or pressure node) and a displacement node (or pressure antinode) is equal to an *odd* number of *quarter*-wavelengths. As a result, $\lambda_n = 4L / n$ and $f_n = nv / 4L$, where n (which is still called the harmonic) is an *odd* number.

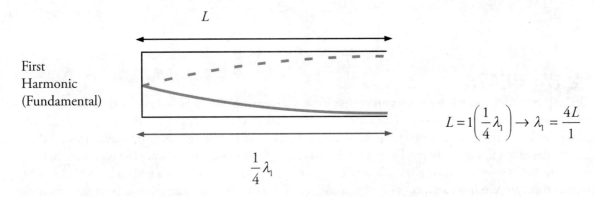

12.3

Third
Harmonic

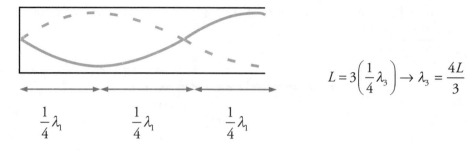

$$L = 3\left(\frac{1}{4}\lambda_3\right) \rightarrow \lambda_3 = \frac{4L}{3}$$

$\frac{1}{4}\lambda_1$ $\qquad$ $\frac{1}{4}\lambda_1$ $\qquad$ $\frac{1}{4}\lambda_1$

Note that for all types of resonance, $f_n = nf_1$ and $\lambda_n = \lambda_1 / n$.

Example 12-6: An organ pipe that is closed at one end has a length of 3 m. What is the second-longest harmonic wavelength for sound waves in this pipe?

 A. 3 m
 B. 4 m
 C. 6 m
 D. 9 m

Solution: Because one end of the pipe is closed, the length of the pipe, L, must be an *odd* number of *quarter*-wavelengths: $L = 1(\lambda/4)$, $3(\lambda/4)$, $5(\lambda/4)\dots$, in order to support standing waves. Therefore, the possible harmonic wavelengths are $\lambda = 4L/1$, $4L/3$, $4L/5$, and so on. The second longest is $\lambda = 4L/3 = 4(3\text{ m})/3 = 4$ m, choice B.

Example 12-7: An organ pipe that is open at both ends has a length of 3 m. What is the second-longest harmonic wavelength for sound waves in this pipe?

 A. 3 m
 B. 4 m
 C. 6 m
 D. 9 m

Solution: Because both ends of the pipe are open, the length of the pipe, L, must be a whole number of half-wavelengths: $L = 1(\lambda/2)$, $2(\lambda/2)$, $3(\lambda/2)\dots$, in order to support standing waves. Therefore, the possible harmonic wavelengths are $\lambda = 2L/1$, $2L/2$, $2L/3$, and so on. The second longest is $\lambda = 2L/2 = L = 3$ m, choice A.

12.3 BEATS

In the previous chapter, it was mentioned that if two waves with different frequency interfere, the resultant wave will be complicated. If the two waves are sound waves with slightly different frequencies (the difference is less than about 10 Hz), the product is a pulsating, "wobbling" resultant wave. This produces the phenomenon known as **beats**. Because the frequencies don't match, sometimes the waves are in phase and sometimes they're out of phase. When they're in phase, their amplitudes add; when they're out of phase, their amplitudes subtract. The combined waveform reaches its maximum amplitude when the waves interfere constructively and its minimum amplitude when they interfere destructively, and these points alternate. Maximum amplitude sounds loud and minimum amplitude sounds soft, so we hear loud, soft, loud, soft, etc. The resulting equally spaced moments of constructive interference (the loud moments) are the beats.

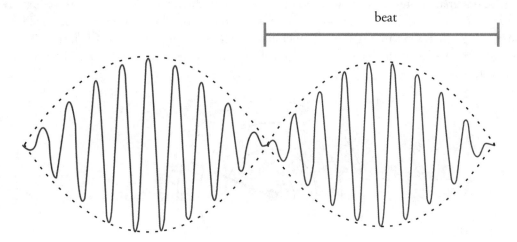

The frequency at which the beats are heard (the **beat frequency**) is equal to the difference between the frequencies of the two original sound waves. Therefore, if one of these waves has frequency f_1 and the other has frequency f_2, then $f_{\text{beat}} = |f_1 - f_2|$.

Beat Frequency

$$f_{\text{beat}} = |f_1 - f_2|$$

Example 12-8: A piano tuner strikes a tuning fork at the same time he strikes a piano key with a note of similar pitch. If he hears 3 beats per second, and the tuning fork produces a standard 440 Hz tone, then what must be the frequency produced by the struck piano string?

- A.   437 Hz
- B.   443 Hz
- C.   437 Hz or 443 Hz
- D.   434 Hz or 446 Hz

Solution: If $f_{\text{beat}} = 3$ Hz, then the frequencies of the tuning fork and piano string are "off" by 3 Hz. The frequency produced by the piano string might be 3 Hz lower or 3 Hz higher than the tuning fork; without more information, we don't know which one. If the tuning fork produces a tone of frequency 440 Hz, the piano string produces a frequency of either 440 − 3 = 437 Hz or 440 + 3 = 443 Hz. Choice C is the answer.

12.4 INTENSITY AND INTENSITY LEVEL

Intensity and intensity level are closely related quantities. The **intensity** of a sound wave (or, indeed, any wave) is the energy it transmits per second (the power) per unit area. It is measured in W/m^2. For a point source (i.e., one that creates waves that travel uniformly in all directions), the area in the equation is the surface area of a sphere, which equals $4\pi r^2$. Each wavefront in the figure below can be thought of as a bundle of energy that is expanding in size, much like a balloon being blown up. The farther a detector is from the source, the larger the bundle of energy will be, and therefore the detector will receive a smaller fraction of it.

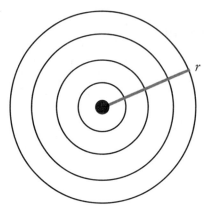

Mathematically, the important fact to remember is that, for a point source, intensity varies inversely as the square of the distance r from that source: $I \propto 1/r^2$. If the detector of a wave doubles his distance from the source, the power produced by the wave will spread out over an area that is $2^2 = 4$ times larger, causing the detector to receive ¼ as much. Intensity is also proportional to the square of the amplitude of a wave.

Since the intensity that we can hear spans an impressively large range (about twelve orders of magnitude!), we use logarithms to make the numbers easier to handle. The **threshold of hearing**, which is roughly the lowest intensity the human ear can perceive as sound at the common middle frequencies, is equal to 10^{-12} W/m^2; this intensity is denoted by I_0. The **intensity level** (or **sound level**) of a sound wave whose intensity is I is equal to the base-10 logarithm of the ratio I/I_0. The unit of intensity level is the **bel**, abbreviated **B**. Usually, we multiply this by 10 to get the intensity level, β, in **decibels** (dB):

Intensity Level in Decibels

$$\beta = 10\log_{10}\frac{I}{I_0}$$

The most important relationship to get from this equation can be summarized as follows:

Every time we *multiply* I by 10, we *add* 10 to β.

Every time we *divide* I by 10, we *subtract* 10 from β.

For example, if the intensity is multiplied by 10,000, which is $10 \times 10 \times 10 \times 10$, the intensity level in decibels is increased by adding $10 + 10 + 10 + 10 = 40$. If we divide by the intensity by, say, $100,000 = 10^5$, then the decibel level decreases by 50.

Example 12-9: At a distance of 1 m, the intensity level of a soft whisper is about 30 dB, while a normal speaking voice is about 60 dB. How many times greater is the power delivered per unit area by a normal-speaking voice than by a whisper?[1]

   A. 2.5
   B. 30
   C. 1000
   D. 3000

Solution: The normal speaking voice has an intensity level that's 30 dB greater than the whisper. Therefore, the intensity must be $10 \times 10 \times 10 = 10^3 = 1000$ times greater. Since "power delivered per unit area" *is* intensity, the answer is C.

Example 12-10: A person listening to music on a stereo system experiences a sound level of 70 dB. If the volume dial is turned up to increase the intensity by a factor of 500, what sound level would this person hear now?

   A. 97 dB
   B. 105 dB
   C. 115 dB
   D. 120 dB

Solution: If the intensity had increased by a factor of 100, which is 10×10, the sound level would have increased by $10 + 10 = 20$ dB. If the intensity had increased by a factor of 1000, which is $10 \times 10 \times 10$, the sound level would have increased by $10 + 10 + 10 = 30$ dB. The fact that the intensity increased by a factor of 500, which is between 100 and 1000, means that the sound level increased by between 20 dB and 30 dB. If the original sound level was 70 dB, then the new sound level must be between $70 + 20 = 90$ dB and $70 + 30 = 100$ dB. Only choice A falls in this range.

Example 12-11: Suppose one moves 10 times further away from a loud siren of constant power. What is the resultant decrease in sound level?

   A. 10 dB
   B. 20 dB
   C. 40 dB
   D. 100 dB

Solution: Increasing distance by a factor of 10 decreases intensity by a factor of 100, which is 10×10. Therefore, sound level will be reduced by $10 + 10 = 20$ dB, choice B.

---

[1] Our perception of loudness is completely different from both intensity and intensity level. Roughly speaking, a difference in intensity level of 10 dB (and therefore a factor of 10 in intensity) corresponds to a perceived loudness difference of a factor of 2.

12.5   THE DOPPLER EFFECT

Suppose a train that is loudly sounding its horn is approaching a passenger waiting on a platform. As the train is approaching, the person hears the pitch at a higher frequency than does the engineer on the train. As the train is moving away, the person on the platform hears a lower frequency than does the engineer. These differences in frequency are the result of the **Doppler effect**, which arises whenever a source of waves is moving relative to the detector. The result is that the perceived or *detected* frequency will be different from the frequency of the sound that was emitted from the *source*.

Normally when a sound is emitted from a source, the rate of the compressions (or frequency, f) emitted from the source is the same as the rate received at the detector. The most important fact to remember is that if the source and detector are moving *closer* together (no matter which is moving), the detected frequency with be *higher* than the emitted frequency. Similarly, if the source and detector are moving *farther apart,* the detected frequency will be *lower* than the emitted frequency.

> **Doppler Effect**
>
> approaching ↔ higher detected frequency
>
> receding ↔ lower detected frequency

For sound, if the detector moves toward the source or if the source moves toward the detector, the detected frequency will be higher than the emitted frequency. But the reasons are different.

If a detector moves toward (or away from) a stationary source, the *relative* speed of sound changes. As an example, if a sound wave is moving toward the detector at 340 m/s and the detector moves toward the source at 20 m/s, the wave will appear to be moving at 360 m/s in the detector's frame of reference. Similarly, if the detector is moving away from the source at 20 m/s, the wave will appear to moving at 320 m/s. The wavelength (i.e., the spacing between wavefronts) will not change. According to the wave equation, $v = \lambda f$, an increase (or decrease) in perceived wave speed with a constant wavelength will cause an increase (or decrease) in perceived frequency.

If the source moves, the waves themselves become distorted. Say a source emits a pulse that spreads out in all directions. The wavefront is a sphere, though in 2 dimensions it looks like a circle. If the source moves to the right the next pulse it emits would again look like a circle, but whose center is to the right of the previous pulse's center. The wavefronts bunch up on the right and spread out on the left. The wavelength has therefore changed. If the detector is at rest, then the speed of the wave hasn't changed. According to the wave equation, $v = \lambda f$, an increase (or decrease) in wavelength with a constant wave speed will result in a decrease (or increase) in frequency.

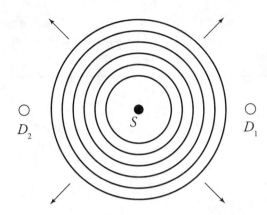

No relative motion between the source (S) and detectors (D_1 and D_2)

Each wave compression emitted by S arrives at the same speed when perceived by D_1 and D_2. The perceived frequency is the same.

No Doppler shifts.

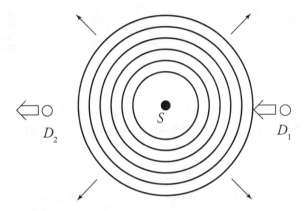

Here, there *is* relative motion between the source (S) and detectors (D_1 and D_2).

D_1 is approaching S, so each compression of the wave emitted from S requires less time to reach D_1. The perceived wave speed at D_1 is faster, and thus the frequency at D_1 is higher.

D_2 is receding from S, so each compression of the wave requires more time to reach D_2. The perceived wave speed at D_2 is slower, and thus the perceived frequency is lower.

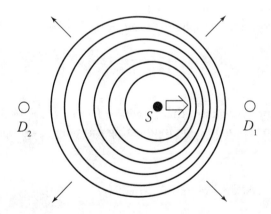

Here, there *is* relative motion between the source (S) and detectors (D_1 and D_2).

S is approaching D_1, so the compressions of the wave emitted from S are closer together. The perceived wavelength at D_1 is shorter, and thus the frequency at D_1 is higher.

S is receding from D_2, so the compressions of the wave emitted from S are farther apart. The perceived wavelength at D_2 is longer, and thus the frequency at D_2 is lower.

To predict exactly what the perceived frequency will be, we need an equation. Despite the fact that there are lots of individual cases to consider (whether the source and/or the detector are stationary or in motion), we can summarize everything in a single equation:

Doppler Effect

$$f_D = f_S \frac{v \pm v_D}{v \mp v_S}$$

In this equation:

f_D = the frequency heard by the detector
f_S = the frequency emitted by the source
v_D = the speed at which the detector is moving
v_S = the speed at which the source is moving
v = the speed of the wave

What we need to do to make this one equation fit all the possible cases is use the conceptual relationships given in the box on the previous page to decide whether to use the + or − in the numerator and whether to use + or − in the denominator.

Notice that we have written ± in the numerator and ∓ in the denominator; one way to memorize the sign conventions for this equation is by the mnemonic "top sign is toward." When the motion of the detector is toward the source, you use the top of ±, or the "+" sign, in the numerator. When the motion of the source is toward the detector, you use the top of ∓, or the "−" sign, in the denominator.

For example, suppose the source is stationary and the detector is moving toward it. Because $v_S = 0$, there's no decision to make in the denominator. Now, we know that f_D will be higher than f_S in this case. Therefore, we choose the + in the numerator, to make the fraction multiplying f_S bigger, to give the higher f_D we expect:

$$f_D = f_S \frac{v + v_D}{v} \text{ (adding } v_D \text{ makes the numerator bigger)}$$

If the detector is moving away from the stationary source, we know that f_D will be lower than f_S in this case. Therefore, we choose the − in the numerator to make the fraction multiplying f_S smaller, to give the lower f_D we expect:

$$f_D = f_S \frac{v - v_D}{v} \text{ (subtracting } v_D \text{ makes the numerator smaller)}$$

Now, suppose the detector is stationary and the source is moving toward it. Since $v_D = 0$, there's no decision to make in the numerator. We know that f_D will be higher than f_S in this case. Therefore, we choose the—in the denominator, to make the denominator smaller, and thus make the fraction multiplying f_S bigger, to give the higher f_D we expect:

$$f_D = f_S \frac{v}{v - v_S} \text{ (subtracting } v_S \text{ makes the denominator smaller)}$$

If the source is moving away from the stationary detector, we know that f_D will be lower than f_S in this case. Therefore, we choose the + in the denominator, to make the denominator bigger, and thus make the fraction multiplying f_S smaller, to give the lower f_D we expect:

$$f_D = f_S \frac{v}{v + v_S} \text{ (adding } v_S \text{ makes the denominator bigger)}$$

If both the source and the detector are moving, we have two decisions to make (one in the numerator and one in the denominator). The key is to make the two decisions separately. For example, let's say you're the detector, driving in your car following a police car whose siren is wailing. In this case, both the source (the police car) and the detector (you) are moving. To decide what to do in the numerator, ask yourself: *what's the detector doing?* It's approaching the source, so its "contribution" to the Doppler effect should be an increase in frequency. Therefore, we'd choose the + in the numerator. Now, *what's the source doing?* It's receding from the detector, so its "contribution" to the Doppler effect should be a *decrease* in frequency. Therefore, we'd choose the + in the denominator.

$$f_D = f_S \frac{v + v_D}{v + v_S}$$

If your speed is greater than that of the police car, you're gaining on it, so the relative motion is motion *toward.* We'd expect f_D to be greater than f_S. If $v_D > v_S$, then the fraction multiplying f_S is bigger than 1, so f_D will indeed be greater than f_S. On the other hand, if your speed is less than that of the police car, it's pulling away from you, so the relative motion is motion *away.* In this case, we'd expect f_D to be lower than f_S. Further, if $v_D < v_S$, then the fraction multiplying f_S is less than 1, so f_D will indeed be lower than f_S. Finally, it's important to notice what happens if your speed is the same as the police car's speed. If $v_D = v_S$, then the fraction multiplying f_S is equal to 1, so $f_D = f_S$. Therefore, even though you're both moving, there's no Doppler shift because there's no *relative* motion between you.

The Doppler effect also applies to electromagnetic waves, such as visible light. The same qualitative relationships continue to hold: motion *toward* results in a frequency shift upward, while motion *away* results in a frequency shift downward. An astronomer observing a star moving away from the earth observes the light emitted as being shifted downward in frequency, toward the red end of the visible spectrum (in fact, this is known as the **redshift**). Furthermore, by measuring the shift, the astronomer can calculate how fast the star is moving away from us.[2]

Example 12-12: A speaker emitting a sound with a constant frequency approaches a detector. Which of the following wave characteristics will have a greater value at the detector than at the source?

   I.   Frequency
  II.   Wavelength
 III.   Speed

---

[2] For light waves, the equation that is used to calculate the magnitude of the Doppler effect is different. This is because of a postulate of special relativity: the speed of light is the same in all frames of reference. The detector, therefore, cannot perceive the speed of light to be faster or slower than 3×10^8 m/s. Another way of saying this is that we can always treat the detector as being at rest while the source may move.

12.5

Solution: Since the source is approaching the detector, the detected frequency will be higher than the emitted frequency. The wavelength will be shorter, and the wave speed will be the same. Therefore, only characteristic I will have a greater value at the detector than at the source.

12.5

Example 12-13: When you push the "star" key on your cell phone, a tone whose frequency is about 1080 Hz is emitted. However, the button gets stuck and the tone is continuous. Exasperated, you drop the broken phone off a bridge. What is the frequency of the tone you hear at the instant the phone's speed is 20 m/s (speed of sound in air = 340 m/s)?

Solution: Since you (the detector) are stationary, $v_D = 0$. Now, because the source of the sound (the broken phone) is moving away from you, we use the plus sign on v_S in the denominator of the Doppler effect equation to find that

$$f_D = f_S \frac{v}{v + v_S} = (1080 \text{ Hz}) \cdot \frac{340 \text{ m/s}}{340 \text{ m/s} + 20 \text{ m/s}} = (1080 \text{ Hz}) \cdot \frac{340}{360} = (3 \text{ Hz}) \cdot 340 = 1020 \text{ Hz}$$

Note that, because the phone is *accelerating* away from you, the magnitude of v_S is increasing as the phone falls, and thus the frequency you detect is *decreasing* as a function of time.

Example 12-14: As a high-speed chase begins, a police car travels at a speed of 40 m/s directly toward the suspect's getaway car, which is traveling at a speed of 70 m/s, trying to outrun the pursuing police. The frequency that the suspect hears will be what percentage of the frequency of the police car's siren? (speed of sound = 340 m/s)

Solution: Use the Doppler effect equation, choosing the signs carefully. The suspect in the getaway car is the detector (so $v_D = 70$ m/s), moving *away* from the source. The source is the police car ($v_S = 40$ m/s), moving *toward* the detector. Therefore,

$$f_D = f_S \frac{v \pm v_D}{v \mp v_S} = f_S \frac{340 \text{ m/s} - 70 \text{ m/s}}{340 \text{ m/s} - 40 \text{ m/s}} = f_S \frac{270}{300} = f_S \frac{90}{100} = (90\%) f_S$$

In order to find the correct value of f_D, it was necessary to plug in the values for v_D and v_S, and to change the top and the bottom of the equation separately; we couldn't just use the relative velocity of 30 m/s. However, if all the problem had asked for was the qualitative effect (i.e., whether the detected frequency was higher or lower than that of the source), then we could have worked out that the frequency was lower simply by noticing that the detector was getting farther away from the source.

Example 12-15: A technician is using his ultrasound scanner to detect a fetal heartbeat. The scanner emits short pulses of frequency 5 MHz, which then bounce off the beating heart and return to the scanner (functioning as a detector). The detector compares the final received frequency, f_2, with the original emitted frequency, f_1, and converts the difference in frequency into the speed and direction of the heart's motion. The difference in frequency, $\Delta f = f_2 - f_1$, is equal to $\pm 2vf_1/v_{sound}$, where v is the speed of the heart and $v_{sound} = 1500$ m/s is the speed of the ultrasound pulses. If $\Delta f = -100$ Hz, then the observed heart is:

- A.   expanding at 1.5 cm/s.
- B.   contracting at 1.5 cm/s.
- C.   expanding at 7.5 cm/s.
- D.   contracting at 7.5 cm/s.

Solution: First, the fact that Δf is negative means that f_2 is lower than f_1, and if the final detected frequency is *lower* than the frequency emitted by the source, then the heart surface must be moving *away from* the source (i.e., contracting). This eliminates choices A and C. Now, to figure out the value of the heart's speed, v, we just use the given formula:

$$\Delta f = -\frac{2vf_1}{v_{sound}} \rightarrow v = -\frac{v_{sound}\Delta f}{2f_1} = -\frac{(1,500 \text{ m/s})(-100 \text{ Hz})}{1 \times 10^7 \text{ Hz}} = 1.5 \times 10^{-2} \text{ m/s}$$

This is equal to 1.5 cm/s, and choice B is correct.

Summary of Formulas

Standing Waves in a Tube:

Both ends open: $\lambda_n = \dfrac{2L}{n}$

$$f_n = \dfrac{n}{2L}v \ (n = 1, 2, 3, ...)$$

One end closed: $\lambda_n = \dfrac{4L}{n}$

$$f_n = \dfrac{n}{4L}v \ (n = 1, 3, 5, ...; \text{odd } n \text{ only})$$

Beats, Intensity, Doppler Effect:

Beat frequency: $f_{beat} = |f_1 - f_2|$

Intensity: $I = \dfrac{\text{power}}{\text{area}}$

I is inversely proportional to r^2 (where r = distance from source), and directly as the square of the wave amplitude.

Sound intensity level (in decibels, dB): $\beta = 10\log_{10}\dfrac{I}{I_0}$

(where $I_0 = 10^{-12} \text{ W/m}^2$ = 0 threshold of hearing)

multiply *I* by 10 $\leftrightarrow$ *add* 10 to β.

divide *I* by 10 $\leftrightarrow$ *subtract* 10 from β.

Doppler effect: describes the change in frequency between a source and a detector due to relative motion of both

relative motion toward $\leftrightarrow$ frequency increase ($f_D > f_S$)

relative motion away $\leftrightarrow$ frequency decrease ($f_S > f_D$)

For constant velocities, this shift is constant. The frequency is not increasing or decreasing with time, but is simply a higher or lower constant at the detector than at the source. Relative acceleration creates an increasing or decreasing frequency.

Doppler effect (for waves other than light): $f_D = f_S \dfrac{v \pm v_D}{v \mp v_S}$

CHAPTER 12 FREESTANDING PRACTICE QUESTIONS

1. When all the finger holes on a clarinet are closed, it can be approximated as a hollow tube with one closed end (mouthpiece) and one open end. When all the finger holes on a clarinet are closed, the lowest pitch that can be produced corresponds to the G-flat below middle C (185 Hz). How long is the clarinet? (assume the speed of sound in air is 340 m/s).

A) 90 cm
B) 70 cm
C) 45 cm
D) 30 cm

2. A 37.5 cm glass pipe that is open at both ends is placed next to a student a cappella group. It was observed that the pipe first resonates when the choir produces a note at 450 Hz. At which subsequent frequencies will resonance again be observed? (The speed of sound through the pipe is 340 m/s.)

A) 675 Hz and 900 Hz
B) 675 Hz and 1350 Hz
C) 900 Hz and 1350 Hz
D) 900 Hz and 1800 Hz

3. The engine of a small and unmanned airplane produces a known and specific sound frequency (not given). A stationary sound detection device observes that the known emitted sound frequency is 90% of the perceived sound frequency. Relative to the detection device, in which direction and at what velocity is the plane moving?

A) Towards the detector, at 34 m/s
B) Away from the detector, at 34 m/s
C) Towards the detector, at 64 m/s
D) Away from the detector, at 64 m/s

4. An airplane is traveling 157 m/s north on a runway and is producing a sound of frequency f. A woman is seated in a car moving 43 m/s to the south, away from the airplane. What frequency will she observe? (assume the speed of sound in air is 343 m/s)

A) $1/2\,f$
B) $3/5\,f$
C) f
D) $2\,f$

5. A man standing 1 m away from an omnidirectional speaker is exposed to a sound of 140 dB. How far would he have to travel in order to no longer be in pain (the threshold of pain is about 120 dB), given $I = P/A$ and $\beta = 10\log(I\,/\,I_0)$, where $I_0 = 10^{-12}\,\text{W/m}^2$.

A) 9 m
B) 10 m
C) 20 m
D) 100 m

6. A stationary cat is purring. Which of the following correctly explains why its owner hears a frequency that is higher than that which is produced by the cat?

A) The owner is moving towards the cat.
B) The owner is moving away from the cat.
C) Both are on an accelerating train.
D) Both are on a decelerating boat.

7. A herpetologist studying alligators at the Kennedy Space Center is 1000 m from the launch pad, when a siren sounds, signaling 30 minutes to launch. After running away for 4000 m, the herpetologist turns to watch the launch. How does the intensity of sound produced by the siren at his new location compare to the original intensity, I_1, given $I = P/A$?

A) $5\,I_1$
B) $1/5\,I_1$
C) $1/25\,I_1$
D) $1/50\,I_1$

CHAPTER 12 PRACTICE PASSAGE

Sound waves propagate away from a source in spherical wavefronts, lines that connect the points on a sound wave that were emitted at the same time. When the source is stationary, these wave fronts are concentric spheres centered about the source. However, when the source begins to move with a velocity v_0, the wavefronts get closer together in the direction of v_0 and are spread farther apart in the opposite direction.

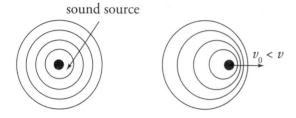

Figure 1 Wavefronts generated by sound sources that are stationary and moving with a speed less than the speed of sound.

As a result of the change in the distance between wavefronts, a listener standing ahead of or behind the object will hear a frequency different from the original emitted frequency, a phenomenon known as the Doppler effect, according to the equation:

$$f_D = f_S \frac{v \pm v_D}{v \mp v_S}$$

Equation 1

where f_D and f_S are the detected and emitted frequencies, respectively, v is the speed of sound, and v_D and v_S are the velocities of the detector and the source, respectively.

Some jets have been designed to fly at speeds greater than the speed of sound. There speeds are usually given as a Mach number, $M = v_0/v$, which indicates the jet's speed relative to the speed of sound in the surrounding air. Because the speed of sound in air increases as the temperature increases, the jets flying with the same Mach number can be travelling at different speeds. When a jet flies at exactly Mach 1, the wavefronts build up just in front of the object, creating an intense shock wave. Flight at this speed is incredibly turbulent. Interestingly, in this case an observer ahead of the jet would not hear it until the jet itself arrived, since the first wavefront and the jet arrive at the same time. Jets can also fly faster than the speed of sound, at supersonic speeds. When this happens, the jet actually advances ahead of the shock wave it creates. The intense sound heard when a shockwave passes by an observer is known as a sonic boom.

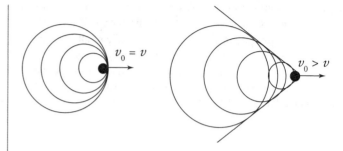

Figure 2 Wavefronts created by a jet flying at the speed of sound and at a supersonic speed.

1. Two jets are flying at Mach 3, one close to sea level, the other at 50,000 ft where the air temperature is cooler. Compared to the jet at sea level, the one flying at 50,000 ft is travelling:

A) at the same speed.
B) at a lower speed because the speed of sound decreases at altitude due to the lower air temperature.
C) at a greater speed because the speed of sound decreases at altitude due to the lower air temperature.
D) at a greater speed because the speed of sound increases at altitude due to the greater air temperature.

2. While driving down the road at 10 m/s, a driver hears 330 Hz siren from police car approaching from behind. If the frequency emitted by the siren is 300 Hz, how fast is the police car going?

A) 9 m/s
B) 10 m/s
C) 20 m/s
D) 40 m/s

3. A stationary observer is standing on a sidewalk when a police car emitting a 300 Hz siren passes by on the road at 20 m/s. Just as the police car passes her, what is the frequency she hears?

A) 283 Hz
B) 300 Hz
C) 318 Hz
D) 340 Hz

4. If the sonic boom that the jet produces when it goes supersonic is 60 dB louder than acceptable limits for the people on the base below, at minimum how many times farther away should it be from the base when it goes supersonic?

A) 10^3
B) 10^4
C) 10^5
D) 10^6

5. As a siren approaches an observer at a constant velocity, the observer hears a sound that is:

A) increasing in frequency.
B) at a constant frequency that is higher than the emitted frequency.
C) at a constant frequency that is lower than the emitted frequency.
D) decreasing in frequency.

6. What is a possible explanation for why flying at Mach 1 results in incredibly turbulent flight?

A) The transverse motion of the air molecules of the sound wave jostle the vessel up and down.
B) The transverse motion of the air molecules of the sound wave make it difficult for the pilot to steer.
C) The build-up of sound waves in front of the jet creates an extreme pressure front.
D) Jets are increasingly structurally unstable the faster they travel.

7. A jet flying at Mach 2 flies directly over a ship in the ocean. When the observers on the ship hear the jet, the jet is:

A) approaching the ship.
B) directly overhead.
C) already past the ship.
D) somewhere in the vicinity of the ship, but it is impossible know where it is in its path over the ship.

SOLUTIONS TO CHAPTER 12 FREESTANDING QUESTIONS

1. **C**   The clarinet with all its finger holes closed approximates a hollow tube with one closed end and one open end, and can be diagrammed as below:

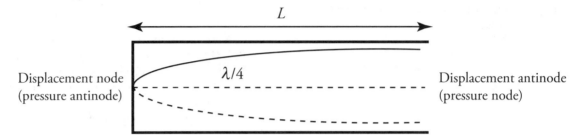

Displacement node (pressure antinode) $\lambda/4$ Displacement antinode (pressure node)

There is only one quarter (not one half) of a wavelength, and so the length of the pipe must be one-quarter the wavelength of the sound wave. The first (or fundamental) harmonic of a pipe with one closed end is $f_1 = v/4L$, where L is the length of the pipe. Rearranging this formula: $L = v/4\,f_1 = 340 \text{ m/s} / [(4)(185)]) = 0.46 \text{ m}$.

2. **C**   If the pipe first resonated at 450 Hz, then the fundamental frequency (f_1) of the standing wave in the pipe is 450 Hz. The subsequent frequencies that will produce resonance are $f_2, f_3, f_4, \ldots f_n$. These can be calculated using the equation $f_n = nf_1$. Since f_1 is given to us, the next resonance will be at $f_2 = (2)(450) = 900$ Hz, and the resonance after that will be $f_3 = (3)(450) = 1350$ Hz.

3. **A**   The Doppler effect is measured using the equation $f_D = f_S[v \pm v_D]/[v \mp v_S]$. The prompt tells us that the emitted sound frequency (f_S) is 90% of the perceived sound frequency (f_D), therefore $f_D/f_S = 10/9$. Since the detected sound frequency is greater than the perceived sound frequency ($f_D/f_S > 1$), and the sound detector is stationary ($v_D = 0$), then the Doppler effect dictates that the source must be moving towards the detector ($v - v_S$), eliminating choices B and D. To calculate the velocity of the sound source, we must solve for v_S using the Doppler effect:

$f_D/f_S = v/(v - v_S)$

$(f_D/f_S)(v - v_S) = v$

$(f_D/f_S) \times v - (f_D/f_S) \times v_S = v$

$[(f_D/f_S) - 1] \times v = (f_D/f_S) \times v_S$

$v_S = (f_S/f_D) \times v \times [(f_D/f_S) - 1]$

$v_S = (340 \text{ m/s}) \times (9/10) \times [(10/9) - 1] = 340 / 10 = 34 \text{ m/s}$

4. **B** This is a Doppler shift question, and thus begins with using the Doppler equation:

$$f_D = f_S \frac{v \pm v_D}{v \mp v_S}$$

The speed of the detector (v_D) is subtracted in the numerator because the car is moving away from the source, and thus the frequency observed will be lower than that produced. Addition is used in the denominator because the source, the airplane, is moving away from the detector and thus the frequency needs to be decreased. Subsequently plugging into the equation yields

$$f_D = f_S \frac{343 \text{ m/s} - 43 \text{ m/s}}{343 \text{ m/s} + 157 \text{ m/s}} \approx f_S \frac{300 \text{ m/s}}{500 \text{ m/s}} \approx \frac{3}{5} f$$

which gives choice B as correct. Both choices C and D can be eliminated because when two objects are moving apart, the frequency needs to decrease. (Note that if addition were used in the numerator and subtraction in the denominator, thus reversing the relationship and causing the frequency to increase, the answer would approximate 390/190 or approximately $2 f$, which is choice D.)

5. **A** A difference of 20 dB means a decrease in intensity of 10^2. This can either be gathered from the given logarithmic equation [$20 = 10 \log(I/I_0) \rightarrow 2 = \log(I/I_0)$ and therefore $I = 10^2$)] or by remembering that for every time 10 is added or subtracted from β, 10 is multiplied or divided from I, respectively. Knowing that I decreased by a factor of 100 means that the area would have had to increase by a factor of 100, since the power stays constant (from $I = P/A$). Since $A \propto r^2$, the radius must increase by a a factor of 10. Since the man was already 1 m from the source, he will have to travel 9 m. Choice B is a trap answer which ignores the original 1 m. Choice C is simply the number of dB dropped. Choice D is a trap which is equal to the factor that intensity is reduced.

6. **A** Choices C and D are both incorrect; they will have no effect on the frequency heard since the action is occurring to both the observer and the source. Choice B is backwards, because approaching objects will experience an increase in frequency (choice A is correct).

7. **C** Since the new radius is 5 times the original radius, the area will increase by 25 times (remembering that A is proportional to r^2). Since the area will increase by a factor of 25, the intensity will decrease by that factor (they are inversely proportional), giving choice C. Choice A can be eliminated because it assumes a direct, rather than inverse, relationship between the intensity and the area. Choice B is a trap; it is the correct answer if one forgets to square the multiple of the radius.

SOLUTIONS TO CHAPTER 12 PRACTICE PASSAGE

1. **B**   Since $M = v_0/v$, for a given Mach number, v_0 and v are directly related. The passage indicates that the speed of sound increases with increasing air temperature. Thus, at 50,000 ft where the air is cooler, the speed of sound is lower than at sea level. As a result the jet flying at 50,000 ft must be flying more slowly than the jet flying at sea level, even though they are travelling at the same Mach number.

2. **D**   Since the detected frequency is greater than the emitted frequency, choices A and B be eliminated since these velocities would not result in the siren approaching the observer. Using the fact that the detector is moving away from the source and that the source is approaching the detector, we obtain the equation $f_D = f_S (v - v_D)/(v - v_S)$. Plugging the given values into the equation yields 330 Hz = 300 Hz (340 m/s − 10 m/s)/(340 m/s − v_S) → 330 = 300 (330)/(340 −v_S) → 340 − v_S = 300 → v_S = 40 m/s.

3. **B**   As the siren is passing the observer, the siren is neither moving towards nor away from the listener. As a result, there is no difference between the detected and the emitted frequencies.

4. **A**   In order to decrease the sound by 60 dB, the intensity of the sonic boom must be decreased by a factor 10^6. Although this result makes choice D a tempting answer choice, it must be remembered that intensity is proportional to $1/r^2$. As a result, in order to decrease the intensity by a factor of 10^6, the radius only has to increase by a factor of 10^3.

5. **B**   If a sound source is approaching the observer, the frequency should increase, which eliminates choices C and D. If the siren is moving at a constant velocity, then as it approaches, the fraction $(v - v_D)/(v - v_S)$, which indicates the frequency shift, is constant, not continually increasing, which eliminates choice A.

6. **C**   Since sound is a pressure wave, a buildup of many sound waves does create an extreme pressure front. Choices A and B cannot be correct since sound is not a transverse wave. Although there may be some regime in which jets do become more structurally unstable the faster they fly, it does not answer the question since the passage mentions that the extreme turbulence is felt at exactly Mach 1, not at all speeds greater than Mach 1, indicating that choice D cannot explain this particular phenomenon.

7. **C**   As indicated by the passage, a supersonic jet flies ahead of the shockwave it creates. Therefore, when the observers hear the shockwave as it passes, the jet has already passed by.

Chapter 13
Light and Geometrical Optics

13.1 ELECTROMAGNETIC WAVES

We've seen that if we oscillate one end of a long rope, we generate a wave that travels down the rope and whose frequency is the frequency with which we oscillate.

You can think of an electromagnetic wave in a similar way: An oscillating electric charge generates an **electromagnetic (EM)** wave, which is composed of oscillating electric and magnetic fields. These fields oscillate with the same frequency at which the electric charge that created the wave oscillated. The fields oscillate in phase with each other, perpendicular to each other and to the direction of propagation. For this reason, electromagnetic waves are transverse waves. The direction in which the wave's electric field oscillates is called the direction of **polarization** of the wave.

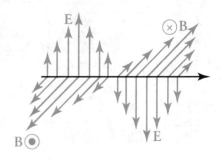

Most EM waves have electric fields oscillating in all perpendicular directions to propagation equally and are thus *unpolarized*.

Unlike waves on a rope or sound waves, electromagnetic waves do not require a material medium to propagate; they can travel through empty space (vacuum). When an EM wave travels through vacuum, its speed is a constant. It is one of the fundamental constants of nature and a value you should memorize for the MCAT:

Speed of Light in Vacuum

$$c = 3 \times 10^8 \, \tfrac{m}{s}$$

All electromagnetic waves, regardless of frequency, travel through vacuum at this speed. The most important equation for waves, $v = \lambda f$, is also true for electromagnetic waves. For EM waves traveling through vacuum, $v = c$, so the equation becomes $c = \lambda f$.

The frequencies for electromagnetic waves span a huge range, and different ranges have been given specific names. This assignment of names to specific regions based on frequency (or wavelength) is known as the **electromagnetic spectrum** and is shown here.

Notice that visible light occupies only a small part of the electromagnetic spectrum. When waves from all over the visible spectrum are mixed together, the resulting light is perceived as white. You should memorize the order of the colors of the visible spectrum from lowest frequency (longest wavelength) to highest frequency (shortest wavelength): ROYGBV ("Roy-Gee-Biv"), which stands for <u>r</u>ed, <u>o</u>range, <u>y</u>ellow, <u>g</u>reen, <u>b</u>lue, and <u>v</u>iolet. In terms of wavelengths, violet light has a wavelength (in vacuum) of about 400 nm and red light has a wavelength of about 700 nm; the other colors are in between.

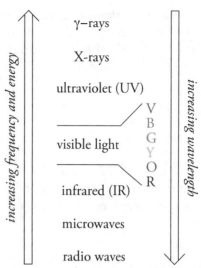

Photons

When electromagnetic radiation interacts with matter (absorption and emission), we find that it carries energy, and that the energy is quantized. That is, the energy associated with EM radiation is absorbed or emitted by matter in "packets"; individual bundles. Each such bundle of energy is called a **photon**, and the energy of a photon is directly proportional to the frequency:

Photon Energy

$$E = hf = h\frac{c}{\lambda}$$

The constant of proportionality, h, is called **Planck's constant**. (In SI units, its value is about 6.6×10^{-34} J·s.)

The fact that electromagnetic radiation carries energy in packets (photons), which we can think of as "particles of light", gives rise to the idea of **wave-particle duality** for electromagnetic radiation: EM radiation travels like a wave but interacts with matter like a particle. One peculiarity of this duality is that, for waves, energy is proportional to the square of amplitude (recall the intensity relation from the previous chapter), whereas for particles (photons), energy is proportional to frequency. In Chapter 11, we noted that these two properties were independent of one another. Thus, the wave and particle models for light differ significantly in their predictions, and yet each is sometimes true.

Example 13-1: Which one of the following statements is true regarding red photons and blue photons traveling through vacuum?

A. Red light travels faster than blue light and carries more energy.
B. Blue light travels faster than red light and carries more energy.
C. Red light travels at the same speed as blue light and carries more energy.
D. Blue light travels at the same speed as red light and carries more energy.

Solution: All electromagnetic waves, regardless of frequency, travel through vacuum at the same speed, *c*. This eliminates choices A and B. Now, because blue light has a higher frequency than red light (remember ROYGBV, which lists the colors in order of increasing frequency), photons of blue light have higher energy than photons of red light. Therefore, the answer is D.

13.2 REFLECTION AND REFRACTION

When a beam of light strikes the boundary between two transparent media, some of the light will be reflected from the surface. In the figure below, some of the sunlight will be reflected off the water in the tank.

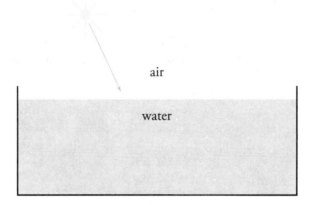

When a ray of light passing through one medium is reflected from the surface of another, the angle at which it bounces off the new medium is equal to the angle at which it strikes. In other words, *the angle of reflection is equal to the angle of incidence*. This fact is known as the **law of reflection**. Notice that, by definition, the angles of incidence and reflection are measured with reference to a line that's perpendicular to the plane of interface between the two media; that is, the angle of incidence and the angle of reflection are the angles that the incident and reflected rays make with *the normal*, not with the surface.

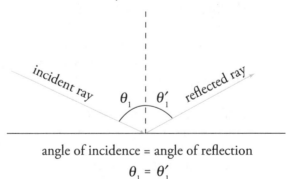

angle of incidence = angle of reflection

$$\theta_1 = \theta_1'$$

Example 13-2: In the figure above, assume that a ray of sunlight strikes the water, making an angle of 60° with the surface. What is the angle of reflection?

    A. 15°
    B. 30°
    C. 60°
    D. 90°

Solution: Be careful. If the incident ray makes an angle of 60° with the surface, then it makes an angle of 30° with the normal. Therefore, the angle of incidence is 30°. By the law of reflection, the angle of reflection is 30° also. Choice B is the answer.

In the figure below, not all of the sunlight that encounters the surface of the water is reflected; some is transmitted into the water. Unless the angle of incidence is 0°, the light will be *bent* as it enters the water. The bending is called **refraction**. The **angle of refraction** is the angle that the **transmitted** (or **refracted**) ray makes with the line that's perpendicular to the plane of interface between the two media.

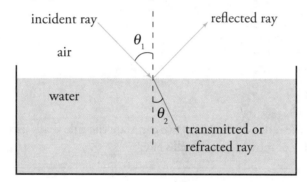

If $\theta_1 = 0°$ (that is, if the incident ray is perpendicular to the boundary), then $\theta_2 = 0°$. However, if θ_1 is any other angle, then θ_2 will be different from θ_1; that is, the ray bends as it's transmitted. In order to figure out the angle of refraction, we first need to discuss a medium's index of refraction.

Index of Refraction

Light travels at speed $c = 3 \times 10^8$ m/s when traveling in a vacuum. However, when light travels through a material medium such as water or glass, its transmission speed is less than c. Every medium, in fact, has an **index of refraction** that tells us how much slower light travels through that medium than through empty space.

> ### Index of Refraction
>
> $$\text{index of refraction} = \frac{\text{speed of light in vacuum}}{\text{speed of light in medium}}$$
>
> $$n = \frac{c}{v}$$

The index of refraction of vacuum is, by definition, exactly equal to 1. Because the index for air is very close to 1, we simply use $n = 1$ for air as well. (The MCAT will use this approximation unless otherwise specified.) Notice that n has no units, it's never less than 1, and the greater the value of n for a medium, the slower light travels through that medium. For most materials, the value of n is between 1 and 2.5. Glass has an index of refraction of about 1.5 (but varies depending on the type of glass) while diamond has a particularly high value of n, about 2.4. Values of n above 2.5 are rare.

Example 13-3: Light travels through water at an approximate speed of 2.25×10^8 m/s. What is the refractive index of water?

   A. 0.75
   B. 1.33
   C. 1.50
   D. 2.25

Solution: First, eliminate choice A: The index of refraction is never less than 1. Now, by definition,

$$n = \frac{c}{v} = \frac{3 \times 10^8 \text{ m/s}}{2.25 \times 10^8 \text{ m/s}} = \frac{3}{2.25} = \frac{3}{2\frac{1}{4}} = \frac{3}{\frac{9}{4}} = 3 \cdot \frac{4}{9} = \frac{4}{3} \approx 1.33$$

Therefore, the answer is B.

Now that we know about the index of refraction, we can state the rule that's used to figure out the angle of refraction. It's called the law of refraction, or Snell's law:

Law of Refraction (Snell's Law)

$$n_1 \sin \theta_1 = n_2 \sin \theta_2$$

In this equation, n_1 is the refractive index of the medium through which the incident ray is traveling, and n_2 is the refractive index of the medium through which the transmitted (or refracted) ray is traveling.

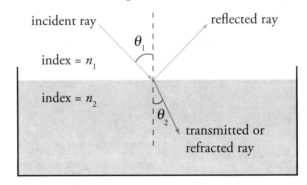

It follows from Snell's law that if $n_2 > n_1$, then $\theta_2 < \theta_1$. That is, if the transmitting medium has a higher index of refraction than the incident medium, then the ray will bend *toward* the normal. Similarly, if $n_2 < n_1$, then $\theta_2 > \theta_1$. That is, if the transmitting medium has a lower index of refraction than the incident medium, then the ray will bend *away from* the normal. You should memorize both of these facts.

Example 13-4: A ray of light traveling through air is incident on a piece of glass whose refractive index is 1.5. If the sine of the angle of incidence is 0.6, what's the sine of the angle of refraction?

Solution: Using the law of refraction, we find that

$$n_1 \sin\theta_1 = n_2 \sin\theta_2 \rightarrow \ (1)(0.6) = (1.5)(\sin\theta_2) \ \rightarrow \ \sin\theta_2 = \frac{0.6}{1.5} = \frac{6}{15} = \frac{2}{5} = 0.4$$

Notice that $\sin\theta_2$ is less than $\sin\theta_1$; this immediately tells us that $\theta_2 < \theta_1$. The light is traveling from air ($n_1 = 1$) into glass, whose refractive index is higher. If the transmitting medium (i.e., the second one) has a higher index of refraction than the incident medium (i.e., the first one), then θ_2 *will* be less than θ_1; that is, the ray will bend toward the normal.

Example 13-5: Consider the diagram below, showing an incident ray, reflected ray, and transmitted ray:

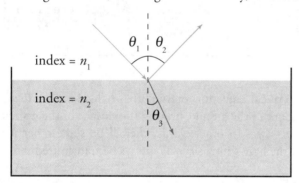

What information is needed to find θ_2?

A. n_1, n_2, and θ_1
B. n_1, n_2, and θ_3
C. n_1 only
D. θ_1 only

Solution: The angle labeled θ_2 is the angle of reflection. To find it, all we need to know is the angle of incidence, θ_1. (By the law of reflection, we find that $\theta_2 = \theta_1$.) The answer is D. (This unconventional labeling of the angles is a common MCAT tactic, by the way.)

Total Internal Reflection

When a light ray traveling in a medium of high refractive index approaches a medium of lower refractive index (for example, a light ray traveling in water towards the interface with the air), it may or may not escape into the second medium. If the ray's angle of incidence exceeds a certain **critical angle**, the light ray will undergo **total internal reflection**: All of the incident ray's energy will be reflected back into its original medium; there will be no refracted ray.

> ### Critical Angle for Total Internal Reflection
>
> $$\sin \theta_{crit} = \frac{n_2}{n_1}$$

In this equation, n_1 is the refractive index of the medium through which the incident ray is traveling, and n_2 is the refractive index of the medium on the other side of the boundary. The angle θ_{crit} is the critical angle. What this means is that if the angle of incidence, θ_1, is greater than θ_{crit}, then total internal reflection will occur.[1] However, if θ_1 is less than θ_{crit}, then total internal reflection will not occur. (If θ_1 just happens to equal θ_{crit}, then the refracted beam skims along the boundary with $\theta_2 = 90°$.)

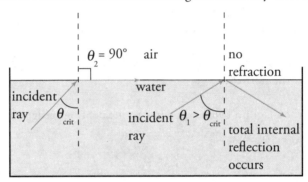

Notice that there can be a critical angle for total internal reflection *only if n_1 is greater than n_2*. For example, a beam of light incident in the air and striking the surface of the water can never experience total internal reflection because $n_1 < n_2$. In other words, there'll be some reflection and some refraction, as usual. In this case, some of the light's intensity will always be transmitted into the water.

Example 13-6: A beam of light is incident on the boundary between air and a piece of glass whose index of refraction is $\sqrt{2}$. When would total internal reflection (TIR, for short) of this beam occur?

Solution: First, in order to have TIR, the beam would have to start in the glass, trying to exit into the air. (If the beam were traveling in the air and incident on the glass, then TIR could not occur.) Furthermore, the angle of incidence would have to be greater than the critical angle, which we calculate as follows:

$$\sin \theta_{crit} = \frac{n_2}{n_1} = \frac{1}{\sqrt{2}} = \frac{\sqrt{2}}{2} \rightarrow \theta_{crit} = 45°$$

Total internal reflection is a vital technology for medicine because it is the underlying principle of fiber optics, used in endoscopy for laparoscopic and arthroscopic surgeries. Without the ability to see clearly inside the body with a thin, flexible tube through which light travels both into and out of the body (after reflecting off of organs and other tissues), many surgical procedures would still require large incisions and long recovery times.

---

[1] If you forget the formula for the critical angle, there's another way to know that total internal reflection occurs: If you plug numbers into the law of refraction and find that $\sin \theta > 1$ (which is impossible), that tells you there is no angle of refraction, so there must be total internal reflection.

13.3   WAVE EFFECTS

Diffraction

Simply put, waves, whether they're water waves, sound waves, EM waves, etc., don't always travel in a single direction when they encounter an obstruction. This redistribution of the wave's intensity is known as **diffraction**. Water waves bend around a rock sticking up out of the water, for example. The "obstruction" can even be a hole. For example, water or light incident on a hole in a barrier will pass through and *spread out* beyond the barrier. These effects are observed when the size of the object or opening is comparable to the wavelength of the waves.

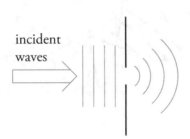

Polarization

Normally, the electric-field components of the waves in a beam of light vibrate in *all* planes. **Polarized** light is light whose direction of polarization has been restricted somehow. For example, all the waves in a beam of **plane-polarized** light have their electric-field components vibrating in a single plane.

It is possible to transform unpolarized light into polarized light by several methods. One method is the use of a *polarizing filter.* The filter has a polarization axis, so that when unpolarized light strikes the filter, only the portion of the waves vibrating in that direction pass through while the portion of the waves vibrating perpendicular to the axis is absorbed. The light that emerges is now polarized in in direction of the axis and has half the intensity of the original unpolarized light.

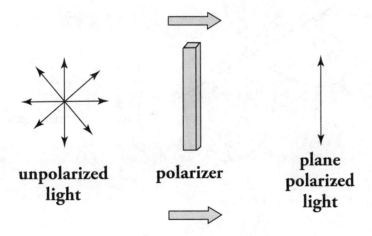

If polarized light passes through a second polarizer, the amount of light that passes through or is absorbed depends on the angle between the direction of polarization of the incident light and the axis of the polarizer. As an example, if vertically polarized light is incident upon a horizontally polarizing filter, none of the light will pass through.

13.3

If two light waves of equal amplitude vibrate perpendicular to each other and have a 90° phase difference (the "crest" of one wave interferes with the "0" of the other), the light is *circularly polarized*.

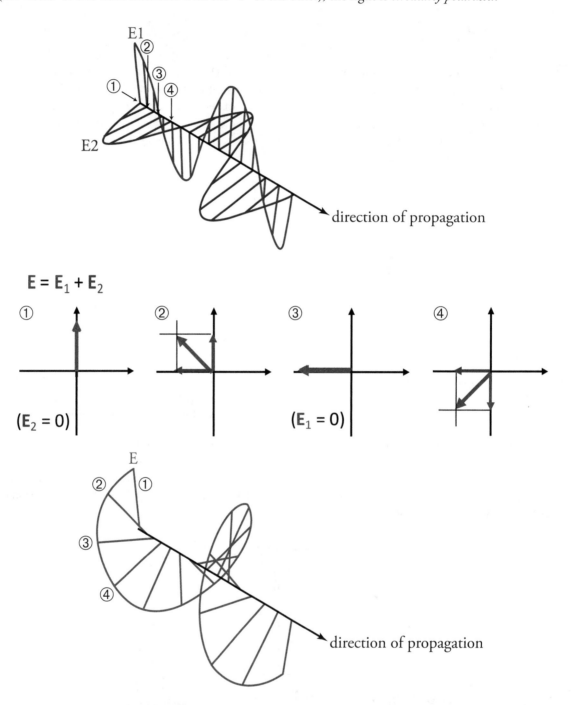

As a result, the electric field appears to be rotating.

Dispersion

When light moves from one medium to another, some wavelengths are bent more than others. The reason for this is that electromagnetic waves of different frequencies travel at slightly different speeds when traveling through a material medium like glass or water. Although Big Rule 1 for waves states that the speed of a wave is determined by the medium, not by the wave's frequency, light waves traveling through a material medium are an exception to this rule.[2] (In fact, they're the only exception that's at all likely to appear on the MCAT.) When light travels through a material (not vacuum), different frequencies will have different speeds. Thus, when we say that the index of refraction for a piece of glass is 1.5, what is really true is that the index varies slightly as the color of the light varies. For example, the index of refraction of the glass could be 1.47 for red light but 1.54 for violet light.[3] Because different colors have different refractive indexes, they will have different angles of refraction. This is why when white light passes through a prism, the beam is broken into its component colors. Each color leaves the prism at its own angle of refraction.[4] We call this variation in wave speed for different frequencies (and the effects this variation produces) **dispersion**.

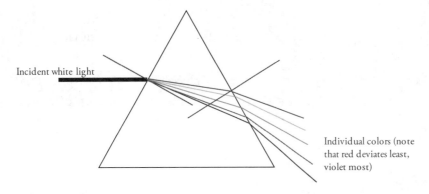

Incident white light

Individual colors (note that red deviates least, violet most)

13.4 MIRRORS

A **mirror** is a surface, usually made of glass or metal, that forms an image of an object by *reflecting* light.

Plane Mirrors

A **plane** mirror is an ordinary flat mirror. If you put an object in front of a plane mirror, the image will appear to be behind the mirror. The image will be the same size as the object and will appear to be as far behind the mirror's surface as the object is in front of it. The image will also appear upright; it won't be inverted.

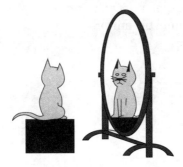

---

[2] This isn't the case when electromagnetic waves travel through vacuum, where *all* frequencies travel at the same speed, *c*.

[3] In general, as in this example, the higher the frequency of the light, the lower the speed. However, there are complicated exceptions to this rule of thumb, and there's no need to memorize it or learn about the exceptions for the MCAT.

[4] The greater the index of refraction, the more the light will be bent on entering the medium from air or vacuum, so high-frequency violet light will generally bend more than red light.

Curved Mirrors

We all have experience with plane mirrors, but a **curved** mirror presents us with images that are less familiar. The purpose of this section is to find a systematic way to describe the images formed by curved mirrors.

There are essentially two types of curved mirrors: concave and convex. The shiny (reflecting) surface of a **concave** mirror appears like the entrance to a "cave" from the point of view of the object. The reflecting surface of a **convex** mirror bends away from the object. As a simple demonstration of the difference, imagine holding a polished spoon. If you look into the spoon, you're looking at a concave surface; if you turn it around and look at the back of the spoon, you're looking at a convex surface.

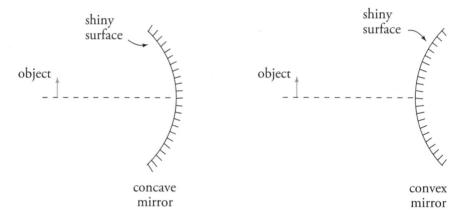

The curved mirrors we'll consider could be termed **spherical** mirrors, because near the center of the mirror, the surface is spherical (that is, part of a sphere).

When light parallel to the central **axis** of a concave mirror strikes the surface, it's reflected through a point called the **focus** (or **focal point**), denoted by F. This point is halfway to the **center of curvature**, C, of the mirror, which is the center of the sphere that the mirror is "cut from." The distance between the center of curvature and the mirror is called the **radius of curvature**, r. (The radius of curvature is also sometimes denoted by RC.) Because the focal point is halfway between the mirror and C, the distance from the mirror to the focal point, the all-important **focal length**, f, is half the radius of curvature: $f = \frac{1}{2}r$.

When light parallel to the central axis of a *convex* mirror strikes the surface, it's reflected directly *away from* the "imaginary" **focal point** behind the mirror.

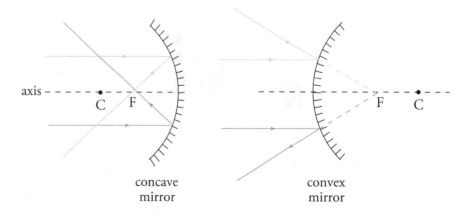

We see an image in a mirror at the point where the rays reflected off the mirror intersect *or* at the point from where the reflected rays seem to intersect (and therefore emanate from) behind the mirror. When a very distant object is placed in front of a mirror, the light rays that strike the mirror are approximately parallel, like the rays shown above. This illustrates the significance of the focal point. *The image of a distant object will appear at the focal point, for all curved mirrors.* This turns out to be true for thin lenses as well. But what if the object is not distant?

The following figures illustrate the process of image formation by curved mirrors:

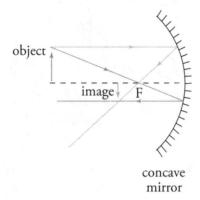

concave
mirror

The ray diagram for the concave mirror shows two incident rays reflecting off the mirror. One ray, parallel to the axis, is reflected through the focal point. Another ray, which goes through the focal point, is reflected parallel to the axis. The intersection point of these reflected rays determines the location of the image.

Note that the light rays still cross after reflecting off the mirror, but the image is located behind the focal point. If the object is moved closer to the mirror (i.e., inside the focal point), the reflected rays no longer cross and the image forms behind the mirror.

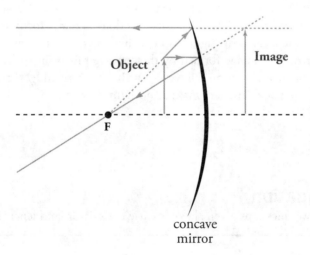

concave
mirror

One ray, parallel to the axis, is again reflected through the focal point. Another ray, which is directed as if it came from the focal point, is reflected parallel to the axis.

The ray diagram for the convex mirror also shows two incident rays reflecting off the mirror. One ray, parallel to the axis, is reflected directly away from the focal point. Another ray, which hits the center of the mirror (the point where its axis of symmetry intersects the mirror surface), is reflected at the same angle below the axis. Following these reflected rays back behind the mirror, their intersection point determines the location of the image.

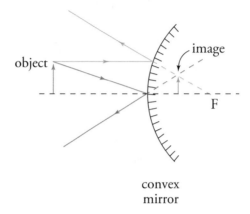

convex
mirror

Ray diagrams (like the ones drawn in the figures above) can be used to determine the approximate location of the image, but they usually can't give precise answers to all the questions we may be asked about the image formed by a mirror. What we want is a systematic way to get precise answers to these four questions:

1. Where is the image?
2. Is the image real or is it virtual?
3. Is the image upright or is it inverted?
4. How tall is the image (compared to the object)?

Before we discuss how to answer these questions, let's first define the terms *real* and *virtual*. An image is said to be **real** if light rays actually focus at the position of the image. A real image can be projected onto a surface. An image is said to be **virtual** if lights rays don't actually focus at the apparent location of the image. For example, look back at the figures above, showing the formation of images by a concave mirror and by a convex mirror. The image formed by the concave mirror in the first diagram is real: light rays actually intersect at the image location. However, the images formed by the concave mirror in the second diagram and by the convex mirror are virtual: no light rays intersect at its location; they just seem to come from that location.

The Mirror Equation

To answer the first two questions given above, we use the mirror (and lens) equation:

> **Mirror (and Lens) Equation**
>
> $$\frac{1}{o} + \frac{1}{i} = \frac{1}{f}$$

Here, o stands for the object's distance from the mirror, and is always positive. The value of f represents the focal length of the mirror. The value of i that satisfies this equation gives us the image's distance from the mirror. Both f and i are positive if they are on the same side as the human observer in relation to the mirror or lens. In the case of a mirror, the human observer is on the same side as the object. In the case of a lens, the human observer is on the opposite side of the object. Using the mirror (and lens) equation, we can find the location of the image, answering the first question.

The second question is also answered using the mirror equation. If we get a *positive* value for i, that tells us that the image is in front of the mirror and it's *real*; a *negative* value for i means the image is behind the mirror and is *virtual*. For example, let's say that $o = 2$ cm and $f = 6$ cm. Substituting these values into the mirror equation, we find that $i = -3$ cm. Therefore, the image is 3 cm behind the mirror and it's virtual. Note that you can use any unit for the measurement of distance, as long as it is the same unit for o, i, and f.

The Magnification Equation

To answer the last two questions, we then use the magnification equation:

Magnification Equation

$$m = -\frac{i}{o}$$

The value of m is the **magnification factor**; multiplying the height of the object by m gives us the height of the image. The sign of m tells us whether the image is upright or inverted. If m is *positive*, the image is *upright*; if m is *negative*, the image is *inverted*. To illustrate this, let's continue our example above, with $o = 2$ cm and $f = 6$ cm. We found that $i = -3$ cm. Therefore, the magnification factor is $m = -(-3 \text{ cm})/(2 \text{ cm}) = +1.5$. This tells us that the height of the image is 1.5 times the height of the object, and (because m is positive) the image is upright.

The object distance, o, is always positive. If i is positive, then m is negative; if i is negative, then m is positive. In other words,

Real images are inverted, and virtual images are upright.

Now, the only thing that's left to do is to find the way to "tell" the mirror equation whether we have a concave mirror or a convex mirror. The rule is simple: When using the mirror equation, we write the focal length of a *concave* mirror as a *positive* number, and we write the focal length of a *convex* mirror as a *negative* number. Here's a summary of mirrors:

Mirrors

Concave mirror   Convex mirror
f is positive f is negative

$$\frac{1}{o} + \frac{1}{i} = \frac{1}{f}$$

i positive $\longrightarrow$ real image (in front of mirror)

i negative $\longrightarrow$ virtual image (behind mirror)

$$m = -\frac{i}{o}$$

m positive $\longrightarrow$ image upright

m negative $\longrightarrow$ image inverted

- Concave mirrors can create real and virtual images
- Convex mirrors can only create virtual images

Example 13-7: Describe the image formed in a plane mirror.

A. Real and upright
B. Real and inverted
C. Virtual and upright
D. Virtual and inverted

Solution: First, eliminate choices A and D; *real* always goes with *inverted*, and *virtual* always goes with *upright*. We know from common experience that the image formed in a flat mirror is upright, so the answer must be C.

Example 13-8: If an object is placed very far from a concave mirror, where will the image be formed?

A. Halfway between the focal point and the mirror
B. At the focal point
C. At the center of curvature
D. At infinity

Solution: Use the mirror equation. "The object is placed very far from a mirror" means that we take $o = \infty$, so $1/o = 0$. The mirror equation then says $1/i = 1/f$, so $i = f$. That is, the image is formed at the focal point of the mirror, choice B.

Example 13-9: An object is placed 40 cm in front of a concave mirror with a radius of curvature of 60 cm. Locate and describe the image.

Solution: Because $f = \dfrac{1}{2}r$, we know that $f = 30$ cm. The mirror equation now gives

$$\frac{1}{40 \text{ cm}} + \frac{1}{i} = \frac{1}{30 \text{ cm}} \rightarrow \frac{1}{i} = \frac{1}{30} - \frac{1}{40} = \frac{4-3}{120} = \frac{1}{120} \rightarrow \therefore i = 120 \text{ cm}$$

(Be careful: The MCAT often gives the radius of curvature, r. What you want is f, the focal length, which is half of r.) Since i is positive, we know the image is real; also, it's located 120 cm from the mirror on the same side of the mirror as the object. (*Virtual* images are located *behind* the mirror.) Since $m = -i/o = -(120 \text{ cm})/(40 \text{ cm}) = -3$, we know that the image is 3 times the height of the object and inverted.

Example 13-10: An object is placed 40 cm in front of a convex mirror with a radius of curvature of -60 cm. Locate and describe the image.

Solution: Because $f = \dfrac{1}{2}r$, we know that $f = -30$ cm. The mirror equation now gives

$$\frac{1}{40 \text{ cm}} + \frac{1}{i} = \frac{1}{-30 \text{ cm}} \rightarrow \frac{1}{i} = \frac{1}{-30} - \frac{1}{40} = \frac{-4-3}{120} = \frac{-7}{120} \rightarrow \therefore i = -\frac{120}{7} \text{ cm}$$

Since i is negative, we know the image is virtual; also, it's located $120/7 \approx 17$ cm from the mirror on the opposite side of the mirror from the object. Since $m = -i/o = -(-\frac{120}{7} \text{ cm})/(40 \text{ m}) = +3/7$, we know that the image is 3/7 times the height of the object and upright. Comparing this example to the preceding one, notice how critical the sign of f was. It changed everything about the image.

Example 13-11: A convex mirror forms an upright image 12 cm behind the mirror when an object of height 15 cm is placed 20 cm in front of it. What is the height of the image?

Solution: To find the height of the image, we need the magnification. We're given that $o = 20$ cm and $i = -12$ cm. (We know that i is negative because not only do convex mirrors only form virtual images [a good fact to remember, by the way] but the question also says that the image is formed "behind the mirror." Images formed behind the mirror are virtual.) Therefore, $m = -i/o = -(-12 \text{ cm})/(20 \text{ cm}) = 3/5$. Multiplying the height of the object by the magnification gives the height of the image. Therefore, the height of the image is $(3/5)(15 \text{ cm}) = 9$ cm.

13.5 LENSES

A **lens** is a thin piece of clear glass or plastic that forms an image of an object by *refracting* light. The purpose of this section is to find a systematic way to describe the images formed by lenses.

There are essentially two types of lenses: converging and diverging. **Converging** lenses are thicker in the middle than they are at the ends, and they refract light rays that are parallel to the axis *toward* the focal point on the other side of the lens. **Diverging** lenses are thinner in the middle than they are at the ends, and they refract light rays that are parallel to the axis *away from* the "imaginary" focal point that's in front of the lens.

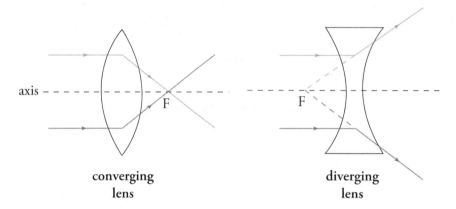

converging
lens

diverging
lens

We want to be able to answer the same four questions for lenses as we did for mirrors. Fortunately, *virtually everything we did for mirrors carries over unchanged to lenses.* For example, the mirror equation is also the lens equation, and the magnification equation is also the same. The conventions for positive and negative i and m are also the same for lenses as they are for mirrors.

We distinguish between the two types of lenses in the same way we distinguished between the two types of mirrors. When using the lens equation, we write the focal length of a *converging* lens as a *positive* number, and we write the focal length of a *diverging* lens as a *negative* number.

Here's an important note. The MCAT uses the terms *concave* and *convex* to refer to different mirrors and lenses. The diagrams above show us that the surfaces of a converging lens are convex, and the surfaces of a diverging lens are concave. Thus, a concave lens is the same as a diverging lens, and a convex lens is the same as a converging lens. Now for a warning: For a concave *mirror*, f is positive; and for a convex *mirror*, f is negative. When these terms are applied to lenses, things necessarily switch: For a concave *lens*, f is negative; and for a convex *lens*, f is positive. *Be careful* when you see the words *concave* or *convex*. Whether these terms describe a mirror or a lens will make a critically important difference in whether you write the focal length as a positive or as a negative number.

Besides the fact the lenses form images by refracting light (rather than by reflecting light, as is the case for mirrors), there's really only one difference: For lenses, *real* images are formed on the *opposite* side of the lens from the object while *virtual* images are formed on the *same* side of the lens as the object.

13.5

Here's a summary of lenses:

Lenses

Converging lens   Diverging lens
(convex lens)   (concave lens)
f is positive f is negative

$$\frac{1}{o} + \frac{1}{i} = \frac{1}{f}$$

i positive $\Rightarrow$ real image (other side of lens)
i negative $\Rightarrow$ virtual image (same side of lens as object)

$$m = -\frac{i}{o}$$

m positive $\Rightarrow$ image upright
m negative $\Rightarrow$ image inverted

- Converging (convex) lenses can create real and virtual images.
- Diverging (concave) lenses can create only virtual images.

Example 13-12: If an object is placed 10 cm in front of a diverging lens with a focal length of –40 cm, then the image will be located:

     A.   5 cm in front of the lens
     B.   5 cm behind the lens
     C.   8 cm in front of the lens
     D.   8 cm behind the lens

Solution: We use the lens equation to find i:

$$\frac{1}{10 \text{ cm}} + \frac{1}{i} = \frac{1}{-40 \text{ cm}} \rightarrow \frac{1}{i} = \frac{1}{40} - \frac{1}{10} = \frac{-1-4}{40} = \frac{-5}{40} = -\frac{1}{8} \rightarrow \therefore i = -8 \text{ cm}$$

This eliminates choices A and B. Because i is negative, the image is virtual, and for lenses, virtual images are formed on the same side of the lens as the object. Therefore, the answer is C.

Example 13-13: An object of height 10 cm is held 50 cm in front of a convex lens with a focal length of magnitude 40 cm. Describe the image.

Solution: The fact that the lens is convex means that it's a converging lens with a *positive* focal length; therefore, $f = +40$ cm. The lens equation now gives us i:

$$\frac{1}{50 \text{ cm}} + \frac{1}{i} = \frac{1}{40 \text{ cm}} \rightarrow \frac{1}{i} = \frac{1}{40} - \frac{1}{50} = \frac{5-4}{200} = \frac{1}{200} \rightarrow \therefore i = 200 \text{ cm}$$

Because i is positive, we know the image is real; also, it's located 200 cm from the lens on the *opposite* side of the lens from the object. Because $m = -i/o = -(200 \text{ cm})/(50 \text{ cm}) = -4$, we know that the image is 4 times the height of the object and inverted.

Lens Power

13.5

A lens with a short focal length refracts light more (i.e., through larger angles) than a lens with a longer focal length. We say that the lens of short focal length has a greater *power* than a lens with a longer focal length.

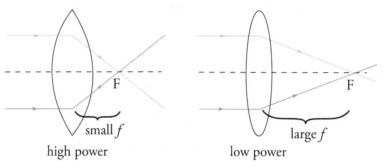

The **power** of a lens is defined to be the reciprocal of f, the focal length. When f is expressed in *meters*, the unit of lens power is called the **diopter** (abbreviated **D**).

Lens Power

$$P = \frac{1}{f} \text{ where } f \text{ is in meters}$$

For example, to find the power of a lens whose focal length is 40 cm, we first write f in meters: $f = 0.4$ m. Since $0.4 = 2/5$, the reciprocal of 0.4 is $5/2 = 2.5$. Therefore, the power of this lens is 2.5 diopters. Since the focal length of a converging lens is positive, the power of a converging lens is positive. Similarly, since the focal length of a diverging lens is negative, the power of a diverging lens is negative.

If two (or more) lenses are placed side by side, the power of the lens combination is equal to the sum of the powers of the individual lenses. In the case of two lenses, $P = P_1 + P_2$. For example, if we place a converging lens with a power of 3 D right next to a converging lens with a power of 1 D, then the power of the lens combination will be 4 D.

Example 13-14: A lens has a focal length of −20 cm. Is the lens converging or diverging? What is the power of this lens?

Solution: The fact that the lens has a negative focal length means that it's a diverging (or concave) lens. Rewriting f in meters, we have $f = -\frac{1}{5}$ m . Therefore, the power of this lens is

$$P = \frac{1}{f} = \frac{1}{-\frac{1}{5}\text{ m}} = -5\text{ D}$$

The Basics of Eyesight Correction

Let's now look at the fundamental use of auxiliary lenses to correct the two most common types of eye defects: myopia and hyperopia. **Myopia** is the technical name for *nearsightedness*; myopic individuals cannot focus clearly on distant objects. **Hyperopia** (or **hypermetropia**) is the technical name for *far-sightedness*; in contrast to myopes, hyperopic individuals cannot focus clearly on objects that are near the eye. (As we age, most of us will be afflicted with *presbyopia*, in which the eyes' ability to *accommodate* is compromised by the loss of elasticity in the lens of the eye. **Accommodation** refers to the ability to focus on nearby objects through the action of the ciliary muscles, which essentially squeeze the lens of the eye, increasing its curvature and decreasing its focal length. However, the correction for presbyopia is the same as that for hyperopia.)

Correcting Myopia: Light rays from objects whose distance from the eye is greater than about 6 m are essentially parallel to the axis of the lens of the eye, so a relaxed eye will focus these rays at the focal point. Because the diameter of a myopic eye is greater than the focal length of the lens of the eye, the image of the object is focused not on the retina but in front of it. As a result, a myopic individual receives a blurred image of distant objects. To correct this defect, a lens that "delays" the focusing is required. In essence, what is needed is a lens to diverge the parallel rays before they enter the lens of the eye so that they will focus beyond the focal point of the unaided eye, specifically on the retina. Because diverging lenses have negative focal lengths, they have negative powers (this follows from the definition $P = 1/f$). The greater the distance between the focal point of the lens of the myopic eye and the retina, the more the auxiliary lens must diverge the incoming parallel rays; that is, the more powerful the corrective lens (and the more negative the lens power).

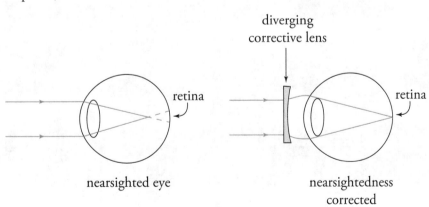

Correcting Hyperopia or Presbyopia: In these cases, light rays would be focused beyond the retina, either due to the diameter of the eye being smaller than the focal length of the lens of the eye or the inability of the ciliary muscles to decrease the focal length of the lens of the eye. To correct this defect, a lens that "accelerates" the focusing is required. In essence, what is needed is a lens to converge the rays before they enter the lens of the eye so that they will focus in front of the focal point of the unaided eye, specifically, on the retina. Because converging lenses have positive focal lengths, they have positive powers. (This follows from the definition $P = 1/f$.) The greater the distance between the focal point of the lens of the hyperopic eye and the retina, the more the auxiliary lens must converge the incoming rays; that is, the more powerful the corrective lens (and the more positive the lens power).

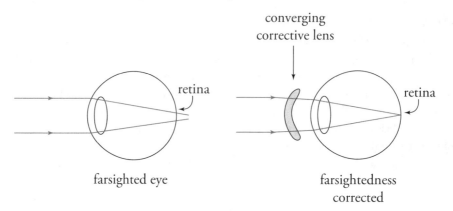

farsighted eye

farsightedness corrected

If you wear eyeglasses or contacts, check the prescription. If you have trouble seeing faraway objects, then you're nearsighted (myopic), and your corrective lenses are diverging and will have a negative power. On the other hand, if you have trouble seeing objects that are close-up, then you're farsighted (hyperopic), and your corrective lenses are converging and will have a positive power. Also, if the power of your left corrective lens is different from the power of your right corrective lens, the lens with the power of greater *absolute value* corresponds to the weaker eye. For example, if your left eye requires a lens of power –3.5 D while your right eye requires a lens of power –3.25 D, then your left eye is weaker because 3.5 > 3.25.

Summary of Formulas

Light acts as both a wave and a particle depending on the circumstance. In the former, energy is a function of amplitude; in the latter, energy is a function of frequency.

$$c = 3 \times 10^8 \text{ m/s for light in a vacuum}$$

-   All angles for reflection and refraction formulas are measured from the normal to the surface.

Photon energy: $E = hf = h\dfrac{c}{\lambda}$

Law of reflection: $\theta_1 = \theta_1'$

Index of refraction: $n = \dfrac{c}{v}, n \geq 1$

Law of refraction (Snell's law): $n_1 \sin\theta_1 = n_2 \sin\theta_2$

Total internal reflection: If $n_1 > n_2$ and $\theta_1 > \theta_{crit}$, where $\sin\theta_{crit} = \dfrac{n_2}{n_1}$

Total internal reflection (meaning no light is transmitted from the incident medium through the boundary) can occur for incident angles greater than θ_{crit} and only when the incident medium has a larger index of refraction (n) than that of the medium beyond the boundary.

Mirror/lens equation: $\dfrac{1}{o} + \dfrac{1}{i} = \dfrac{1}{f}$

Magnification: $m = -\dfrac{i}{o}$

Converging mirror or lens (concave mirror or convex lens) $\leftrightarrow$ f positive

Diverging mirror or lens (convex mirror or concave lens) $\leftrightarrow$ f negative

Note o is always positive.

Real, inverted image $\leftrightarrow$ positive i

Virtual, upright image $\leftrightarrow$ negative i

Lens power: $P = \dfrac{1}{f}$ (P in diopters when f is expressed in meters)

CHAPTER 13 FREESTANDING PRACTICE QUESTIONS

1. In optics, spontaneous parametric down conversion is often used to create two photons from one photon. Thus, it is possible for a blue photon with a frequency of 700 THz to be split into two identical red photons when incident on a nonlinear crystal. What is the wavelength of the red photons with respect to the blue photon, λ_B, given that energy is conserved?

A) $2\lambda_B$
B) $4\lambda_B$
C) $1/2\lambda_B$
D) $1/4\lambda_B$

2. If the magnification of a mirror is 2, where are the focal point and the image?

A) The image is on the same side of the mirror as the object and the focal point is twice as far from the mirror as the object.
B) The image is on the same side of the mirror as the object and the focal point is half as far from the mirror as the object.
C) The image is on the opposite side of the mirror as the object and the focal point is twice as far from the mirror as the object.
D) The image is on the opposite side of the mirror as the object and the focal point is half as far from the mirror as the object.

3. Glasses that correct for nearsightedness have a negative power associated with them. Are these lenses diverging or converging, and do they have a focal length that is positive or negative?

A) Diverging lens with positive focal length
B) Converging lens with negative focal length
C) Diverging lens with negative focal length
D) Converging lens with positive focal length

4. A physics student looking into a carnival funhouse mirror sees that his image is upright but his head appears twice as big as normal and his feet look half as big as normal. Let o represent the distance from the student to the mirror, f_{top} represent the focal length of the top of the mirror (where the student's head appears), and f_{bottom} represent the focal length of the bottom of the mirror (where the student's feet appear). What combination of curved mirrors is necessary to create the illusion?

A) The mirror top is concave with $f_{top} = 2o$ and the mirror bottom is convex with $f_{bottom} = -(1/2)o$.
B) The mirror top is concave with $f_{top} = 2o$ and the mirror bottom is convex with $f_{bottom} = -o$.
C) The mirror top is concave with $f_{top} = 3o$ and the mirror bottom is convex with $f_{bottom} = -(1/3)o$.
D) The mirror top is convex with $f_{top} = -o$ and the mirror bottom is concave with $f_{bottom} = (1/2)o$.

5. For a plane mirror, the object distance from the mirror is o, the image distance from the mirror is i, the focal point distance from the mirror is f, and the magnification of the mirror is m. Which of the following is true of the plane mirror?

I. Since f approaches infinity, then $i = -o$.
II. Since $f = 0$, then $i = -o$.
III. Since $i = -o$, then $m = 1$ and the image is the same size as the object.

A) I only
B) II only
C) I and III
D) II and III

6. An object is placed in front of a convex mirror. If the object is moved closer to the mirror, the image will move:

A) farther from the mirror and become smaller.
B) farther from the mirror and become larger.
C) closer to the mirror and become smaller.
D) closer to the mirror and become larger.

7. A beam of light passing through crown glass ($n = 1.5$) strikes the surface between the glass and air and experiences Total Internal Reflection. Which of the following changes to the experiment would ensure that the beam of light continues to experience this phenomenon?

A) Have the light originate in air
B) Decrease the angle of incidence
C) Immerse the glass in water ($n = 1.33$)
D) Decrease the wavelength of light

CHAPTER 13 PRACTICE PASSAGE

Optical instruments, such as mirrors and lenses, are often used to converge or diverge light. When more than one optical instrument bends light in succession, it is sometimes useful to consider the image produced by the first mirror or lens to be the object from which the light comes to the second mirror or lens. In such cases, the virtual object for the second instrument is sometimes on the opposite side of the instrument as the incoming light. The convention for these objects is that their distances are negative in optics equations.

One example of the use of multiple optical instruments together can be found in vision correction. For an object to appear in focus, light from that object must converge on the retina at the back of the eye, roughly 2 cm away from the front in most humans. Normally, the cornea and crystalline lens (together effectively constituting one converging lens, with an index of refraction of about 1.4) at the front of the eyeball do this. When this does not occur, eyeglasses can often be used to fix the problem. Eyeglasses are made of converging or diverging lenses in frames, and they change the angle of the incoming light that reaches the lens at the front of the eye, which then is able to focus the differently angled light at the retina.

A lens bends light by refraction, so the refractive index of the lens material is one of the determinants of the focal length of the lens. For a lens with circular curvatures on either side, the radius of curvature of each side is another determinant. In a vacuum or air, the thin lens equation gives the focal length of a lens of minimal thickness, index of refraction n, radius of curvature of the side nearest the source of light R_1, and radius of curvature of the side opposite the source of light R_2:

$$\frac{1}{f} = (n-1)(\frac{1}{R_1} - \frac{1}{R_2})$$

Equation 1

1. If a certain eye can only focus on objects at least 50 cm away, which of the following lenses, if placed in front of the eye, would allow it to focus on an object 25 cm away?

A) A converging lens with focal length 17 cm
B) A diverging lens with focal length 17 cm
C) A diverging lens with focal length 50 cm
D) A converging lens with focal length 50 cm

2. Which of the following is true of a nearsighted eye's native lens?

A) Its lens power is too small, causing the light rays to converge before they reach the retina.
B) Its lens power is too small, causing the light rays not to have converged even when they reach the retina.
C) Its lens power is too great, causing the light rays to converge before they reach the retina.
D) Its lens power is too great, causing the light rays not to have converged even when they reach the retina.

3. Which of the following describes the image formed in a typical human eye from light rays from an object 10 cm away?

A) The image is virtual and 0.4 cm away from the lens.
B) The image is real and 2 cm away from the lens.
C) The image is real and 2.5 cm away from the lens.
D) The image is virtual and 2.5 cm away from the lens.

4. Which of the following is true of images created with optical instruments by virtual objects with negative object distances?

A) Real images are always upright, and virtual images are always inverted.
B) Real images are always inverted, and virtual images are always upright.
C) Both real and virtual images are always upright.
D) Both real and virtual images are always inverted.

5. What is the speed of light in the lens of the eye?

A) 1.5×10^8 m/s
B) 2.1×10^8 m/s
C) 3.0×10^8 m/s
D) 4.2×10^8 m/s

6. A person notices that an object at a given distance is clearly in focus when viewed in air, but when the same object at the same distance is viewed in clear water, it appears blurry. Which of the following best explains this phenomenon?

A) The water absorbs much of the light energy coming from the object.

B) The index of refraction of water is different from that of air.

C) Dispersion in the water causes only a few of the light rays from the object to reach the eyes.

D) The water acts as a polarizing filter.

7. How will the lens power of a thin lens with a greater index of refraction compare to that of a thin lens with a smaller index of refraction, if the two lenses have all the same radii of curvatures?

A) It will be greater.

B) It will be equal.

C) It will be less.

D) It cannot be determined.

SOLUTIONS TO CHAPTER 13 FREESTANDING QUESTIONS

1. **A** The energy of a photon is $E = hf = hc/\lambda$. Since $E_B = 2E_R$ we know that $f_B = 2f_R$, and consequently, $\lambda_R = 2\lambda_B$.

2. **C** The magnification equation is $m = -i/o$. Since $m = 2$, i is negative, which tells us the image is on the opposite side of the mirror as the object, a virtual image. This question is a two-by-two, meaning that we need two pieces of information to answer correctly. The fact that the image is virtual eliminates choices A and B. Using the mirror equation we find that $f = 2o$. Therefore, the focal point is twice as far from the mirror as the object.

3. **C** For lenses, negative focal length is a property of a diverging lens and a positive focal length is a property of a converging lens. This eliminates choices A and B. The second piece of information comes from the fact that the power of nearsighted corrective glasses is negative, indicating a negative focal length since $P = 1/f$.

4. **B** Since the image is always upright, the magnification, m, is always positive. For the top of the mirror, $m = 2 = -i/o$ and $i = -2o$. Plugging this into the mirror equation $1/f = 1/i + 1/o = 1/(-2o) + 1/o = 1/(2o)$ and $f = 2o$. A positive focal length corresponds to a concave mirror. For the bottom of the mirror, $m = 1/2$ and $i = -(1/2)o$. Plugging this into the mirror equation $1/f = 1/i + 1/o = -2/o + 1/o = -1/o$ and $f = -o$. A negative focal length corresponds to a convex mirror. The correct answer is choice B.

5. **C** For a plane mirror, the image size is the same as the object size, and the object is upright. So $m = -i/o = 1$ and $i = -o$. So Item III is true, eliminating choices A and B. Both Items I and II have $i = -o$, so plugging this into the mirror equation gives $1/f = 1/i + 1/o = 1/(-o) + 1/o = 0$ and $f =$ something very large. So Item I is true, eliminating choice D. Notice that Item II cannot be true because if $f = 0$ then $1/f = 1/0$ which is not defined. The correct answer is choice C.

6. **D** Ray tracing is not necessary to solve this problem. The mirror and the magnification equations can be used, but without numbers they could be time consuming. A simple method would be to choose the initial object distance to be very large ($o \approx \infty$). For any mirror (except the plane mirror) or lens, the image of a distant object forms at the focal point (Note: the mirror equation, $1/o + 1/i = 1/f$, backs this up; for large o, $1/o \approx 0$, so $i \approx f$). It also stands to reason that the image of a very distant object will be very small (by the magnification equation, $m = -i/o \approx 0$). The final object distance can be chosen as almost 0 (i.e., when the object is pressed up against the mirror). From experience, if an object is pressed up against any mirror, the image will also be pressing up against the mirror and appear to be the same size as the object. The image therefore moves from the focal point to the mirror, eliminating choices A and B, and goes from being very small to the size of the object, eliminating choice C.

7. **D** For light to experience total internal reflection, two conditions must be met. First, the light must originate in the slower medium (i.e., the one with the larger index of refraction), which eliminates choice A; second, the angle of incidence must be greater than the critical

angle. While decreasing the angle of incidence may result in total internal reflection, it is not guaranteed since the angle could be smaller than or equal to the critical angle. This eliminates choice B. The formula for the *critical angle* is given by $\theta_c = \sin^{-1}(n_2 / n_1)$. Immersing the glass in water would increase n_2, which would increase the critical angle. This may cause the angle of incidence to be less than the critical angle, eliminating choice C. Due to *dispersion*, the shorter the wavelength of light, the slower it travels in glass, and therefore the more it will bend. Another way of thinking about this is that n_1 slightly increases for shorter wavelength. This would decrease the critical angle, and therefore make it impossible for refraction to occur.

SOLUTIONS TO CHAPTER 13 PRACTICE PASSAGE

1. **D** According to the first paragraph, the lens needs to create an image where the object ought to be (50 cm away from the eye), and then the image becomes the "object" for the eye's lens, which converges the light on the retina. In other words, the object is at a distance of 25 cm and the image at a distance of 50 cm, and since the image is going to be on the same side of the lens as the object, the image will be virtual. Next, apply $\dfrac{1}{f} = \dfrac{1}{o} + \dfrac{1}{i}$ and plug in: $\dfrac{1}{f} = \dfrac{1}{25} + \dfrac{1}{(-50)} = \dfrac{1}{50}$, so the focal length is 50 cm.

2. **C** In this question, one can eliminate two answers by deciding whether the lens power is too great or too small and eliminate the final wrong answer by determining whether the light rays converge too soon or too late. Nearsighted eyes can see near things well (the light of which is already diverging: look back at the diagram for correcting myopia), but cannot focus on faraway things (the light of which is arriving in parallel rays). This suggests that the eyes converge too strongly, which is a too-great lens power (eliminate choices A and B). Second, if the lens converges too strongly, the light rays must converge before they reach the retina (eliminate choice D). Note: This question can be answered without any information from the passage.

3. **B** According to the second paragraph, the retina is about 2 cm away from the lens in most humans. Also, the light rays actually converge on the retina. That describes the formation of a real image. Thus, the image is real (eliminate choices A and D) and is about 2 cm away from the lens (eliminate choice C). Be careful not to select choice C! This would be the correct answer if the distance between the retina and the lens were the focal length, but this does not match the passage's description; the position of the light rays actually converging (or where they would be traced back to converge, for a virtual image) is the image distance, not the focal length.

4. **A** Recall $m = -\dfrac{i}{o}$. If o is negative, then its negative sign cancels with the negative sign already in the equation, and the sign of m matches the sign of i: a positive i implies a positive m, and a negative i implies a negative m. Thus, real images (positive i) are upright (positive m), and virtual images (negative i) are inverted (negative m). Choice B is normally true on the MCAT, but that is because the object distance is normally positive.

5. **B** Apply $n = \dfrac{c}{v}$. According to the second paragraph, in the lens, the index of refraction is 1.4, so $v = \dfrac{c}{n} \approx \dfrac{3 \times 10^8}{1.4} \approx 2.1 \times 10^8$ m/s. Note that light cannot travel faster than c, so choice D can be eliminated immediately.

6. **B** The lens in the eye works by refraction (like all lenses). If the eye does not change, but the medium from which the light is coming changes, then the angle of refraction will change (as in $n_1 \sin \theta_1 = n_2 \sin \theta_2$: modify n_1 while holding n_2 and θ_1 constant, and θ_2 will change). If the angle of refraction changes, then the light will not focus on the retina anymore. Note: This could be determined without reference to the passage, but if necessary, the fact that the light must converge on the retina can be found in the second paragraph, and the fact that refraction is involved is in the third paragraph.

   Alternatively, use process of elimination. Even if choice A were true, it would mean that less light energy would reach the eye, reducing the intensity of light; that dims the image but does not blur it. In choice C, dispersion refers to differences in a material's index of refraction for different frequencies of light (different colors); this can blur an image as different colors have slightly different focal lengths, but it would not significantly diminish the total amount of light reaching the eye. In choice D, polarization does not blur light, and water does not normally polarize light.

7. **A** Recall that lens power is given by $P = \dfrac{1}{f}$, and combining this with Equation 1 yields $P = (n-1)(\dfrac{1}{R_1} - \dfrac{1}{R_2})$. Thus, P is directly proportional to $(n-1)$, and when n increases, so does P.

Chapter 14
Quantum Physics

14.1 QUANTIZATION

In the previous chapter, we learned that electromagnetic radiation can behave as a wave or as a particle called a photon. The discovery of this wave-particle duality of light was one of the first important results of the new **quantum physics** around the turn of the twentieth century. The word "quantum" refers to a specific amount of something measurable, like mass, charge, wavelength, momentum, energy, etc. Quantum physics, then, is the physics associated with discrete values and changes in the values of such quantities; that is, their **quantization**. We've already encountered an example of this phenomenon with charge: only charges that are integer multiples of the elementary charge $e = 1.6 \times 10^{-19}$ coulombs will ever be observed, because you can't have half a proton or two thirds of an electron. Thus charge is **quantized**.

Quantum physics is a complex and fascinating field that describes myriad strange phenomena and underlies many of our most important technological advances, such as computers, MRIs, and lasers. For MCAT purposes, you will need to understand the basic quantum model of the atom and the Pauli exclusion principle, the quantization of EM energy and the photoelectric effect, and the Heisenberg uncertainty principle.

14.2 THE BOHR MODEL OF THE ATOM

When a diffuse elemental gas is energized by heating or passing a current through it, the gas glows with a particular hue. If that light is passed through a prism, then dispersion will cause the light to separate into its component colors, corresponding to frequencies and wavelengths. This pattern of distinct bright lines of color is called the element's **emission spectrum**.

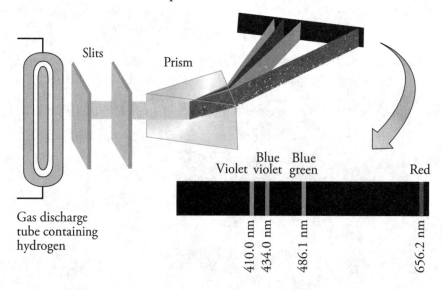

Recall that the energy of a photon is given by

$$E_{photon} = hf = hc \,/\, \lambda$$

where h is Planck's constant, 6.63×10^{-34} joule-seconds. Thus, one can use the measured wavelengths of light to determine the energies of the atomic transitions that produced the light. The assumption is that the particular frequencies of photons emitted by the atoms in the gas correspond to the energy losses of the atoms as their electrons transition from higher to lower energy states. Because only these characteristic frequencies are observed for a given element under normal conditions, this indicates that only certain electron transitions can occur.

Example 14-1: The wavelength of the red Hα spectral line characteristic of the visible hydrogen spectrum is 656 nm. How much energy does a hydrogen atom lose when it emits an Hα photon? Use $h = 6.63 \times 10^{-34}$ J·s.

Solution: Use the equation for the energy of a photon in terms of wavelength:

$$E_{photon} = \frac{hc}{\lambda} = \frac{\left(6.63 \times 10^{-34}\ \text{J} \cdot \text{s}\right)\left(3 \times 10^{8}\ \text{m/s}\right)}{656 \times 10^{-9}\ \text{m}} \approx 3 \times 10^{-19}\ \text{J}$$

The energy of the emitted photon corresponds exactly to the energy lost by the hydrogen atom.

Danish physicist Niels Bohr explained these discrete and characteristic emission spectra by modifying the classical Rutherford atomic model, which depicted the atom as a planetary system, with a tiny but massive central positive charge orbited by distant electrons. The Rutherford model explained many experimental results, but it failed to account for the discrete emission spectra. Scientists knew that accelerating charges emitted EM waves, but because there were no restrictions on the orbital radii of the electrons in the Rutherford model, there was no reason that the emission spectra shouldn't include all wavelengths instead of the discrete few actually observed. To fix this problem, Bohr's model proposed that the angular momentum of the orbiting electrons was quantized, restricted to multiples of the Planck constant:

Quantization of Angular Momentum

$$mvr = nh \,/\, 2\pi$$

where $n = 1, 2, 3 \ldots$

Note that this angular momentum for a circular orbit is simply the familiar linear momentum $p = mv$ multiplied by the orbital radius r.

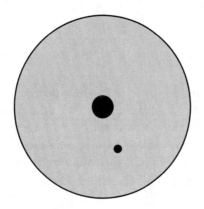
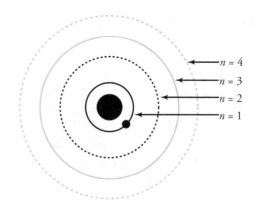

Rutherford Model
Electrons assume arbitrary orbits

Bohr Model
Electrons assume quantized orbits

The Bohr model assumes that atoms have electron orbitals with quantized energy levels and that a transition between levels requires the absorption or emission of a photon:

Energy of a Photon Emitted or Absorbed under the Bohr Model

$$E_{photon} = |\Delta E_{atom}|$$

Bohr's model retained two classical assumptions built into the Rutherford model: conservation of energy and the idea that the Coulomb force provided the centripetal acceleration for the electrons. For the sake of simplicity, the equations below apply to a hydrogen atom with a single proton and electron.

Total orbital energy: $E = KE + PE = \frac{1}{2}mv^2 - k\dfrac{e^2}{r}$

Centripetal force: $F_c = \dfrac{mv^2}{r} = k\dfrac{e^2}{r^2}$

Example 14-2: Find the orbital radius of an electron in the nth orbital of a hydrogen atom.

Solution: First solve for the orbital speed v using the angular momentum quantization equation

$$mvr = \frac{nh}{2\pi} \rightarrow v = \frac{nh}{2\pi mr}$$

Now substitute this value for v into the centripetal force equation and solve the resulting equation for r

$$\frac{mv^2}{r} = k\frac{e^2}{r^2} \rightarrow \frac{m\left(n^2h^2\right)}{r\left(4\pi^2m^2r^2\right)} = \frac{n^2h^2}{4\pi^2mr^3} = \frac{ke^2}{r^2}$$

$$r_n = \frac{n^2h^2}{4\pi^2km_{electron}e^2}$$

Example 14-3: What is the diameter of a hydrogen atom in the ground state according to the Bohr model? Use 9×10^{-31} kg for the mass of the electron.

Solution: The ground state of an atom corresponds to a value of $n = 1$, and the diameter is just twice the radius. Thus we can substitute values into the equation for the radius found in Example 14-2 above.

$$r_1 = \frac{h^2}{4\pi^2 k m_{electron} e^2} = \frac{\left(6.63 \times 10^{-34}\right)^2}{4\left(\pi\right)^2 \left(9 \times 10^9\right)\left(9 \times 10^{-31}\right)\left(1.6 \times 10^{-19}\right)^2} \approx$$

$$\frac{44 \times 10^{-68}}{4 \times 9 \times 9 \times 9 \times 2.5 \times 10^{-60}} \approx \frac{10^{-68}}{200 \times 10^{-60}} = 5 \times 10^{-11} \text{ m}$$

Thus the diameter of the hydrogen atom in the ground state is about 1×10^{-10} meters (also called one angstrom).

Example 14-4: What is the energy of the nth orbital of a hydrogen atom in terms of n and known constants?

Solution: Solve the centripetal force equation for mv^2 and substitute into the energy equation:

$$\frac{mv^2}{r} = \frac{ke^2}{r^2} \rightarrow mv^2 = \frac{ke^2}{r}$$

$$E = KE + PE = \tfrac{1}{2}mv^2 - k\frac{e^2}{r} = \frac{1}{2}\frac{ke^2}{r} - \frac{ke^2}{r} = -\frac{ke^2}{2r}$$

Now substitute the expression for r_n into the result:

$$E_n = -\frac{ke^2}{2r_n} = -\frac{ke^2}{2n^2 h^2} \times 4\pi^2 k m_{electron} e^2 = -\frac{2\pi^2 k^2 m_{electron} e^4}{n^2 h^2}$$

If you plug in values for the constants, you find that $E_n = -2.17 \times 10^{-18}$ J$/n^2$. More commonly, the energy of the atomic energy levels is expressed in terms of electron-volts (eV), that is, the product of the elementary charge e with volts V. Because the elementary charge is equal to 1.6×10^{-19} C, converting from joules to eV requires dividing by this number. This yields

Energy Level of a Hydrogen Atom

$$E_n = -13.6 \text{ eV} / n^2$$

where $n = 1, 2, 3 \ldots$

Be sure you understand why this energy is negative. Electrons orbiting a nucleus are energetically bound to it and must absorb more energy to move further from that nucleus or to escape (thereby ionizing the atom). Thus the energy of the orbital has to become increasingly positive as n increases, up to zero as n approaches infinity (which means ionization has occurred).

Bohr's model thus explains the emission spectra of hydrogen and, by extension, the other elements: any single change in n entails a discrete change in energy according to

$$\Delta E = -13.6 \text{ eV} \left(\frac{1}{n_{final}^2} - \frac{1}{n_{initial}^2} \right)$$

This change in energy between two states will correspond to the emission (if the change is negative) or absorption (if the change is positive) of a photon. The energy of that photon will therefore be given by

The Energy of a Photon Emitted or Absorbed by a Hydrogen Atom

$$hf = |\Delta E| = \left| 13.6 \text{ eV} \left(\frac{1}{n_{final}^2} - \frac{1}{n_{initial}^2} \right) \right|$$

Example 14-5: What is the frequency of a photon that, when absorbed, will ionize a hydrogen atom that begins in the $n = 2$ state? Planck's constant is $h = 4.14 \times 10^{-15}$ eV·s

Solution: When an atom is ionized, its final state is $n \to \infty$, so applying the preceding equation yields

$$hf = \left| 13.6 \text{ eV} \left(0 - \frac{1}{2^2} \right) \right| = 3.4 \text{ eV}$$

$$f = \frac{3.4 \text{ eV}}{4.14 \times 10^{-15} \text{ eV} \cdot \text{s}} \approx 8 \times 10^{14} \text{ Hz}$$

Example 14-6: The red Hα line has a wavelength of 656 nm. If the final state in the atomic transition that produces this line is $n = 2$, what was the initial state?

Solution: According to the solution to Example 14-1, the energy of the Hα photon is roughly 3×10^{-19} J. First convert this value to eV by dividing by $e = 1.6 \times 10^{-19}$ C to get about 2 eV. Then apply the equation for the energy change associated with a hydrogen energy-level transition:

$$|\Delta E| = 2 \text{ eV} = \left| 13.6 \text{ eV} \left(\frac{1}{2^2} - \frac{1}{n_{initial}^2} \right) \right|$$

$$\frac{2}{13.6} = \frac{1}{4} - \frac{1}{n_{initial}^2} \to \frac{1}{7} - \frac{1}{4} = -\frac{1}{n_{initial}^2}$$

$$\frac{4}{28} - \frac{7}{28} = -\frac{3}{28} \approx -\frac{1}{9} = -\frac{1}{n_{initial}^2}$$

$$n_{initial}^2 = 9 \to n_{initial} = 3$$

14.3   THE PAULI EXCLUSION PRINCIPLE

A few years after Bohr refined his model, Wolfgang Pauli devised an explanation for the fact that the elements exhibited patterns of chemical behavior related to the number of electrons. For example, atoms with even numbers of electrons are in general more chemically stable than those with odd numbers. Pauli determined that these groupings of elements and their behaviors could be explained that so long as only one electron was allowed to occupy a particular *quantum state*, defined not only by the principal quantum number *n* but three additional quantum numbers. For MCAT purposes, understanding the **Pauli exclusion principle** usually means recognizing that each atomic orbital can hold only two electrons of opposite *spin*, a quantum number that defines the intrinsic angular momentum of the electron. However, the Pauli exclusion principle applies to protons and neutrons as well, and asserts more broadly that there is a limit to how many such particles can be confined in a small space.

14.4   THE PHOTOELECTRIC EFFECT

In the late nineteenth century, long before Bohr's quantum atomic model, it was noticed that a spark would jump between two charged plates when a strong light was shone on the negative plate, and that the spark would diminish or disappear altogether when a filter was used to block the ultraviolet component of the light. Because the light is giving rise to an electric current, the effect is called the **photoelectric effect**. Below is a picture of the apparatus used to measure this effect.

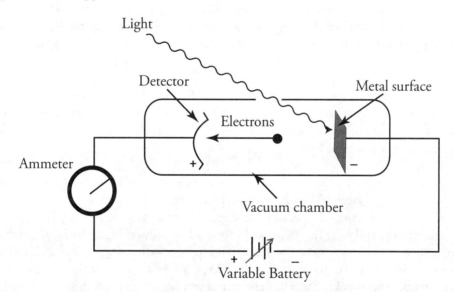

The ammeter will register a current only when *photoelectrons* (that is, electrons ejected by the incident light) pass from the metal surface to the detector. Note that the voltage of the battery can be varied and that its polarity can be reversed.

According to the classical theory of light as a wave, the energy absorbed by the metal surface depends only upon the amplitude of the light wave, i.e., the light's brightness. The energy delivered by this continuous wave increases with time; the longer a light of a given intensity shines on a surface, the more energy will be absorbed. It was also well known by the time the photoelectric effect was first observed that some of the electrons normally bound to a metal would be ejected when the metal was heated. This is analogous to a pot of water on the stove: individual water molecules are bound to the volume of liquid water, but due to thermal effects, some will occasionally evaporate off the surface. This effect increases as the water is heated to boiling. The binding energy of the metal for its surface electrons (the ones most likely to be ejected) is called the metal's **work function**, ϕ.

Based upon the wave theory and the thermal ejection of electrons, one would expect the following:

- a brighter light would yield a stronger current than a dimmer one, regardless of color/frequency;
- because the light takes some time to heat the metal, there would be a delay between the time the light first shines on the metal and when a current is detected; and
- if the polarity of the battery were reversed, so that electrons ejected from the metal surface were repelled by the detector and only the more energetic among them would reach the detector, increasing the brightness of the light would increase the maximum potential difference the ejected electrons could overcome to reach the detector. In other words, when light of a certain brightness is shone on the metal surface, there will be some negative potential at the detector at which the measured current drops to zero. This is called the **stopping voltage**, V_{stop}. According to the wave theory of light, increasing the brightness of the light should increase the magnitude of this stopping voltage.

Surprisingly, each of these expectations was contradicted by experimental results. Though increasing the brightness of the light did yield more current when there was a current to begin with, light below a certain frequency would not generate *any* current, regardless of brightness. Current was detected instantaneously when the light illuminated the metal surface. Finally, the intensity of the light had no effect on the measured stopping voltage, but the frequency of the light did affect V_{stop}. The wave theory of light was at an impasse.

In 1905, Einstein published the paper that explained these findings (the paper for which he later won the Nobel Prize). Einstein's explanation of the photoelectric effect developed the photon model of light previously mentioned. There are three important points in this model that explain the experimental results better than does the wave model of light.

- Electromagnetic radiation (i.e., light) of a certain frequency is made up of discrete bundles of energy (now called "photons"), each with energy $E = hf$.
- Photons of light are absorbed or emitted as single instantaneous interactions (as opposed to the mechanism provided by the wave model for gradually absorbing or emitting energy).
- When a photon strikes the surface of a metal, it interacts with a single electron, imparting all of its energy in the form of increased kinetic energy for the electron. If this energy is greater than the work function of the metal, the electron will be ejected from the metal with kinetic energy given by the following expression (note the subscript indicating that this is the maximum kinetic energy for an ejected electron: many electrons ejected will be "deeper" in the metal and thus will lose more energy in the process of ejection).

Kinetic Energy of a Photoelectron

$$KE_{max} = hf - \phi$$

Let's consider how the photon model resolves the three problems with the experiment previously described. First, if the individual photons interact with individual electrons, then a single photon must provide enough energy for the electron to overcome the work function of the metal, or that electron will remain bound and no photoelectric current will be measured. A brighter light means there are more photons, but the energy of *each individual photon remains the same unless the frequency/color of the light is changed.* Therefore, as was observed, making the light brighter will increase the measured current if there is some current to being with, but a frequency of light that doesn't create any current of photoelectrons will never do so, no matter how bright it is.

The photon-electron interaction also explains why the photoelectric current is measured instantaneously instead of after a delay for the metal to absorb enough light energy. Photons deliver their energy all at once instantaneously, so as soon as photons of sufficient energy hit the metal, some electrons will be ejected and will begin to strike the detector.

To understand the relevance of Einstein's explanation for the determination of the stopping voltage, it helps to consider the requirements for a photoelectron to reach the detector. When the detector is connected to the positive terminal of the battery and there is a positive voltage difference between the metal surface and the detector (as shown in the figure), it will attract all the photoelectrons ejected from the metal surface. On the other hand, when the polarity of the battery is reversed so that the detector is connected to the negative terminal of the battery, then the detector repels the photoelectrons. In that case, in order for the ammeter to measure a current, the detected photoelectrons must overcome the negative voltage difference between the metal surface and the detector. As that negative voltage is increased in magnitude, eventually it will be large enough that no photoelectrons will reach the detector. At that point, the current will drop to zero.

Stopping Voltage for the Photoelectric Effect

$$-eV_{stop} = KE_{max}$$

Remember that we've defined V_{stop} as a negative voltage, so the term on the left must have an additional negative sign to equal a necessarily positive kinetic energy.

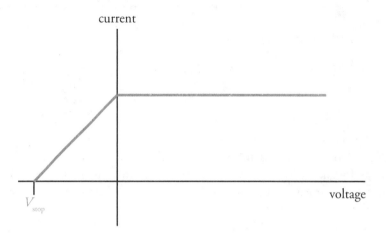

Current through the Ammeter as a Function of Applied Voltage

Example 14-7: The photon model of light is necessary to explain each of the following experimentally observed effects EXCEPT:

A. The ejection of electrons from a metal surface with light shining upon it
B. The stopping voltage as a function of light frequency
C. The instantaneous detection of a current following the application of light to the metal surface
D. The fact that an intense infrared light may result in no measured current where a dim ultraviolet light results in measured current

Solution: Refer back to the list of three expected outcomes of the photoelectric experiment given the wave theory of light. The wave theory of light predicts that the stopping voltage should be a function of intensity, not frequency, eliminating choice B. It also predicts a delay between the application of light to the metal surface and a detection of a current (providing adequate time for the plate to energize and eject electrons). This eliminates choice C. Moreover, the wave theory predicts that the ejection of electrons at all depends purely upon the intensity of the light applied to the metal surface, not on its frequency. This eliminates choice D. Choice A is correct because the ejection of electrons by the application of light is perfectly predictable according to the classical wave theory: it's just the *manner* in which they are ejected that requires the photon theory.

Example 14-8: Almost all modern medical imaging (that doesn't rely on actual film) relies on a simple principle: translating electromagnetic or ionizing radiation signals from the imaging device into electrical signals, which can then be translated into an image on a screen. In the operation of a positron emission tomography (*PET*) scan, for example, a radioactive tracer is injected into a patient. The tracer undergoes β^+ decay, and the positrons annihilate electrons in their vicinity in a matter-antimatter interaction that releases gamma radiation. The gamma radiation is then picked up by a so-called "gamma camera" composed of an array of scintillating crystals (which absorbs the gamma photon and reemits a photon of lower energy) and *photomultiplier tubes* (which absorb these secondary photons). The principle of operation of the photomultiplier tubes is the photoelectric effect: incident photons are converted to photoelectrons, which are absorbed and amplified as a cascading electric current measured and recorded by a computer. These flashes of current are eventually composed into an image.

Suppose the photomultiplier tubes in a gamma camera use cesium to absorb the incident photons. Cesium has a work function of 2.1 eV. What is the maximum wavelength of incident light that would eject a photoelectron from cesium?

Solution: First, recognize that the *maximum* wavelength of light will correspond to the *minimum* frequency and therefore energy. The minimum kinetic energy an electron could have when ejected would be 0, meaning the electron just barely overcame the work function of the metal. Applying the equation for the kinetic energy of the ejected photoelectron yields

$$0 = hf_{min} - \phi = \left(4.1 \times 10^{-15} \text{ eV}\right) f_{min} - 2.1 \text{ eV}$$

$$f_{min} = \frac{2.1}{4.1 \times 10^{-15}} \approx 5 \times 10^{14} \text{ Hz}$$

Now convert this minimum frequency into a maximum wavelength:

$$c = f\lambda \rightarrow \lambda_{max} = \frac{c}{f_{min}} = \frac{3 \times 10^8}{5 \times 10^{14}} = 6 \times 10^{-7} \text{ m}$$

Example 14-9: Suppose a photoelectric experiment is conducted and the applied voltage is varied over a range of values to generate a graph of current versus voltage similar to that shown above. If the intensity of the light is increased but all other aspects of the experiment are kept the same, which of the following aspects of the generated graph would change?

  I.   The slope of the line from V_{stop} to $V = 0$
 II.   The location of V_{stop}
III.   The maximum value of the current

  A.   I only
  B.   II only
  C.   I and III only
  D.   I, II, and III

Solution: The stopping voltage depends upon the maximum kinetic energy of the photoelectrons, which in turn depends upon the *frequency* of the incident light and the work function of the metal target. Therefore, changing the *intensity* of the incident light will not alter the stopping voltage, so Item II is false, eliminating choices B and D. Increasing the intensity will, however, increase the number of photons striking the target, and therefore will increase the number of photoelectrons and therefore the maximum current, meaning Item III is true, eliminating choice A. Choice C is correct, and Item I is true because if the stopping voltage stays the same but the maximum current increases, the slope of the line from V_{stop} up to the now higher *y*-intercept must be greater.

Example 14-10: Now suppose the experiment were repeated and both the applied voltage and frequency of the incident light were varied by the experimenter (but not the intensity of the light). For each set frequency, the experimenter would increase the negative voltage of the variable battery until no current was measured in the ammeter (sufficiently low frequencies would produce zero current even for positive voltages). What would the experimenter's graph of stopping voltage versus incident frequency look like?

14.5

Solution: Consider that only electrons that have at least as much kinetic energy as the potential energy gap they must cross can be detected as current. This is analogous to tossing balls in the air in a room with a high ceiling: you can weakly toss up a million balls, but none of them will be detected as a "current" of thumps against the ceiling unless you toss some with enough energy to reach the height of the ceiling. Mathematically, this means:

$$KE_{max} = -\Delta PE \rightarrow hf - \phi = -eV_{stop} \rightarrow -V_{stop} = \frac{h}{e}f - \frac{\phi}{e}$$

Note that we've solved for $-V_{stop}$: that is simply because we are more accustomed to reading graphs predominantly in the first quadrant (this just means that values above the horizontal axis indicate negative voltages of the variable battery). The graph of this function looks like this (note the dashed line below the horizontal, representing a linear extrapolation of the work function: no data points could be discovered below the threshold frequency):

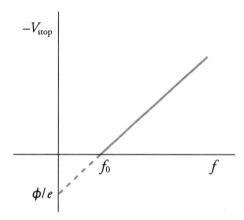

14.5 THE HEISENBERG UNCERTAINTY PRINCIPLE

In 1927, Werner Heisenberg was working with Niels Bohr in Copenhagen to further develop the new quantum physics. While Bohr was away skiing, Heisenberg recognized a surprising but critical consequence of wave-particle duality: uncertainty. To measure the position of a particle extremely accurately, one had to shine a very short wavelength light on it, because the wavelength itself is a limitation on the determination of position. A short wavelength corresponds to a high frequency and high energy, and when a high energy photon interacts with a particle like an electron, it imparts some of its energy and momentum to the particle. (The relation between energy and momentum is given by $E = p^2/2m$, which you should confirm to yourself using the classical formulas for kinetic energy and momentum.) This means the momentum of the particle changes, which introduces an uncertainty into the measure of the momentum. Conversely, a longer wavelength, lower energy light beam would allow one to measure the momentum of the particle it interacted with to greater precision, but the long wavelength means a greater uncertainty in the position of the particle. Using capital deltas to represent the uncertainty in a quantity, Heisenberg's uncertainty relation can be written as

> **The Heisenberg Uncertainty Relation**
>
> $$\Delta x \Delta p \geq h/2\pi$$

where x represents to the position of the particle (or object more generally) and h is Planck's constant.

Example 14-11: Driving through M-k-sopolis, you are pulled over by a policeman for doing 30 m/s in a 25 m/s speed limit zone. Trying to talk your way out of the ticket, you ask the officer how he knows you were in 25 m/s zone. He replies that he used a high frequency laser detector to determine your position to within 10^{-7} m. Given this precision in position, is the minimum uncertainty in his measurement of your momentum large enough that you can argue you might have been going 25 m/s? Assume your car has a mass of 1000 kg, and use $h = 6.63 \times 10^{-34}$ J·s.

Solution: The uncertainty in the position of your car is $\Delta x = 10^{-7}$ m. Plugging this into the Heisenberg uncertainty relation yields

$$\Delta x \Delta p \geq \frac{h}{2\pi} \rightarrow \Delta p \geq \frac{6.63 \times 10^{-34}}{2\pi \times 10^{-7}} \approx 10^{-27} \text{ kg} \cdot \text{m/s}$$

The uncertainty in velocity is thus $\Delta p = m\Delta v \rightarrow \Delta v = 10^{-27}/10^3 = 10^{-30}$ m/s. Since this is much, MUCH less than 5 m/s (the difference between your measured speed and the speed limit), you'll have to bite the bullet and pay the ticket!

Heisenberg's uncertainty relation has far-reaching consequences. For one, though it is often explained using the language of measurement, you should not interpret it to mean that a particle like an electron *really* has an exact position and momentum, but we just can't find out what they are. The reality is far stranger than that: uncertainty isn't just a matter of what we can *know*, but rather a matter of *what really is the case!* In quantum physics, quantities like position and momentum, energy and time, are fundamentally probabilistic. This means that they have most likely values, but not exact values; if one attempted to determine the exact value of one of the quantities, the other would become entirely uncertain. In other words, if you were to describe *exactly* how fast an electron was moving, the uncertainty in its position would be the entire universe: it could be anywhere with equal likelihood! Practically speaking, this would be impossible, because to measure any quantity requires using a beam that has wave properties, and no wave can have a wavelength of 0 or infinity. This uncertainty affects biomedical research into very small objects, because it limits the extent to which microscopic structures can be imaged by light but also opens up possibilities for imaging them with particles like electrons. More theoretically, Heisenberg's uncertainty relation explains, for example, why the ground state of a hydrogen atom is the smallest orbital, i.e., why there can't be a smaller one. This is something that the Bohr model did not explain.

Example 14-12: Determine the uncertainty of the momentum of an electron in the $n = 1$ state.

Solution: We previously determined that the diameter of the hydrogen atom in the ground state was about 10^{-10} m. An electron in the $n = 1$ state therefore could be found anywhere within that diameter, meaning $\Delta x = 10^{-10}$ m. The uncertainty of its momentum is therefore given by

$$\Delta x \Delta p \geq \frac{h}{2\pi} \rightarrow \Delta p \geq \frac{6.63 \times 10^{-34}}{2\pi \times 10^{-10}} \approx 10^{-24} \text{ kg} \cdot \text{m/s}$$

Though the math is slightly beyond the level of the MCAT, it is straightforward to show using the relation $E = p^2/2m$ that, given this uncertainty in momentum, were the electron to be confined to a smaller radius, the uncertainty in its energy would necessarily be greater than 13.6 eV, the energy of the hydrogen ground state. In other words, a "lower" state than the ground state would, according to the Heisenberg uncertainty principle, have to have a *higher* energy. This is a contradiction, proving that the ground state in the Bohr model of hydrogen indeed must be the lowest energy state.

SUMMARY OF FORMULAS

Energy of a photon: $E_{photon} = hf = hc/\lambda$

Bohr model of the atom assumes:

> The atom is made up of a dense, massive positive nucleus orbited by negative electrons (like the Rutherford model)

> The energy levels of an atom are quantized. They are determined by the discrete orbital states of the electrons, numbered $n = 1, 2, 3....$ The higher numbered states correspond to higher energies. The lowest state, $n = 1$, is the *ground* state, and is stable over time.

> Atoms can change quantized energy states by absorbing or emitting a photon. The energy of the photon must correspond exactly to the energy difference between the two states: $E_{photon} = |\Delta E_{atom}|$

> Atoms can also change energy states thermally by interacting with other particles. As with the case of photon absorption, though, the changes in atomic energy are quantized, and excited atoms will tend to return to the ground state by emitting photons (this is why a heated metal glows, for example).

Bohr model of the hydrogen atom: $E_n = -13.6 \text{ eV} / n^2$, where $n = 1, 2, 3...$

Photons absorbed or emitted by a hydrogen atom: $hf = \left| 13.6 \text{ eV} \left(\dfrac{1}{n_{final}^2} - \dfrac{1}{n_{initial}^2} \right) \right|$

> The Pauli exclusion principle states that no two electron, protons, or neutrons can occupy the same quantum state (have the same quantum numbers) within a small space.

> The photoelectric effect occurs when light incident upon a metal surface causes electrons to be ejected by that surface. Individual photons provide energy hf to individual electrons, and if that energy is enough to overcome the binding energy of the metal, the electrons are ejected.

The maximum kinetic energy of the ejected electrons is $KE_{max} = hf - \phi$.

The stopping voltage necessary to prevent the most energetic electrons from reaching a negatively-charged plate is given by $-eV_{stop} = KE_{max}$

The Heisenberg uncertainty principle sets a limit on the precision with which position and momentum are determined: $\Delta x \Delta p \geq h/2\pi$

CHAPTER 14 FREESTANDING QUESTIONS

1. A red photon and a blue photon both strike a piece of unknown material at the same acute angle of incidence. Any of the following could happen EXCEPT:

A) The blue photon ejects an electron but the red photon does not.
B) The blue photon passes through the material at a faster speed than does the red photon.
C) The blue photon is reflected while the red photon is transmitted.
D) Both photons eject electrons from the material.

2. An electromagnetic beam with wavelength λ_0 is incident upon an unknown metal. If electrons are ejected with maximum kinetic energy K, what is the work function of the metal?

A) hc/λ_0
B) $h\lambda_0/c$
C) $hc/\lambda_0 - K$
D) $h\lambda_0/c - K$

3. According to the *de Broglie hypothesis*, wave-particle duality extends to all particles, not just photons. The wavelength of any particle is a function of the particle's momentum p according to the equation $\lambda = h/p$. An electron orbiting a proton can thus be considered a standing wave that forms a closed loop around the nucleus: only modes producing integer wavelengths are permitted. What is the wavelength of the ground state, fundamental mode of the electron in this simple Bohr atom (let m_e represent the mass of the electron)?

A) $\dfrac{h^2}{4\pi^2 m_e ke^2}$

B) $\dfrac{h^2}{2\pi m_e ke^2}$

C) $\dfrac{h^2}{\pi m_e ke^2}$

D) $\dfrac{2\pi m_e ke^2}{h^2}$

4. A series of trials are conducted using the standard photoelectric experiment set up, with the variable voltage at the detector set to a high positive difference from the target metal surface. In each trial, a filter is used to allow only light of a certain frequency to shine on the metal target's surface. Over the course of five trials, five different frequencies of increasing value are allowed to strike the target. If we assume that the intensity of the light striking the target remains constant over all the trials, which of the following graphs represents the most likely outcome of measured current as a function of frequency?

A)
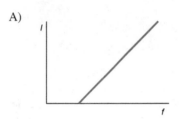

B)
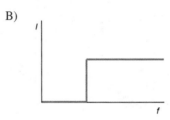

C)
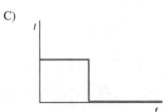

D)
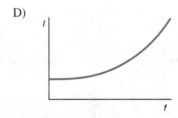

5. Which of the following changes to the photoelectric experiment could change the value of the stopping voltage?

    I. Increasing the duration of the experiment
    II. Changing the wavelength of the incident light
    III. Changing the material used for the metal target

A) I only
B) II only
C) I and III only
D) II and III only

6. A singly ionized helium atom behaves the same way as a hydrogen atom, the important difference being that there are two protons in the nucleus instead of one. What would be the energy of the photon released by an He^+ ion as it transitioned from the $n = 2$ state to the $n = 1$ state?

A) 10.2 eV
B) 13.6 eV
C) 20.4 eV
D) 40.8 eV

7. When you breathe in, oxygen molecules from the atmosphere enter small sacs in your lungs called alveoli. These sacs have an average diameter of 250 μm when inflated. If an oxygen molecule has a mass of about 5.3×10^{-26} kg, what is the minimum uncertainty in the speed of an O_2 molecule confined in an alveolus?

A) 8×10^{-9} m/s
B) 8×10^{-6} m/s
C) 8×10^{-3} m/s
D) 8 m/s

CHAPTER 14 PRACTICE PASSAGE

Cells of malignant tumors may be destroyed by various types of radiation or particles, including X-rays, protons and positrons (the positively-charged antiparticle of the electron). Ultimately, the mechanism of cell destruction is the photon or particle transferring energy to a molecule, breaking a bond in the molecule. As this occurs, the photon or particle loses energy.

For high-energy charged particles (such as protons and positrons, but *not* X-rays) moving through matter, the rate at which they lose energy to atoms in the matter was worked out by Hans Bethe and Felix Bloch in the 1930s, soon after the discovery of quantum mechanics. For protons the rate is given in Figure 1 as a function of proton momentum. (This is actually $\Delta E/\rho\Delta x$, the energy loss per centimeter divided by the density of the matter through which the particle passes.) As the proton loses energy, its momentum decreases and it moves along the curve to the left.

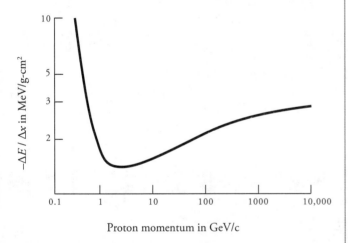

Figure 1

X-rays are created by accelerating electrons to high energy and then slamming them into a high-density metal. As the electrons decelerate rapidly, about 1% of their energy is radiated as X-ray photons, and the remainder heats the metal.

In the following, h represents Planck's Constant, with a value of 6.6×10^{-34} J-s.

1. Compared to a lower-energy X-ray photon, a higher-energy X-ray photon will have:

A) higher frequency and higher wavelength.
B) higher frequency and lower wavelength.
C) lower frequency and higher wavelength.
D) lower frequency and lower wavelength.

2. Using the Bethe-Bloch formula, a radiation technician can calculate the energy of a proton that would *range out* (its momentum would reach zero) after traversing enough body tissue to reach an interior tumor. An advantage of using protons of this energy is:

A) the proton will disintegrate in the tumor, causing more damage to the tumor.
B) the proton will deposit more energy (thus causing more damage) in the tumor than in the material in front of the tumor.
C) the proton will deposit less energy (thus causing more damage) in the tumor than in the material in front of the tumor.
D) the proton has the minimum possible energy when it enters the body, causing less damage to healthy tissue.

3. Suppose 400 kJ/mole is required to break a bond, disintegrating a particular molecule. What is the lowest possible frequency of a single photon that could possibly break the bond?

A) 10^9 Hz
B) 10^{12} Hz
C) 10^{15} Hz
D) 6×10^{39} Hz

4. An electron knocked out of a molecule by passing radiation may bind to a neutral hydrogen atom making H⁻, with one proton and two electrons. In the ground state, will both electrons have the same energy?

A) No, because the Pauli exclusion principle forbids two electrons having the same energy.
B) Yes, because the Pauli exclusion principle allows a maximum of two electrons with the same energy.
C) Yes, but the two electrons must have opposite spin to satisfy the Pauli exclusion principle.
D) No, the Pauli exclusion principle makes both energies uncertain, so they cannot be equal.

5. A proton has a certain momentum as it passes through a certain cell. For which momentum will the proton cause the least damage to molecules in the cell?

A) 0.8 GeV/c
B) 3.0 GeV/c
C) 52 GeV/c
D) 1000 GeV/c

6. A photon is most effective at breaking molecules if it is not much bigger than the molecules; that is to say, if its positional uncertainty is on the same scale as the molecule. If a 1.7×10^{-22} kg protein has a linear dimension of about 6 nm, what is the minimum *transverse momentum* (i.e., momentum in a direction perpendicular to the main direction of propagation) of a photon that could be small enough to break the protein?

A) 2.2×10^{-20} cm/s
B) 1.6×10^{8} GeV/c
C) 3×10^{-15} kg-m/s
D) 3.3×10^{-25} kg-m/s

7. Suppose a positron with momentum p_1 disintegrates a stationary molecule, and continues on in its original direction with a new, lower momentum of p_2. What is the summed momentum of the fragments of the disintegrated molecule?

A) $(p_1 - p_2)/h$
B) $(p_1 + p_2)/h$
C) $p_1 - p_2$
D) $\sqrt{p_1^2 - p_2^2}$

SOLUTIONS TO CHAPTER 14 FREESTANDING QUESTIONS

1. **B** According to the explanation of the photoelectric effect, an electron can be ejected from a material by a photon whenever the photon energy hf is greater than the work function of the material. In this case, where the work function is unknown, all we can assume is that a more energetic, higher frequency photon is more likely to eject an electron than is a less energetic, lower frequency photon. Because blue light is higher frequency than red light, the blue photon is more likely to eject an electron. This is consistent with choices A and D, eliminating them. The phenomenon of dispersion entails that blue light experiences a higher index of refraction than does red light when it moves through a material. This means that blue light is more likely to undergo total internal reflection when it strikes the interface between two materials than red light: $\sin \theta_{crit} = n_2 / n_1$, where n_2 is the index of refraction of the unknown material and n_1 would be the index for the medium of incidence (which would have to have a higher index than the unknown material for any TIR to occur). This eliminates choice C. Choice B is correct because a higher index of refraction for blue light means that the blue photon will travel slower than the red one.

2. **C** The principle of conservation of energy tells us that the initial energy of the photon, $hf = hc/\lambda$, must equal the final energy of the system, which is the sum of the potential energy represented by the work function ϕ and the kinetic energy of the electron, K.

$$\frac{hc}{\lambda_0} = \phi + K \rightarrow \phi = \frac{hc}{\lambda_0} - K$$

3. **B** The key to answering this question is to realize that, if integer multiples of wavelengths are required for the de Broglie electron standing waves, then the ground state, the fundamental mode, must have a wavelength equal to the circumference of that circular orbit: $\lambda_1 = 2\pi r_1$. The value for r_n was found in example 14-2: we follow the same procedure here. Beginning with the equation for quantized angular momentum yields

$$mvr = \frac{nh}{2\pi} \rightarrow v_1 = \frac{(1)h}{2\pi m r_1}$$

Now substitute this value for v into the centripetal force equation and solve the resulting equation for r_1

$$\frac{mv^2}{r} = k\frac{e^2}{r^2} \rightarrow \frac{m_{electron}\left(h^2\right)}{r_1\left(4\pi^2 m_{electron}^2 r_1^2\right)} = \frac{h^2}{4\pi^2 m_{electron} r_1^3} = \frac{ke^2}{r_1^2}$$

$$r_1 = \frac{h^2}{4\pi^2 k m_{electron} e^2}$$

Finally, substitute this equation into the formula for λ_1:

$$\lambda_1 = 2\pi\left(\frac{h^2}{4\pi^2 k m_{electron} e^2}\right) = \frac{h^2}{2\pi k m_{electron} e^2}$$

4. **B** In the photoelectric experiment, when the frequency of the incident light is too low, no photoelectrons will be ejected. In this case, no current will be measured: this eliminates choice C. As the frequency increases, the energy of the incident photons increases, until at some point it is sufficient to begin ejecting photoelectrons. At that point, because the detector is positively polarized, all the ejected electrons will be collected, which will be represented in the current measured. The question also states that the intensity of the light is kept constant, so the number of photons remains basically the same, as therefore does the number of photoelectrons. This means the current will remain constant for all frequencies so long as the frequency is sufficiently high to eject any photoelectrons, which is shown by graph B.

5. **D** The photoelectric effect is essentially instantaneous, so increasing the duration of the experiment should not affect the determination of the stopping voltage, which depends upon the maximum kinetic energy of the ejected photoelectrons. $eV_{stop} = KE_{max}$. Thus I is false, eliminating choices A and C. The remaining choices are distinguished entirely by whether III is true, so you should focus on that. Changing the material used for the target will change the work function, ϕ. Because the maximum kinetic energy of ejected photoelectrons depends upon this value according to $KE_{max} = hf - \phi$, this would indeed affect the value of the stopping voltage, meaning III is true and the correct choice is D.

6. **D** The important difference between a hydrogen atom and a singly ionized helium ion is the charge of the nucleus: it is twice as great for the He⁺. Without repeating the calculations shown in examples 14-2 and 14-4, it should be evident that the expression for the energy levels in hydrogen

$$E_n = -\frac{ke^2}{2r_n} = -\frac{ke^2}{2n^2h^2} \times 4\pi^2 km_{electron}e^2$$

will introduce two additional factors of 2 when accounting for the two protons in the He⁺ ion. The e^2 in the numerator of the first energy expression will be $2e^2$, and the second e^2 from the radius term will also be $2e^2$. Thus the energy levels for He⁺ will be equal to four times the equivalent levels for hydrogen:

$$E_n = 4(-13.6 \text{ eV}/n^2) = -54.4 \text{ eV}/n^2$$

And therefore the equation for photon energies emitted by He⁺ as it transitions between energy levels is

$$\Delta E = hf = \left|54.4 \text{ eV}\left(\frac{1}{n_{final}^2} - \frac{1}{n_{initial}^2}\right)\right| \rightarrow \Delta E_{2-1} = \left|54.4 \text{ eV}\left(\frac{1}{1^2} - \frac{1}{2^2}\right)\right| = 54.4 \times \frac{3}{4} = 40.8 \text{ eV}$$

Note that there is a short cut: if you remember that 10.2 eV is the energy difference for the hydrogen atom transitioning between $n = 2$ and $n = 1$, multiplying that by four for the reasons explained above yields the answer.

7. **B** Apply the Heisenberg uncertainty principle:

$$\Delta x \Delta p = \frac{h}{2\pi} \rightarrow \Delta p = \frac{h}{2\pi\Delta x} \rightarrow \Delta v = \frac{h}{2\pi\Delta x \times m} = \frac{6.63 \times 10^{-34}}{2\pi\left(250 \times 10^{-6}\right)\left(5.3 \times 10^{-26}\right)} \approx$$

$$\frac{1}{1300} \times 10^{2} \approx 8 \times 10^{-6} \text{ m/s}$$

Note that the answer choices all have the same coefficient, so you're really just trying to figure out the order of magnitude. In such cases, don't stress over the numbers, make quick estimations!

SOLUTIONS TO CHAPTER 14 PRACTICE PASSAGE

1. **B** We know immediately that frequency energy corresponds to higher energy, according to the relation $E = hf$. So the answer must be either choice A or choice B. Because the speed of the wave is fixed at c, the frequency and wavelength are inversely proportional, according to the relation $f\lambda = c$. So as the frequency increases, the wavelength must decrease.

2. **B** According to Figure 1, as a proton approaches the end of its passage through tissue (toward the left side of the curve), the less momentum a proton has, the more energy it loses per unit length. This means that, per centimeter, the amount of energy the proton gives to the matter (and hence the amount of molecular damage it can cause, eliminating choice C) increases as the proton nears stopping. Choice A cannot be right because protons are stable; they do not disintegrate. Choice D is not right because, depending on the exact numbers, a lower-energy proton (which would necessarily have less momentum as well) may do more damage than a higher-energy proton.

3. **C** If it takes a certain amount of energy to break a mole of bonds, we must divide by Avogadro's number to get the energy needed to break a single bond. The lowest-energy photon that could break the bond would be one that gives up all of its energy to the molecule, giving just enough energy to break the bond. From the relation $E = hf$, the frequency corresponding to this minimum-energy photon is

$$f_{min} = \frac{E_{binding}}{N_A \times h} = \frac{4 \times 10^{5} \dfrac{\text{J}}{\text{mol}}}{\left(6 \times 10^{23} \dfrac{1}{\text{mol}}\right)\left(6.63 \times 10^{-34} \text{ J} \cdot \text{s}\right)} \approx \frac{4}{40} \times 10^{16} = 10^{15} \text{ Hz}$$

4. **C** The Pauli exclusion principle allows states with two electrons in which at least one quantum number is different, which is consistent with choice C. This is the case for a filled $n = 1$ shell; the principle doesn't expressly forbid any two electrons from having the same energy, so choice A is wrong. Choice B is incorrect for basically the same reason; recall from chemistry that for a given $n > 1$, there are more than two states at the same energy because there are more than two electrons per shell. Choice D is incorrect because the Pauli exclusion principle does not deal with uncertainty.

5. **B** Damage to cells happens when molecular bonds are broken by energy transferred from the proton. Figure 1 shows a minimum in energy loss, i.e., energy transferred to molecules in the cell, of around 3 to 4 GeV/c.

6. **D** When a question mentions a linear dimension, then asks about a momentum, this should make you think of the uncertainty principle. If the momentum were known to precision Δp, the location of the photon would be smeared out over a length $\Delta x = h/2\pi\Delta p$. So we actually want more momentum uncertainty to get enough position certainty to match the size of the molecule. The momentum must be at least as large as its uncertainty, so the momentum must be at least

$$\Delta p = \frac{h}{2\pi\Delta x} = \frac{6.63 \times 10^{-34}}{2\pi \times 3 \times 10^{-9}} \approx 3.3 \times 10^{-26} \ \text{kg} \cdot \text{m/s}$$

Although A and B have different units than C and D, only choice A can be eliminated due to having the wrong dimension. The units in choices B, C and D all have dimensions of momentum.

7. **C** Momentum is conserved in the collision, so the total momentum after must equal the total momentum before. With the molecule at rest, the total momentum before is the momentum of the positron, p_1; Because we are only considering motion in one direction, we can use scalars. After the collision,

$p_2 + p_{frag} = p_1$

$p_{frag} = p_1 - p_2$

Choices A and B can be eliminated, both because they have the wrong units to be momentum and because conservation of momentum is a classical fact that does not involve Planck's constant.

Glossary

After each definition, the section of the *MCAT Physics* text where the term is discussed is given.

acceleration
The rate of change of velocity: $\bar{\mathbf{a}} = \Delta\mathbf{v}/\Delta t$.
[**Section 3.2**]

action-reaction pair
The two forces described by Newton's third law:
If Object 1 exerts a force, $\mathbf{F}_{1\text{-on-}2}$, on Object 2,
then Object 2 exerts a force, $\mathbf{F}_{2\text{-on-}1}$, on Object
1. These forces—known as an action-reaction
pair—have the same magnitude but point in
opposite directions, so $\mathbf{F}_{2\text{-on-}1} = -\mathbf{F}_{1\text{-on-}2}$, and act
on different objects. [**Section 4.1**]

adiabatic
Describes a thermodynamic process in which
there is no heat exchange. [**Section 7.3**]

alternating current (AC)
Current whose direction reverses (usually many
times per second) during the operation of the
circuit. [**Section 10.3**]

ammeter
A device for measuring current in a circuit.
[**Section 10.1**]

ampere (or amp)
The SI unit of current: 1 ampere (amp) = 1 A = 1
coulomb per second = 1 C/s. [**Section 10.1**]

amplitude
The maximum displacement of an oscillator
from its equilibrium position, or the maximum
displacement of a wave from equilibrium.
[**Section 11.1, 11.2**]

angles of incidence, reflection, and refraction
In optics, the angles that the incident beam,
reflected beam, and transmitted beam make with
the normal to the boundary between the two
media. [**Section 13.2**]

angular momentum
The rotational analog of linear momentum,
equal to $\ell m v$, where ℓ is the distance, measured
perpendicularly, from the reference point to the
line containing the velocity v of the object whose
mass is m. [**Section 6.8**]

antinode
A point where a standing wave has its maximum
amplitude. [**Section 11.4**]

Archimedes' principle
The magnitude of the buoyant force on an object
is equal to the weight of the fluid displaced. So,
if the density of the fluid is ρ_{fluid} and the volume
of the object that is submerged is V_{sub}, then the
magnitude of the buoyant force is given by $F_{\text{Buoy}} = \rho_{\text{fluid}} V_{\text{sub}} g$. [**Section 8.1**]

beats
The variation in amplitude of the resultant
wave created by the interference of two waves
with different frequencies. If f_1 and f_2 are the
frequencies of the two waves, then the beat
frequency is given by $f_{\text{beat}} = \left| f_1 - f_2 \right|$.
[**Section 12.3**]

Bernoulli effect
The lowering of fluid pressure as the flow speed
increases; also known as the *Venturi effect*.
[**Section 8.2**]

Bernoulli's equation
The statement that follows from the
Conservation of Mechanical Energy applied to
ideal fluid flow. [**Section 8.2**]

Bohr model of the atom
The description of the atom as having quantized
orbitals associated with discrete energies and
energy level transitions. [**Section 14.2**]

buoyant force
The upward force exerted by a fluid on an object partly or completely submerged in it. If the density of the fluid is ρ_{fluid} and the volume of the object that is submerged is V_{sub}, then the magnitude of the buoyant force is given by $F_{Buoy} = \rho_{fluid}V_{sub}g$. [**Section 8.1**]

capacitance
The ratio of charge to voltage for a capacitor: $C = Q/V$. [**Section 10.2**]

center of gravity
For an extended object or system, the point where the gravitational force acts. In a uniform gravitational field, the center of gravity is the same as the center of mass. [**Section 5.1**]

center of mass
The point that behaves as if all of an object's mass were concentrated there. [**Section 5.1**]

centripetal acceleration
The acceleration of an object that undergoes uniform circular motion; if the speed of the object is v and the radius of its circular path is r, then its centripetal acceleration points toward the center of the circle and has magnitude $a_c = v^2 / r$. [**Section 5.2**]

centripetal force
The net force on an object that undergoes uniform circular motion: $\mathbf{F}_c = m\mathbf{a}_c$, where $\mathbf{a}_c$ is the object's centripetal acceleration. Its magnitude is $F_c = mv^2 / r$ if the speed of the object is v and the radius of the circular path is r. [**Section 5.2**]

coefficient of friction
A positive unitless number that describes the strength of the friction force between two surfaces in contact. The coefficient of kinetic friction is usually denoted μ_k, and the coefficient of static friction by μ_s; in virtually all cases, $\mu_s > \mu_k$ for a given pair of surfaces. [**Section 4.3**]

completely inelastic collision
A completely (or perfectly) inelastic collision is an inelastic collision in which the colliding objects stick together afterwards and thus have a single velocity after the collision. [**Section 6.7**]

compression
1. A type of stress applied to an object that decreases its length. [**Section 8.3**]

2. A compression is also a region where the local density and pressure is momentarily increased from standard due to the passage of a sound wave. [**Section 12.1**]

concave
1. A concave mirror is a mirror whose reflecting surface is curved toward the object so that its center is furthest away from the object; it has a positive focal length. [**Section 13.4**]

2. A concave lens is a diverging lens; it has a negative focal length. [**Section 13.5**]

conduction
A mode of heat transfer in which the medium does not move during the transfer of thermal energy. [**Section 7.2**]

conductor
A material with a very low resistivity, which therefore allows charge to flow through it easily. Metals are conductors. [**Section 9.3**]

conservative force
If the work done by a force depends only on the initial and final positions of the object that the force is acting on, and not on the particular path between the positions, the force is said to be conservative. The gravitational and electric forces are examples of conservative forces; friction is non-conservative. [**Section 6.4**]

continuity equation

For ideal fluid flow, the amount of fluid per unit time (the flow rate) passing one point in a flow tube must be the same as the amount passing through another point: $f_1 = f_2$ (or $A_1v_1 = A_2v_2$). [**Section 8.2**]

convection

A mode of heat transfer in which the medium moves during the transfer of thermal energy. [**Section 7.3**]

converging lens

A lens that is thicker in the middle than at its edges. A converging lens causes incident parallel rays of light to converge to the focal point after passing through the lens. [**Section 13.5**]

convex

1. A convex mirror is a mirror whose reflecting surface is curved away from the object; it has a negative focal length. [**Section 13.4**]

2. A convex lens is a converging lens; it has a positive focal length. [**Section 13.5**]

coulomb

The SI unit of electric charge, abbreviated C; the fundamental electric charge (the charge on a proton or the magnitude of the charge on an electron) is defined to be $e = 1.6 \times 10^{-19}$ C. Therefore, one coulomb is equal to the total charge on 6.25×10^{18} protons. [**Section 9.1**]

Coulomb's law

The law that gives the magnitude of the electric force between two charged objects: $F_E = k|q_1q_2|/r^2$. [**Section 9.2**]

critical angle

The angle at which an incident beam of light refracts at an angle of 90°. If n_1 is the refractive index of the incident medium and n_2 is the index of the refracting medium (and $n_1 > n_2$), then the critical angle, θ_{crit}, is defined by the equation $\sin \theta_{crit} = n_2 / n_1$. [**Section 13.2**]

current

A net flow of electric charge; more precisely, it's the net amount of charge that passes a given point per unit time: $I = Q/t$. [**Section 10.1**]

decibel

A unit of sound level. If I is the intensity of a sound wave, then the sound level (in decibels, dB) is defined as $\beta = 10 \log (I/I_0)$, where I_0 is the threshold of hearing (a reference intensity, 10^{-12} W/m²). [**Section 12.4**]

density

The ratio of an object's mass to its volume: density = $\rho = m/V$. [**Section 8.1**]

dielectric

An insulating material sandwiched between the plates of a capacitor; a capacitor always has a higher capacitance when a dielectric is present. [**Section 9.3, 10.2**]

diffraction

The redistribution of a wave's energy as it encounters and moves beyond an obstruction (or hole). [**Section 13.3**]

diopter

The unit of lens power: 1 diopter = 1 D = 1 m⁻¹. [**Section 13.5**]

direct current

Current whose direction remains steady during the operation of an electric circuit. [**Section 10.1, 10.3**]

dispersion

The variation of the speed of a wave as the frequency changes. For the MCAT, the only example of dispersion you should know is the variation of the speed of light through a material medium, such as glass. The colorful spectrum that is seen exiting a glass prism is an example of this dispersion. [**Section 13.3**]

displacement

The change in position of an object. The magnitude of an object's displacement gives the net distance traveled by the object. [**Section 3.2**]

diverging lens
A lens that is thinner in the middle than at its edges. A diverging lens causes incident parallel rays of light to diverge away from the focal point after passing through the lens. [**Section 13.5**]

Doppler effect
The perceived change in frequency of a wave due to relative motion between the source of a wave and the detector. When the source and detector are in relative motion toward each other, the detected frequency is higher than the emitted frequency; when the source and detector are in relative motion away from each other, the detected frequency is lower than the emitted frequency. [**Section 12.5**]

efficiency
The percentage of the useful work that a machine does in comparison to its theoretical maximum, or W_{output}/Energy$_{input}$. [**Section 6.7**]

elastic collision
A collision for which total kinetic energy is conserved. [**Section 6.7**]

elastic potential energy
The energy stored in a stretched or compressed spring: $PE_{elastic} = \frac{1}{2}kx^2$, where k is the spring constant. [**Section 11.1**]

electric field
A force field created by one or more electric charges. [**Section 9.3**]

electric force
The force exerted by an electric field; if a charge q is in an electric field **E**, then the electric force on q is given by the equation $F_E = q$E. [**Section 9.2, 9.3**]

electric potential
The electric potential at a point P is equal to the work required to bring a unit charge from infinity to P, divided by that charge. If P is a distance r away from a point charge Q, then the electric potential at P is a scalar quantity given by $\phi = kq/r$ where k is Coulomb's constant. [**Section 9.4**]

electric potential energy
The energy stored in the field surrounding a configuration of charged objects. A charge q experience and electric potential ϕ has an electric potential energy given by $PE = q\phi$. [**Section 9.4**]

electromagnetic (EM) spectrum
The full range of electromagnetic radiation, where different ranges of frequencies (and wavelengths) are categorized. Such categories include (in order of increasing frequency): radio waves, microwaves, infrared (IR) light, visible light, ultraviolet light, x-rays, and gamma rays. [**Section 13.1**]

electron
A fundamental subatomic particle with a negative electric charge (equal to $-e$, the negative of the elementary electric charge) that orbits the nucleus of an atom. [**Section 9.1**]

entropy
The measure of disorder of a thermodynamic system. [**Section 7.4**]

equilibrium
An object or system is said to be in translational equilibrium if the net force on it is zero. An object or system is said to be in rotational equilibrium if the net torque on it is zero. An object or system is said to be in equilibrium if it is in both translational and rotational equilibrium. [**Section 5.4**]

For an oscillator, the equilibrium position is the point at which the restoring force is zero [**Section 11.1**]

equipotential
A curve or surface on which the electric potential remains constant. [**Section 9.4**]

equivalent resistance
The single resistance that provides the same overall resistance as a combination of resistors. [**Section 10.1**]

farad
The SI unit of capacitance: 1 farad = 1 coulomb per volt = 1 C/V. [**Section 10.2**]

flow rate
The amount of fluid that flows per unit time; it is equal to the cross-sectional area of the flow tube multiplied by the flow speed: $f = Av$. [**Section 8.2**]

fluid
A substance that can flow, or more precisely, a substance that cannot withstand a shear stress. Both liquids and gases are fluids. [**Section 8.1**]

focal length
The distance from a mirror or lens to its focal point along the axis of curvature. Concave mirrors and converging lenses have positive focal lengths; convex mirrors and diverging lenses have negative focal lengths. [**Section 13.4, 13.5**]

focal point (or focus)
The point where any curved mirror or lens focuses the image of a distant object. For a concave mirror or a converging lens, the focal point (or focus) is the point *to* which rays of light that are initially parallel to the optical axis are focused after contact with the mirror or lens. For a convex mirror or a diverging lens, the focal point is the point *from* which rays of light that are initially parallel to the optical axis are diverged after contact with the mirror or lens. [**Section 13.4, 13.5**]

force
Intuitively, a push or pull exerted by one object on another. This may result in an acceleration if the forces on the object are not balanced [**Section 4.1**]

frequency
The number of oscillations (or cycles) per second. [**Section 11.1, 11.2, 12.1, 13.1**]

friction
The friction force is the parallel component of the contact force exerted by a surface on an object. [**Section 4.3**]

fundamental frequency
The lowest permissible frequency, or longest permissible wavelength, of a standing wave; also referred to as the *first harmonic*. [**Section 11.4**]

gravitational acceleration
The acceleration produced by the gravitational pull of a body, directed toward the center of the body. The magnitude of the gravitational acceleration, g, produced by the earth is approximately 10 m/s^2 near the surface. [**Section 3.5**]

gravitational force
In Newton's theory of gravitation, every object exerts a force, a gravitational pull, on every other object. If the masses of the two object are m_1 and m_2, and if their centers of mass are separated by a distance r, then the magnitude of the gravitational force between them is given by $F_{grav} = Gm_1m_2 / r^2$. [**Section 4.1, 4.2**]

heat
The transfer of thermal energy between a system and its environment. [**Section 7.1**]

Heisenberg uncertainty principle
The quantum physics principle that restricts the precision with which position and momentum of a particle can be defined: $\Delta x \Delta p \geq h / 2\pi$ [**Section 14.5**]

hertz
The SI unit of frequency; 1 hertz = 1 Hz = 1 cycle (or oscillation) per second. [**Section 11.1**]

Hooke's law
The magnitude of the force exerted by a stretched or compressed object or spring is proportional to the distance by which it is stretched or compressed from equilibrium: $F_{rest} = -kx$. [**Section 11.1**]

hydrostatic gauge pressure
The pressure at a point below the surface of a fluid at rest, due to the weight of the fluid above it: $P_{gauge} = \rho_{fluid} g D$, where D is the depth. [**Section 8.1**]

impulse
The product of force and the time during which it acts: impulse = $\mathbf{J} = \mathbf{F}\Delta t$. [**Section 6.7**]

impulse-momentum theorem
The total impulse delivered to an object is equal to its change in momentum: $\mathbf{J}_{total} = \Delta\mathbf{p}$. [**Section 6.7**]

index of refraction
The index of refraction for a medium is equal to the ratio of the speed of light in vacuum to the speed of light through the medium: $n = c/v$. [**Section 13.2**]

inelastic collision
A collision in which total momentum is conserved, but total kinetic energy is not. [**Section 6.7**]

inertia
1. Resistance to acceleration; an object's inertia is measured by its mass and is the ratio of the net force on an object to its acceleration: inertia = $m = F_{net} / a$. [**Section 4.1**]

2. Rotational inertia (also known as moment of inertia) is resistance to rotational acceleration. [**Section 5.5**]

insulator
A material with a very high resistivity that does not permit charge to flow through it easily. Glass and wood are examples of insulators. [**Section 9.3**]

intensity
The intensity of a wave is the power it transmits per unit area; the units of I are therefore W/m². Intensity is related directly to the wave's amplitude and diminishes with the square of the distance from the source. [**Section 12.4**]

interference
The combination of two or more waves. When the waves are in phase (crest meets crest, trough meets trough), this is *constructive* interference, and the amplitude of the resultant wave is equal to the sum of the individual amplitudes; when the waves are *out of phase* (crest meets trough, trough meets crest), this is *destructive* interference, and the amplitude of the resultant wave is equal to the difference between the individual amplitudes. [**Section 11.3**]

isobaric
Describes a thermodynamic process in which pressure is held constant. [**Section 7.3**]

isochoric
Describes a thermodynamic process in which volume is held constant. [**Section 7.3**]

isothermal
Describes a thermodynamic process in which temperature is held constant. [**Section 7.3**]

joule
The SI unit of work and energy; 1 joule = 1 J = 1 N·m = 1 kg·m²/s². [**Section 6.1**]

kinetic energy
The energy due to motion; for an object of mass m and speed v, the kinetic energy is $KE = \frac{1}{2}mv^2$. [**Section 6.3**]

kinetic friction
Also known as sliding friction, it is the friction that results when there is relative motion between the two surfaces; that is, when one surface slides across the other. If F_N is the magnitude of the normal force and μ_k is the coefficient of kinetic friction between the two surfaces, then the force of kinetic friction is directed opposite to the direction of the sliding and its magnitude is $F_f = \mu_k F_N$. [**Section 4.3**]

Kirchhoff's laws
1. The total amount of current entering a junction in a circuit must be equal to the total amount of current leaving the junction.

2. The sum of the voltages around a closed loop in a circuit must be zero. [Section 10.1]

lens
A thin piece of glass or plastic that forms an image by refracting light. [Section 13.5]

lever arm
Denoted by ℓ, it is the perpendicular distance from the pivot (reference) point to the line of action of a force. [Section 5.3]

longitudinal wave
A wave in which the oscillations of the medium are parallel to the direction of propagation of the wave. Sound waves are longitudinal. [Section 12.1]

magnetic field
The force field created by a *moving* electric charge. [Section 10.4]

magnetic force
The force exerted by a magnetic field on a moving charge. If a charge q moves with velocity $\mathbf{v}$ through a magnetic field $\mathbf{B}$, then the magnetic force on q is given by $\mathbf{F} = q(\mathbf{v} \times \mathbf{B})$. The magnitude of $\mathbf{F}$ is $|q|vB\sin\theta$ (where θ is the angle between $\mathbf{v}$ and $\mathbf{B}$), and the direction of $\mathbf{F}$ is given by the right-hand rule if q is positive and by the left-hand rule if q is negative. [Section 10.4]

magnification
The ratio of the height of the image to the height of the object; a negative value for the magnification means that the image is inverted relative to the object. For a mirror or lens, the magnification is given by the equation $m = -i / o$, where i and o are the distances from the mirror or lens to the image and the object, respectively. [Section 13.4, 13.5]

mass
The quantitative measure of an object's inertia; intuitively, we think of mass as measuring the amount of matter in an object. In SI units, mass is expressed in kilograms (kg) and is the ratio of the net force on an object to its acceleration: mass $= m = F_{net} / a$. [Section 4.1]

mechanical advantage
The factor by which a machine or mechanism multiplies the input or effort force. This term is applied to simple machines such as inclined planes, pulley systems, and levers. [Section 6.6]

mirror
A surface that forms an image by reflecting light. [Section 13.4]

moment of inertia
Also known as rotational inertia, an object's moment of inertia measures its resistance to rotational acceleration (just as an object's mass measures its resistance to translational acceleration). [Section 5.5]

momentum
The product of an object's mass and velocity: momentum $= \mathbf{p} = m\mathbf{v}$. [Section 6.7]

net force
The sum of all the forces that act on an object. [Section 4.1]

neutron
A subatomic particle with zero electric charge that is a constituent of atomic nuclei. [Section 9.1]

newton
The SI unit of force: 1 newton $= 1\ \text{N} = 1\ \text{kg·m/s}^2$. [Section 4.1]

Newton's laws of motion

1. If $F_{net} = 0$, then the object's velocity will not change.

2. $F_{net} = m\mathbf{a}$

3. If Object 1 exerts a force, $F_{1\text{-}on\text{-}2}$, on Object 2, then Object 2 exerts a force, $F_{2\text{-}on\text{-}1}$, on Object 1. These forces (known as an action-reaction pair) have the same magnitude but point in opposite directions, so $F_{2\text{-}on\text{-}1} = -F_{1\text{-}on\text{-}2}$, and act on different objects. [**Section 4.1**]

node
A point where a standing wave has zero amplitude. [**Section 11.4**]

normal
As an adjective, it means *perpendicular*. As a noun, a normal is a line that's perpendicular to a surface. [**Section 4.3, 13.2**]

normal force
For an object in contact with a surface, the normal force is the component of the force exerted by the surface that is perpendicular to the surface. [**Section 4.3**]

north pole of magnet
The pole from which the magnetic field lines emerge from a magnet. [**Section 10.4**]

ohm
The unit of resistance: 1 ohm = 1 Ω = 1 volt per amp = 1 V/A. [**Section 10.1**]

Ohm's law
A material is said to obey Ohm's law if its resistance remains constant as the voltage across it varies; thus, for such a material, $V = IR$, where R is a constant. [**Section 10.1**]

parallel resistors
Resistors in a circuit are said to be in parallel if they provide alternate routes for current to flow from one point in the circuit to another; parallel resistors always share the same voltage drop. [**Section 10.1**]

pascal
The unit of pressure: 1 pascal = 1 Pa = 1 newton per square meter = 1 N/m². [**Section 8.1**]

Pascal's law
A confined fluid transmits an externally applied change in pressure to all parts of the fluid equally. [**Section 8.1**]

Pauli exclusion principle
The quantum physics rule that restricts the number of particles that can occupy the same quantum state within a small proximity; the principle that explains how electron orbitals fill in the elements. [**Section 14.3**]

period
The time required for one complete oscillation (or cycle). [**Section 11.1, 11.2**]

periodic (or harmonic) motion
Any motion that regularly repeats, such as uniform circular motion or oscillatory motion. [**Section 11.1**]

photoelectric effect
The effect wherein photons eject individual electrons from a metal. [**Section 14.4**]

photon
Light travels as a wave, but interacts with matter as a stream of particles; these "particles," each an indivisible quantum of energy, are photons. Photons have no mass and move at the speed of light. The energy carried by each photon is proportional to the frequency of the light: $E_{photon} = hf$, where h is a constant of nature known as Planck's constant. [**Section 13.1, 14.2**]

polarized

1. A transverse wave is polarized if the direction of its oscillations is constant (or is confined to vary in a particular way). For a plane-polarized electromagnetic wave, the direction of polarization is the direction of oscillation of the electric field.

2. Circular polarization is the result of two perpendicular waves with a 90° phase difference interfering, and resulting in the apparent rotation of the electric field. [Section 13.1, 13.3]

potential energy

The energy of an object (or system) due to its position or configuration. There are different forms of potential energy, depending on the force involved; for the MCAT, the three most important forms are gravitational PE, electrical PE, and elastic PE. [Section 6.4, 9.4, 11.1]

power

1. In mechanics, power is the rate at which work is done or energy is used. Power is thus equal to work (or energy) divided by time, and its SI unit is the watt, where 1 watt = 1 W = 1 J/s. [Section 6.2]

2. In optics, lens power is a measure of the focusing strength of a lens. By definition, lens power is equal to the reciprocal of the focal length of the lens: $P = 1/f$. If f is expressed in meters, then lens power has units of diopters, where 1 diopter = $1 D = 1 m^{-1}$. [Section 13.5]

pressure

A scalar quantity equal to the magnitude of the perpendicular force per unit area. [Section 7.2, 7.3, 8.1]

projectile motion

The motion of a particle moving under the influence of uniform (constant) acceleration; if the object's initial velocity is not purely vertical, the path of the object will be a parabola. [Section 3.6]

proton

A subatomic particle with a positive electric charge (equal to the elementary electric charge, $+e$) that is a constituent of atomic nuclei. [Section 9.1]

quantized

A quantity is said to be quantized if it exists only in discrete amounts. Examples: (1) Electric charge on an object can only be an integer multiple of the basic unit of electric charge, e. (2) Electromagnetic radiation of frequency f can be absorbed only in whole number multiples of the photon energy, hf. [Sections 9.1, 14.1]

quantum physics

The physics associated with discrete values and changes in the values of such quantities; associated strongly with wave-particle duality. [Section 14.1]

radiation

1. Energy emitted or absorbed due to propagation of waves (electromagnetic waves, unless a different kind of wave is specially mentioned). [Section 13.1]

2. A mode of heat transfer via electromagnetic waves. [Section 7.2]

rarefaction

A region where the local density and pressure is momentarily decreased from standard due to the passage of a sound wave. [Section 12.1]

real image

An image formed by a mirror or lens where light rays actually do intersect. Unlike a virtual image, a real image can be projected onto a screen. [Section 13.4]

reflection

When waves or particles "bounce off" a surface on which they are incident, the return of these waves or particles is called reflection. [Section 13.2]

refraction

The change in direction of a wave when it passes from one medium into another. [Section 13.2]

resistance
The ratio of the voltage to current: $R = V/I$. [Section 10.1]

resistivity
The intrinsic resistance of a material. [Section 10.1]

resistor
A component of an electrical circuit that provides resistance to the flow of current. [Section 10.1]

restoring force
For an object undergoing oscillation, the force on the object that is directed toward equilibrium. [Section 11.1]

series resistors
Resistors in a circuit are said to be in series if current must flow through each of them, one after the other; series resistors always share the same current. [Section 10.1]

shear stress
The magnitude of the shearing force exerted on an object divided by the area parallel to which it acts. [Section 8.3]

simple harmonic motion
Periodic (oscillatory) movement where the period and frequency of the oscillations do not depend on the amplitude, caused by a restoring force that is proportional to the displacement from equilibrium. [Section 11.1]

Snell's law
The law of refraction in optics, $n_1 \sin \theta_1 = n_2 \sin \theta_2$, where n_1 and n_2 are the refractive indexes of the incident and refracting media (respectively), and θ_1 is the angle of incidence and θ_2 the angle of refraction. [Section 13.1, 13.2]

sound level
A measurement, in decibels, of the intensity of a sound wave. The sound-level for a wave of intensity I is given by the equation $\beta = 10 \log_{10} (I/I_0)$, where I_0 is the threshold of hearing. [Section 12.4]

south pole of magnet
The pole into which the magnetic field lines enter a magnet. [Section 10.4]

specific gravity
The unitless ratio of the density of a substance to the density of water: sp. gr. = $\rho_{\text{substance}}/\rho_{\text{water}}$. [Section 8.1]

speed
The magnitude of an object's velocity. [Section 3.2]

standing wave
A wave caused by the superposition of two oppositely directed traveling waves, for which the resulting crests and troughs do not travel. [Section 11.4]

state function or state variable
The measure of an intrinsic, macroscopic property of a thermodynamic system that defines the present attributes of the system, independent of past processes. [Section 7.2]

static friction
The friction that results when there is no relative motion between the two surfaces; that is, when neither slides across the other. If F_N is the magnitude of the normal force and μ_s is the coefficient of static friction between the two surfaces, then the force of static friction is directed opposite to the direction of the intended motion and its *maximum* magnitude is $F_{f, \text{max}} = \mu_{s, \text{max}} F_N$. [Section 4.3]

stopping voltage
In the photoelectric experiment, the negative voltage necessary to prevent the most energetic photoelectrons ejected from the metal surface from reaching the detector. [Section 14.4]

strain

The ratio of the change in one of an object's dimensions to the original, caused by an applied stress. For a compressive or tensile stress, the strain is equal to (the magnitude of) the change in the object's length divided by the original length. For a shear stress, the strain is equal to the distance the object is deformed perpendicular to the shear stress divided by the length perpendicular to the direction of the bend. [**Section 8.3**]

stress

The magnitude of the force acting on an object, divided by the area over which it acts. [**Section 8.3**]

superposition

The addition principle that applies to several different physical phenomena, such as electric forces, fields, potentials, and waves, where the result is simply equal to the sum of the individual vector or scalar values. [**Section 9.2, 9.3, 9.4, 11.3**]

system

The object or substance—or objects or substances and the interactions among them—that are the focus of study. Contrasted with the environment, which is everything else. [**Section 7.1**]

temperature

A thermodynamic state function that corresponds to the internal, random kinetic energy of the constituent particles of a system. [**Section 7.1, 7.2**]

tension

A type of force applied to a solid object that tends to increase its length. Tension is also used to describe the pulling force exerted by a stretched string, rope, chain, or spring. [**Section 4.1, 4.5, 8.3**]

tesla

The SI unit of magnetic field strength: 1 tesla = 1 T = 1 newton per amp-meter = 1 N/A·m. [**Section 10.4**]

thermodynamics

The study of how macroscopic systems transfer or transform energy. [**Section 7.1**]

Thermodynamic laws

0th law: Two objects in thermal equilibrium with the same third object are in thermal equilibrium with each other. Defines temperature as a state function. [**Section 7.2**]

1st law: The total quantity of energy in the universe is conserved. more specifically, the energy into and out of a system equals its change in internal energy; $\Delta E = Q - W$ [**Section 7.3**]

2nd law: The entropy of a closed system will either stay the same or increase. [**Section 7.4**]

threshold of hearing

The lowest intensity the human ear can detect; denoted I_0, it is defined as 10^{-12} W/m². [**Section 12.4**]

torque

A quantity associated with a force that measures how effective the force is at producing rotational acceleration. If **r** is the vector from the pivot point to the point of application of a force **F**, and the angle between **r** and **F** is θ, then the torque of the force is defined to be $\tau = rF\sin\theta$. [**Section 5.3**]

Torricelli's result

The equation giving the speed of efflux for a static fluid from a small hole in a large open container: $v = \sqrt{2gD}$, where D is the depth of the hole below the surface of the fluid. [**Section 8.2**]

total internal reflection

When an incident beam of light strikes the surface of a medium with a lower index of refraction, the beam will experience total internal reflection (TIR) if the angle of incidence is greater than the critical angle. In this case, none of the beam's energy is transmitted to the other medium; it is only reflected. [**Section 13.2**]

total mechanical energy
The sum of an object's kinetic energy and potential energy: $E = KE + PE$. [Section 6.5]

transverse wave
A wave in which the oscillations that make up the wave are perpendicular to the direction of the wave's propagation. Waves on a rope and electromagnetic waves are transverse. [Section 11.2]

velocity
The rate of change of an object's position: $\bar{\mathbf{v}} = \Delta \mathbf{s}/\Delta t = \mathbf{d}/\Delta t$. An object's velocity gives both the speed and the direction of motion of the object. [Section 3.2]

virtual image
An image formed by a mirror or lens where light rays don't actually intersect. Unlike a real image, a virtual image cannot be displayed on a screen. Convex mirrors and diverging (concave) lenses form only virtual images. [Section 13.4]

viscosity
The internal friction of a fluid; an ideal fluid is one whose viscosity is negligible. [Section 8.2]

volt
The SI unit of electric potential and voltage; 1 volt = 1 V = 1 joule per coulomb = 1 J/C. [Section 9.4]

voltage
The difference in electric potential between two points. [Section 9.4, 10.1]

voltmeter
A device for measuring the voltage across a circuit element. [Section 10.1]

watt
The SI unit of power; 1 watt = 1 W = 1 joule per second = 1 J/s. [Section 6.2]

wave
A disturbance that carries energy and momentum from one position to another. [Section 11.2]

wavelength
The distance (denoted by λ) between consecutive crests (or between consecutive troughs) of a wave. [Section 11.2]

weight
The gravitational force exerted on an object: $\mathbf{w} = m\mathbf{g}$. [Section 4.2]

work
The work done by a constant force $\mathbf{F}$ as it acts through a displacement $\mathbf{d}$ is given by the equation $W = Fd \cos\theta$, where θ is the angle between $\mathbf{F}$ and $\mathbf{d}$. For an ideal gas in a container, work can be expressed as the product of its change in volume and its pressure, $W = P\Delta V$. Work is a scalar quantity, and its SI unit is the joule, where 1 joule = 1 J = 1 kg-m^2/s^2. [Section 6.1, 7.3]

work-energy theorem
The total amount of work done on an object is equal to the change in the object's kinetic energy: $W = \Delta KE$. [Section 6.3]

work function
The binding energy of a metal for its free electrons, overcome during the photoelectric effect. [Section 14.4]

MCAT Physics
Formula Sheet

KINEMATICS

The Big Five

if a is constant:

1. $d = vt = \dfrac{1}{2}(v_0 + v)t$

2. $v = v_0 + at$

3. $d = v_0 t + \dfrac{1}{2}at^2$

4. $d = vt - \dfrac{1}{2}at^2$

5. $v^2 = v_0^2 + 2ad$

Projectile Motion

Horizontal	Vertical
$x = v_{0x} t$	$y = v_{0y} t - \dfrac{1}{2}gt^2$
$v_x = v_{0x}$	$v_y = v_{0y} - gt$
$a_x = 0$	$a_y = -g$

$$v_{0x} = v_0 \cos\theta_0$$
$$v_{0y} = v_0 \sin\theta_0$$

DYNAMICS

Newton's Laws

1. $\mathbf{F}_{net} = 0 \rightarrow \mathbf{v} = $ constant
2. $\mathbf{F}_{net} = m\mathbf{a}$
3. $\mathbf{F}_{2\text{-on-}1} = -\mathbf{F}_{1\text{-on-}2}$

GRAVITY

$$F_{grav} = w = mg$$

$$F_{grav} = G\frac{Mm}{r^2}$$

$$g = G\frac{M}{r^2}$$

$$g_{Earth} \approx 10\,\frac{m}{s^2}$$

θ	0°	30°	45°	60°	90°	120°	135°	150°	180°
$\cos\theta$	$\sqrt{4}/2$	$\sqrt{3}/2$	$\sqrt{2}/2$	$\sqrt{1}/2$	$\sqrt{0}/2$	$-\sqrt{1}/2$	$-\sqrt{2}/2$	$-\sqrt{3}/2$	$-\sqrt{4}/2$
$\sin\theta$	$\sqrt{0}/2$	$\sqrt{1}/2$	$\sqrt{2}/2$	$\sqrt{3}/2$	$\sqrt{4}/2$	$\sqrt{3}/2$	$\sqrt{2}/2$	$\sqrt{1}/2$	$\sqrt{0}/2$

$\sqrt{2} \approx 1.4$ $\sqrt{3} \approx 1.7$

INCLINED PLANE

θ = incline angle to horizontal

Force due to gravity parallel to ramp = $mg\sin\theta$

Force due to gravity perpendicular to ramp = $mg\cos\theta (= F_N)$

CENTER OF MASS (= CENTER OF GRAVITY)

$$x_{CM} = \frac{m_1 x_1 + ... + m_n x_n}{m_1 + ... + m_n} = \frac{w_1 x_1 + ... + w_n x_n}{w_1 + ... + w_n} = x_{CG}$$

WORK, ENERGY, POWER

Work: $W = Fd\cos\theta$

Kinetic energy: $KE = \dfrac{1}{2}mv^2$

Work-Energy theorem: $W_{total} = \Delta KE$

Power: $P = \dfrac{W}{t}$, $P = Fv$ if $\mathbf{F} \parallel \mathbf{v}$, and $\mathbf{v}$ is constant.

Potential energy: $PE_{grav} = mgh$ (if $h \ll r_{Earth}$)

Mechanical energy: $E = KE + PE$

Conservation of Mechanical Energy: $E_i = E_f$ or $KE_i + PE_i = KE_f + PE_f$

If non-conservative (nc) forces—like friction—act during the motion:

$E_i + W_{by\ nc\ forces} = E_f$

FRICTION

F_N = magnitude of normal force

$F_{f,static,max} = \mu_s F_N$

$F_{f,kinetic} = \mu_k F_N$

UNIFORM CIRCULAR MOTION

Centrepital acceleration: $a_c = \dfrac{v^2}{r}$

Centrepital force: $F_c = ma_c = m\dfrac{v^2}{r}$

TORQUE

$\tau = rF\sin\theta = lF$

MOMENTUM

$\mathbf{p} = m\mathbf{v}$

Impulse: $\mathbf{J} = \mathbf{F}t$

Impulse-Momentum theorem: $\mathbf{J} = \Delta\mathbf{p}$

Conservation of Momentum: total $\mathbf{p}_i = $ total $\mathbf{p}_f$

STRESS AND STRAIN

Stress = $\dfrac{F}{A}$

Strain = $\dfrac{\Delta L}{L}$

Hooke's law: $\Delta L = \dfrac{FL}{EA}$

THERMODYNAMICS

First law: $\Delta E = Q - W$

Work: $W = P\Delta V$

Temp. of monatomic ideal gas:
$$\frac{1}{2}mv_{avg}^2 = \frac{3}{2}k_B T$$

Heat and Temp for an ideal gas:
$Q = nC_V \Delta T$ (constant volume) or
$Q = nC_P \Delta T$ (constant pressure)

FLUIDS

Density: $\rho = \dfrac{m}{V}$, $\rho_{H_2O} = 1000 \dfrac{kg}{m^3}$

Specific gravity: sp. gr. $= \dfrac{\rho}{\rho_{H_2O}}$

Pressure: $P = \dfrac{F_\perp}{A}$

Total Hydrostatic pressure: $P = P_0 + \rho g D = P_{atm} + \rho g D$ (if $P_0 = P_{atm}$)

Gauge pressure: $P_{gauge} = P - P_{atm}$

Archimedes' principle: $F_{Buoyant} = \rho_{fluid} V_{sub} g$

Pascal's law: $\dfrac{F_1}{A_1} = \dfrac{F_2}{A_2}$

Volume flow rate: $f = Av$

Continuity equation: $A_1 v_1 = A_2 v_2$

Bernoulli's equation: $P_1 + \rho g y_1 + \dfrac{1}{2}\rho v_1^2 = P_2 + \rho g y_2 + \dfrac{1}{2}\rho v_2^2$

ELECTRIC CIRCUITS

Current: $I = \dfrac{Q}{t}$

Resistance: $R = \dfrac{V}{I}$ ("Ohm's law": $V = IR$)

Resistance: $R = \rho \dfrac{L}{A}$

Resistors in series: $R_S = R_1 + R_2 + \ldots$

Resistors in parallel: $\dfrac{1}{R_P} = \dfrac{1}{R_1} + \dfrac{1}{R_2} + \ldots$

Power in circuit: $P = IV = I^2 R = \dfrac{V^2}{R}$

Power in AC circuit: $\bar{P} = I_{rms} V_{rms} = \dfrac{I_{max}}{\sqrt{2}} \cdot \dfrac{V_{max}}{\sqrt{2}}$

OSCILLATIONS AND WAVES

Hooke's law: $\mathbf{F}_S = -k\mathbf{x}$

$PE_S = \dfrac{1}{2}kx^2$

frequency and period: $f = \dfrac{1}{T}, T = \dfrac{1}{f}$

$f = \dfrac{1}{2\pi}\sqrt{\dfrac{k}{m}}, T = 2\pi\sqrt{\dfrac{m}{k}}$

$f_{simple\ pendulum} = \dfrac{1}{2\pi}\sqrt{\dfrac{g}{L}}$

$\lambda f = v$

$v = \sqrt{\dfrac{F_T}{\mu}} = \sqrt{\dfrac{F_T}{m/L}}$

Harmonic frequencies: $f_n = n\dfrac{v}{2L}, f_n = nf_1$

Harmonic wavelengths: $\lambda_n = \dfrac{2L}{n}, \lambda_n = \dfrac{1}{n}\lambda_1$

CAPACITORS

Capacitance: $C = \dfrac{Q}{V}$

$C_{parallel\text{-}plate} = \varepsilon_0 \dfrac{A}{d}$

$C_{with\ dielectric} = K \cdot C_{without}$

electric field between plates: $E = \dfrac{V}{d}$

$PE_E = \dfrac{1}{2}QV = \dfrac{1}{2}CV^2 = \dfrac{Q^2}{2C}$

Capacitors in series: $\dfrac{1}{C_S} = \dfrac{1}{C_1} + \dfrac{1}{C_2} + \ldots$

Capacitors in parallel: $C_P = C_1 + C_2 + \ldots$

SOUND

$v = \sqrt{\dfrac{B}{\rho}}$

Intensity: $I = \dfrac{Power}{Area}$

Intensity-level (in dB): $\beta = 10\log\dfrac{I}{I_0}$

Harmonic f's and λ's:

Open ends: $f_n = \dfrac{nv}{2L}$, $\lambda_n = \dfrac{2L}{n}$

Closed ends: $f_n = \dfrac{nv}{4L}$, $\lambda_n = \dfrac{4L}{n}$ (odd n)

$f_{beat} = |f_1 - f_2|$

Doppler effect: $f_D = \dfrac{v \pm v_D}{v \mp v_S}f_S$

Approaching $\leftrightarrow$ higher f
Receding $\leftrightarrow$ lower f

ELECTROSTATICS AND MAGNETISM

Coulomb's law: $F_E = k\dfrac{|Q||q|}{r^2}$

Electric field due to Q: $E = k\dfrac{|Q|}{r^2}$

Electric force by field: $\mathbf{F}_E = q\mathbf{E}$

Electric potential due to Q: $\phi = k\dfrac{Q}{r}$

$\Delta PE_E = q\Delta\phi = qV$

magnetic force: $\mathbf{F}_M = q(\mathbf{v} \times \mathbf{B})$

$F_M = qvB\sin\theta$

LIGHT AND OPTICS

$E_{photon} = hf = \dfrac{hc}{\lambda}$; $c = 3.0 \times 10^8$ m/s

index of refraction: $n = \dfrac{c}{v}$

Law of reflection: $\theta_1 = \theta_1'$

Law of refraction (Snell's law): $n_1 \sin\theta_1 = n_2 \sin\theta_2$

TIR: if $\theta_1 > \theta_{crit}$, where $\sin\theta_{crit} = \dfrac{n_2}{n_1}$

Mirror-Lens equation: $\dfrac{1}{o} + \dfrac{1}{i} = \dfrac{1}{f}$

Focal length: $f = \dfrac{R}{2}$

Magnification: $m = -\dfrac{i}{o}$

Lens power: $P = \dfrac{1}{f}$; $P_{combination} = P_1 + P_2$

QUANTUM PHYSICS

Photoelectron Energy: $KE_{max} = hf - \phi$

Stopping Voltage: $-eV_{stop} = KE_{max}$

Heisenberg Uncertainty Principle:

$\Delta x \Delta p \geq h/2\pi$

CONSTANTS AND UNITS

Constants

magnitude of gravitational acceleration near the surface of Earth: $\quad g = 9.8 \text{ m/s}^2 \approx 10 \text{ m/s}^2$

density of water: $\quad \rho_{water} = 1000 \text{ kg/m}^3 = 1 \text{ g/cm}^3$

elementary electric charge: $\quad e = 1.6 \times 10^{-19} \text{ C}$

Coulomb's constant: $\quad k_0 = 9 \times 10^9 \text{ N·m}^2 / \text{C}^2$

threshold of hearing: $\quad I_0 = 10^{-12} \text{ W/m}^2$

speed of light in vacuum: $\quad c = 3 \times 10^8 \text{ m/s}$

atmospheric pressure: $\quad P_{atm} = 10^5 \text{ Pa}$

speed of sound in air: $\quad v_{sound} = 340 \text{ m/s}$

visible light wavelengths: $\quad$ 400 nm to 700 nm

SI Units

distance: $\qquad [d] = \text{meters} = \text{m}$

mass: $\qquad [m] = \text{kilograms} = \text{kg}$

time: $\qquad [t] = \text{seconds} = \text{s}$

velocity, speed: $\qquad [v] = \text{meters per second} = \text{m/s}$

acceleration: $\qquad [a] = \text{meters per second squared} = \text{m/s}^2$

force: $\qquad [F] = \text{newtons} = \text{kg·m/s}^2$

torque: $\qquad [\tau] = \text{newton-meters} = \text{N·m}$

momentum: $\qquad [p] = \text{kg·m/s}$

impulse: $\qquad [J] = \text{newton-seconds} = \text{N·s}$

work: $\qquad [W] = \text{joules} = \text{J} = \text{kg·m}^2/\text{s}^2$

energy: $\qquad [KE] = [PE] = [E] = \text{joules} = \text{J} = \text{kg·m}^2/\text{s}^2$

power: $\qquad [P] = \text{watts} = \text{W} = \text{J/s}$

pressure: $\qquad [P] = \text{pascals} = \text{Pa} = \text{N/m}^2$

density: $\qquad [\rho] = \text{kilograms per cubic meter} = \text{kg/m}^3$

flow rate: $\qquad [f] = \text{m}^3/\text{s}$

electric charge: $\qquad [q] = \text{coulombs} = \text{C}$

electric field: $\qquad [E] = \text{newtons per coulomb} = \text{N/C (or volts per meter} = \text{V/m)}$

electric potential: $\qquad [\phi] = \text{volts} = \text{V} = \text{J/C}$

voltage: $\qquad [V] = \text{volts} = \text{V} = \text{J/C}$

current: $\qquad [I] = \text{amps} = \text{A} = \text{C/s}$

resistance: $\qquad [R] = \text{ohms} = \Omega = \text{V/A}$

resistivity: $\qquad [\rho] = \text{ohm-meters} = \Omega\text{·m}$

capacitance: $\qquad [C] = \text{farads} = \text{F} = \text{C/V}$

magnetic field: $\qquad [B] = \text{teslas} = \text{T} = \text{N/A·m}$

frequency: $\qquad [f] = \text{hertz} = \text{Hz} = \text{s}^{-1}$

period: $\qquad [T] = \text{seconds} = \text{s}$

sound level: $\qquad [\beta] = \text{decibels} = \text{dB}$

lens power: $\qquad [P] = \text{diopters} = \text{D} = \text{m}^{-1}$

MCAT Math for Physics

PREFACE

The MCAT is primarily a conceptual exam, with little actual mathematical computation. Any math that is on the MCAT is fundamental: just arithmetic, algebra, and trigonometry. There is absolutely no calculus. The purpose of this section of the book is to go over some math topics with which you may feel a little rusty.

This text is intended for reference and self-study. Therefore, there are lots of examples, all completely solved. Practice working through these examples and master the fundamentals!

Chapter 15
Arithmetic, Algebra, and Graphs

15.1 THE IMPORTANCE OF APPROXIMATION

Since you aren't allowed to use a calculator on the MCAT, you need to practice doing arithmetic calculations by hand again. Fortunately, the amount of calculation you'll have to do is small, and you'll also be able to approximate. For example, let's say you were faced with simplifying this expression:

$$\frac{\sqrt{5 \times 10^{-7}}}{(3.1 \times 10^{-2})^2}$$

Our first inclination would be to reach for our calculator, but we don't have one available. Now what? Realize that on the Chemical and Physical Foundations of Biological Systems section of the MCAT, 95 minutes for 67 questions, or approximately 1.4 minutes per question, so there simply cannot be questions requiring lengthy, complicated computation. Instead, we'll figure out a reasonably accurate (and fast) approximation of the value of the expression above:

$$\frac{\sqrt{5 \times 10^{-7}}}{(3.1 \times 10^{-2})^2} = \frac{\sqrt{50 \times 10^{-8}}}{(3.1)^2 \times (10^{-2})^2} \approx \frac{\sqrt{50} \times \sqrt{10^{-8}}}{10 \times 10^{-4}} \approx \frac{7 \times 10^{-4}}{10 \times 10^{-4}} = \frac{7}{10} = 0.7$$

So, if the answer to an MCAT question was the value of the expression above, and the four answer choices were, say, 0.124, 0.405, 0.736, and 1.289, we'd know right away that the answer is 0.736. The choices are far enough apart that even with our approximations, we were still able to tell which choice was the correct one. Just as importantly, we didn't waste time trying to be more precise; it was unnecessary, and it would have decreased the amount of time we had to spend on other questions.

If you find yourself writing out lengthy calculations on your scratch paper when you're working through MCAT questions that contain some mathematical calculation, it's important that you recognize that you're not using your time efficiently. Say to yourself, "I'm wasting valuable time trying to get a precise answer, when I don't need to be precise." Which of the following calculations for figuring out the value of 23.6×72.5 is faster?

$$\begin{array}{r} 23.6 \\ \times\ 72.5 \\ \hline 1180 \\ 472 \\ \hline 1652 \\ \hline 1711.00 \end{array}$$
or
$$\begin{array}{r} 25 \\ \times\ 70 \\ \hline 1750 \end{array}$$

In the one-step calculation on the right, we approximated: $23.6 \approx 25$ and $72.5 \approx 70$, and the answer we got in just a few seconds differs from the precise answer by only 2%. For the MCAT, you should always strive to make such approximations so that you can do the math quickly.

Try this one: What's 1583 divided by 32.1? (You have five seconds. Go.)

For the previous practice exercise, you should have written (or done in your head):

$$\frac{1500}{30} = 50$$

15.2 SCIENTIFIC NOTATION, EXPONENTS, AND RADICALS

It's well known that very large or very small numbers can be handled more easily when they're written in **scientific notation**, that is, in the form $\pm m \times 10^n$, where $1 \le m < 10$ and n is an integer. For example:

$$602,000,000,000,000,000,000,000 = 6.02 \times 10^{23}$$

$$-35,000,000,000 = -3.5 \times 10^{10}$$

$$0.000000004 = 4 \times 10^{-9}$$

Quantities like these come up all the time in physical problems, so you must be able to work with them confidently. Since a power of ten (the term 10^n) is part of every number written in scientific notation, the most important rules for dealing with such expressions are the Laws of Exponents:

Laws of Exponents

		Illustration (with $b = 10$ or a power of 10)
Law 1	$b^p \times b^q = b^{p+q}$	$10^5 \times 10^{-9} = 10^{5+(-9)} = 10^{-4}$
Law 2	$b^p/b^q = b^{p-q}$	$10^5/10^{-9} = 10^{5-(-9)} = 10^{14}$
Law 3	$(b^p)^q = b^{pq}$	$(10^{-3})^2 = 10^{(-3)(2)} = 10^{-6}$
Law 4	$b^0 = 1$ (if $b \ne 0$)	$10^0 = 1$
Law 5	$b^{-p} = 1/b^p$	$10^{-7} = 1/10^7$
Law 6	$(ab)^p = a^p b^p$	$(2 \times 10^4)^3 = 2^3 \times (10^4)^3 = 8 \times 10^{12}$
Law 7	$(a/b)^p = a^p/b^p$	$[(3 \times 10^{-6})/10^2]^2 = (3 \times 10^{-6})^2/(10^2)^2 = 9 \times 10^{-16}$

Example 15-1: Simplify each of the following expressions, writing your answer in scientific notation:
a) $(4 \times 10^{-3})(5 \times 10^9)$
b) $(4 \times 10^{-3})/(5 \times 10^9)$
c) $(3 \times 10^{-4})^3$
d) $[(1 \times 10^{-2})/(5 \times 10^{-7})]^2$

Solution:
a) $(4 \times 10^{-3})(5 \times 10^9) = (4)(5) \times 10^{-3+9} = 20 \times 10^6 = 2 \times 10^7$
b) $(4 \times 10^{-3})/(5 \times 10^9) = (4/5) \times 10^{-3-9} = 0.8 \times 10^{-12} = 8 \times 10^{-13}$
c) $(3 \times 10^{-4})^3 = 3^3 \times (10^{-4})^3 = 27 \times 10^{-12} = 2.7 \times 10^{-11}$
d) $[(1 \times 10^{-2})/(5 \times 10^{-7})]^2 = (1 \times 10^{-2})^2/(5 \times 10^{-7})^2 = (1 \times 10^{-4})/(25 \times 10^{-14}) = (1/25) \times 10^{-4-(-14)}$
    $= (4/100) \times 10^{10} = 4 \times 10^8$

Another important skill involving numbers written in scientific notation involves changing the power of 10 (and compensating for this change so as not to affect the original number). The approximation carried out in the very first example in this chapter is a good example of this. To find the square root of 5×10^{-7}, it is much easier to first rewrite this number as 50×10^{-8}, because then the square root is easy:

$$\sqrt{50 \times 10^{-8}} = \sqrt{50} \times \sqrt{10^{-8}} \approx 7 \times 10^{-4}$$

Other examples of this procedure are found in Example 15-1 above; for instance,

$$20 \times 10^{6} = 2 \times 10^{7}$$
$$0.8 \times 10^{-12} = 8 \times 10^{-13}$$
$$27 \times 10^{-12} = 2.7 \times 10^{-11}$$

In writing $\sqrt{50 \times 10^{-8}} = \sqrt{50} \times \sqrt{10^{-8}} \approx 7 \times 10^{-4}$, I used a familiar law of square roots, that the square root of a product is equal to the product of the square roots. Here's a short list of rules for dealing with radicals:

Laws of Radicals

Illustration

Law 1 $\sqrt{ab} = \sqrt{a} \cdot \sqrt{b}$ $\sqrt{9 \times 10^{12}} = \sqrt{9} \times \sqrt{10^{12}} = 3 \times 10^{6}$

Law 2 $\sqrt{a/b} = \sqrt{a} / \sqrt{b}$ $\sqrt{(4 \times 10^{-6})/10^{-18}} = \sqrt{(4 \times 10^{-6})} / \sqrt{10^{-18}} = (2 \times 10^{-3})/10^{-9} = 2 \times 10^{6}$

Law 3 $\sqrt[q]{a^{p}} = a^{p/q}$ $\sqrt[3]{(8 \times 10^{6})^{2}} = (8 \times 10^{6})^{2/3} = 8^{2/3} \times 10^{(6)(2/3)} = 4 \times 10^{4}$

A couple of remarks about this list: First, Laws 1 and 2 illustrate how to handle square roots, which are the most common. However, the same laws are true even if the index of the root is not 2. (The **index** of a root [or radical] is the number that indicates the root that's to be taken; it's indicated by the little q in front of the radical sign in Law 3. Cube roots are index 3 and written $\sqrt[3]{}$; fourth roots are index 4 and written $\sqrt[4]{}$; and square roots are index 2 and written $\sqrt[2]{}$, although we hardly ever write the little 2.) Second, Law 3 provides the link between exponents and radicals.

Example 15-2: Approximate each of the following expressions, writing your answer in scientific notation:

a) $\sqrt{3.5 \times 10^{9}}$

b) $\sqrt{8 \times 10^{-11}}$

c) $\sqrt{\dfrac{1.5 \times 10^{-5}}{2.5 \times 10^{-17}}}$

Solution:

a) $\sqrt{3.5 \times 10^9} = \sqrt{35 \times 10^8} = \sqrt{35} \times \sqrt{10^8} \approx \sqrt{36} \times \sqrt{10^8} = 6 \times 10^4$

b) $\sqrt{8 \times 10^{-11}} = \sqrt{80 \times 10^{-12}} = \sqrt{80} \times \sqrt{10^{-12}} \approx \sqrt{81} \times \sqrt{10^{-12}} = 9 \times 10^{-6}$

c) $\sqrt{\dfrac{1.5 \times 10^{-5}}{2.5 \times 10^{-17}}} = \dfrac{\sqrt{1.5 \times 10^{-5}}}{\sqrt{2.5 \times 10^{-17}}} = \dfrac{\sqrt{15 \times 10^{-6}}}{\sqrt{25 \times 10^{-18}}} \approx \dfrac{\sqrt{16} \times \sqrt{10^{-6}}}{\sqrt{25} \times \sqrt{10^{-18}}} = \dfrac{4 \times 10^{-3}}{5 \times 10^{-9}} = 0.8 \times 10^6 = 8 \times 10^5$

Example 15-3: Approximate each of the following expressions, writing your answer in scientific notation:

a) The mass (in grams) of 4.7×10^{24} molecules of CCl_4: $\dfrac{(4.7 \times 10^{24})(153.8)}{6.02 \times 10^{23}}$

b) The electrostatic force (in newtons) between the proton and electron in the ground state of hydrogen:

$$\dfrac{(8.99 \times 10^9)(1.6 \times 10^{-19})^2}{(5.3 \times 10^{-11})^2}$$

c) The diameter (in cm) of a 1 kg sphere of gold: $200\sqrt[3]{\dfrac{3}{4\pi} \dfrac{1}{19,300}}$

Solution:

a) $\dfrac{(4.7 \times 10^{24})(153.8)}{6.02 \times 10^{23}} \approx \dfrac{5(150)}{6} \times 10^{24-23} = 5(25) \times 10 = 1.25 \times 10^3$

b) $\dfrac{(8.99 \times 10^9)(1.6 \times 10^{-19})^2}{(5.3 \times 10^{-11})^2} \approx \dfrac{9(1.6)^2 \times 10^{9+(-19)(2)}}{(5.3)^2 \times 10^{(-11)(2)}} \approx \dfrac{(9)3 \times 10^{-29}}{27 \times 10^{-22}} = 1 \times 10^{-7}$

c) $200\sqrt[3]{\dfrac{3}{4\pi} \dfrac{1}{19,300}} \approx 200\sqrt[3]{\dfrac{1}{4} \dfrac{1}{20,000}} = \dfrac{200}{\sqrt[3]{80 \times 10^3}} = \dfrac{200}{\sqrt[3]{80} \times 10} \approx \dfrac{200}{4 \times 10} = 5$

Two notes about the approximation in part (c). First, we canceled the 3 and the π in the first fraction; this is fine since $\pi \approx 3.14$. Second, we had to approximate $\sqrt[3]{80}$. Since 80 is between $64 = 4^3$ and $125 = 5^3$, the cube root of 80 is between 4 and 5. And, since 80 is closer to 64 than it is to 125, the cube root of 80 is closer to 4. In general, to approximate the nth root of a number that isn't an nth power, simply locate the given number between successive n^{th} powers and approximate from there. For example, $\sqrt{42}$ is not an integer since 42 is not a perfect square. However, 42 is between $36 = 6^2$ and $49 = 7^2$, so $\sqrt{42}$ is between 6 and 7. And since 42 is about halfway between 36 and 49, the square root of 42 is about halfway between 6 and 7: $\sqrt{42} \approx 6.5$.

15.3 FRACTIONS, RATIOS, AND PERCENTS

A **fraction** indicates a division; for example, 3/4 means 3 divided by 4. The number above (or to the left of) the fraction bar is the numerator, and the number below (or to the right) of the fraction bar is called the denominator.

$$\frac{3}{4} \quad \begin{array}{l} \leftarrow \text{ numerator} \\ \leftarrow \text{ denominator} \end{array} \quad 3/4$$

Our quick review of the basic arithmetic operations on fractions begins with the simplest rule: the one for multiplication:

$$\frac{a}{b} \times \frac{c}{d} = \frac{ac}{bd}$$

In words, just multiply the numerators and then, separately, multiply the denominators.

Example 15-4: What is 4/9 times 2/5?

Solution: $\dfrac{4}{9} \times \dfrac{2}{5} = \dfrac{4 \times 2}{9 \times 5} = \dfrac{8}{45}$

The rule for dividing fractions is based on the reciprocal. If $a \neq 0$, then the **reciprocal** of a/b is simply b/a; that is, to form the reciprocal of a fraction, just flip it over. For example, the reciprocal of 3/4 is 4/3; the reciprocal of –2/5 is –5/2; the reciprocal of 3 is 1/3; and the reciprocal of –1/4 is –4. (The number 0 has no reciprocal.) As a result of this definition, we have the following basic fact: The product of any number and its reciprocal is 1.

Example 15-5: Find the reciprocal of each of these numbers:

   a)   2.25

   b) 5×10^{-4}

   c) 4×10^{5}

Solution:

   a)   2.25 is equal to 2 + (1/4), which is 9/4. The reciprocal of 9/4 is 4/9.

   b) $\dfrac{1}{5 \times 10^{-4}} = \dfrac{1}{5} \times \dfrac{1}{10^{-4}} = 0.2 \times 10^{4} = 2 \times 10^{3}$

   c) $\dfrac{1}{4 \times 10^{5}} = \dfrac{1}{4} \times \dfrac{1}{10^{5}} = 0.25 \times 10^{-5} = 2.5 \times 10^{-6}$

Now, in words, the rule for dividing fractions reads: *multiply by the reciprocal of the divisor.* That is, flip over whatever you're dividing by, and then multiply:

$$\frac{a}{b} \div \frac{c}{d} = \frac{a}{b} \times \frac{d}{c}$$

Example 15-6: What is 4/9 divided by 2/5?

Solution: $\dfrac{4}{9} \div \dfrac{2}{5} = \dfrac{4}{9} \times \dfrac{5}{2} = \dfrac{4 \times 5}{9 \times 2} = \dfrac{20}{18} = \dfrac{10}{9}$

Finally, we turn to addition and subtraction. In elementary and junior-high school, you were probably taught to find a common denominator (preferably, the *least* common denominator, known as the LCD), rewrite each fraction in terms of this common denominator, then add or subtract the numerators. If a common denominator is easy to spot, this may well be the fastest way to add or subtract fractions:

$$\frac{1}{2} + \frac{3}{4} = \frac{2}{4} + \frac{3}{4} = \frac{2+3}{4} = \frac{5}{4}$$

However, there is an efficient method for adding and subtracting fractions by making use of the following rules:

Here's what the arrows in the top line represent: "Multiply *up* (*d* times *a* gives *ad*), multiply *up* again (*b* times *c* gives *bc*), do the adding or subtracting of these products, and place the result over the product of the denominators (*bd*)." The length of this last sentence hides the simplicity of the rule, but it describes the recipe to follow. For example,

$$\frac{4}{9} + \frac{2}{5} = \frac{20+18}{45} = \frac{38}{45} \qquad\qquad \frac{4}{9} - \frac{2}{5} = \frac{20-18}{45} = \frac{2}{45}$$

Example 15-7:
a) Approximate the sum $\dfrac{1}{2.4 \times 10^5} + \dfrac{1}{6 \times 10^4}$

b) What is the reciprocal of this sum?

c) Simplify: $\dfrac{1}{2 \times 10^{-8}} - \dfrac{2}{5 \times 10^{-7}}$

Solution:

a) Using the rule illustrated above, we find that

$$\frac{1}{2.4 \times 10^5} + \frac{1}{6 \times 10^4} = \frac{(6 \times 10^4) + (2.4 \times 10^5)}{(2.4 \times 10^5)(6 \times 10^4)} = \frac{(6 \times 10^4) + (24 \times 10^4)}{(2.4 \times 10^5)(6 \times 10^4)} = \frac{(6 + 24) \times 10^4}{(2.4)(6) \times 10^{5+4}} \approx \frac{30 \times 10^4}{15 \times 10^9} = 2 \times 10^{-5}$$

b) The reciprocal of this result is $\frac{1}{2 \times 10^{-5}} = \frac{1}{2} \times \frac{1}{10^{-5}} = 0.5 \times 10^5 = 5 \times 10^4$.

c)

$$\frac{1}{2 \times 10^{-8}} - \frac{2}{5 \times 10^{-7}} = \frac{(5 \times 10^{-7}) - (2 \times 10^{-8})(2)}{(2 \times 10^{-8})(5 \times 10^{-7})} = \frac{(50 \times 10^{-8}) - (4 \times 10^{-8})}{(2)(5) \times 10^{-8 + (-7)}} = \frac{(50 - 4) \times 10^{-8}}{10 \times 10^{-15}} = 46 \times 10^6$$

$$= 4.6 \times 10^7$$

Let's now move on to ratios. A **ratio** is another way of saying *fraction*. For example, the ratio of 3 to 4, written 3:4, is equal to the fraction 3/4. Here's an illustration using isotopes of chlorine: The statement *the ratio of ^{35}Cl to ^{37}Cl is 3:1* means that there are 3/1 = 3 times as many ^{35}Cl atoms as there are ^{37}Cl atoms.

A particularly useful way to interpret a ratio is in terms of parts of a total. A ratio of a:b means that there are $a + b$ total parts, with a of them being of the first type and b of the second type. Therefore, *the ratio of ^{35}Cl to ^{37}Cl is 3:1* means that if we could take all ^{35}Cl and ^{37}Cl atoms, we could partition all them into 3 + 1 = 4 equal parts such that 3 of these parts will all be ^{35}Cl atoms, and the remaining 1 part will all be ^{37}Cl atoms. We can now restate the original ratio as a ratio of these parts to the total. Since ^{35}Cl atoms account for 3 parts out of the 4 total, the ratio of ^{35}Cl atoms to all Cl atoms is 3:4; that is, 3/4 of all Cl atoms are ^{35}Cl atoms. Similarly, the ratio of ^{37}Cl atoms to all Cl atoms is 1:4, which means that 1/4 of all Cl atoms are ^{37}Cl atoms.

Example 15-8: The formula for the compound TNT (trinitrotoluene) is $C_7H_5N_3O_6$.
a) What fraction of the atoms in this compound are nitrogen atoms?
b) If the molar masses of C, H, N, and O are 12 g, 1 g, 14 g, and 16 g, respectively, what is the ratio of the mass of all the nitrogens to the total mass?

Solution:

a) There are a total of 7 + 5 + 3 + 6 = 21 atoms per molecule. The ratio of N atoms to the total is 3:21, or, more simply, 1:7. Therefore, 1/7 of the atoms in this compound are nitrogen atoms.

b) The desired ratio of masses is calculated like this:

$$\frac{\text{mass of all N atoms}}{\text{total mass of molecule}} = \frac{3(14)}{7(12) + 5(1) + 3(14) + 6(16)} = \frac{42}{227} \approx \frac{40}{220} = \frac{2}{11}$$

Example 15-9: In a simple hydrocarbon (molecular formula C_xH_y), the ratio of C atoms to H atoms is 5:4, and the total number of atoms in the molecule is 18. Find x and y.

Solution: Since the ratio of C atoms to H atoms is 5:4, there are 5 parts C atoms and 4 parts H atoms, for a total of 9 equal parts. These 9 equal parts account for 18 total atoms, so each part must contain 2 atoms. Thus, C (which has 5 parts) has 5 × 2 = 10 atoms, and H (which has 4 parts) has 4 × 2 = 8 atoms. Therefore, x = 10 and y = 8.

Example 15-10: The ratio of O atoms to C atoms in each molecule of triethylene glycol is 2:3, and the ratio of O atoms to the total number of C atoms and H atoms is 1:5. If there are 24 atoms (C, H, and O only) per molecule, find the formula for this compound.

Solution: The ratio of O to C atoms is 2:3, which tells us there are 2 parts O atoms and 3 parts C atoms, for a total of 5 parts C and O. Since the ratio of O to (C *and* H) atoms is 1:5, there are 5 times as many C and H atoms as there are O atoms. But, we have found that there are 2 parts O atoms, so C and H must account for 5 times as many: 10 parts. And, because there are 3 parts C atoms, there must be 10 − 3 = 7 parts H atoms. We therefore have 2 + 3 + 7 = 12 parts total, accounting for 24 atoms, which means 2 atoms per part. So, there must be 2 × 2 = 4 O atoms, 3 × 2 = 6 C atoms, and 7 × 2 = 14 H atoms. The formula is $C_6H_{14}O_4$.

The word **percent**, symbolized by %, is simply an abbreviation for the phrase "out of 100". Therefore, a percentage is represented by a fraction whose denominator is 100. For example, 60% means 60/100, or 60 out of 100. The three main question types involving percents are as follows:

1. What is y% of z?
2. x is what percent of z?
3. x is y% of what?

Fortunately, all three question types fit into a single form and can all be answered by one equation. Translating the statement *x is y% of z* into an algebraic equation, we get

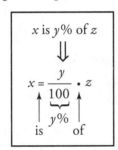

So, if you know any two of the three quantities x, y, and z, you can use the equation above to figure out the third.

Example 15-11:
a) What is 25% of 200?
b) 30 is what percent of 150?
c) 400 is 80% of what?

Solution:
a) Solving the equation $x = (25/100) \times 200$, we get $x = 25 \times 2 = 50$.
b) Solving the equation $30 = (y/100) \times 150$, we get $y = (30/150) \times 100 = (1/5) \times 100 = 20$.
c) Solving the equation $400 = (80/100) \times z$, we get $z = (100/80) \times 400 = 100 \times 5 = 500$.

It's also helpful to think of a simple fraction that equals a given percent, which can be used in place of $y/100$ in the equation above. For example, 25% = 1/4, 50% = 1/2, and 75% = 3/4. Other common fractional equivalents are: 20% = 1/5, 40% = 2/5, 60% = 3/5, and 80% = 4/5; 33.3% = 1/3 and 66.7% = 2/3; and 10n% = n/10 (for example, 10% = 1/10, 30% = 3/10, 70% = 7/10, and 90% = 9/10).

Example 15-12:
- a) What is 60% of 35?
- b) 12 is 75% of what?
- c) What is 70% of 400?

Solution:
- a) Since 60% = 3/5, we find that $x = (3/5) \times 35 = 3 \times 7 = 21$.
- b) Because 75% = 3/4, we solve the equation $12 = (3/4) \times z$, and find $z = 12 \times (4/3) = 16$.
- c) Since 70% = 7/10, we find that $x = (7/10) \times 400 = 7 \times 40 = 280$.

Example 15-13:
- a) What is the result when 50 is increased by 50%?
- b) What is the result when 80 is decreased by 40%?

Solution:
- a) "Increasing 50 by 50%" means adding (50% of 50) to 50. Since 50% of 50 is 25, increasing 50 by 50% gives us 50 + 25 = 75.
- b) "Decreasing 80 by 40%" means subtracting (40% of 80) from 80. Since 40% of 80 is 32, decreasing 80 by 40% gives us 80 – 32 = 48.

Example 15-14:
- a) What is 250% of 60?
- b) 2400 is what percent of 500?

Solution:
- a) Solving the equation $x = (250/100) \times 60$, we get $x = 25 \times 6 = 150$.
- b) Solving the equation $2400 = (y/100) \times 500$, we get $2400 = 5y$, so $y = 2400/5 = 480$.

Example 15-15: There are three stable isotopes of magnesium: ^{24}Mg, ^{25}Mg, and ^{26}Mg. The relative abundance of ^{24}Mg is 79%. Consider a sample of natural magnesium containing a total of 8×10^{24} atoms.
- a) About how many atoms in the sample are ^{24}Mg atoms?
- b) If the number of ^{25}Mg atoms in the sample is 8×10^{23}, what is the relative abundance (as a percentage) of ^{25}Mg?
- c) What's the relative abundance of ^{26}Mg?

Solution:
- a) Since the question is asking, *What is 79% of 8×10^{24}?*, we have

$$x = \frac{79}{100} \times (8 \times 10^{24}) \approx \frac{80}{100} \times (8 \times 10^{24}) = 6.4 \times 10^{24}$$

- b) The question is asking, *8×10^{23} is what percent of 8×10^{24}?*, so we write

$$8 \times 10^{23} = \frac{y}{100} \times (8 \times 10^{24}) \Rightarrow \frac{y}{100} = \frac{8 \times 10^{23}}{8 \times 10^{24}} = \frac{1}{10} \Rightarrow y = 10 \Rightarrow \text{ relative abundance } = 10\%$$

- c) Assuming that these three isotopes account for all naturally-occurring magnesium, the sum of the relative abundance percentages should be 100%. Therefore, we need only solve the equation 79% + 10% + Y% = 100%, from which we find that Y = 11.

Example 15-16: What is the percentage by mass of carbon in $C_7H_5N_3O_6$? (Given: Molar mass of compound = 227 g.)

A. 26%
B. 37%
C. 49%
D. 62%

Solution: Once the fraction of the total molar mass of the compound that's contributed by carbon is calculated, we obtain a percentage by multiplying this fraction by 100%. Since the molar mass of carbon is 12 g, and the molecule contains 7 C atoms, we have

$$\text{\%C, by mass} = \frac{7(12)}{227} = \frac{84}{227} \approx \frac{100}{250} = \frac{2}{5} = \frac{2}{5} \times 100\% = 40\%$$

Therefore, choice B is best.

15.4 EQUATIONS AND INEQUALITIES

You may have several questions on the MCAT that require you to solve—or manipulate—an algebraic equation or inequality. Fortunately, these equations and inequalities won't be very complicated.

When manipulating an algebraic equation, there's basically only one rule to remember: *Whatever you do to one side of the equation, you must do to the other side.* (Otherwise, it won't be a valid equation anymore.) For example, if you add 5 to the *left*-hand side, then add 5 to the *right*-hand side; if you multiply the *left*-hand side by 2, then multiply the *right*-hand side by 2, and so forth.

Inequalities are a little more involved. While it's still true that whatever you do to one side of an inequality you must also do the other side, there are a couple of additional rules, both of which involve flipping the inequality sign—that is, changing > to < (or vice versa) or changing ≥ to ≤ (or vice versa).

1. *If you multiply both sides of an inequality by a negative number, then you must flip the inequality sign.*
   For example, let's say you're given the inequality $-2x > 6$. To solve for x, you'd multiply both sides by $-1/2$. Since this is a negative number, the inequality sign must be flipped: $x < -3$.

2. *If both sides of an inequality are positive quantities, and you take the reciprocal of both sides, then you must flip the inequality sign.*
   For example, let's say you're given the inequality $2/x \leq 6$, where it's known that x must be positive. To solve for x, you can take the reciprocal of both sides. Upon doing so, the inequality sign must be flipped: $x/2 \geq 1/6$, so $x \geq 1/3$.

Example 15-17:

a) Solve for T: $PV = nRT$

b) Solve for t (given that t is positive): $y = (1/2)gt^2$

c) Solve for x (given that x is positive): $4x^2 = 2.4 \times 10^{-11}$

d) Solve for B: $h = k + \log(B/A)$

e) If $mg = GMm/r^2$ and r is positive, solve for r in terms of g, G, and M.

f) If $f = \pi r^2 v$, solve for r in terms of f and v.

g) If $\lambda f = c$ and $n\lambda = 2L$, solve for n in terms of L, f, and c.

h) If $1/f = (1/o) + (1/i)$, solve for i in terms of o and f.

i) Assume that $p = p_0 + 10\rho D$, where p_0 and ρ are constants. If $p = 300$ when $D = 10$ and $p = 400$ when $D = 15$, find the value of p when $D = 30$.

j) Solve for x: $3(2 - x) < 18$

k) Find all positive values of λ that satisfy $\dfrac{2 \times 10^{-25}}{\lambda} \geq 4 \times 10^{-19}$

Solution:

a) Dividing both sides by nR, we get $T = PV/(nR)$.

b) Multiply both sides $2/g$, then take the square root: $t = \sqrt{\dfrac{2y}{g}}$.

c) $4x^2 = 2.4 \times 10^{-11} \Rightarrow x^2 = 6 \times 10^{-12} \Rightarrow x = \sqrt{6} \times 10^{-6} \approx 2.5 \times 10^{-6}$

d) $h = k + \log\dfrac{B}{A} \Rightarrow \log\dfrac{B}{A} = h - k \Rightarrow 10^{h-k} = \dfrac{B}{A} \Rightarrow B = 10^{h-k} A$ [see Section 19]

e) $mg = G\dfrac{Mm}{r^2} \Rightarrow g = G\dfrac{M}{r^2} \Rightarrow r^2 = G\dfrac{M}{g} \Rightarrow r = \sqrt{G\dfrac{M}{g}}$

f) $f = \pi r^2 v \Rightarrow r^2 = \dfrac{f}{\pi v} \Rightarrow r = \sqrt{\dfrac{f}{\pi v}}$

g) Since $\lambda = c/f$, we get $n\dfrac{c}{f} = 2L \Rightarrow n = \dfrac{2Lf}{c}$.

h) $\dfrac{1}{f} = \dfrac{1}{o} + \dfrac{1}{i} \Rightarrow \dfrac{1}{i} = \dfrac{1}{f} - \dfrac{1}{o} = \dfrac{o-f}{fo} \Rightarrow i = \dfrac{fo}{o-f}$

i) Let's plug in the given information: $300 = p_0 + 100\rho$ and $400 = p_0 + 150\rho$. If we subtract the first equation from the second one, the p_0's cancel and we get $100 = 50\rho$, so $\rho = 2$. Plugging $\rho = 2$ back into either one of the equations, we find that $p_0 = 100$. Therefore, $p = 100 + 20D$. So, when $D = 30$, we get $p = 100 + (20)(30) = 700$.

j) $3(2 - x) < 18 \Rightarrow 2 - x < 6 \Rightarrow -x < 4 \Rightarrow x > -4$

k) $\dfrac{2 \times 10^{-25}}{\lambda} \geq 4 \times 10^{-19} \Rightarrow \dfrac{\lambda}{2 \times 10^{-25}} \leq \dfrac{1}{4 \times 10^{-19}} \Rightarrow \lambda \leq \dfrac{2 \times 10^{-25}}{4 \times 10^{-19}} = 0.5 \times 10^{-6} \Rightarrow \lambda \leq 5 \times 10^{-7}$

15.5   THE X-Y PLANE, LINES, AND OTHER GRAPHS

The figure below shows the familiar *x-y* **plane**, which we use to plot data and draw lines and curves showing how one quantity is related to another one:

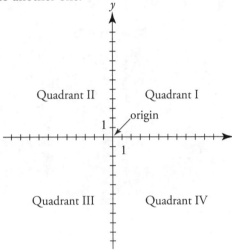

The *x-y* plane is formed by intersecting two number lines perpendicularly at the origins. The horizontal axis is generically referred to as the *x*-**axis** (although the quantity measured along this axis might be named by some other letter, such as time, *t*), and the vertical axis is generically known as the *y*-**axis**. The axes split the plane into four **quadrants**, which are numbered consecutively in a counterclockwise fashion. Quadrant I is in the upper right and represents all points (x, y) where x and y are both positive; in Quadrant II, x is negative and y is positive; in Quadrant III, x and y are both negative; and in Quadrant IV, x is positive and y is negative.

Suppose that two quantities, x and y, were related by the equation $y = 2x^2$. We would consider x as the **independent variable**, and y as the **dependent variable**, since for each value of x we get a unique value of y (that is, y *depends* uniquely on x). The independent variable is plotted along the horizontal axis, while the dependent variable is plotted along the vertical axis. Constructing a graph of an equation usually consists of plotting specific points (x, y) that satisfy the equation—in this case, examples include $(0, 0)$, $(1, 2)$, $(2, 8)$, $(-1, 2)$, $(-2, 8)$, etc.—and then connecting these points with a line or other smooth curve. The first coordinate of each point—the x coordinate—is known as the **abscissa**, and the second coordinate of each point—the y coordinate—is known as the **ordinate**.

15.5

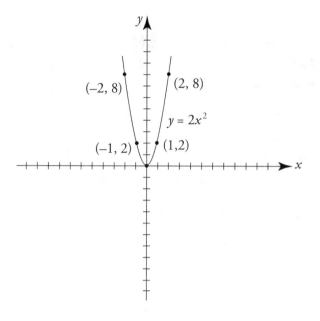

Lines

One of the simplest and most important graphs is the (straight) **line**. A line is determined by its slope—its steepness—and one specific point on the line, such as its intersection with either the x- or y-axis. The **slope** of a line is defined to be a change in y divided by the corresponding change in x ("rise over run"). Lines with positive slope rise to the right; those with negative slope fall to the right. And the greater the magnitude (absolute value) of the slope, the steeper the line.

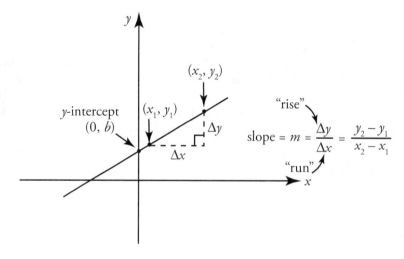

Perhaps the simplest way to write the equation of a line is in terms of its slope and the y-coordinate of the point where it crosses the y-axis. If the slope is m and the y-intercept is b, the equation of the line can be written in the form

$$y = mx + b$$

The only time this form doesn't work is when the line is vertical, since vertical lines have an undefined slope and such a line either never crosses the y-axis (no b) or else coincides with the y-axis. The equation of every vertical line is simply $x = a$, where a is the x-intercept.

Example 15-18:
   a)   Where does the line $y = 3x - 4$ cross the y-axis? the x-axis? What is its slope?
   b)   Find the equation of the line that has slope -2 and crosses the y-axis at the point $(0, 3)$.
   c)   Find the equation of the line that has slope 4 and crosses the y-axis at the origin.
   d)   A *linear* function is a function whose graph is a line. Let's say it's known that some quantity p is a linear function of x. If $p = 50$ when $x = 0$ and $p = 250$ when $x = 20$, find an equation for p in terms of x. Then use the equation to find the value of p when $x = 40$.

Solution:
   a)   The equation $y = 3x - 4$ matches the form $y = mx + b$ with $m = 3$ and $b = -4$. Therefore, this line has slope 3 and crosses the y-axis at the point $(0, -4)$. To find the x-intercept, we set y equal to 0 and solve for x: $0 = 3x - 4$ implies that $x = 4/3$. Therefore, this line crosses the x-axis at the point $(4/3, 0)$.
   b)   We're given $m = -2$ and $b = 3$, so the equation of the line is $y = -2x + 3$.
   c)   We're given $m = 4$ and $b = 0$, so the equation of the line is $y = 4x$.
   d)   Since p is a linear function of x, it must have the form $p = mx + b$ for some values of m and b. Because $p = 50$ when $x = 0$, we know that $b = 50$, so $p = mx + 50$. Now, since $p = 250$ when $x = 20$, we have $250 = 20m + 50$, so $m = 10$. Thus, $p = 10x + 50$. Finally, plugging in $x = 40$ into this formula, we find that the value of p when $x = 40$ is $(10)(40) + 50 = 450$.

Example 15-19: An insulated 50 cm^3 sample of water has an initial temperature of $T_i = 10°C$. If Q calories of heat are added to the sample, the temperature of the water will rise to T, where $T = kQ + T_i$. When the graph of T vs. Q is sketched (with Q measured along the horizontal axis), it's found that the point $(Q, T) = (200, 14)$ lies on the graph.
   a)   What is the value of k?
   b)   How much heat is required to bring the water to 20°C?
   c)   If $Q = 2200$ cal, what will be the value of T?

Solution:
   a)   The equation $T = kQ + T_i$ matches the form $y = mx + b$, so k is the slope of the line. To find the slope, we evaluate the *rise-over-run* expression—which in this case is $\Delta T/\Delta Q$—for two points on the line. Using $(Q_1, T_1) = (0, 10)$ and $(Q_2, T_2) = (200, 14)$, we find that

$$k = \text{slope} = \frac{\Delta T}{\Delta Q} = \frac{T_2 - T_1}{Q_2 - Q_1} = \frac{14 - 10}{200 - 0} = \frac{1}{50}$$

   b)   We set T equal to 20 and solve for Q:

$$T = kQ + T_i \Rightarrow T = \frac{1}{50}Q + 10 \Rightarrow 20 = \frac{1}{50}Q + 10 \Rightarrow Q = 500 \text{ (cal)}$$

   c)   Here we set $Q = 2200$ and evaluate T:

$$T = kQ + T_i \Rightarrow T = \frac{1}{50}Q + 10 \Rightarrow T = \frac{1}{50}(2200) + 10 = 44 + 10 = 54 \text{ (°C)}$$

(Technical note: The equation for the temperature of the water, $T = kQ + T_i$, is valid as long as no phase change occurs.)

Besides lines, there are a few other graphs and features you should be familiar with.

The equation $y = kx^2$, where $k \neq 0$, describes the basic **parabola**, one whose turning point (**vertex**) is at the origin. It has a U shape, and opens upward if k is positive and downward if k is negative. The graph of the related equation $y = k(x - a)^2$ is obtained from the basic parabola by shifting it horizontally so that its vertex is at the point $(a, 0)$. The graph of the equation $y = kx^2 + b$ is obtained from the basic parabola by shifting it vertically so that its vertex is at the point $(0, b)$. Finally, the graph of the equation $y = k(x - a)^2 + b$ is obtained from the basic parabola in two shifting steps: First, shift the basic parabola horizontally so that its vertex is at the point $(a, 0)$; next, shift this parabola vertically so that the vertex is at the point (a, b). These parabolas are illustrated below for positive a, b, k, and x:

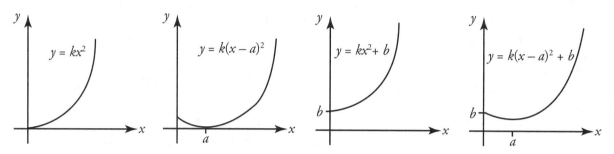

The equation $y = k/x$, where $k \neq 0$, describes a **hyperbola**. It is the graph of an inverse proportion (see Section 18.2). For small values of x, the values of y are large; and for large values of x, the values of y are small. Notice that the graph of a hyperbola approaches—but never touches—both the x- and y-axes. These lines are therefore called **asymptotes**.

The equation $y = k/x^2$, where $k \neq 0$, has a graph whose shape is similar to a hyperbola but it approaches its horizontal asymptote faster and vertical asymptote slower than a hyperbola does (because of the square in the denominator).

The graph of the equation $y = Ae^{-kx}$ (where k is positive) is an **exponential decay curve**. It intersects the y-axis at the point $(0, A)$, and, as x increases, the value of y decreases. Here, the x-axis is an asymptote.

The graph of the equation $y = A(1 - e^{-kx})$, where k is positive, contains the origin, and as x increases, the graph rises to approach the horizontal line $y = A$. This line is an asymptote.

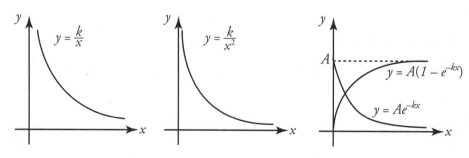

Chapter 16
Trigonometry

16.1 INTRODUCTION

Let me begin by saying that you will *not* need to know the countless identities that pervade this subject, equations you may have studied in high school like $\sin^2 \theta = (1 - \cos 2\theta)/2$. The MCAT requires only that you know the important basics. The term **trigonometry** literally means *triangle measurement*, and this is where the basics start.

Consider a *right* triangle; that is, a triangle with a 90° (right) angle. Let's call the triangle ABC and let C be the vertex of the right angle. Then sides AC and BC are called the **legs**, and side AB is called the **hypotenuse**. If the lengths of sides BC, AC, and AB are a, b, and c, respectively, then the *Pythagorean theorem* tells us that $a^2 + b^2$ must be equal to c^2.

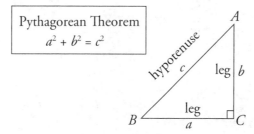

Pythagorean Theorem
$$a^2 + b^2 = c^2$$

Three positive numbers a, b, and c that satisfy the Pythagorean theorem and can therefore be the lengths of the sides of a right triangle, are known as a **Pythagorean triple**. The most familiar of these is the triple 3, 4, 5. (It's easy to check that $3^2 + 4^2 = 5^2$.) The legs have lengths 3 and 4, and the hypotenuse (which is always the longest side of any right triangle) has length 5. Other examples of Pythagorean triples are 5, 12, 13 and 7, 24, 25, but the list is endless. An important and useful fact about Pythagorean triples is this: Any multiple of a Pythagorean triple is another Pythagorean triple. For example, since 3, 4, 5 is such a triple, so are 6, 8, 10 (obtained from 3, 4, 5 by multiplying the lengths by 2) and 9, 12, 15 (by multiplying by 3) and 1.5, 2, 2.5 (by multiplying by one-half).

Example 16-1:

a) Is 5, 6, 8 a Pythagorean triple?

b) If a, 16, 20 is a Pythagorean triple and $a < 20$, what is a?

Solution:

a) Since $5^2 + 6^2 = 25 + 36 = 61$ but $8^2 = 64$, the sum $5^2 + 6^2$ does *not* equal 8^2. Therefore, 5, 6, 8 is not a Pythagorean triple. No right triangle could have sides whose lengths are 5, 6, and 8.

b) Because $a < 20$, we know that a is not the length of the longest side of the triangle, so it's not the hypotenuse. The hypotenuse must be 20. Therefore, we want to solve the equation $a^2 + 16^2 = 20^2$. Since $16^2 = 256$ and $20^2 = 400$, we find that $a^2 = 400 - 256 = 144$, so $a = 12$. Notice that the Pythagorean triple 12, 16, 20 is just four times the triple 3, 4, 5.

We can also use a right triangle to make a crucial observation. Consider a magnified version of right triangle ABC. Each angle of the larger triangle (let's call it DBE) is equal to the corresponding angle in the smaller one. These triangles are said to be **similar**, and each side of the larger triangle is the *same* multiple of the corresponding side in the smaller triangle. For example, if leg BE is twice the length of leg BC, then leg DE is twice the length of leg AC, and hypotenuse DB is twice the length of hypotenuse AB. One of the consequences of this is that certain ratios of the lengths of the sides of the triangle are the same, regardless of the size of the triangle. For example, let's say that each side of triangle DBE is k times the corresponding side of triangle ABC, so BE = $k \cdot$ BC, DE = $k \cdot$ AC, and DB = $k \cdot$ AB. Now consider, for example, AC/AB, the ratio of leg AC to the hypotenuse AB. It will be equal to the ratio DE/DB, because

$$\frac{DE}{DB} = \frac{k \cdot AC}{k \cdot AB} = \frac{AC}{AB}$$

Similarly, we'll have

$$\frac{BE}{DB} = \frac{BC}{AB} \quad \text{and} \quad \frac{DE}{BE} = \frac{AC}{BC}$$

These three ratios are therefore uniquely determined by the *angles* of the triangle, regardless of the size of the triangle, and they're given special names: **sine**, **cosine**, and **tangent** (respectively).

Triangle DBE is a magnified version of triangle ABC, which means:

$$\frac{DE}{AC} = \frac{BE}{BC} = \frac{DB}{AB}$$

Therefore,

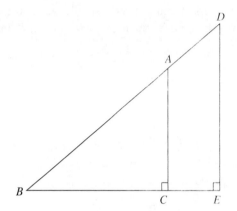

$$\frac{AC}{AB} = \frac{DE}{DB} \qquad \leftarrow \text{this ratio is the sine of angle B}$$

$$\frac{BC}{AB} = \frac{BE}{DB} \qquad \leftarrow \text{this ratio is the cosine of angle B}$$

$$\frac{AC}{BC} = \frac{DE}{BE} \qquad \leftarrow \text{this ratio is the tangent of angle B}$$

So, for an arbitrary acute angle θ in a right triangle, we have the following definitions:

sine of θ: $\qquad \sin\theta = \dfrac{\text{opp}}{\text{hyp}} = \dfrac{b}{c}$

cosine of θ: $\qquad \cos\theta = \dfrac{\text{adj}}{\text{hyp}} = \dfrac{a}{c}$

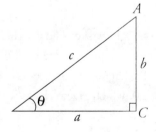

tangent of θ: $\qquad \tan\theta = \dfrac{\text{opp}}{\text{adj}} = \dfrac{b}{a}$

The abbreviation *opp* stands for *opposite*, *adj* stands for *adjacent*, and *hyp* stands for *hypotenuse*. So, for example, the sine of an acute angle in a right triangle, opp/hyp, is equal to the length of the side opposite the angle divided by the length of the hypotenuse. Some people remember the definitions of the sine, co-sine, and tangent of an acute angle in a right triangle by this mnemonic:

SOH CAH TOA

where the letters stand for the following: <u>S</u>ine = <u>O</u>pp/<u>H</u>yp, <u>C</u>osine = <u>A</u>dj/<u>H</u>yp, <u>T</u>angent = <u>O</u>pp/<u>A</u>dj.

Example 16-2: In a 3-4-5 right triangle ABC, let A be the smaller acute angle and let B be the larger acute angle.
   a)   What are $\sin A$, $\cos A$, and $\tan A$?
   b)   What are $\sin B$, $\cos B$, and $\tan B$?

Solution: Because A is the smaller acute angle, the side opposite A is the shorter leg (of length 3); therefore, the side opposite the larger acute angle, B, has length 4.

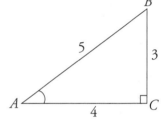

   a)   By definition, $\sin A = 3/5$, $\cos A = 4/5$, and $\tan A = 3/4$
   b)   By definition, $\sin B = 4/5$, $\cos B = 3/5$, and $\tan B = 4/3$

Example 16-3: In right triangle ABC, the right angle is at C. If $\sin A = 1/3$ and $AB = 6$, what are the lengths of the legs of the triangle?

Solution: The triangle is sketched to the right. By defini-tion, $\sin A = BC/AB$; from this equation, we immediately get $BC = AB \cdot \sin A = 6 \cdot (1/3) = 2$. Now, by the Pythagorean the-orem, $AC^2 + BC^2 = AB^2$, so $AC^2 = 6^2 - 2^2 = 32$, which gives $AC = \sqrt{32} = 4\sqrt{2}$.

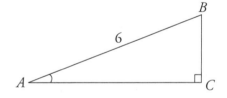

Example 16-4: In right triangle DEF, the right angle is at F. If $\tan E = 2$ and $EF = 2$, what's the length of the hypotenuse?

Solution: The triangle is sketched to the right. By definition, $\tan E = DF/EF$; from this equation, we get $DF = EF \cdot \tan E = 2 \cdot 2 = 4$. Now, by the Pythagorean theorem, $DF^2 + EF^2 = DE^2$, so $DE^2 = 4^2 + 2^2 = 20$, which gives $DE = \sqrt{20} = 2\sqrt{5}$.

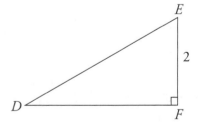

How would you find the sine of an angle whose measure is, say, 20°? Here's a way that only requires the definitions we've gone over so far, plus a protractor and a ruler:

Step 1: Draw a horizontal line segment, AC.
Step 2: Place a protractor so that its center is at the left endpoint (A) of the line segment drawn in Step 1.
Step 3: Draw a line from A through the 20° mark on the protractor.
Step 4: Draw a line segment up from C that's perpendicular to AC. Let B be the point where it intersects the line drawn in Step 3.
Step 5: Use a ruler to measure the lengths of BC and AB.
Step 6: sin 20° = sin A = BC/AB

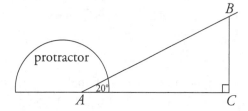

If you try this with a horizontal line segment AC whose length is 3 inches, you'll find that BC ≈ 1 1/16″ and AB ≈ 3 3/16″ , so

$$\sin A = \sin 20° \approx \frac{1\frac{1}{16}}{3\frac{3}{16}} = \frac{1}{3}$$

But what if you don't have a protractor and ruler? Then without some fancy (and time-consuming) math, it's going to be pretty tough. But the MCAT won't require you to know the sine of 20°. The MCAT will expect that you'll know the values of the sine, cosine, and tangent of angles that are multiples of 30° and 45° only.

If we take a square of side length 1 and cut it in half down a diagonal, we end up with a pair of isosceles right triangles.

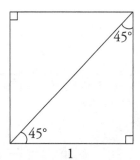 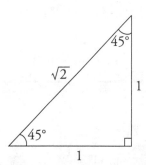

In each triangle, both acute angles are 45°. By the Pythagorean theorem, the hypotenuse has length

$$\sqrt{1^2 + 1^2} = \sqrt{2}$$

It's now easy to apply the definitions to find that

> **Memorize**
>
> $$\sin 45° = \frac{1}{\sqrt{2}} = \frac{\sqrt{2}}{2} \qquad \cos 45° = \frac{1}{\sqrt{2}} = \frac{\sqrt{2}}{2} \qquad \tan 45° = \frac{1}{1} = 1$$

If we take an equilateral triangle of side length 2 and cut it from a corner into two equal pieces, we end up with a pair of 30°-60° right triangles.

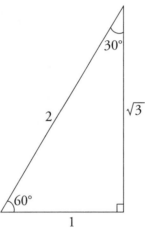

The shorter leg in each right triangle has length 1 (half the length of the hypotenuse), so by the Pythagorean theorem, the length of the longer leg is

$$\sqrt{2^2 - 1^2} = \sqrt{3}$$

It's now easy to apply the definitions to find that

> **Memorize**
>
> $$\sin 30° = \frac{1}{2} \qquad\qquad \sin 60° = \frac{\sqrt{3}}{2}$$
>
> $$\cos 30° = \frac{\sqrt{3}}{2} \qquad\qquad \cos 60° = \frac{1}{2}$$
>
> $$\tan 30° = \frac{1}{\sqrt{3}} = \frac{\sqrt{3}}{3} \qquad\qquad \tan 60° = \frac{\sqrt{3}}{1} = \sqrt{3}$$

Example 16-5: In right triangle *ABC*, the right angle is at *C* and angle *A* = 60°. If BC = 2, what are AB and AC?

Solution: The triangle is sketched to the right. By definition, sin *A* = BC/AB; from this equation, we immediately get

$$AB = \frac{BC}{\sin A} = \frac{2}{\sin 60°} = \frac{2}{\frac{1}{2}\sqrt{3}} = \frac{4\sqrt{3}}{3}$$

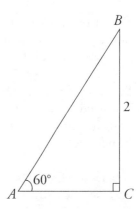

To find the other leg, AC, we now have several options. Here's one: Since cos *A* = AC/AB, we get

$$AC = AB \cdot \cos A = \frac{4\sqrt{3}}{3} \cdot \cos 60° = \frac{4\sqrt{3}}{3} \cdot \frac{1}{2} = \frac{2\sqrt{3}}{3}$$

16.2   EXTENDING THE DEFINITIONS

In the preceding section, we gave the definitions of the trig functions sine, cosine, and tangent only for an *acute* angle (that is, an angle whose measure is between 0° and 90°) in a right triangle. However, for many important uses of trig, we won't want such a restriction. The purpose of this section is to extend the definitions of these trig functions to an angle of *any* measure.

Consider the usual *x-y* coordinate system and imagine a ray starting at the origin and lying along the positive *x*-axis. We can generate an angle, *θ*, of any size we want by rotating this ray about the origin. If we rotate it counterclockwise, we'll call the generated angle positive; if we rotate clockwise, we'll call it negative. To figure out the values of the trig functions of this angle, we choose any point P (other than the origin) on the terminal side of the angle—that is, on the final position of the rotated ray—and then drop a perpendicular from P to the *x*-axis. Let (*x, y*) denote the coordinates of the point P, and let *r* be the distance from the origin to P. The trig functions of *θ* are then defined in terms of *x, y,* and *r* as follows:

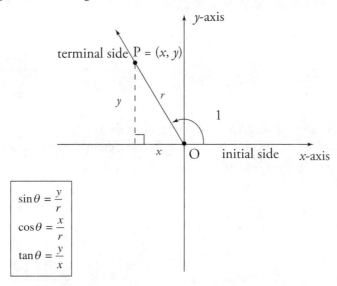

Notice that if θ is a positive, acute angle, then these definitions in terms of x, y, and r give the same values as those involving the lengths designated adjacent, opposite, and hypotenuse in a right triangle. The advantage of the definitions above is that they apply to *any* angle, not just to acute angles in right triangles.

The terminal side of the angle θ pictured above lies in Quadrant II, so we say the angle itself is in Quadrant II. So, for the point P, the x coordinate is negative and the y coordinate is positive. (The value of r is *always* positive.) Therefore, the value of $\sin \theta$ is positive, but the values of $\cos \theta$ and $\tan \theta$ are negative.

Similarly, if θ lies in Quadrant III, then both x and y will be negative, so $\tan \theta$ will be positive, but both $\sin \theta$ and $\cos \theta$ will be negative. If θ lies in Quadrant IV, then x is positive and y is negative, so $\cos \theta$ is positive, but $\sin \theta$ and $\tan \theta$ will be negative. If θ lies in Quadrant I, then $\sin \theta$, $\cos \theta$, and $\tan \theta$ will all be positive.

If θ lies on either the x- or y-axis, then either y or x will be zero. For example, if $\theta = 90°$, then θ lies on the positive y axis, so $x = 0$. In this case, we can see right away that $\cos \theta = \cos 90° = x/r = 0/r = 0$, $\sin 90° = y/r = y/y = 1$, and $\tan 90°$ is undefined (because we can't divide by 0). Any angle—like 90°, 180°, etc.—whose terminal side lies along either the x- or the y-axis is called a **quadrantal** angle.

Example 16-6: Find $\sin \theta$, $\cos \theta$, and $\tan \theta$ for each of the following angles:
  a) $\theta = 120°$
  b) $\theta = 180°$
  c) $\theta = 225°$
  d) $\theta = 330°$

Solution:
  a) The figure below shows an angle of 120°. Since the right triangle that's formed by dropping a perpendicular to the x-axis is a 30°-60° right triangle, we know that we can take $x = -1$, $y = \sqrt{3}$, and $r = 2$. Therefore,

$$\sin 120° = \frac{y}{r} = \frac{\sqrt{3}}{2}; \quad \cos 120° = \frac{x}{r} = \frac{-1}{2} = -\frac{1}{2};$$

$$\tan 120° = \frac{y}{x} = \frac{\sqrt{3}}{-1} = -\sqrt{3}$$

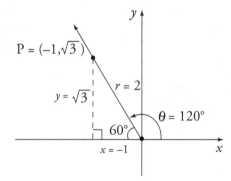

  b) The figure below shows an angle of 180°. Here, no triangle is formed, but that doesn't matter. We simply choose a point P on the terminal side of the angle, say, P = (−1, 0). Since $x = -1$, $y = 0$, and $r = 1$, we have

$$\sin 180° = \frac{y}{r} = \frac{0}{1} = 0; \quad \cos 180° = \frac{x}{r} = \frac{-1}{1} = -1;$$

$$\tan 180° = \frac{y}{x} = \frac{0}{-1} = 0$$

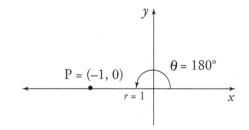

c) The figure at the right shows an angle of 225°. Since the right triangle that's formed by dropping a perpendicular to the *x*-axis is a 45°-45° right triangle, we know that we can take $x = -1$, $y = -1$, and $r = \sqrt{2}$. Therefore,

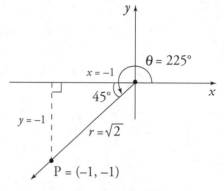

$$\sin 225° = \frac{y}{r} = \frac{-1}{\sqrt{2}} = -\frac{\sqrt{2}}{2}; \quad \cos 225° = \frac{x}{r} = \frac{-1}{\sqrt{2}} = -\frac{\sqrt{2}}{2};$$

$$\tan 225° = \frac{y}{x} = \frac{-1}{-1} = 1$$

d) The figure at the right shows an angle of 330°. Since the right triangle that's formed by dropping a perpendicular to the *x*-axis is a 30°-60° right triangle, we know that we can take $x = \sqrt{3}$, $y = -1$, and $r = 2$. Therefore,

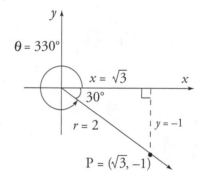

$$\sin 330° = \frac{y}{r} = \frac{-1}{2} = -\frac{1}{2}; \quad \cos 330° = \frac{x}{r} = \frac{\sqrt{3}}{2};$$

$$\tan 330° = \frac{y}{x} = \frac{-1}{\sqrt{3}} = -\frac{\sqrt{3}}{3}$$

Example 16-7: Find sin θ, cos θ, and tan θ for each of the following angles:

a) $\theta = 270°$
b) $\theta = 420°$
c) $\theta = -150°$

Solution:

a) The figure below shows an angle of 270°. Here, no triangle is formed, but that doesn't matter. We simply choose a point P on the terminal side of the angle, say, P = (0, –1). Since $x = 0$, $y = -1$, and $r = 1$, we have

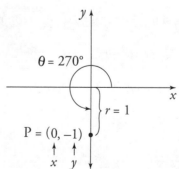

$$\sin 270° = \frac{y}{r} = \frac{-1}{1} = -1; \quad \cos 270° = \frac{x}{r} = \frac{0}{1} = 0;$$

$$\tan 270° = \frac{y}{x} = \frac{-1}{0} \text{ is undefined}$$

b) The figure at the right shows an angle of 420°. Notice that the angle is formed by making one complete revolution (360°) plus an additional 60°. Since the right triangle that's formed by dropping a perpendicular to the x-axis is a 30°-60° right triangle, we know that we can take $x = 1$, $y = \sqrt{3}$, and $r = 2$. Therefore,

$$\sin 420° = \frac{y}{r} = \frac{\sqrt{3}}{2}; \quad \cos 420° = \frac{x}{r} = \frac{1}{2};$$

$$\tan 420° = \frac{y}{x} = \frac{\sqrt{3}}{1} = \sqrt{3}$$

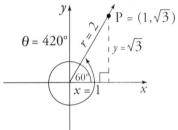

c) The figure at the right shows an angle of –150°. Because the angle is *negative*, we must perform a *clockwise* rotation (rather than a counterclockwise one) to generate it. Since the right triangle that's formed by dropping a perpendicular to the x-axis is a 30°-60° right triangle, we know that we can take $x = -\sqrt{3}$, $y = 1$, and $r = 2$. Therefore,

$$\sin (-150°) = \frac{y}{r} = \frac{-1}{2} = -\frac{1}{2}; \quad \cos (150°) = \frac{x}{r} = \frac{-\sqrt{3}}{2} = -\frac{\sqrt{3}}{2};$$

$$\tan (150°) = \frac{y}{x} = \frac{-1}{-\sqrt{3}} = \frac{\sqrt{3}}{3}$$

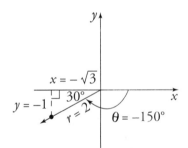

Example 16-8: If $\sin \theta = -\sqrt{3}/2$ and $\cos \theta = 1/2$, what is the value of $\tan \theta$?

Solution: One way to answer this question is to try to find θ. Since $\sin \theta$ is negative and $\cos \theta$ is positive, the terminal side of θ must lie in Quadrant IV. A quick sketch will show that $\theta = 300°$, where we take the point P = $(1, -\sqrt{3})$ on the terminal side. Therefore, $\tan \theta = \tan 300° = y/x = -\sqrt{3}$). Another solution is to notice the simple and important identity $\tan \theta = (\sin \theta)/(\cos \theta)$ [which is true because $y/x = \frac{y}{r} / \frac{x}{r}$], so

$$\tan \theta = -\frac{\sqrt{3}}{2} / \frac{1}{2} = -\sqrt{3} \, .$$

16.3 INVERSE TRIGONOMETRY FUNCTIONS

Given an angle θ, we can use the methods of the preceding sections to find, say, its sine, and we get some number. For example, the sine of 30° is 1/2. Now let's turn the question around: Given a number, can we find an angle whose sine is that number? For example, if we were asked to find an angle whose sine is 1/2, we could say 30°. This is the essence of the inverse trig functions; given a number, can we find an angle whose sine (or cosine or tangent) is that number? Here's another example: Give an angle whose tangent is 1. One correct answer would be 45°.

To specify an angle whose sine is a given number, we use the following symbol: $\sin^{-1}$, which is read *inverse sine*. (Be careful: The –1 is *not* an exponent here; it's merely the mathematical abbreviation for an inverse function.) The expression $\sin^{-1} z$ stands for an angle whose sine is the number z. So, for example, since $\sin 30° = 1/2$, we could write $\sin^{-1}(1/2) = 30°$. Similarly, the inverse cosine is written $\cos^{-1}$, and the inverse tangent is written $\tan^{-1}$. Based on the last example in the preceding paragraph, we could write $\tan^{-1} 1 = 45°$.

If you've memorized the boxed equations above, and if you remember the quadrants in which sine, cosine, or tangent can be negative

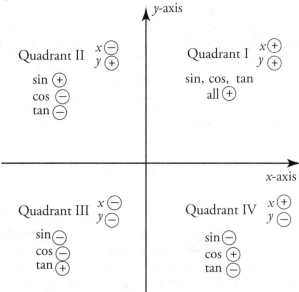

then you'll have the tools you'll need to simplify expressions involving inverse trig functions on the MCAT.

One important point to remember: For a given number z, there are usually infinitely many angles whose sine is z. For example, can you think of an angle besides 30° whose sine is 1/2? The angle 150° would work; its sine is also 1/2. And what about 390° (which is just 360° plus 30°)? And since 30° is a possible angle, so is –330°. And since 150° is a possible angle, so is –210°. In fact, any angle, positive or negative, whose terminal side is the same as that of 30° or 150° has a sine of 1/2, so any of these angles would be possible values for the expression $\sin^{-1}(1/2)$. To know which value to choose, the question will have to restrict the possible answers in some way, either directly in the question or by looking at the available answer choices. Usually, though, you want the smallest positive or negative angle.

Example 16-9:

16.3

a) Give at least three possible values for $\sin^{-1}(\sqrt{3}/2)$.

b) What is the smallest negative angle that equals $\sin^{-1}(-\sqrt{3}/2)$?

c) Find the two smallest positive values of $\cos^{-1}(1/2)$.

d) Find the smallest positive angle and the smallest negative angle each of which equals $\tan^{-1}(-\sqrt{3}/3)$.

e) Find the smallest positive value of $\cos^{-1}0$.

f) Find the smallest negative value of $\tan^{-1}(-1)$.

g) What's the positive value of $\cos[\sin^{-1}(1/2)]$?

h) What's wrong with this expression: $\sin^{-1}2$?

Solution:

a) We're asked for angles whose sine is $\sqrt{3}/2$. One we know right away: 60°. Another one is 120° (look back at Examples 16-6a). Any other angle whose terminal side is the same as that of 60° or 120° will also work. Examples of angles whose terminal side matches that of 60° include 420° (look back at Example 16-7b), 780°, 1140°, etc., as well as –300°, –660°, –1020°, etc. Examples of angles whose terminal side matches that of 120° include 480°, 840°, 1200°, etc., as well as –240°, –600°, –960°, etc.

b) We want the smallest negative angle whose sine is $-\sqrt{3}/2$. The answer is –60°.

c) We're being asked to find positive angles whose cosine is 1/2. One we know right away: 60°. Another one is 300°, a Quadrant IV angle. These are the two smallest positive values of $\cos^{-1}(1/2)$.

d) First, let's find the smallest positive angle whose tangent is $-\sqrt{3}/3$. Tangent is negative in Quadrants II and IV only, so the smallest positive angle whose tangent is $-\sqrt{3}/3$ will be a Quadrant II angle. The answer is 150°. The smallest negative angle is –30°. You can check both of these answers by sketching the angles, just as we did in Examples 16-6 and 16-7.

e) Since $\cos\theta = x/r$, we know that $\cos\theta$ will be equal to 0 when $x = 0$. The smallest positive value of θ for which a point P on its terminal side has $x = 0$ is $\theta = 90°$.

f) The smallest negative angle whose tangent is –1 is $\theta = -45°$.

g) Let $\theta = \sin^{-1}(1/2)$. Then we know we can take $\theta = 30°$. The question is asking for $\cos\theta$, so we have $\cos 30° = \sqrt{3}/2$. (If we had taken $\theta = 150°$, we would have gotten a negative value for $\cos\theta$, but the question specifically asked for the *positive* value of $\cos\theta$.)

h) The expression $\sin^{-1}2$ is undefined; that is, there is *no* angle whose sine is 2. In fact, the sine of any angle must be between –1 and +1 (inclusive). The reason is simple: By definition, $\sin\theta = y/r$, and y can never be greater in magnitude than r. So, the ratio y/r can never be greater than 1 or less than –1. The same is true for the cosine of an angle; it, too, must always be between –1 and +1 (inclusive). Therefore, the expressions $\sin^{-1}z$ and $\cos^{-1}z$ are meaningless if $z < -1$ or if $z > 1$. (However, the expression $\tan^{-1}z$ is defined for *any* value of z, positive, negative, or zero, no matter how big or small.)

16.4 RADIAN MEASURE

So far we've been measuring angles in degrees. By definition, a complete rotation (revolution) is equal to 360°, or, equivalently, a right angle has a measure of 90°. But why should a complete rotation be equal to 360 units? Why not, say, 100?

Actually, the ancient Babylonians started this system (called the sexagesimal system) basing angle measurement on the number 60. A degree can be split into 60 equal parts, each called a *minute*, and each minute can be further divided into 60 equal parts called *seconds*. (For example, an angle whose measure is 20° 30′ is 20.5° [the prime denotes minutes]; an angle whose measure is 20° 30′ 15″ is equal to 20° 30 1/4′ [the double prime denotes seconds].) One theory is that a complete revolution was called 360° because a year (one revolution around the Sun, although the Babylonians didn't know about the earth orbiting the sun) is approximately 360 days. So, each day of the year corresponded to 1 degree. Whatever the reason, it's clear that 360 was an arbitrary choice with no real mathematical basis. But what of an ancient civilization on another planet, whose year has 500 days? They might have started measuring angles in some other unit, *reegeds*, where a complete revolution is equal to 500 reegeds (500^{∂}), and a right angle would have a measure of 125^{∂}. If we were to communicate with this civilization, our angle measurements would be incompatible. What we'd want is a truly universal unit for measuring angles, one which is natural in the sense that an intelligent civilization on another planet will devise the same system (without regard to, say, how many days their year is). This universal unit for measuring angles is called the **radian**.

Draw a circle and construct an angle whose vertex is at the center such that when the sides of the angle hit the circle, the length of the subtended arc is equal to the radius of the circle. The measure of such an angle is, by definition, one radian.

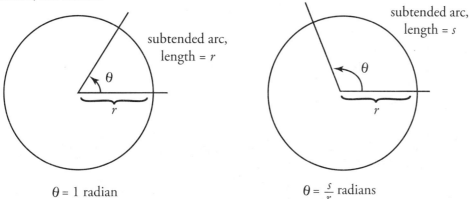

For a general angle, if s is the length of the subtended arc and the radius of the circle is r, then the radian measure of the angle is the ratio s/r. The size of a radian is not arbitrary and it doesn't even depend on the size of the circle you draw. It's a natural unit for measuring angles.

So, what is the connection between degrees and radians? A complete rotation is 360°. What is a complete rotation in radians? The length of the arc subtended by a complete rotation is equal to the entire circumference of the circle, which is $s = 2\pi r$. Dividing this by r to get the radian measure, we see that a complete rotation is equal to 2π (or about 6.3) radians. (By the way, this means that 1 radian is equal to $360°/2\pi \approx 57.3°$.) So, the conversion between radians and degrees is this: 2π radians = 360°, or, if you prefer, divide both sides of this equation by 2 to get

$$\pi \text{ radians} = 180°$$

This way, every time you see an angle written in radians and there's a π there, just mentally substitute $180°$ for the π and you're back in degree mode. For example, an angle whose radian measure is $\pi/3$ is equal to $180°/3 = 60°$. Since angles that are multiples of $30°$ and $45°$ are so common, it's useful to memorize the following conversions between degrees and radians:

$$30° \leftrightarrow \frac{\pi}{6} \quad 45° \leftrightarrow \frac{\pi}{4} \quad 60° \leftrightarrow \frac{\pi}{3} \quad 90° \leftrightarrow \frac{\pi}{2} \quad 180° \leftrightarrow \pi$$

When faced with an angle in radian measure like $2\pi/3$, just think of it as $2(\pi/3)$, which is $2(60°) = 120°$. Similarly, if you needed to convert an angle like $150°$ to radians, think of it this way: $150° = 5(30°) = 5(\pi/6)$. In general, here are the formulas for converting between degrees and radians:

$$(\theta \text{ in radians}) \times \frac{180°}{\pi} = (\theta \text{ in degrees}) \qquad (\theta \text{ in degrees}) \times \frac{\pi}{180°} = (\theta \text{ in radians})$$

Finally, notice that in the definition of radian measure, $\theta = s/r$, we're dividing a length by a length. Therefore, the ratio θ has no units. Radian measure is actually unitless. So, if you see an equation like $\theta = 2$ (no units), you'll know that the "2" means 2 radians. If you want to express the measure of an angle in degrees, you *must* put in the degree sign; $\theta = 2°$ means an angle of measure 2 degrees. But if you want to express the measure of an angle in radians, no unit is required; writing the word *radians* after the number is optional. In fact, because radian measure is unitless, we can interpret an expression like $\sin \pi/6$ either as the sine of an angle whose measure is $\pi/6$ radians, or simply as the sine of the *number* $\pi/6$.

Example 16-10:
a) Convert from radians to degrees: $3\pi/4$; $3\pi/2$; $4\pi/3$; 2
b) Convert from degrees to radians: $180°$; $210°$; $225°$; $300°$
c) Evaluate: $\sin (\pi/6)$; $\cos \pi$; $\tan (7\pi/4)$
d) Evaluate: $\sin (-5\pi/6)$; $\cos (2\pi/3)$; $\tan 3\pi$
e) Find the smallest positive value of $\cos^{-1} (\sqrt{2}/2)$, in radians.
f) Find the smallest negative value of $\tan^{-1} (-1)$, in radians.

Solution:
a) $3\pi/4 = 3(\pi/4) = 3(45°) = 135°$; $3\pi/2 = 3(\pi/2) = 3(90°) = 270°$;
    $4\pi/3 = 4(\pi/3) = 4(60°) = 240°$; $2 \ (180°/\pi) = (360/\pi)° \approx 115°$
b) $180° = \pi$ radians; $210° = 7(30°) = 7(\pi/6) = 7\pi/6$ radians;
    $225° = 5(45°) = 5(\pi/4) = 5\pi/4$ radians; $300° = 5(60°) = 5(\pi/3) = 5\pi/3$ radians
c) $\sin (\pi/6) = \sin 30° = 1/2$; $\cos \pi = \cos 180° = -1$ (look back at Example 16-6b)
    $\tan (7\pi/4) = \tan [7(45°)] = \tan 315° = -1$
d) $\sin (-5\pi/6) = \sin [-5(30°)] = \sin (-150°) = -1/2$ (look back at Example 16-7c)
    $\cos (2\pi/3) = \cos [2(60°)] = \cos 120° = -1/2$ (look back at Example 16-6a)
    $\tan 3\pi = \tan [3(180°)] = \tan 540° = 0$ (look back at Example 16-6b)
e) $\cos^{-1} (\sqrt{2}/2) = 45° = \pi/4$
f) $\tan^{-1} (-1) = -45° = -\pi/4$

Chapter 17
Vectors

17.1 SCALARS AND VECTORS

Some quantities are completely described simply by a number (possibly with units). Examples include constants (like –2, 9.8, 0, and π) and physical quantities such as mass, length, time, speed, energy, power, density, volume, pressure, temperature, charge, potential, resistance, capacitance, frequency, sound level, and refractive index. All of these quantities are known as **scalars**, which you can think of as just a fancy word for *numbers*.

On the other hand, there are other quantities which are completely specified only when they're described by a number *and a direction*. Examples include displacement, velocity, acceleration, force, momentum, and electric and magnetic fields. All of these quantities are known as **vectors**. A vector is a quantity that involves *both* a number (its magnitude, which is a scalar) *and* a direction.

Here's an example: If I say the wind is blowing at 5 m/s, I'm giving the wind's *speed*, which is a *scalar*. However, if I say the wind is blowing at 5 m/s to the east, I'm giving the wind's *velocity*, which is a *vector*. (By the way, the distinction between speed and velocity is easy to remember: <u>s</u>peed is a <u>s</u>calar, while <u>v</u>elocity is a <u>v</u>ector.)

Since a vector is determined by a number and a direction, we represent a vector by an arrow. The length of the arrow we draw represents the number, and the direction of the arrow represents the direction of the vector. For example, the wind velocity *5 m/s to the east* might be drawn as an arrow like this:

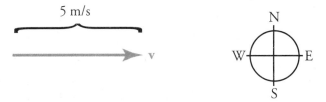

The symbol **v** is the name of this vector. In books, vector names are written as boldface letters; in handwritten work, we'd put a small arrow over the letter—like this: $\vec{v}$ or $\vec{v}$ —to signify that the quantity is a vector.

The number (or scalar) associated with a vector is its **magnitude**; it's the length of the arrow. For instance, for the vector **v** = 5 m/s to the east, the magnitude would be the scalar 5 m/s. Here's another example: If we push on something with a force of 10 N to the left,

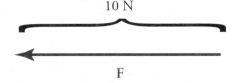

then the magnitude of the vector **F** = *10 N to the left* would be 10 N. Magnitudes are never negative.

There are two common ways to denote the magnitude of a vector. The first is to change the bold letter for the vector to an italic letter. Using this notation, the magnitude of the vector **v** would be written as *v*. As another example, the magnitude of the vector **F** would be written as *F*. The second way to denote the magnitude of a vector is to put absolute-value signs around the letter name of the vector. In this notation, the magnitude of the vector **v** would be written as $|\mathbf{v}|$ (or, in handwritten work, as $|\vec{v}|$) and the magnitude of the vector **F** would be $|\mathbf{F}|$.

17.2 OPERATIONS WITH VECTORS

For the MCAT, the three most important operations we perform with vectors are (1) addition of vectors, (2) subtraction of vectors, and (3) multiplication of a vector by a scalar.

Vector Addition

To add one vector to another vector, we use the **tip-to-tail method**. The **tail** of a vector is the starting point of the arrow, and the **tip** of a vector is the ending point (the sharp point of the arrow head):

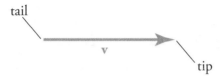

To add two vectors, we first put the tip of one of the vectors at the tail of the other one (tip-to-tail). Then we connect the exposed tail to the exposed tip; that vector is the sum of the vectors. The following figure shows this process for adding the vectors **A** and **B** to get their sum, **A + B**:

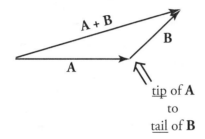

We could have put the tip of **B** at the tail of **A**, and the answer would have been the same:

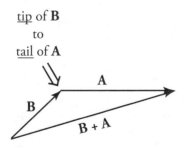

We can see from these two figures that the vector **A + B** has the same length *and* the same direction as the vector **B + A**. Therefore, the vectors are the same: **A + B = B + A**. We say that vectors obey the *commutative law for addition*; this means we can add them in either order, and the result is the same. (Actually, vectors *automatically* obey the commutative law for addition, by definition; that is, if **A** and **B** are vectors, then **A + B** will always be the same as **B + A**. There actually are quantities that are specified by a number and a direction but which do not obey the law **A + B = B + A**. Because of this failure, these quantities are not called vectors. However, you won't have to worry about such peculiar quantities for the MCAT.)

Vector Subtraction

To subtract one vector from another vector, we use the familiar *scalar* equation $a - b = a + (-b)$ as motivation. That is, for any two vectors **A** and **B**, we say that **A** − **B** is equal to **A** + (−**B**). So, we first have to answer the question: Given a vector **B**, how do we form the vector −**B**? By definition, the vector −**B** has the same magnitude as **B** but the opposite direction:

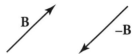

Therefore, to form the vector difference **A** − **B**, we just add −**B** to **A**:

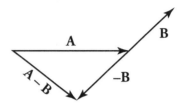

The following figure shows how to form the vector difference **B** − **A**, which is **B** + (−**A**):

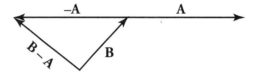

Notice that **B** − **A** is *not* the same as **A** − **B**, because their directions are not the same. That is, in general, **B** − **A** ≠ **A** − **B**; vector *subtraction* is generally *not* commutative. In fact, **B** − **A** will always be the *opposite* of **A** − **B** (same magnitude, opposite direction): **B** − **A** = −(**A** − **B**).

Another procedure you can use to subtract the vectors **A** and **B** is to put the tail of **A** at the tail of **B**, then connect the tips. (Vector *addition* uses the *tip*-to-tail method; vector *subtraction* (by this alternate procedure) uses the *tail*-to-tail method.) If you draw the resulting vector from the tip of **B** to the tip of **A**, you've constructed the vector **A** − **B**. On the other hand, if you draw the resulting vector from the tip of **A** to the tip of **B**, you've drawn the vector **B** − **A**.

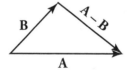 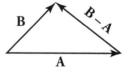

Notice that the figure on the left also illustrates the tip-to-tail vector addition **B** + (**A** − **B**) = **A**, while the figure on the right illustrates the tip-to-tail vector addition **A** + (**B** − **A**) = **B**.

Scalar Multiplication

To multiply a vector by a scalar, we consider three cases: that is, whether the scalar is positive, negative, or zero.

If k is a positive scalar, then $k\mathbf{A}$, the product of k and some vector $\mathbf{A}$, is a vector whose magnitude is k times the magnitude of $\mathbf{A}$ and whose direction is the same as that of $\mathbf{A}$. In short, multiplying a vector by a positive scalar k just changes the magnitude by a factor of k (but leaves the direction of the vector unchanged). If k is less than 1, the scalar multiple $k\mathbf{A}$ is shorter than $\mathbf{A}$; if k is greater than 1, then $k\mathbf{A}$ is longer than $\mathbf{A}$.

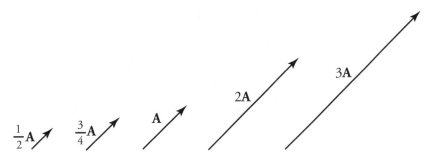

If k is a negative scalar, then $k\mathbf{A}$, the product of k and some vector $\mathbf{A}$, is a vector whose magnitude is the *absolute value* of k times the magnitude of $\mathbf{A}$ and whose direction is *opposite* the direction of $\mathbf{A}$. In short, multiplying a vector by a negative scalar k changes the magnitude by a factor of $|k|$ and reverses the direction of the vector.

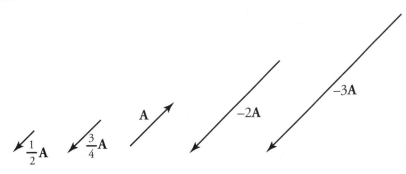

If k is zero, then the product $k\mathbf{A}$ gives $\mathbf{0}$, the **zero vector**. This unique vector has magnitude 0 and has no direction. Rather than being pictured as an arrow, the zero vector is simply pictured as a dot.

$$\mathbf{A} \quad \bullet \; 0\mathbf{A} = \mathbf{0}$$

Example 17-1: Consider the vectors **A**, **B**, and **C** shown below:

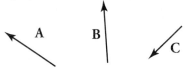

Construct each of the following vectors:

  a)   **A** + **B**

  b)   **A** − 2**C**

  c) $\frac{1}{2}$**A** − **B** + 3**C**

Solution:

  a)   Using the tip-to-tail method for vector addition gives

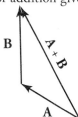

  b)   Since **A** − 2**C** = **A** + (−2**C**), we first multiply **C** by −2, then add the result to **A**:

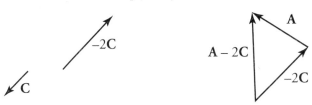

  c)   We multiply **A** by 1/2, then **B** by −1, then **C** by 3, and add the three results:

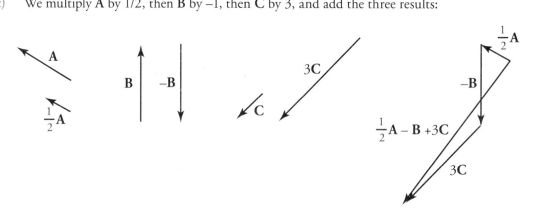

Example 17-2: Consider the vectors **A**, **B**, and **C** shown below:

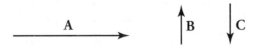

Construct each of the following vectors:
  a) −**A** + **B**;
  b) **B** + **C**;
  c) **A** + 2**B**

Solution:
  a) Multiplying **A** by −1 then using the tip-to-tail method to add the result to **B**, we get

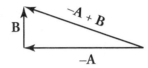

  b) Since **C** has the same length as **B** but the opposite direction, **C** is equal to −**B**. So, adding
      B + **C** gives us **B** + (−**B**), which is **0**, the zero vector. You can also see that the sum of **B** and **C**
      will be **0** using the tip-to-tail method for vector addition: If we put the tip of **B** at the tail of
      C, then the tail of **B** *coincides* with the tip of **C**, so the vector sum is **0**.
  c) Multiplying **B** by 2 then using the tip-to-tail method to add the result to **A**, we get

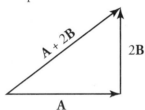

Example 17-3: Add these four vectors:

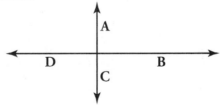

Solution: The vectors **A** and **C** have equal magnitudes but opposite directions, so **A** + **C** is **0**; that is, **A**
and **C** cancel each other out. Now, since **D** points in the direction opposite to **B**, if we place the tail
of **D** at the tip of **B**, then connect the tail of **B** to the tip of **D**, we get **B** + **D**, which is a vector in the
same direction as **B**, but much shorter. This vector is **B** + **D**, which is also the sum **A** + **B** + **C** + **D** (since
A + **C** = **0**):

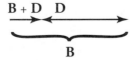

17.3 VECTOR PROJECTIONS AND COMPONENTS

In the preceding section, we performed the basic vector operations geometrically. In this section, we'll see how we can perform these operations with algebra and trig.

Let's imagine a vector **A** in a standard *x-y* coordinate system, with the tail of **A** at the origin. We construct perpendicular segments from the tip of **A** to the *x*-axis and to the *y*-axis. The resulting **vector projections** of **A** are denoted by A_x and A_y; the vector A_x is the horizontal projection of **A**, and A_y is the vertical projection. Notice that $A = A_x + A_y$. Therefore, *any vector A in the x-y plane can be written as the sum of a horizontal vector and a vertical vector (namely, its horizontal and vertical projections).*

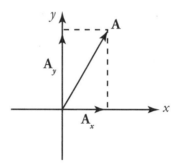

We now want to find a way to write A_x and A_y algebraically. Since any vector is specified by giving its magnitude and its direction, we need an algebraic way of describing the directions of these vectors. We do this by constructing two special vectors, one of which points in the horizontal direction, the other in the vertical direction. These two vectors are called **i** and **j**, and each has length 1:

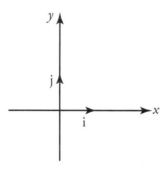

Any horizontal vector is some multiple of **i** ($A_x = A_x$**i**), and any vertical vector is some multiple of **j** ($A_y = A_y$**j**). Therefore, *any vector A in the x-y plane can be written as the sum of a multiple of **i** plus a multiple of **j**:*

$$A = A_x\mathbf{i} + A_y\mathbf{j}$$

These multiples, A_x and A_y, are called the **components** of **A**. Notice that projections are vectors, while components are scalars.

For example, the horizontal vector of magnitude 3 that points to the right is 3**i**, and the horizontal vector of magnitude 3 that points to the left is 3(–**i**) or –3**i**. The vertical vector of magnitude 4 that points upward is 4**j**, and the vertical vector of magnitude 4 that points downward is 4(–**j**) or –4**j**. For the vector **A** = –3**i** + 4**j**, we would say that its horizontal projection is –3**i** and its horizontal component is –3; similarly, its vertical projection is 4**j** and its vertical component is 4.

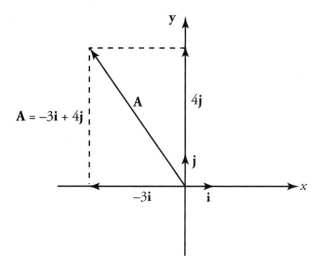

The great advantage of writing vectors algebraically is that it gives us the ability to perform vector operations quickly and precisely without having to draw the vectors (and using such procedures as the tip-to-tail method).

Magnitude

The magnitude of a vector can be found from its horizontal and vertical components using the Pythagorean theorem:

$$A = \sqrt{(A_x)^2 + (A_y)^2}$$

For example, the magnitude of the vector **A** = –3**i** + 4**j** is $A = \sqrt{(-3)^2 + 4^2} = 5$.

Direction

The direction of a vector can be described by giving the angle, θ, which the vector makes with positive x-axis. Since the components of a vector **A** are given by the formulas

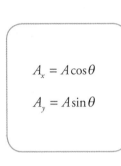

$$A_x = A\cos\theta$$

$$A_y = A\sin\theta$$

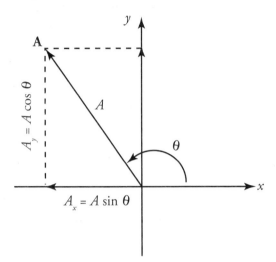

we see that

$$\frac{A_y}{A_x} = \frac{A\sin\theta}{A\cos\theta} = \tan\theta \;\rightarrow\; \theta = \tan^{-1}\frac{A_y}{A_x}$$

Vector Addition and Subtraction

The operations of addition and subtraction of vectors is made especially easy by the use of components. To add the vector $\mathbf{A} = A_x\mathbf{i} + A_y\mathbf{j}$ to the vector $\mathbf{B} = B_x\mathbf{i} + B_y\mathbf{j}$, we simply add the horizontal components and add the vertical components; and to subtract the vectors, we just subtract their components:

$$\mathbf{A} + \mathbf{B} = (A_x + B_x)\mathbf{i} + (A_y + B_y)\mathbf{j}$$
$$\mathbf{A} - \mathbf{B} = (A_x - B_x)\mathbf{i} + (A_y - B_y)\mathbf{j}$$

Scalar Multiplication

To multiply a vector by a scalar, just multiply each component by the scalar:

$$k\mathbf{A} = (kA_x)\mathbf{i} + (kA_y)\mathbf{j}$$

Example 17-4: Let **A** = −22**i** + 16**j**, **B** = 30**j**, and **C** = −10**i** − 10**j**.
Find each of the following vectors:

a)   **A** + **B**

b)   **A** − 2**C**

c) $\dfrac{1}{2}$**A** − **B** + 3**C**

Solution:

a)   **A** + **B** = (−22 + 0)**i** + (16 + 30)**j** = −22**i** + 46**j**

b)   Since 2**C** = 2(−10**i** − 10**j**) = −20**i** − 20**j**, we get:

$\quad$ **A** − 2**C** = [−22 − (−20)]**i** + [16 − (−20)]**j** = −2**i** + 36**j**

c)   Since $\dfrac{1}{2}$**A** = $\dfrac{1}{2}$(−22)**i** + $\dfrac{1}{2}$(16)**j** = −11**i** + 8**j** and 3**C** = 3(−10**i** − 10**j**) = −30**i** − 30**j**, we find that

$$\frac{1}{2}\mathbf{A} - \mathbf{B} + 3\mathbf{C} = (-11 - 0 - 30)\mathbf{i} + (8 - 30 - 30)\mathbf{j} = -41\mathbf{i} - 52\mathbf{j}$$

Compare this example (and its results) with Example 17-1.

Example 17-5: What's the magnitude and direction of the vector **A** = 3**i** − 3**j**?

Solution: If we draw the vector starting at the origin, then

the vector points down into Quadrant IV. Its magnitude is

$A = \sqrt{3^2 + (-3)^2} = 3\sqrt{2}$, and its direction is given by

$$\theta = \tan^{-1}\frac{A_y}{A_x} = \tan^{-1}(\frac{-3}{3}) = \tan^{-1}(-1) = 315° \text{ or } -45°$$

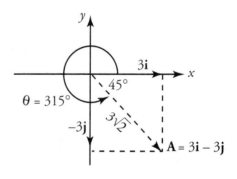

Example 17-6: Let **A** be the vector of magnitude 6 that makes an angle of 150° with the positive *x*-axis.
Sketch this vector, determine its components, and write **A** in terms of **i** and **j**.

Solution: The figure at the right is a sketch of this vector.
Its components are

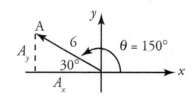

$$A_x = A\cos\theta = 6\cos 150° = 6(-\frac{\sqrt{3}}{2}) = -3\sqrt{3}$$

$$A_y = A\sin\theta = 6\sin 150° = 6(\frac{1}{2}) = 3$$

Therefore, since for any vector **A** we have **A** = A_x**i** + A_y**j**, we can write

$$\mathbf{A} = -3\sqrt{3}\mathbf{i} + 3\mathbf{j}$$

17.3

Example 17-7: Any vector whose magnitude is 1 is called a **unit vector**. (For example, both **i** and **j** are examples of unit vectors.) Let **C** be the unit vector that makes an angle of 225° with the positive x-axis. Sketch this vector, determine its components, and write **C** in terms of **i** and **j**.

Solution: The figure at the right is a sketch of this vector. Its components are

$$C_x = C\cos\theta = 1\ \cos 225° = -\frac{\sqrt{2}}{2}$$

$$C_y = C\sin\theta = 1\ \sin 225° = -\frac{\sqrt{2}}{2}$$

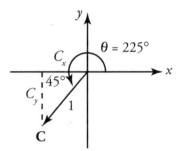

Therefore, since for any vector **C** we have **C** = C_x**i** + C_y**j**, we can write

$$\mathbf{C} = -\frac{\sqrt{2}}{2}\mathbf{i} - \frac{\sqrt{2}}{2}\mathbf{j}$$

Example 17-8: The figure below shows a vector **W** of magnitude 100 and its projections, **W**₁ and **W**₂, onto two mutually perpendicular directions, such that **W** = **W**₁ + **W**₂. Find the magnitudes of **W**₁ and **W**₂.

Solution: By definition of the sine and cosine, we have

$$W_1 = W\cos\theta = 100\cos 60° = 100(\frac{1}{2}) = 50$$

$$W_2 = W\sin\theta = 100\sin 60° = 100(\frac{\sqrt{3}}{2}) = 50\sqrt{3}$$

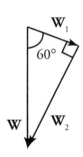

Chapter 18
Proportions

The concept of proportionality is fundamental to analyzing the behavior of many physical phenomena and is a common topic for MCAT questions.

18.1   DIRECT PROPORTIONS

If one quantity is always equal to a constant times another quantity, we say that the two quantities are **proportional** (or **directly proportional**, if emphasis is desired). For example, if k is some nonzero constant and the equation $A = kB$ is always true, then A and B are proportional, and k is called the **proportionality constant**. We express this fact mathematically by using this symbol: $\propto$, which means *is proportional to*. So, if $A = kB$, we'd write $A \propto B$. Of course, if $A = kB$, then $B = (1/k)A$, so we could also say that $B \propto A$.

Here are a few examples:

Example 18-1: The circumference of a circle is equal to π times the diameter: $C = \pi d$. Therefore, $C \propto d$.

Example 18-2: The gravitational potential energy of an object of weight w can be written as $PE = wh$, where h is the altitude of the object (if it's much smaller than the radius of the earth). Therefore, $PE \propto h$.

Example 18-3: The force exerted on a particle of charge q moving with speed v through a magnetic field of magnitude B is $F = qvB$, if the velocity **v** is perpendicular to **B**. Therefore, $F \propto v$.

The most important fact about direct proportions is this:

> If $A \propto B$, and B is multiplied by a factor of b, then A will also be multiplied by a factor of b.

After all, if $A = kB$, then $bA = k(bB)$.

Example 18-4: Since the circumference of a circle is proportional to its diameter, $C \propto d$, then, if the diameter is doubled, so is the circumference. If the diameter is cut in half, so is the circumference. If the diameter is tripled, so is the circumference.

Example 18-5: Since the gravitational potential energy of an object of weight w is proportional to its altitude, $PE \propto h$, then if the altitude is doubled, so is the potential energy. If the altitude is quadrupled, so is the potential energy. If the altitude is divided by 3 (which is the same as saying it's multiplied by 1/3), then the potential energy will also decrease by a factor of 3.

Example 18-6: Since the force exerted on a particle of charge q moving with speed v perpendicular to a magnetic field of magnitude B is $F = qvB$, we know that $F \propto v$. If the particle's speed is decreased by a factor of 2, the force F it feels will also be decreased by a factor of 2. If the speed is increased by a factor of 5, the force F will also increase by a factor of 5.

It's important to notice that the actual numerical value of the proportionality constant was irrelevant in the statements made above. For example, the fact that π is the proportionality constant in the equation $C = \pi d$ did not affect the conclusions made above. If C and d were some other quantities and C happened to always be equal to $(17,000)d$, we'd still say $C \propto d$, and all the conclusions made in Example 18-4 above would still be correct.

Graphically, proportions are easy to spot. If the horizontal and vertical axes are labeled linearly (as they usually are), then *the graph of a proportion is a straight line through the origin*. Be careful not to make the common mistake of thinking that any straight line is the graph of a proportion. If the line doesn't go through the origin, then it's *not* the graph of a proportion.

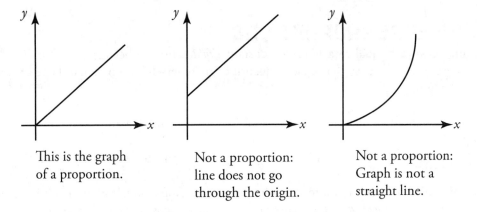

This is the graph of a proportion.

Not a proportion: line does not go through the origin.

Not a proportion: Graph is not a straight line.

The examples we've seen so far have been the equations $C = \pi d$, $PE = wh$, and $F = qvB$. Notice that in all of these equations, all the variables are present to the first power. But what about an equation like this: $KE = \frac{1}{2}mv^2$? This equation gives the kinetic energy of an object of mass m moving with speed v. So, if m is constant, KE is proportional to v^2. Now, what if v were multiplied by, say, a factor of 3, what would happen to KE? Because $KE \propto v^2$, if v increases by a factor of 3, then KE will increase by a factor of 3^2, which is 9. (By the way, this does not mean that if we graph KE versus v, we'll get a straight line through the origin. KE is not proportional to v; it's proportional to v^2. If we were to graph KE vs. v^2, *then* we'd get a straight line through the origin.) Here's another example using the same proportion, $KE \propto v^2$: If v were decreased by a factor of 2, then KE would decrease by a factor of $2^2 = 4$.

Here are a few more examples:

Example 18-7: The volume of a sphere of radius r is given by the equation $V = \frac{4}{3}\pi r^3$. Therefore, the volume is proportional to the radius cubed: $V \propto r^3$. So, for example, if r were doubled, then V would increase by a factor of $2^3 = 8$. If r were decreased by a factor of 3, then V would decrease by a factor of $3^3 = 27$.

Example 18-8: Consider an object starting from rest and accelerating at a constant rate of a in a straight line. Let the distance it travels be x and its final velocity be v. Then it's known that $x = v^2/2a$, which means x is proportional to v squared: $x \propto v^2$. If v were quadrupled, then x would increase by a factor of $4^2 = 16$. If v were reduced by a factor of 5, then x would be reduced by a factor of $5^2 = 25$. Now, how about this: What if x were increased by a factor of 9, what would happen to v? Since x is proportional to v^2, if x increases by a factor of 9, then v^2 also increases by a factor of 9; this means that v increases by a factor of 3.

Example 18-9: The intensity of energy radiated by an object of absolute temperature T is given by the formula $I = \sigma T^4$, where σ is a constant. Therefore, $I \propto T^4$. If T were increased by a factor of 3, then I would increase by a factor of $3^4 = 81$. In order to reduce I to 1/16 its original value, the temperature T would have to be reduced by a factor of 2, since $\dfrac{1}{16} = (\dfrac{1}{2})^4$.

18.2 INVERSE PROPORTIONS

If one quantity is always equal to a nonzero constant *divided* by another quantity (that is, if $A = k/B$, where k is some constant), we say that the two quantities are **inversely proportional**. Here are two equivalent ways of saying this:

(i) If the product of two quantities is a constant ($AB = k$), then the quantities are inversely proportional.

(ii) If A is proportional to $1/B$ [that is, if $A = k(1/B)$], then A and B are inversely proportional.

In fact, we'll use this final description to symbolize an inverse proportion. That is, if A is inversely proportional to B, then we'll write $A \propto 1/B$. (There's no commonly-accepted single symbol for *inversely proportional to*.) Of course, if $A = k/B$, then $B = k/A$, so we could also say that $B \propto 1/A$.

Here are a few examples:

Example 18-10: The electric potential, ϕ, at a distance r from a point charge q is given by the equation $\phi = kq/r$, where k is a constant. Therefore, ϕ is inversely proportional to r. $\phi \propto 1/r$.

Example 18-11: The pressure P and volume V of a sample containing n moles of an ideal gas at a fixed temperature T is given by the equation $PV = nRT$, where R is a constant. Therefore, the pressure is inversely proportional to the volume: $P \propto 1/V$.

Example 18-12: For electromagnetic waves traveling through space, the wavelength λ and frequency f are related by the equation $\lambda f = c$, where c is the speed of light (a universal constant). Therefore, wavelength is inversely proportional to frequency: $\lambda \propto 1/f$.

The most important fact about inverse proportions is this:

> If $A \propto 1/B$, and B is multiplied by a factor of b, then A will be multiplied by a factor of $1/b$.

After all, if $A = k/B$, then $(1/b)A = k/(bB)$. Intuitively, if one quantity is *increased* by a factor of b, the other quantity will *decrease* by the same factor, and vice versa.

Example 18-13: Since the electric potential is inversely proportional to the distance from the source charge, $\phi \propto 1/r$, then, if the distance is doubled, the potential is cut in half. If the distance is cut in half, the potential is doubled. If the distance is tripled, the potential is multiplied by 1/3.

Example 18-14: Since the pressure of an ideal gas at constant temperature is inversely proportional to the volume, $P \propto 1/V$, then if the volume is doubled, the pressure is reduced by a factor of 2. If the volume is quadrupled, the pressure is reduced by a factor of 4. If the volume is divided by 3 (which is the same as saying it's multiplied by 1/3), then the pressure will increase by a factor of 3.

Example 18-15: Because for electromagnetic waves traveling through space, the wavelength is inversely proportional to frequency, $\lambda \propto 1/f$, if f is increased by a factor of 10, λ will decrease by a factor of 10. If the frequency is decreased by a factor of 2, the wavelength will increase by a factor of 2.

The graph of an inverse proportion is a *hyperbola*. In the graph below, $xy = k$, so x and y are inversely proportional to each other.

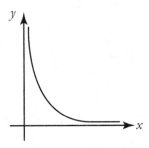

This is the graph of
an inverse proportion.

The examples we've seen so far have been where one quantity is inversely proportional to the first power of another quantity. But what about an equation like this:

$$F = G\frac{Mm}{r^2}$$

This equation gives the gravitational force between two objects of masses M and m separated by a distance r. (G is the universal gravitational constant.) So, if M and m are constant, F is inversely proportional to r^2. Now, what if r were increased by, say, a factor of 3, what would happen to F? Because $F \propto 1/r^2$, if r increases by a factor of 3, then F will decrease by a factor of 3^2, which is 9. Here's another example using the same proportion, $F \propto 1/r^2$: If r were decreased by a factor of 2, then F would increase by a factor of $2^2 = 4$.

Example 18-16: The electrostatic force between two charges Q and q separated by a distance r is given by the equation $F = kQq/r^2$, where k is a constant. Therefore, the electrostatic force is inversely proportional to the distance squared: $F \propto 1/r^2$. So, for example, if r were doubled, then F would decrease by a factor of $2^2 = 4$. If r were decreased by a factor of 3, then F would increase by a factor of $3^2 = 9$.

Example 18-17: The frequency of a simple harmonic oscillator consisting of a block of mass m attached to a spring of force constant k is given by the formula $f = 1/2\pi \sqrt{k/m}$. Therefore, the frequency is inversely proportional to the square root of the block's mass: $f \propto 1/\sqrt{m}$. So, if m were multiplied by 4, f would be multiplied by 1/2, since $1/\sqrt{4} = 1/2$. If m were increased by a factor of 36, then f would decrease by a factor of 6. If we wanted f to increase by a factor of 3, we'd have to decrease m by a factor of 9.

Example 18-18: An object starting from rest travels a distance given by $d = at^2/2$ in a time t if it undergoes a constant acceleration a.
   a)   If t is doubled, then what happens to d?
   b)   If t is tripled, what happens to d?

Solution:
   a)   Since $d \propto t^2$, if t increases by a factor of 2, then d increases by a factor of $2^2 = 4$.
   b)   Since $d \propto t^2$, if t increases by a factor of 3, then d increases by a factor of 9.

Example 18-19: The kinetic energy of an object of mass m traveling with speed v is given by the formula $KE = mv^2/2$.
   a)   If v is increased by a factor of 6, what happens to KE?
   b)   In order to increase KE by a factor of 6, what must happen to v?

Solution:
   a)   Since $KE \propto v^2$, if v increases by a factor of 6, then KE increases by a factor of $6^2 = 36$.
   b)   Since $KE \propto v^2$, it follows that $\sqrt{KE} \propto v$. So, if KE is to increase by a factor of 6, then v must be increased by a factor of $\sqrt{6}$.

Example 18-20: The area of a circle of radius r is given by $A = \pi r^2$.
   a)   If r is halved, then what happens to A?
   b)   If r increases by 50%, by what percentage will A increase?
   c)   If the *diameter* of the circle is halved, what happens to A?

Solution:
   a)   Since $A \propto r^2$, if r decreases by a factor of 2, then A will decrease by a factor of $2^2 = 4$.
   b)   If r increases by $r/2$ (which is 50% of r) to $3r/2$, then r increases by a factor of 3/2. Therefore, A increases to $(3/2)^2 = 9/4 = 225\%$ times its original value. This represents an increase of $225\% - 100\% = 125\%$.
   c)   Since $d = 2r$, we know that $d \propto r$. Therefore, if d is halved, then so is r, and A decreases by a factor of 4 [just as in part (a)]. Alternatively, we could first write the formula for the area of a circle in terms of d, its diameter, as follows:

$$A = \pi r^2 = \pi(\frac{1}{2}d)^2 = \frac{1}{4}\pi d^2$$

Therefore, $A \propto d^2$, so if d is decreased by a factor of 2, then A will be decreased by a factor of $2^2 = 4$.

Example 18-21: A metal rod of length L will be stretched by a distance $\Delta L = mgL/EA$ when a weight $w = mg$ is suspended from it.

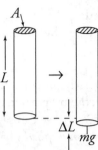

In this formula, E is a constant (depending on the material of which the rod is made) and $A = \pi r^2$ is the rod's cross-sectional area.

   a)   How will ΔL change if the mass m is doubled?
   b)   If identical weights are suspended from two metal rods of the same initial length and made of the same material, but with the radius of Rod #1 being twice that of Rod #2, which rod will be stretched more, and by what factor?

Solution:

   a)   Since $\Delta L \propto m$, if m increases by a factor of 2, then so does ΔL.

   b)   Because $A \propto r^2$, it follows that $\Delta L \propto 1/r^2$. Since the radius of Rod #2 is half the radius of Rod #1, the stretch of Rod #2 will be $\dfrac{1}{\left(\frac{1}{2}\right)^2}$ = 4 times that of Rod #1.

Example 18-22: Newton's law of gravitation states that the force between two objects is given by $F = GMm/r^2$, where M and m are the masses of the objects, r is the distance between them, and G is the universal gravitational constant.

   a)   If both masses are doubled, and the distance between them is also doubled, what happens to F?
   b)   If r is decreased by 50%, what happens to F?

Solution:

   a)   If both masses are doubled, then the product Mm increases by a factor of $(2)(2) = 4$. If the distance r is doubled, then r^2 increases by a factor of 4. Since $F \propto Mm/r^2$ and both Mm and r^2 increase by the same factor (in this case, 4), F will remain unchanged:

$$F' = G\frac{(2M)(2m)}{(2r)^2} = G\frac{4Mm}{4r^2} = G\frac{Mm}{r^2} = F$$

   b)   If r decreases by 50%, then r changes to $r - (r/2) = r/2$; that is, r decreases by a factor of 2. Since $F \propto 1/r^2$, if r decreases by a factor of 2, F will increase by a factor of $2^2 = 4$.

Example 18-23: Consider the equation $xy = z$.
   a)   If z is a constant, how are x and y related?
   b)   If x is constant, how are y and z related?
   c)   If x is a positive constant, and we increase y by adding 2, by what factor does z increase?

Solution:
   a)   If z is a constant, then x and y are inversely proportional: $x \propto 1/y$.
   b)   If x is constant, then y and z are (directly) proportional: $z \propto y$.
   c)   If x is constant, then $z \propto y$. If we add 2 to y, we can say that z will increase by some amount, but we cannot say by what factor. If we *multiplied* y by 2, *then* we could say that z will increase by a factor of 2. But *adding* 2 to y does not allow us to say by what *factor z* will increase. Predictions can be made with proportions only when we're told the factor by which some quantity changes (that is, what the quantity is *multiplied* by).

Chapter 19
Logarithms

19.1   THE DEFINITION OF A LOGARITHM

A **logarithm** (or just **log**, for short) is an exponent.

For example, in the equation $2^3 = 8$, 3 is the exponent, so 3 is the logarithm. More precisely, since 3 is the exponent that gives 8 when the base is 2,

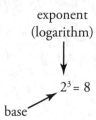

we say that the base-2 log of 8 is 3, symbolized by the equation $\log_2 8 = 3$.

Here's another example: Since $10^2 = 100$, the base-10 log of 100 is 2; that is, $\log_{10} 100 = 2$. The logarithm of a number to a given base is the exponent the base needs to be raised to give the number. What's the log, base 3, of 81? It's the exponent we'd have to raise 3 to in order to give 81. Since $3^4 = 81$, the base-3 log of 81 is 4, which we write as $\log_3 81 = 4$.

The exponent equation $2^3 = 8$ is equivalent to the log equation $\log_2 8 = 3$; the exponent equation $10^2 = 100$ is equivalent to the log equation $\log_{10} 100 = 2$; and the exponent equation $3^4 = 81$ is equivalent to the log equation $\log_3 81 = 4$. For every exponent equation, $b^x = y$, there's a corresponding log equation: $\log_b y = x$, and vice versa. To help make the conversion, use the following mnemonic, which I call the *two arrows method*:

$$\log_2 8 = 3 \iff 2^3 = 8$$

$$\log_b y = x \iff b^x = y$$

You should read the log equations with the two arrows like this:

$$\log_2 8 = 3 \iff 2 \xrightarrow{\text{to the}} 3 \xrightarrow{\text{equals}} 8 \iff 2^3 = 8$$

$$\log_b y = x \iff b \xrightarrow{\text{to the}} x \xrightarrow{\text{equals}} y \iff b^x = y$$

Always remember: The log is the exponent.

19.2 LAWS OF LOGARITHMS

There are only a few rules for dealing with logs that you'll need to know, and they follow directly from the rules for exponents (given earlier, in Chapter 15). After all, logs *are* exponents.

In stating these rules, we will assume that in an equation like $\log_b y = x$, the base b is a positive number that's different from 1, and that y is positive. (Why these restrictions? Well, if b is negative, then not every number has a log. For example, $\log_{-3} 9$ is 2, but what is $\log_{-3} 27$? If b were 0, then only 0 would have a log; and if b were 1, then every number x could equal $\log_1 y$ if $y = 1$, and *no* number x could equal $\log_1 y$ if $y \neq 1$. And why must y be positive? Because if b is a positive number, then b^x [which is y] is always positive, no matter what real value we use for x. Therefore, only positive numbers have logs.)

Laws of Logarithms

Law 1   The log of a product is the sum of the logs:
$$\log_b (yz) = \log_b y + \log_b z$$

Law 2   The log of a quotient is the difference of the logs:
$$\log_b (y/z) = \log_b y - \log_b z$$

Law 3   The log of (a number to a power) is that power times the log of the number:
$$\log_b (y^z) = z \log_b y$$

We could also add to this list that *the log of 1 is 0*, but this fact just follows from the definition of a log: Since $b^0 = 1$ for any allowed base b, we'll always have $\log_b 1 = 0$.

For the MCAT, the two most important bases are $b = 10$ and $b = e$. Base-10 logs are called **common** logs, and the "10" is often not written at all:

$$\log y \quad \text{means} \quad \log_{10} y$$

The base-10 log is useful because we use a *decimal* number system, which is based on the number 10. For example, the number 273.15 means $(2 \cdot 10^2) + (7 \cdot 10^1) + (3 \cdot 10^0) + (1 \cdot 10^{-1}) + (5 \cdot 10^{-2})$. In physics, the formula for the decibel level of a sound uses the base-10 log. In chemistry, the base-10 log has many uses, such as finding values of the pH, pOH, pK_a, and pK_b.

Base-e logs are known as **natural** logs. Here, e is a particular constant, approximately equal to 2.7. This may seem like a strange number to choose as a base, but it makes calculus run smoothly—which is why it's called the *natural* logarithm—because (and you don't need to know this for the MCAT) the only numerical value of b for which the function $f(x) = b^x$ is its own derivative is $b = e = 2.71828....$ Base-e logs are often used in the mathematical description of physical processes in which the rate of change of some quantity is proportional to the quantity itself; radioactive decay is a typical example. The notation "ln" (the abbreviation, in reverse, for **n**atural **l**ogarithm) is often used to mean $\log_e$:

$$\ln y \quad \text{means} \quad \log_e y$$

The relationship between the base-10 log and the base-e log of a given number can be expressed as $\ln y \approx 2.3 \log y$. For example, if $y = 1000 = 10^3$, then $\ln 1000 \approx 2.3 \log 1000 = 2.3 \cdot 3 = 6.9$. You may also find it useful to know the following approximate values:

$\log 2 \approx 0.3$	$\ln 2 \approx 0.7$
$\log 3 \approx 0.5$	$\ln 3 \approx 1.1$
$\log 5 \approx 0.7$	$\ln 5 \approx 1.6$

Example 19-1:
a) What is $\log_3 9$?
b) Find $\log_5 (1/25)$.
c) Find $\log_4 8$.
d) What is the value of $\log_{16} 4$?
e) Given that $\log 5 \approx 0.7$, what is the value for $\log 500$?
f) Given that $\log 2 \approx 0.3$, find $\log (2 \times 10^{-6})$.
g) Given that $\log 2 \approx 0.3$ and $\log 3 \approx 0.5$, find $\log (6 \times 10^{23})$.

Solution:
a) $\log_3 9 = x$ is the same as $3^x = 9$, from which we see that $x = 2$. So, $\log_3 9 = 2$.
b) $\log_5 (1/25) = x$ is the same as $5^x = 1/25 = 1/5^2 = 5^{-2}$, so $x = -2$. Therefore, $\log_5 (1/25) = -2$.
c) $\log_4 8 = x$ is the same as $4^x = 8$. Since $4^x = (2^2)^x = 2^{2x}$ and $8 = 2^3$, the equation $4^x = 8$ is the same as $2^{2x} = 2^3$, so $2x = 3$, which gives $x = 3/2$. Therefore, $\log_4 8 = 3/2$.
d) $\log_{16} 4 = x$ is the same as $16^x = 4$. To find x, you might notice that the square root of 16 is 4, so $16^{1/2} = 4$, which means $\log_{16} 4 = 1/2$. Alternatively, we can write 16^x as $(4^2)^x = 4^{2x}$ and 4 as 4^1. Therefore, the equation $16^x = 4$ is the same as $4^{2x} = 4^1$, so $2x = 1$, which gives $x = 1/2$.
e) $\log 500 = \log (5 \cdot 100) = \log 5 + \log 100$, where we used Law 1 in the last step. Since $\log 100 = \log 10^2 = 2$, we find that $\log 500 \approx 0.7 + 2 = 2.7$.
f) $\log (2 \times 10^{-6}) = \log 2 + \log 10^{-6}$, by Law 1. Since $\log 10^{-6} = -6$, we find that $\log (2 \times 10^{-6}) \approx 0.3 + (-6) = -5.7$.
g) $\log (6 \times 10^{23}) = \log 2 + \log 3 + \log 10^{23}$, by Law 1. Since $\log 10^{23} = 23$, we find that $\log (6 \times 10^{23}) \approx 0.3 + 0.5 + 23 = 23.8$.

Example 19-2: In each case, find y.
a) $\log_2 y = 5$
b) $\log_2 y = -3$
c) $\log y = 4$
d) $\log y = 7.5$
e) $\log y = -2.5$
f) $\ln y = 3$

Solution:
a) $\log_2 y = 5$ is the same as $2^5 = y$, so $y = 32$.
b) $\log_2 y = -3$ is the same as $2^{-3} = y$, which gives $y = 1/2^3 = 1/8$.
c) $\log y = 4$ is the same as $10^4 = y$, so $y = 10,000$.
d) $\log y = 7.5$ is the same as $10^{7.5} = y$. We'll rewrite 7.5 as $7 + 0.5$, so $y = 10^{7+(0.5)} = 10^7 \times 10^{0.5}$. Because $10^{0.5} = 10^{1/2} = \sqrt{10}$, which is approximately 3, we find that $y \approx 10^7 \times 3 = 3 \times 10^7$.
e) $\log y = -2.5$ is the same as $10^{-2.5} = y$. We'll rewrite -2.5 as $-3 + 0.5$, so $y = 10^{-3+(0.5)} = 10^{-3} \times 10^{0.5}$. Because $10^{0.5} = 10^{1/2} = \sqrt{10}$, which is approximately 3, we find that $y \approx 10^{-3} \times 3 = 0.003$.
f) $\ln y = 3$ means $\log_e y = 3$; this is the same as $y = e^3$ (which is about 20).

Example 19-3: If a sound wave has intensity I (measured in W/m^2), then its loudness level, β (measured in decibels), is found from the formula

$$\beta = 10 \log \frac{I}{I_0}$$

where I_0 is a constant equal to 10^{-12} W/m^2. What is the loudness level of a sound wave whose intensity is 10^{-5} W/m^2?

Solution: Using the given formula, we find that

$$\beta = 10 \log \frac{10^{-5}}{10^{-12}} = 10 \log(10^7) = 10 \cdot 7 = 70 \text{ decibels}$$

Example 19-4: The definition of the pH of an aqueous solution is
$$\text{pH} = -\log [H_3O^+] \text{ (or } -\log [H^+])$$

where $[H_3O^+]$ is the hydronium ion concentration (in M).

Part I: Find the pH of each of the following solutions:
 a) coffee, with $[H_3O^+] = 8 \times 10^{-6}$ M
 b) seawater, with $[H_3O^+] = 3 \times 10^{-9}$ M
 c) vinegar, with $[H_3O^+] = 1.3 \times 10^{-3}$ M

Part II: Find $[H_3O^+]$ for each of the following pH values:
 d) pH = 7
 e) pH = 11.5
 f) pH = 4.7

Solution:
 a) pH = $-\log (8 \times 10^{-6}) = -[\log 8 + \log (10^{-6})] = -\log 8 + 6$. We can now make a quick approximation by simply noticing that log 8 is a little less than log 10; that is, log 8 is a little less than 1. Let's say it's 0.9. Then pH $\approx -0.9 + 6 = 5.1$.
 b) pH = $-\log (3 \times 10^{-9}) = -[\log 3 + \log (10^{-9})] = -\log 3 + 9$. We now make a quick approximation by simply noticing that log 3 is about 0.5 (after all, $9^{0.5}$ *is* 3, so $10^{0.5}$ is close to 3). This gives pH $\approx -0.5 + 9 = 8.5$.
 c) pH = $-\log (1.3 \times 10^{-3}) = -[\log 1.3 + \log (10^{-3})] = -\log 1.3 + 3$. We can now make a quick approximation by simply noticing that log 1.3 is just a little more than log 1; that is, log 1.3 is a little more than 0. Let's say it's 0.1. This gives pH $\approx -0.1 + 3 = 2.9$.

---

*Note 1: We can generalize these three calculations as follows: If $[H_3O^+] = m \times 10^{-n}$ M, where $1 \le m < 10$ and n is an integer, then the pH is between $(n-1)$ and n; it's closer to $(n-1)$ if $m > 3$ and it's closer to n if $m < 3$. (We use 3 as the cutoff since log 3 ≈ 0.5.)

d) If pH = 7, then $-\log [H_3O^+] = 7$, so $\log [H_3O^+] = -7$, which means $[H_3O^+] = 10^{-7}$ M.
e) If pH = 11.5, then $-\log [H_3O^+] = 11.5$, so $\log [H_3O^+] = -11.5$, which means $[H_3O^+] = 10^{-11.5}$ $= 10^{(0.5)-12} = 10^{0.5} \times 10^{-12} \approx 3 \times 10^{-12}$ M.
f) If pH = 4.7, then $-\log [H_3O^+] = 4.7$, so $\log [H_3O^+] = -4.7$, which means $[H_3O^+] = 10^{-4.7} = 10^{(0.3)-5} = 10^{0.3} \times 10^{-5} \approx 2 \times 10^{-5}$ M. ($10^{-0.3} \approx 2$ follows from the fact that $\log 2 \approx 0.3$.)

*Note 2: We can generalize these last two calculations as follows: If pH = $n.m$, where n is an integer and m is a digit from 1 to 9, then $[H_3O^+] = y \times 10^{-(n+1)}$ M, where y is closer to 1 if $m > 3$ and closer to 10 if $m < 3$. (We take $y = 5$ if $m = 3$.)

Example 19-5: The definition of the pK_a of a weak acid is
$$pK_a = -\log K_a$$

where K_a is the acid's ionization constant.

Part I: Approximate the pK_a of each of the following acids:
a) HBrO, with $K_a = 2 \times 10^{-9}$
b) HNO_2, with $K_a = 7 \times 10^{-4}$
c) HCN, with $K_a = 6 \times 10^{-10}$

Part II: Approximate K_a for each of the following pK_a values:
d) $pK_a = 12.5$
e) $pK_a = 2.7$
f) $pK_a = 9.2$

Solution:
a) $pK_a = -\log (2 \times 10^{-9}) = -[\log 2 + \log (10^{-9})] = -\log 2 + 9$. We can now make a quick approximation by remembering that $\log 2$ is about 0.3. Then $pK_a = -0.3 + 9 = 8.7$. Because the formula to find pK_a from K_a is exactly the same as the formula for finding pH from $[H^+]$, we could also make use of Note 1 in the solution to Example 19-4. If $K_a = m \times 10^{-n}$ M, where $1 \le m < 10$ and n is an integer, then the pK_a is between $(n - 1)$ and n; it's closer to $(n - 1)$ if $m > 3$ and it's closer to n if $m < 3$. In this case, $m = 2$ and $n = 9$, so the pK_a is between $(n - 1) = 8$ and $n = 9$. And, since $2 < 3$, the pK_a will be closer to 9 (which is just what we found, since we got the value 8.7). Given a list of possible choices for the pK_a of this acid, just recognizing that it's a little less than 9 will be sufficient.
b) With $K_a = 7 \times 10^{-4}$, we have $m = 7$ and $n = 4$. Therefore, the pK_a will be between $(n - 1) = 3$ and $n = 4$. Since $m = 7$ is greater than 3, the value of pK_a will be closer to 3 (around, say, 3.2).
c) With $K_a = 6 \times 10^{-10}$, we have $m = 6$ and $n = 10$. Therefore, the pK_a will be between $(n - 1) = 9$ and $n = 10$. Since $m = 6$ is greater than 3, the value of pK_a will be closer to 9 (around, say, 9.2).
d) If $pK_a = 12.5$, then $-\log K_a = 12.5$, so $\log K_a = -12.5$, which means $K_a = 10^{-12.5} = 10^{(0.5)-13} = 10^{0.5} \times 10^{-13} \approx 3 \times 10^{-13}$. We could also make use of Note 2 in the solution to Example 19-4. If $pK_a = n.m$, where n is an integer and m is a digit from 1 to 9, then $K_a = y \times 10^{-(n+1)}$ M, where y is closer to 1 if $m > 3$ and y is closer to 10 if $m < 3$. In this case, with $pK_a = 12.5$, we

have $n = 12$ and $m = 5$, so the K_a value is $y \times 10^{-(12+1)} = y \times 10^{-13}$, with y closer to 1 (than to 10) since $m = 5$ is greater than 3 (this agrees with what we found, since we calculated that $K_a \approx 3 \times 10^{-13}$).

e) With $pK_a = 2.7$, we have $n = 2$ and $m = 7$. Therefore, the K_a value is $y \times 10^{-(2+1)} = y \times 10^{-3}$, with y close to 1 since $m = 7$ is greater than 3. We can check this as follows: If $pK_a = 2.7$, then $-\log K_a = 2.7$, so $\log K_a = -2.7$, which means $K_a = 10^{-2.7} = 10^{(0.3)-3} = 10^{0.3} \times 10^{-3} \approx 2 \times 10^{-3}$.

f) With $pK_a = 9.2$, we have $n = 9$ and $m = 2$. Therefore, the K_a value is $y \times 10^{-(9+1)} = y \times 10^{-10}$, with y closer to 10 (than to 1) since $m = 2$ is less than 3. We can say that $K_a \approx 6 \times 10^{-10}$.

Example 19-6:
a) If y increases by a factor of 100, what happens to $\log y$?
b) If y decreases by a factor of 1000, what happens to $\log y$?
c) If y increases by a factor of 30,000, what happens to $\log y$?
d) If y is reduced by 99%, what happens to $\log y$?

Solution:
a) If y changes to $y' = 100y$, then the log increases by 2, since
$$\log y' = \log(100y) = \log 100 + \log y = \log 10^2 + \log y = 2 + \log y$$

b) If y changes to $y' = y/1000$, then the log decreases by 3, since
$$\log y' = \log\left(\frac{y}{1000}\right) = \log y - \log 1000 = \log y - \log 10^3 = \log y - 3$$

c) If y changes to $y' = 30,000y$, then the log increases by about 4.5, since
$$\log y' = \log(30000y) = \log 3 + \log 10000 + \log y \approx 0.5 + 4 + \log y = 4.5 + \log y$$

d) If y is reduced by 99%, that means we're subtracting $0.99y$ from y, which leaves $0.01y = y/100$. Therefore, y has decreased by a factor of 100. And if y changes to $y' = y/100$, then the log decreases by 2, since
$$\log y' = \log\left(\frac{y}{100}\right) = \log y - \log 100 = \log y - \log 10^2 = \log y - 2$$

Example 19-7: A radioactive substance has a half-life of 70 hours. For each of the fractions below, figure out how many hours will elapse until the amount of substance remaining is equal to the given fraction of the original amount.
a) 1/4
b) 1/8
c) 1/3

Solution:
a) After one half-life has elapsed, the amount remaining is 1/2 the original (by definition). After another half-life elapses, the amount remaining is now 1/2 of 1/2 the original amount, which is 1/4 the original amount. Therefore, a decrease to 1/4 the original amount requires 2 half-lives, which in this case is 2(70 hr) = 140 hr.
b) The fraction 1/8 is equal to 1/2 of 1/2 of 1/2; that is, $1/8 = (1/2)^3$. In terms of half-lives, a decrease to 1/8 the original amount requires 3 half-lives, which in this case is equal to 3(70 hr) = 210 hr. *In general, a decrease to $(1/2)^n$ the original amount requires n half-lives.*

c) The fraction 1/3 is not a whole-number power of 1/2, so we can't directly apply the fact given in the italicized sentence in the solution to part (b). However, 1/3 is between 1/2 and 1/4, so the time to get to 1/3 the original amount is between 1 and 2 half-lives. Since one half-life is 70 hr, the amount of time is between 70 and 140 hours; the middle of this range (since 1/3 is roughly in the middle between 1/2 and 1/4) is about 110 hours. The most general formula for calculating the elapsed time involves a logarithm: If $x < 1$ is the fraction of a radioactive substance remaining after a time t has elapsed, then

$$t = \frac{\log \frac{1}{x}}{\log 2} \times t_{1/2}$$

where $t_{1/2}$ is the half-life. (If you want to use this formula, remember that $\log 2 \approx 0.3$.)

Appendix: Statistics and Research Methods

The MCAT tests your knowledge of basic research methods and statistical concepts within the context of passages and questions about the social and behavioral sciences. The MCAT will not test your knowledge about statistics, *per se*, but will test whether you are able to *apply* statistical concepts and an understanding of research methodology within the context of answering content-related questions, especially in the Psychological, Social, and Biological Foundations of Behavior section. Application questions might include

- Graphical analysis and interpretation

- Determining whether results are supported by data presented in figures

- Demonstrating an understanding of basic statistics and research methods

- Interpreting data presented in graphs, figures, and tables

- Drawing conclusions about data and methodology

What is statistics?

Statistics is a tool to organize data. On the MCAT, statistics is often employed to organize data sets and present data in a logical manner such that the data can be analyzed and conclusions can be drawn. Data often include numerical information collected through research. The different types of statistical data that you might encounter on the MCAT are described in this Appendix.

DESCRIPTIVE STATISTICS

Descriptive statistics quantitatively describe a population or set of data; in behavioral fields, descriptive statistics will often provide information about the data involved in the study, such as: number of subjects (or sample size), proportion of subjects of each sex, average age (or weight, or height, or IQ...whatever is relevant to the study) of the sample. Descriptive statistics include **measures of central tendency** (such as mean, median, mode) and **measures of variability** (such as range and standard deviation).

A.1 MEASURES OF CENTRAL TENDENCY

Measures of central tendency summarize or describe the entire set of data in some meaningful way.

Mean

The mean is the average of the sample. The average is derived from adding all of the individual components and dividing by the number of components. The mean is not necessarily a number provided in the sample. You should be able to recognize what the mean of a given data set is, and be able to calculate the mean.

Example Mean Question:

Subject	Starting Weight (in pounds)	Final Weight (in pounts)
Subject 1	184	176
Subject 2	200	190
Subject 3	221	225
Subject 4	235	208
Subject 5	244	225

Table 1 Starting and Final Weights for Study Subjects

What is the average amount of weight lost in pounds for all five subjects whose data is represented in Table 1, rounded to the nearest pound?

Solution:

In order to answer this question, you must first calculate how much weight each subject lost, and then divide by the number of subjects (in this case, five).

Subject	Starting Weight (in pounds)	Final Weight (in pounds)	Weight Lost (in pounds)
Subject 1	184	176	8
Subject 2	200	190	10
Subject 3	221	225	-4*
Subject 4	235	208	27
Subject 5	244	225	19

* Subject 3 gained 4 pounds

Total weight lost is 60 pounds (remember to subtract 4 pounds for subject 3, not add), divided by 5 subjects is 12 pounds. The average weight lost is **12 pounds**.

Note: the mean can be both useful and deceptive. Using the example above, what sort of conclusions could be drawn from the fact that the subjects lost an average of 12 pounds? One might conclude that the subjects were successful at losing weight. However, the mean does not reflect the fact that one of the participants, Subject 3, actually gained weight. Nor does it reflect that one the participants, Subject 4, was very successful, losing over twice the mean. Consider another example: if ten people are in a room together and all of them earn salaries at or below minimum wage, but one of them is a billionaire, the mean salary for the ten people might make it seem like they were all quite wealthy. Therefore, use caution when making assumptions about a data set when given just the mean.

Median

The median is the middle number in a data set. The median is determined by putting the numbers in consecutive order and finding the middle number. If there is an odd number of numbers, there will be a single number that is the median. If there is an even number of numbers, the median is determined by averaging the two middle numbers. Therefore, the median is not necessarily one of the numbers in the data set. You should be able to recognize what the median of a given data set is, and be able to calculate the median.

Example Median Question:

Subject	Height (in inches)
Subject 1	67
Subject 2	61
Subject 3	72
Subject 4	70
Subject 5	66
Subject 6	68

Table 2 Height of Study Subjects

Is Subject 6 taller than the median for all subjects whose height is displayed in Table 2?

Solution:

In order to determine the median height for all six subjects, their heights must first be organized in ascending order: 61, 66, 67, 68, 70, 72. The middle two numbers are 67 and 68; when averaged, this produces a median of **67.5 inches**. Subject 6 is taller than the median.

<u>Note:</u> the median can be useful in gauging the midpoint of the data, but will not necessarily tell you much about the **outliers** (a numerical observation that is far removed from the rest of the observations). Using the example where nine people earn salaries at or below minimum wage and the tenth is a billionaire, the median will give you a pretty good idea about the income for most of the people in the room, but will not indicate that one person makes much more than the rest. Therefore, also use caution when making assumptions about a data set when given just the median.

Mode

The mode is the most frequently recurring number in the data set. If there are no numbers that occur more than once, there is no mode. If there are multiple numbers that occurs most frequently, each of those numbers is a mode. The mode must be one of the numbers in the sample, and modes are never averaged. You should be able to recognize what the mode of a given data set is, and be able to calculate the mode.

Example Mode Question:

In the following set of test scores, what is the mode?

Test Scores: 32, 65, 66, 67, 68, 68, 69, 70, 71, 72, 73, 75, 75, 75, 75, 78, 82

Solution:

The most frequently recurring number in the set above is **75**.

<u>Note:</u> like the mean and median, the mode is only useful is describing some types of data sets. Mode is particularly useful for scores (such as test scores). For example, looking at the test scores above, the mean is 69.5 and the median is 71. Using all three measures you could conclude that while the mean was low, most of the students in the class scored above the mean, and the most common score was 75. There was one very low score that brought down the mean, but there were no very high scores.

A.2 MEASURES OF VARIABILITY

Knowing information about the central tendency of a data set can be useful, but it is also useful to know something about the variation in the data set. In other words, how similar or diverse are the data?

Range

The range is the difference between the smallest and largest number in a sample. You should be able to recognize what the range of a given data set is, and be able to calculate the range.

Example Range Question:

In the following set of values, what is the range? Values: –5, 8, 11, –1, 0, 4, 14

Solution:

The smallest value in the set above is –5, and the largest is 14. The difference between these two is the range, which is **19**.

Note: the range only provides limited information about a data set, however. Returning to the example of the ten people in a room, the range of incomes might be 3 billion dollars, but that provides relatively little information about the individual salaries of the people in the room. Knowing just the range does not tell us that the majority of the people in the room all have salaries around minimum wage.

Standard Deviation

The standard deviation is more useful than the range for calculating how much the data vary. It can determine if numbers are packed together or dispersed because it is a measure of how much each individual number differs from the mean. The best way to understand standard deviation is to consider a normal distribution (also called a bell-shaped curve). You will not need to calculate standard deviation, but you should understand what it is and should be able to make assumptions and draw conclusions from standard deviation data.

Normal Distributions

A normal distribution is a very important class of statistical distributions for the study of human behavior, because many psychological, social, and biological variables are normally distributed. Large sets of data (such as heights, weights, test scores, IQ) often form a symmetrical, bell-shaped distribution when graphed by frequency (number of instances). For example, if you took the weight of all 25-year-old males in America and plotted the weight on the *x*-axis and the frequency on the *y*-axis, the results will be normally distributed.

Standard Deviation

Standard deviation describes the degree of variation from the mean. A low standard deviation reflects that data points are all similar and close to the mean, while a high standard deviation reflects that the data are more spread out. For the purposes of the MCAT, you should be familiar with a normal distribution (or bell-shaped curve) and should be able to determine what a standard deviation means for a set of data. You will not be expected to calculate the standard deviation. Figure 3 demonstrates the relationship between a normal distribution and standard deviation.

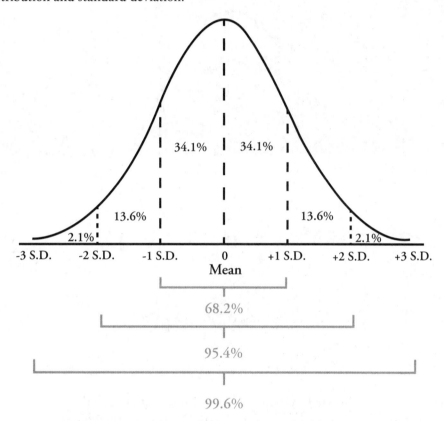

Figure 1 Normal Distribution and Standard Deviation Rules

All normal distributions have the following properties:

- 34.1% of the data will fall within one standard deviation above or below the mean, thus 68.2% of the data will fall within one standard deviation of the mean,
- 13.6% of the data will fall between one and two standard deviations above or below the mean, thus 95.4% of the data will fall within two standard deviations of the mean,
- 2.1% of the data will fall between two and three standard deviations above or below the mean thus 99.6% of the data will fall within three standard deviations of the mean,
- 0.2% of the data will fall beyond three standard deviations above or below the mean, thus 0.4% of the data will fall beyond three standard deviations of the mean.

So for a normal distribution, almost all of the data lie within **3 standard deviations** of the mean.

Example Standard Deviation Question:

Suppose that 1,000 subjects participate in a study on reaction time. The reaction times of the subjects are normally distributed with a mean of 1.3 seconds and a standard deviation of 0.2 seconds. How many subjects had a reaction time between 1.1 and 1.5 seconds? How many participants had reaction times faster than 1.9 seconds? A reaction time of 0.9 seconds is within how many standard deviations of the mean?

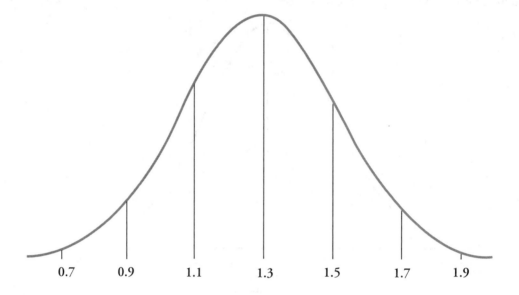

Figure 2   Subjects' Reaction Time

Solution:

Subjects' reaction times would produce a normal distribution like the one above. Reaction times within 1.1 and 1.5 seconds would include all of the data within one standard deviation of the mean (or, in other words, one standard deviation above and below the mean). 68.2% of the data fall within one standard deviation of the mean (34.1% above and 34.1% below), so **682** subjects have a reaction time between 1.1 and 1.5 seconds.

0.2% of the data will fall above 3 standard deviations of the mean, so only **2** subjects will have a reaction time faster than 1.9 seconds.

A reaction time of 0.9 seconds is **two standard deviations below the mean**.

Percentile

Percentiles are often used when reporting data from normal distributions. Percentiles represent the area under the normal curve, increasing from left to right. A percentile indicates the value or score below which the rest of the data falls. For example, a score in the 75th percentile is higher than 75% of the rest of the scores. Each standard deviation represents a fixed percentile as follows:

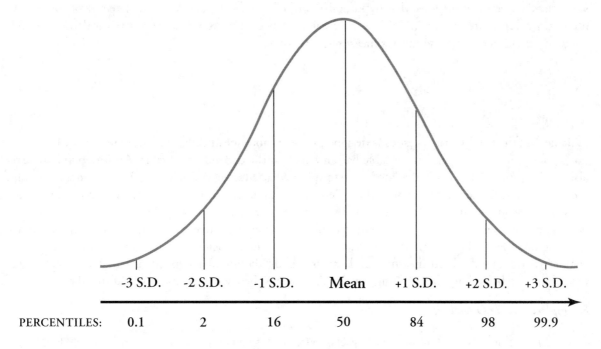

Figure 3 Normal Distribution and Percentiles

- 0.1th percentile corresponds to three standard deviations below the mean
- 2nd percentile corresponds to two standard deviations below the mean
- 16th percentile corresponds to one standard deviation below the mean
- 50th percentile correspond to the mean
- 84th percentile corresponds to one standard deviation above the mean
- 98th percentile corresponds to two standard deviations above the mean
- 99.9th percentile corresponds to three standard deviations above the mean

Example Percentile Question:

> If the scores for an exam are normally distributed, the mean is 20 and the standard deviation is 6, a score of 14 would be what percentile? What score would correspond to the 99.9th percentile?

Solution:

> A score of 14 would be one standard deviation below the mean, which corresponds to the **16th percentile**. The 99.9th percentile is three standard deviations above the mean, which would correspond to a score of **38**.

A.3 INFERENTIAL STATISTICS

Beyond merely describing the data, inferential statistics also allows inferences or assumptions to be made about data. Using inferential statistics, such as a regression coefficient or a *t*-test, you can draw conclusions about the population you are studying. Inferential statistics starts with a hypothesis and checks to see if the data prove or disprove that hypothesis. You will not be expected to calculate any of the following statistical measures on the MCAT, but you will be expected to recognize these statistical analyses and apply information about these various measures.

Variables

Variables are the things that statistics is designed to test; more specifically, statistics measures whether or not a change in the independent variable has an effect on the dependent variable. An **independent variable** is the variable that is manipulated to determine what effect it will have on the dependent variable. A **dependent variable** is a function of the independent variable, as the independent variable changes, so does the dependent variable. Typically, the independent variable is the one altered by the scientist in a behavioral experiment and the dependent variable is the one measured by the scientist. Common independent variables in behavioral sciences include: age, sex, race, socioeconomic status, and other group characteristics. Standardized measures and scores are also common independent variables. Dependent variables could be any number of things, such as test scores, behaviors, symptoms, and the like.

Example Variable Question:

Two scientists want to measure the impact of caffeine consumption on fine motor performance. Therefore, they devise an experiment where a treatment group receives 50 mg of caffeine (in the form of a sugar-free beverage) 20 minutes before performing a standardized motor skills test, and the control group receives an non-caffeinated sugar-free beverage 20 minutes before performing a standardized motor skills test. What is the independent variable in this example? What is the dependent variable?

Solution:

The independent variable is caffeine because the researchers are attempting to determine the impact of this variable on another, the dependent variable (which in this example is performance on the standardized motor skills test).

Sample Size

Sample size refers to the number of observations or individuals measured. Simply enough, if an experiment involves 100 people, the sample size is 100. Sample size is typically denoted with: N (the total number of subjects in the sample being studied) or n (the total number of subjects in a subgroup of the sample being studied). While larger sample sizes always confer increased accuracy, in practicality, particularly for behavioral research where it is likely impossible to test *all* of the people in the country who are clinically depressed, the sample size used in a study is typically determined based on convenience, expense, and the need to have sufficient **statistical power** (which is essentially the likelihood that you have enough subjects to accurately prove the hypothesis is true within an acceptable margin of error). Bigger sample sizes are always better; the larger the sample size, the more likely that you can draw accurate inferences about the population that the sample was drawn from.

Random Samples

In statistics, especially in the behavioral sciences, where (as previously mentioned), it is often not possible to test everyone in the population, it is crucial to select a random sample from the larger population in order to conduct research. A **random sample** is a subset of individuals from within a statistical population that can be used to estimate characteristics of the whole population. A population can be defined as including all of the people with a given condition or characteristic that you wish to study. Except under the rarest of circumstances, it will not be possible to study everyone with a given characteristic or condition, so a subset of the population is selected. If the subset is not selected randomly, then this non-randomness might unintentionally skew the results (which is called **sampling bias**). A classic example of this occurred during the 1948 Presidential Election in the U.S.: a survey was conducted by randomly calling households and asking people who they were planning to vote for, Harry Truman or Thomas Dewey. Based on this phone survey, Dewey was projected to win, but Truman actually did. What could have possibly gone wrong? Well it turns out that in 1948 having a phone was not such a common thing; in fact, only wealthier households were likely to have a telephone. So the "random" selection of telephone numbers was in fact not a representative random sample of the U.S. population, because many people (of whom a large proportion were clearly voting for Truman) did not have telephone numbers. For the purposes of the MCAT, you should be able to identify the following types of sampling biases:

1) The bias of selection from a **specific real area** occurs when people are selected in a physical space. For example, if you wanted to survey college students on whether or not they like their football team, you could stand on the quad and survey the first 100 people that walk by. However, this is not a completely random sample, because people who don't have class that day at that time are unlikely to be represented in the sample.

2) **Self-selection bias** occurs when the people being studied have some control over whether or not to participate. A participant's decision to participate may affect the results. For example, an Internet survey might only elicit responses from people who are highly opinionated and motivated to complete the survey.

3) **Pre-screening** or **advertising** bias occurs often in medical research; how volunteers are screened or where advertising is placed might skew the sample. For example, if a researcher wanted to prove that a certain treatment helps with smoking cessation, the mere act of advertising for people who "want to quit smoking" could provide only a sample of people who are highly motivated to quit and would be likely to quit without the treatment.

4) **Healthy user bias** occurs when the study population is likely healthier than the general population. For example, recruiting subjects from the gym might not be the most representative group.

t-test and p-values

The *t*-test is probably one of the most common tests in the social sciences, because it can be used to calculate whether the means of two groups are significantly different from each other statistically. For example, if you have a control group and a treatment group both take a standardized test, the means of the two groups can be compared statistically. Furthermore, *t*-tests are also often used to calculate the difference between a pre-treatment measure and a post-treatment measure for the same group. For example, you could have a group of subjects take a survey before and after some sort of treatment, and statistically compare the means of the two tests.

The *t*-test is most often applied to data sets that are normally distributed. You will not be required to know how to perform a t-test, but you will need to understand what **significance** is. For the purposes of most experiments, two samples are considered to be significantly different if the *p*-value is below ± 0.05 (the *p*-value

A.3

can be found using a table of values from the *t*-test). If two data sets are determined to be statistically significantly different (the *p*-value is below ± 0.05), then it can be concluded with 95% confidence that the two sets of data are actually different, instead of containing data that could be from the same data set.

Correlation

Expresses a relationship between two sets of data using a single number, the correlation coefficient (if represented at all, the correlation coefficients will usually be represented as *R* or *r*). This value measures the direction and magnitude of linear association between these two variables. A correlation coefficient can have a maximum value of 1 and a minimum value of –1. A **positive correlation** (meaning a coefficient greater than 0) indicates a *positive* association between the two variables; that is, when one variable increases the other also tends to increase as well (similarly, as one variable decreases, the other tends to decrease). A **negative correlation** (meaning a coefficient that is less than 0) indicates a negative association between the two variables; that is, when one increases, the other tends to decrease (or vice versa). A correlation coefficient of exactly 0 indicates that there is no linear relation between the two variables.

Example Correlation Question:

> Psychologists studied 500 male infants from birth to age 16. Infants were measured on "agreeableness" at age one using a standardized questionnaire given to the parents (with scores ranging from 0 to 5). As the infants aged, the psychologists would collect standard measures of behavior problems (including cheating, fighting, getting put in detention, and later delinquency, smoking, and drug use) every two years. Overall behavior problems were summed. The psychologists found a correlation between agreeableness and later behavior problems of – 0.6 (Figure 6). What does a higher "agreeableness" score correlate to? An "agreeableness" score of 4.0 corresponds to roughly how many accumulated behavior problems by age 16? What conclusions can we draw about the causes of behavior problems?

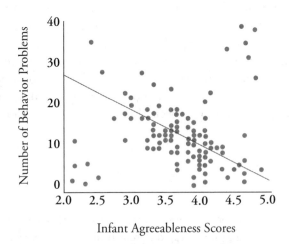

Figure 4   Correlation Between Infant Agreeableness and Later Behavior Problems (R = –0.6)

Solution:

Because the two variables are inversely correlated, as scores for "agreeableness" increase, behavioral problems decrease (this is also demonstrated by Figure 6).

An "agreeableness" score of 4.0 corresponds to approximately 10 accumulated behavior problems by age 16; note that correlations are not best used to make assumptions about people's behavior like this in behavioral psychology and medicine, though they may be used to generalizations.

Note: We can draw no conclusions about behavioral problems based on a correlation! A very important concept in statistics is that **correlation does not imply causation**. A famous example is this one: In New York City, the murder rate is directly correlated to the sale of ice cream (as ice cream sales increase, so do murders). Does this mean that buying ice cream somehow causes murders? Of course not! When two variables are correlated (especially two variables that are as complex as measures of human behavior), there are always a number of other factors that could be influencing either one. In the ice cream/murder example, a logical third factor might be temperature; as the temperature rises, more crimes are committed, but people also tend to eat more cold food, like ice cream.

Reliability

Reliability is the degree to which a specific assessment tool produces stable, consistent, and replicable results. The two types of reliability you should be able to recognize on the exam are test-retest reliability and inter-rater reliability.

- **Test-retest reliability** is a measure of the reliability of an assessment tool in obtaining similar scores over time. In other words, if the same person takes the assessment five times, their scores should be roughly equal, not wildly different.
- **Inter-rater reliability** is a measure of the degree to which two different researchers or raters agree in their assessment. For example, if two different researchers are collecting observational data, their judgments of the same person should be similar, not wildly different.

Validity

Generally, **validity** refers to how well an experiment measures what it is trying to measure. There are three important type of validity: internal, external, and construct. For the purposes of the MCAT, you should know what each type of validity is, and should be able to recognize threats to internal and external validity.

1) **Internal validity** refers to whether the results of the study properly demonstrate a causal relationship between the two variables tested. Highly controlled experiments (with random selection, random assignment to either the control or experimental groups, reliable instruments, reliable processes, and safeguards against confounding factors) may be the only way to truly establish internal validity. **Confounding factors** are hidden variables (those not directly tested for) that correlate in some way with the independent or dependent variable and have some sort of impact on the results.

2) **External validity** refers to whether the results of the study can be generalized to other situations and other people. Generalizability is limited to the independent variable, so the following must be controlled for in order to protect the external validity:
   - sample must be completely random (any of the sampling errors discussed above will threated external validity)
   - all situational variables (treatment conditions, timing, location, administration, investigator) must be tightly controlled
   - cause and effect relationships may not be generalizable to other settings, situations, groups, or people.

3) **Construct validity** is used to determine whether a tool is measuring what it is intended to measure; for example, does a survey ask questions clearly? Are the questions getting at the intended construct? Are the correct multiple choices present? And so on.

A.4 CONDUCTING EXPERIMENTS ON HUMANS

It is complicated to conduct studies on humans because it is infinitely harder to manipulate all of the variables; it is much, much harder to make causal conclusions. Therefore, one of your best tools for questions of this nature (which are likely to show up in the Psychological, Social, and Biological section) will be healthy skepticism; if an answer choice seems too obvious, too general, or too strong, it probably is! Furthermore, the only real type of research conducted on humans that can produce information about the effectiveness of treatment or therapy on a particular disease or condition is a **double-blinded randomized controlled trial**.

In a **randomized controlled trial**, there are two groups: a treatment group and a control group. The treatment group receives the treatment under investigation and the control group either receives no treatment, a placebo, or (in the case of most medical studies) the current standard of care. Randomized controlled trials can answer questions about the effectiveness of different therapies or interventions. Randomization helps avoid selecting a sample that is biased, and having a control group allows for a comparison. However, in human research there are many instances where a randomized controlled trial cannot be utilized; for example, you cannot randomly assign people to different socioeconomic classes, and it would not be ethical to inject healthy subjects with some sort of disease.

Double-blindedness is an especially stringent way of conducting an experiment which attempts to eliminate subjective, unrecognized biases held by the subjects *and* the researchers. In a **double-blind experiment**, neither the participants nor the researchers know which participants belong to the control group, as opposed to the test group. Only after all data have been recorded (and in some cases, analyzed) do the researchers learn which participants were which. Performing an experiment in double-blind fashion can greatly lessen the power of preconceived notions or physical cues (for example, the placebo effect, observer bias, experimenter's bias) to distort the results (by making researchers/participants behave differently than they would in everyday life). Random assignment of test subjects to the experimental and control groups is a critical part of any double-blind research design. The key that identifies the subjects and which group they belonged to is kept by a third party, and is not revealed to the researchers until the study is over. Double-blind methods can be applied to any experimental situation in which there is a possibility that the results will be affected by conscious/unconscious bias on the part of researchers, participants, or both.

NOTES

NOTES

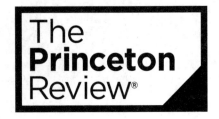
China (Beijing)
1501 Building A,
Disanji Creative Zone,
No.66 West Section of North 4th Ring Road Beijing
Tel: +86-10-62684481/2/3
Email: tprkor01@chol.com
Website: www.tprbeijing.com

China (Shanghai)
1010 Kaixuan Road
Building B, 5/F
Changning District, Shanghai, China 200052
Sara Beattie, Owner: Email: sbeattie@sarabeattie.com
Tel: +86-21-5108-2798
Fax: +86-21-6386-1039
Website: www.princetonreviewshanghai.com

Hong Kong
5th Floor, Yardley Commercial Building
1-6 Connaught Road West, Sheung Wan, Hong Kong
(MTR Exit C)
Sara Beattie, Owner: Email: sbeattie@sarabeattie.com
Tel: +852-2507-9380
Fax: +852-2827-4630
Website: www.princetonreviewhk.com

India (Mumbai)
Score Plus Academy
Office No.15, Fifth Floor
Manek Mahal 90
Veer Nariman Road
Next to Hotel Ambassador
Churchgate, Mumbai 400020
Maharashtra, India
Ritu Kalwani: Email: director@score-plus.com
Tel: + 91 22 22846801 / 39 / 41
Website: www.score-plus.com

India (New Delhi)
South Extension
K-16, Upper Ground Floor
South Extension Part-1,
New Delhi-110049
Aradhana Mahna: aradhana@manyagroup.com
Monisha Banerjee: monisha@manyagroup.com
Ruchi Tomar: ruchi.tomar@manyagroup.com
Rishi Josan: Rishi.josan@manyagroup.com
Vishal Goswamy: vishal.goswamy@manyagroup.com
Tel: +91-11-64501603/ 4, +91-11-65028379
Website: www.manyagroup.com

Lebanon
463 Bliss Street
AlFarra Building - 2nd floor
Ras Beirut
Beirut, Lebanon
Hassan Coudsi: Email: hassan.coudsi@review.com
Tel: +961-1-367-688
Website: www.princetonreviewlebanon.com

Korea
945-25 Young Shin Building
25 Daechi-Dong, Kangnam-gu
Seoul, Korea 135-280
Yong-Hoon Lee: Email: TPRKor01@chollian.net
In-Woo Kim: Email: iwkim@tpr.co.kr
Tel: + 82-2-554-7762
Fax: +82-2-453-9466
Website: www.tpr.co.kr

Kuwait
ScorePlus Learning Center
Salmiyah Block 3, Street 2 Building 14
Post Box: 559, Zip 1306, Safat, Kuwait
Email: infokuwait@score-plus.com
Tel: +965-25-75-48-02 / 8
Fax: +965-25-75-46-02
Website: www.scorepluseducation.com

Malaysia
Sara Beattie MDC Sdn Bhd
Suites 18E & 18F
18th Floor
Gurney Tower, Persiaran Gurney
Penang, Malaysia
Email: tprkl.my@sarabeattie.com
Sara Beattie, Owner: Email: sbeattie@sarabeattie.com
Tel: +604-2104 333
Fax: +604-2104 330
Website: www.princetonreviewKL.com

Mexico
TPR México
Guanajuato No. 242 Piso 1 Interior 1
Col. Roma Norte
México D.F., C.P.06700
registro@princetonreviewmexico.com
Tel: +52-55-5255-4495
+52-55-5255-4440
+52-55-5255-4442
Website: www.princetonreviewmexico.com

Qatar
Score Plus
Office No: 1A, Al Kuwari (Damas)
Building near Merweb Hotel, Al Saad
Post Box: 2408, Doha, Qatar
Email: infoqatar@score-plus.com
Tel: +974 44 36 8580, +974 526 5032
Fax: +974 44 13 1995
Website: www.scorepluseducation.com

Taiwan
The Princeton Review Taiwan
2F, 169 Zhong Xiao East Road, Section 4
Taipei, Taiwan 10690
Lisa Bartle (Owner): lbartle@princetonreview.com.tw
Tel: +886-2-2751-1293
Fax: +886-2-2776-3201
Website: www.PrincetonReview.com.tw

Thailand
The Princeton Review Thailand
Sathorn Nakorn Tower, 28th floor
100 North Sathorn Road
Bangkok, Thailand 10500
Thavida Bijayendrayodhin (Chairman)
Email: thavida@princetonreviewthailand.com
Mitsara Bijayendrayodhin (Managing Director)
Email: mitsara@princetonreviewthailand.com
Tel: +662-636-6770
Fax: +662-636-6776
Website: www.princetonreviewthailand.com

Turkey
Yeni Sülün Sokak No. 28
Levent, Istanbul, 34330, Turkey
Nuri Ozgur: nuri@tprturkey.com
Rona Ozgur: rona@tprturkey.com
Iren Ozgur: iren@tprturkey.com
Tel: +90-212-324-4747
Fax: +90-212-324-3347
Website: www.tprturkey.com

UAE
Emirates Score Plus
Office No: 506, Fifth Floor
Sultan Business Center
Near Lamcy Plaza, 21 Oud Metha Road
Post Box: 44098, Dubai
United Arab Emirates
Hukumat Kalwani: skoreplus@gmail.com
Ritu Kalwani: director@score-plus.com
Email: info@score-plus.com
Tel: +971-4-334-0004
Fax: +971-4-334-0222
Website: www.princetonreviewuae.com

Our International Partners

The Princeton Review also runs courses with a variety of partners in Africa, Asia, Europe, and South America.

Georgia
LEAF American-Georgian Education Center
www.leaf.ge

Mongolia
English Academy of Mongolia
www.nyescm.org

Nigeria
The Know Place
www.knowplace.com.ng

Panama
Academia Interamericana de Panama
http://aip.edu.pa/

Switzerland
Institut Le Rosey
http://www.rosey.ch/

All other inquiries, please email us at internationalsupport@review.com